Hot Topics in Acute Care Surgery and Trauma

Endorsed by the World Society for Emergency Surgery (WSES) and the American Association for Trauma Surgery, the series covers the most debated topics in acute care and trauma surgery, from perioperative management to organisational and health policy issues, to the complex management of acute and trauma surgical patients. It is a valuable resource for both trainees and acute surgical professionals.

Etrusca Brogi • Federico Coccolini
Eric J. Ley • Alex Valadka
Editors

Traumatic Brain Injury

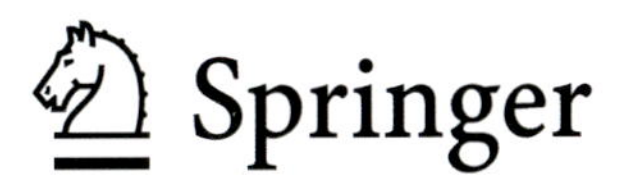

Editors
Etrusca Brogi
Dept. Anesthesia & Intensive Care
Pisa University Hospital
Pisa, Italy

Eric J. Ley
Professor of Trauma
Chief of Critical Care
R Adams Cowley Shock Trauma Center
University of Maryland School of Medicine
Baltimore, Maryland, USA

Federico Coccolini
General, Emergency and Trauma Surgery
Deptartment
Pisa University Hospital
PISA, Pisa, Italy

Alex Valadka
Department of Neurological Surgery
University of Texas Southwestern
Medical Center
Dallas, TX, USA

ISSN 2520-8284 ISSN 2520-8292 (electronic)
Hot Topics in Acute Care Surgery and Trauma
ISBN 978-3-031-50116-6 ISBN 978-3-031-50117-3 (eBook)
https://doi.org/10.1007/978-3-031-50117-3

This Springer imprint is published by the registered company Springer Nature Switzerland AG
The registered company address is: Gewerbestrasse 11, 6330 Cham, Switzerland

Paper in this product is recyclable.

Foreword to the Series

Research is fundamentally altering the daily practice of acute care surgery (trauma, surgical critical care, and emergency general surgery) for the betterment of patients around the world. Management for many diseases and conditions is radically different than it was just a few years previously. For this reason, concise up-to-date information is required to inform busy clinicians. Therefore, since 2011 the World Society of Emergency Surgery (WSES), in a partnership with the American Association for the Surgery of Trauma (AAST), endorses the development and publication of the "Hot Topics in Acute Care Surgery and Trauma," realizing the need to provide more educational tools for young in-training surgeons and for general physicians and other surgical specialists. These new forthcoming titles have been selected and prepared with this philosophy in mind. The books will cover the basics of pathophysiology and clinical management, framed with the reference that recent advances in the science of resuscitation, surgery, and critical care medicine have the potential to profoundly alter the epidemiology and subsequent outcomes of severe surgical illnesses and trauma.

Pisa, Italy — Federico Coccolini
Riverside, CA, USA — Raul Coimbra
Calgary, AB, Canada — Andrew W. Kirkpatrick
San Benedetto del Tronto, Italy — Salomone Di Saverio

Contents

Part I

General Considerations

1 History of Traumatic Brain Injury and the Evolution of Neuromonitoring: An Overview

Leonardo J. M. De Macedo Filho, Buse Sarigul, and Gregory W. J. Hawryluk

1.1 Introduction

Traumatic brain injury (TBI) is a frequent and important wounding mechanism affecting humans now and throughout history. Thanks to medical and technological advancements, even severe brain injury is now survivable in the majority of cases. Although it is often said that the brain injury field has been slow to advance and that it is behind other areas of medicine, the past century has seen tremendous improvement in our understanding of the condition, the resources for patient care, and in patient outcomes. Here we discuss the evolution of brain injury care and the modern neuromonitoring resources that are the end result of these advances.

Key modern advancements include the development of the Glasgow Coma Scale (GCS) and the advent of computed tomography (CT) scanning as well as the development of supportive intensive care. More recently, clinical practice guidelines and neuromonitoring have improved our care of brain-injured patients. Inspired by the landmark Monro-Kellie doctrine, modern therapeutic interventions have focused on decreasing intracranial pressure (ICP) and optimizing cerebral perfusion. This approach and relevant best practices have been central to the Brain Trauma

L. J. M. De Macedo Filho
Department of Neurosurgery, Penn State Health Milton S. Hershey Medical Center, Hershey, PA, USA
e-mail: leonardomacedofilho@edu.unifor.br

B. Sarigul
Department of Neurosurgery, Tuzla Public Hospital, Istanbul, Turkey

G. W. J. Hawryluk (✉)
Neurological Institute, Cleveland Clinic Akron General Hospital, Akron, OH, USA

Uniformed Services University, Bethesda, MD, USA

Brain Trauma Foundation, Palo Alto, CA, USA
e-mail: hawrylg@ccf.org

E. Brogi et al. (eds.), *Traumatic Brain Injury*, Hot Topics in Acute Care Surgery and Trauma, https://doi.org/10.1007/978-3-031-50117-3_1

Foundation's (BTF) influential guidelines first published in 1996. Use of these guidelines, now in their fourth edition, has been associated with improved outcomes. This chapter focuses on the evolution of TBI management from ancient times to recent advances in neurocritical care.

1.2 History of TBI

Historically, moderate and severe TBI (sTBI) were rarely survivable. Efforts to treat TBI date back to antiquity. Trepanation, the oldest known neurosurgical procedure, dates back to at least 10,000 BC. Human skulls with bony flaws that had the same shape as primitive surgical instruments from the same time period are well described [1–4]. Trepanation (from the Greek *trypanon*, drilling, opening a hole) is a surgical procedure that consists of removing a portion of the skull. This technique was widely used in antiquity and in the Middle Ages, continuing into the eighteenth and nineteenth centuries for therapeutic purposes, mainly in TBI. Trepanned skulls have also been found in prehistoric human cultures dating to the Neolithic period [1–4]. Evidence of bone remodeling in some archeologic specimens suggests that these efforts occasionally met with some success.

The *Edwin Smith Surgical Papyrus*, dated to 1700 BC, was discovered in 1862 but remained unpublished until 1930, when the Egyptologist James Breasted published an extensive, annotated translation of its contents. This papyrus is composed of 48 clinical cases, systematically described, starting with the head and descending through the thorax and spine, where the document is interrupted. Some of these cases describe head and skull trauma and injuries in a standardized format that includes a clinical description of the case, diagnosis, and a glossary that seeks to clarify technical terms [2, 4].

Hippocrates, known as "the father of medicine," documented procedures for management of skull fractures and contusions [5]. Three hundred years later, Aulus Aurelius Cornelius Celsus of Alexandria described epidural and subdural hematoma evacuation via trepanation. There is a long pause in the historical record in terms of subsequent descriptions of brain injury management, with the exception of Avicenna's discovery of cerebral vessel blockage in stroke and management modalities for acute stroke [6].

During the ancient and medieval eras, civilizations developed intricate amalgamations of logic and mythical/religious thoughts. Thus, concepts about the body, mind (or soul), illness, and health were intertwined with religious and cultural concepts [2–4, 7]. Moreover, in the medieval era, as a result of the decline of the western Roman Empire, the Arab world preserved the medical knowledge of the Greeks and Romans. Neuroanatomy, neurophysiology, neuropathology, and surgical technique studies returned in the eleventh century with the work of Roger of Salermo during the Renaissance [3, 4]. At the end of the thirteenth century, Lanfrancus (−1310) elaborated the concept of concussion. In the fifteenth century, Berengario da Carpi (1465–1527) divided brain injuries into lacerations, contusions, and perforations. In addition, he described postconcussion headache [8].

Investigations by early Egyptian physicians, Hippocrates, Galen, Aulus Cornelius Celsus, and Paul of Aegina led to a better understanding of neurological anatomy, physiology, and therapeutics [9–11]. Their studies also improved our knowledge about cerebrospinal fluid (CSF). Modern concepts of ICP were first introduced by Monro and Kellie in the eighteenth century [10–13].

CSF is an ultrafiltrate produced by the choroid plexus and is present in the cerebral ventricles and subarachnoid space. It is in close relationship to CNS tissue and meninges [12, 13]. CSF was first identified by Nicola Massa in 1538 [13, 14] and was observed by Domenico Felice Cotugno in 1764 beneath the dura mater, within the brain's ventricles, and around the spinal cord [13, 15]. Moro Secundus (1733–1817) described the intraventricular foramen which provides a connection between the lateral ventricles and the third ventricle [11, 14, 16]. The CSF circulation and the correct direction of the flow were confirmed by Francois Magendie (1783–1855) who discovered that the continuation of CSF flow from the ventricular system to subarachnoid space was through the mid-region of the fourth ventricle [13, 17]. Alexander Bochdalek (1801–1883) described the lateral recesses of the fourth ventricle in 1849 and Hubert von Luschka (1820–1875) discovered the connections with the subarachnoid space—known as the foramina of Luschka—and confirmed the presence of the foramen of Magendie [13, 18]. The explanation of how CSF is secreted by the choroid plexus, flows through the ventricular system, and is reabsorbed via subarachnoid villi and Pacchionian granulations was added by Retzius and Key in 1875 [13, 19]. The link between CSF and ICP was defined by Harvey Cushing when he considered CSF to be the third circulatory system [13].

The Monro-Kellie doctrine established that the brain resides in an inelastic and rigid skull. The total intracranial volume has to remain constant. Moreover, along with the consistent volume of blood inside the cranium, the venous blood should be drained perpetually and replaced via arterial oxygenated blood [10, 13, 16]. An increase in the volume of intracranial CSF, brain tissue, or blood should be compensated by a decrease in other components. Otherwise, an increase in ICP is inevitable [10, 13, 16].

During the nineteenth century three major innovations made possible great advances in neurosurgery: anesthesia, antisepsis and aseptic technique, and brain topography [20]. These innovations resulted primarily from a period of consecutive wars and efforts to treat and reduce morbidity and mortality of TBI [8]. The notable brain injury of Phineas Gage in the 1800s brought attention to the localization of function in the brain after he survived an accident in which an iron rod penetrated his head and destroyed a good portion of his left frontal lobe, leading to marked behavioral change [21]. As the twentieth century began, the "neuron theory" was described by Santiago Ramon y Cajal (1852–1934). He postulated that the nervous system constitutes independent cells and defined the nervous system to include neurons that are in contiguity but not continuity [22]. Cajal was the first to use the term "plasticity" in a Congress held in Rome in 1894 in which he described the potential of the brain to adapt to the environment as a force of internal differentiation and plasticity. Until the 1960s, it was considered that the adult nervous system was incapable of generating new neurons. However, Joseph Altman and Gopal Das used thymidine-H autoradiography to discover newly formed cells, which suggested new neuronal production to the olfactory bulb and the dentate gyrus of the rat hippocampus. These ideas became controversial until two decades later, when Arturo Alvarez-Buylla made his discoveries on neurogenesis and adult neural stem cells via experiments on songbirds and mammals [23]. However, these new discoveries have still not been applied to therapeutic advances in TBI.

The development of neurosurgery accelerated in the first half of the twentieth century. Harvey Cushing (1869–1939) is credited with significant reductions in complications and mortality in cranial surgery. Among his many contributions, he is credited with techniques used to treat head injuries such as subtemporal decompression, which is still frequently used today [8].

Other important developments in the twentieth century were the creation of the GCS and dramatic advances in brain imaging [8, 24]. Also, in the last decades of the twentieth century, the mortality rate for sTBI fell by almost 50% as a result of advancements in supportive care [25].

The BTF, founded in 1986, developed the first evidence-based clinical practice guidelines produced by any surgical specialty. The identification and proliferation of best practices has been repeatedly credited with marked improvement in outcomes from sTBI. The BTF has subsequently produced guidelines on many TBI subtopics including pediatric injuries, prehospital care, prognostication, combat injuries, and concussion. To date, the BTF has published over 15 major guideline projects/editions (Fig. 1.1). Compliance with these guidelines is integral to the American College of Surgeons' trauma center accreditation program and has

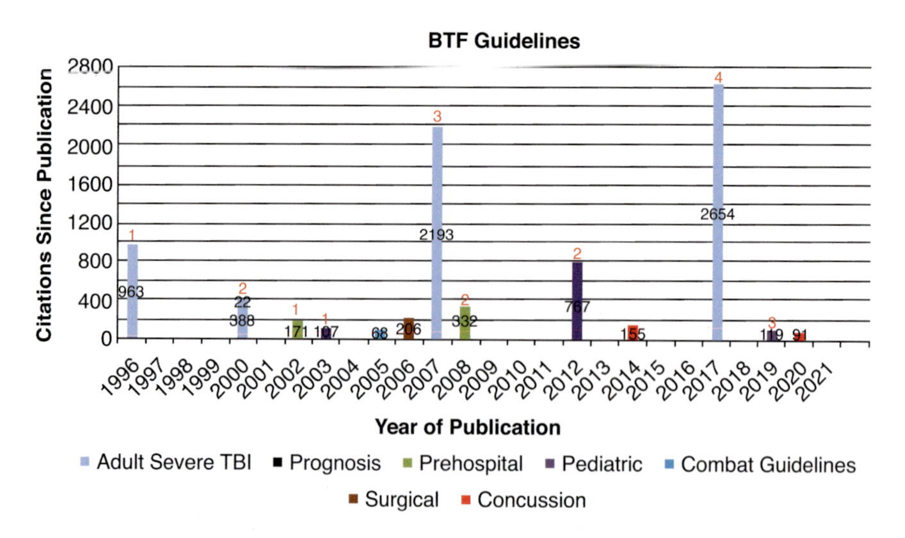

Fig. 1.1 Year of publication and citations of BTF guidelines. The cumulative number of citations calculated by Google Scholar (accessed December 12, 2022). The numbers in red above the bars denote the edition of the guideline. The number within the bars represents the total number of citations

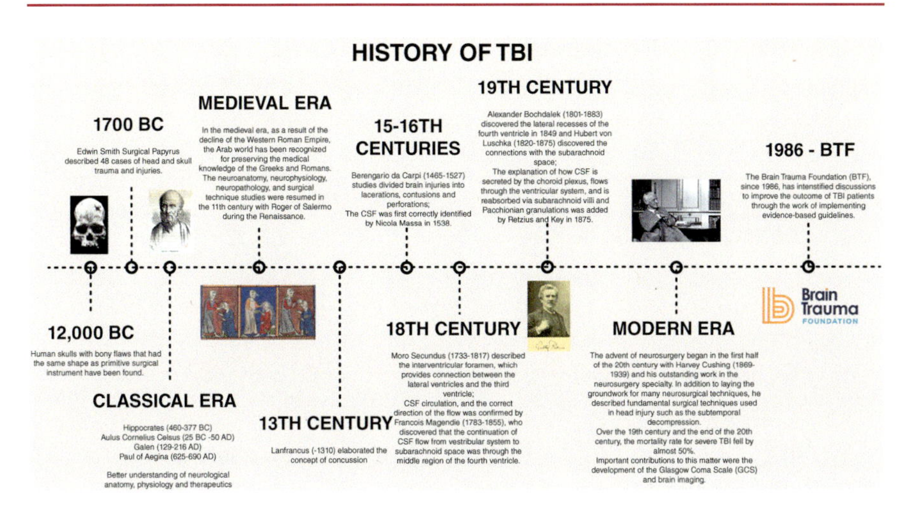

Fig. 1.2 History of TBI—timeline. The x-axis shows important contributions to the understanding of TBI over the centuries and eras, from the Neolithic to the present day, with emphasis on the BTF guidelines and studies on the subject. (Credits: (1) Anterior aspect of Squiers, Inca Skull, showing trephining. Wellcome Collection. Attribution 4.0 International (CC BY 4.0); (2) Les merveilles de l'industrie ou, Description des principales industries modernes/par Louis Figuier. - Paris: Furne, Jouvet, [1873–1877]. - Tome III. PublicDomain; (3) Cranial operation from BL Sloane 1977, Image taken from f. 2 of Chirurgia. Written in French. British Library. Public Domain; (4) Portrait of Gustaf Retzius, extracted from the article Gustaf Retzius som etnograf in Fataburen Kulturhistorisk tidskrift (1919). Nordiska Museet. Public Domain; (5) HarveyWilliams Cushing. Photograph, 1938. Created 1938. Harvey Cushing (1869–1939). Wellcome Collection. Attribution 4.0 International (CC BY 4.0))

intensified discussions on improving the outcome of TBI patients [26–30]. Development and widespread adoption of the BTF guidelines is only a recent advance in the long history of TBI treatment (Fig. 1.2).

1.3 Evolution of Neuromonitoring

1.3.1 Historical Evolution of Intracranial Pressure Monitoring

In 1891, the German physician Heinrich Quincke published the first description of the lumbar puncture technique as well as subsequent investigations of CSF and CSF pressure in relation to various neurological diseases (Fig. 1.3). He determined that a pipette of glass should be affixed to the puncture needle, and through the water column it was possible to measure the CSF pressure [11, 31]. This technique of repetitive CSF opening pressure measurement for assessment of ICP became widely used, becoming the first method for clinical assessment of ICP [11, 31]. However, this method led to the death of some patients with high ICP, presumably by inciting transtentorial herniation [11].

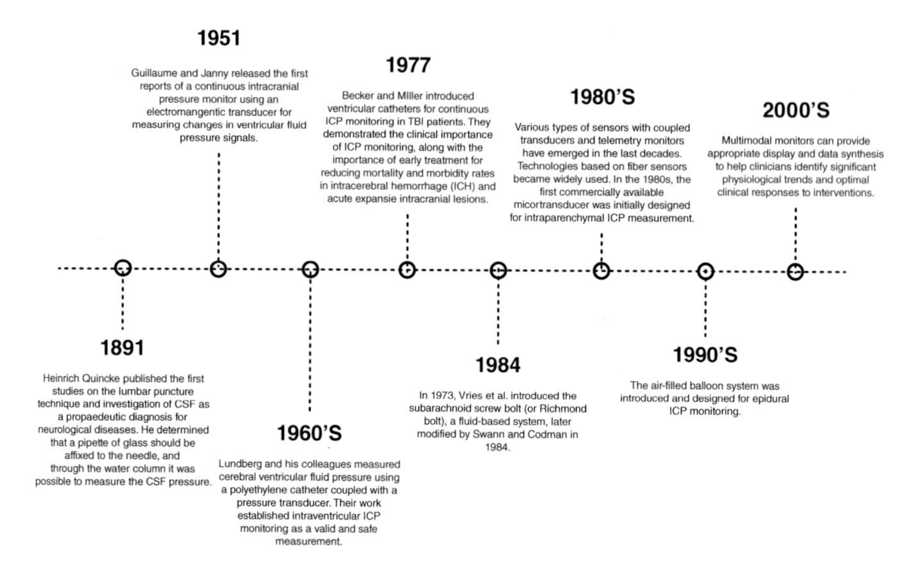

Fig. 1.3 Historical evolution of intracranial pressure monitoring—timeline. The *x*-axis shows contributions from the first studies by Quincke in the nineteenth century to the current multimodal monitors used in TBI

In 1951, Guillaume and Janny released the first reports of a continuous ICP monitor that used an electromagnetic transducer for measuring changes in ventricular fluid pressure signals. They used a U-tube manometer in which the CSF continues to flow until it is equalized by a reverse pressure [10, 11, 13, 32]. ICP monitoring was further advanced in the 1960s by Lundberg and his colleagues, who measured cerebral ventricular fluid pressure using a polyethylene catheter coupled to a pressure transducer. Their work established monitoring of intraventricular pressure as a valid and safe alternative [33–35]. The aim of Lundberg's thesis was to provide a method for ventricular cannulation that was minimally traumatic, feasible, had a low risk of infection and leakage, and facilitated recording with continuous flow of the ICP. In addition, he described three ICP wave patterns associated with intracranial pathologies [11, 33–35]. "A" waves represented increase in ICP to levels of 50 to 100 mmHg that maintained a plateau for 5–20 min, followed by an abrupt drop. "B" waves were abrupt rises in ICP up to 50 mmHg, with a frequency of 0.5–2 waves per minute. These waves could be directly related to cerebral blood flow (CBF) and vessel diameter but were of uncertain origin and relevance. "C" waves, also known as Mayer's wave, represented arterial wave reflexes and were associated with cardiac and respiratory cycles [11, 33–35].

In 1977, Becker and Miller introduced ventricular catheters for continuous ICP monitoring in TBI patients. They demonstrated the clinical importance of ICP monitoring, along with the importance of early treatment for reducing mortality and morbidity rates in intracerebral hemorrhage (ICH) and acute expansile intracranial lesions. The clear evidence of good results among patients in whom ICP elevation could be quickly recognized and treated contributed to the popularization of the method [11, 36, 37]. Between the 1980s and 2000s, ICP monitoring became widespread. However, even today, it is not being used routinely in all ICUs. Also, cost and access limit use in low- and middle-income countries [27–30, 38, 39].

Recommendations that focus on the reduction of ICP and maintenance of adequate cerebral perfusion are central to the BTF guidelines, which review the varying levels of evidence for three types of monitoring in sTBI patients: ICP, cerebral perfusion pressure (CPP), and brain oxygenation [27–30]. Additional monitoring modalities mentioned in the recent guidelines regarding their use for diagnostic, therapeutic, and prognostic purposes include electroencephalography (EEG), partial pressure of brain tissue oxygen ($PbtO_2$), CBF, transcranial Doppler ultrasonography (TCD) for cerebral autoregulatory status, and cerebral microdialysis [11].

1.3.2 ICP Monitoring in Modern Era

1.3.2.1 Invasive ICP Monitoring

ICP can be measured via either invasive or noninvasive methods. Invasive methods include fluid-based systems and implantable microtransducers. Invasive ICP monitoring techniques consist of the insertion of a catheter, which varies in intracranial location and in the pressure transduction method. The devices are typically inserted in the intraventricular or intraparenchymal spaces. Regarding pressure transduction methods, catheters can be connected to an external ventricular drain (EVD) or a microtransducer [11, 13, 40].

The ventricular catheter is traditionally considered as the "gold standard" for reliability in ICP monitoring. The superiority of this technique when compared to others is that it allows CSF drainage for control of the ICP as well as biochemical, cytological, and microbiological CSF sample analysis [11, 13, 40, 41]. In 1973, Vries et al. introduced the subarachnoid screw bolt (or Richmond bolt) [42], a fluid-based system, later modified by Swann and Codman in 1984 [11, 43] in an attempt to reduce the infection rates of ventricular catheters at that time. However, the screw still presented a high risk of infection without allowing CSF drainage. It also had a tendency to underestimate ICP, which inspired the development of newer technologies [11, 13, 41].

Various types of sensors with coupled transducers and telemetry monitors have emerged in the last decades. Technologies based on fiberoptics, strain gauges, and pneumatic sensors are now widely used [11]. In the 1980s, the first commercially available microtransducer was introduced. This was the Honeywell MTC-P5F®, initially designed for intraparenchymal ICP measurement [44]. The first equipment to be used more widely were the Camino [45] and Codman [46] devices. Available technologies for ICP monitoring are made by a relatively small number of manufacturers. Each product or technology has its own benefits and weaknesses related to the technology itself or to the manufacturing process [11, 13, 30, 41, 47–50].

ICP monitoring also affords the opportunity to determine CPP, which represents the vascular pressure gradient that drives oxygen delivery to cerebral tissue. It is calculated as the difference between mean arterial pressure (MAP) and ICP. Decreases in CPP may contribute to secondary brain injury through cerebral hypoperfusion and/or ischemia. The BTF recommends (Level IIB) targeting a CPP between 60 and 70 mmHg—depending upon autoregulatory status—to optimize survival and favorable outcome [11, 27–30].

An ideal monitor for tracking ICP must be easy to use, accurate, reliable, reproducible, inexpensive, and must be associated with minimal infections and bleeding complications. Invasive transducers are reliable and accurate; however, cost and access to the technology are issues that limit its widespread use [11, 13, 50]. EVD catheters are the gold standard for monitoring ICP, despite having a higher risk of hemorrhage and infection than microtransducers [11, 13, 50].

1.3.2.2 Noninvasive ICP Monitoring

A noninvasive ICP monitor can be defined as a technique that provides information on ICP or the neurological consequences of increased ICP, such as reduced CBF and metabolic changes, without penetrating the skin or skull, thus minimizing the risks to the monitored individuals [51, 52]. Noninvasive modalities may represent the future of ICP monitoring because of their lower risk and greater cost efficiency [11, 13, 50–52]. Noninvasive monitoring methods are divided into two groups, those that use physiological parameters related to intracranial compartments, and those based on extracranial compartments that are anatomically connected to intracranial compartments [52].

Since the 1970s, there has been a strong effort to develop noninvasive monitoring to avoid complications associated with invasive ICP monitoring techniques. Consequently, many different noninvasive modalities have been developed in recent decades and are being studied [11, 13, 50]. The most popular noninvasive ICP monitoring techniques in TBI are brain imaging analysis; optic nerve sheath diameter (ONSD); TCD; tympanic membrane displacement; EEG; near-infrared spectroscopy (NIRS); pupillometry; microdialysis; pressure on the anterior fontanelle via fontanometry; venous ophthalmodynamometry; tonometry; acoustoelasticity; and otoacoustic emissions [11, 13, 50, 53, 54].

Fontanometry

Over the 1970s and 1980s, many studies were conducted to investigate the correlation between anterior fontanelle pressure and ICP in children with open fontanelles [50, 54–56]. Fontanometry is a method developed to measure the pressure beneath the fontanelle and thus provide information about ICP. It is based on placing sensors over the patent anterior fontanelle of children younger than 2 1/2 years. Device attachment has been an important and persistent concern with this technique. The best-known of these devices is the Rotterdam® transducer, which has been used in clinical practice [50, 54–56].

Optic Nerve Sheath Diameter

In 1964, Hayreh et al. [57] showed that, due to the communication of the subarachnoid space with the intracranial cavity, changes in CSF pressure can be transmitted along the optic nerve sheath. Therefore, when there is an increase in CSF pressure, the optic nerve sheath diameter (ONSD) can expand [54, 57]. The optic nerve sheath is continuous with the brain dura mater and is surrounded by the subarachnoid space, which contains the CSF [41]. ONSD expansion may be accompanied by papilledema, but unlike papilledema, ONSD expansion occurs almost immediately after an acute increase in ICP [54, 58]. ONSD sonographic measurement is a rapid modality for monitoring ICP increase. However, measuring ONSD is an operator-dependent technique, and conditions including tumors, inflammation, sarcoidosis, and Graves' disease can affect ONSD measurements. It is also difficult to measure ONSD in patients with orbital or optic nerve injuries [50, 54, 59].

Ophthalmodynamometry

Ophthalmodynamometry was originally described by Baurmann [60] in 1925 and consists of measuring the pressure in the ophthalmic artery and vein through an application of known pressure to the eyeball. In 2000, Firsching et al. observed that the venous outlet pressure has a close linear relationship with ICP [61]. The central retinal vein passes through the optic nerve and is surrounded by CSF, and changes in ICP can affect the optic nerve and central retinal vein. Like other ophthalmic ICP monitoring techniques, venous ophthalmodynamometry can be used to screen patients with a suspected increase in ICP before performing an invasive technique. It cannot replace invasive techniques. However, it can be used as a follow-up screening tool in some patients [50, 54, 61].

Tympanic Membrane Displacement

Reid et al. published the first study to compare tympanic membrane displacement (TMD) values with ICP measured via invasive methods in 1990 [62]. Three essential criteria are necessary to perform a tympanometry test: patent cochlear aqueduct, normal middle ear pressure, and intact stapedius reflex. In normal circumstances, the pressure in the intracranial compartment is transmitted to the perilymphatic fluid of the cochlea and thus displaces the stapedius, changing the acoustic reflex. Changes in ICP are thus transmitted through the cochlea, allowing indirect measurement of ICP. When a baseline ICP is established, TMD is useful to calculate normal or raised ICP, and repeated TMD measurements could be used to find changes in ICP [50, 54, 62, 63].

Brain Imaging

A variety of brain CT scan findings, such as loss of gray and white matter differentiation, midline shift, and basal cistern and ventricular effacement, have been associated with elevated ICP, and CT still remains the most-used diagnostic modality in the evaluation of patients with TBI. However, present evidence suggests that CT is not a very sensitive tool in the sense that CT may remain normal even with a raised

ICP [50, 63, 64]. Conversely, Rotterdam and Marshall criteria including midline shift, presence of space-occupying lesions, and status of basal cisterns have been suggested to be predictive of ICP increase [65, 66].

The current role of brain MRI as a diagnostic and monitoring tool in neurosurgery far outweighs its role as a purely noninvasive technique for assessing ICP. MRI techniques for the assessment of ICP are based on the relationship between intracranial compliance and pressure. MRI has also been used to assess optic nerve sheath diameter as a marker of elevated ICP and appears to be more accurate than ultrasound in assessing the CSF-filled subarachnoid space surrounding the optic nerve [63, 67, 68].

Tissue Resonance Analysis

The tissue resonance technique was developed by Michaeli [69] in 2002. It is based on the premise that different tissues vibrate at different frequencies when exposed to a particular sound wave in order to digitally obtain an echopulsogram, which shows a good correlation with invasive ICP. This method is a promising technique for noninvasive ICP monitoring, but it requires further validation [50, 54, 69].

EEG

The EEG represents the spontaneous electrical activity of the cerebral cortex recorded through electrodes placed on the scalp. These electrical signals are then amplified, filtered, and displayed in an 8- or 16-channel system [50, 54]. Aside from the importance of detecting the seizures and subclinical seizures that are common after TBI, many studies show that neurophysiological changes precede ICP changes [70, 71]. Moreover, certain components of EEG spectrum analysis are useful in correlating with ICP. EEG power spectrum analysis was reported in 2012 by Chen. Power spectral analysis allows a graphical representation of EEG readings over time and produces an ICP index (IPI) which correlates to ICP. However, more studies are needed to establish the correlation of EEG spectrum analysis with changes in ICP [50, 72].

Pupillometry

Examination of the pupils has long been a part of neurological assessment. Advances in technology have resulted in development of infrared pupillometry to quantitatively measure subtle changes in pupil size in response to light stimuli, establishing that the velocity of pupillary constriction is sensitive to increases in ICP and that a 10–20% reduction in pupil size is associated with intracranial hypertension [73–75]. In 2003 Taylor et al. suggested a new point-and-shoot hand-held pupillometer for quantitative evaluation of pupillary function. Their study enrolled 404 subjects. It was concluded that pupillary changes may suggest subtle changes in ICP, and the velocity of pupillary constriction was sensitive to increased ICP. A reduction of pupillary size by 10% was associated with ICP levels higher than 22 mmHg [74].

In 2011, Chen [76] introduced the concept of the pupillary neurological index using an algorithmic approach to predict changes in ICP with pupillary reactivity. This algorithm is produced by combining such parameters as minimum and maximum pupillary diameter, the latency of the light reflex, and constriction and dilation velocity. The index includes a scale ranging from 0 to 5 points, and <3 is considered as abnormal. Quantitative pupillometry is shown to be more precise and more consistent than standard flashlight pupil assessment, especially in neurological intensive care units. Conversely, pupillometry has limitations. Evaluation of agitated or confused patients and patients with scleral edema, periorbital edema, intraocular lens replacement, and prior ocular surgery may be challenging. Moreover, the measurements may be affected by the light of the environment [77]. Although promising, the clinical applicability of this technique requires further investigation [50, 54].

TCD

In 1982, Aaslid [78] described TCD as a technique for evaluating cerebral hemodynamics, and since then, it has been used to measure the blood flow velocities and the cerebral vasoreactivity in the basal brain arteries and in the Circle of Willis, albeit mainly in the context of aneurysmal subarachnoid hemorrhage and vasospasm. The most commonly evaluated parameters using the arterial waveform are peak systolic and diastolic velocity, mean velocity, resistance index, and pulsatility index [50, 54, 69, 79, 80].

The measurement is made over regions of the skull with the thinnest bone windows (temporal, transorbital, or back of head). TCD is best suited to provide a qualitative estimate (low, normal, or high) of ICP. It appears to be a promising modality for noninvasive ICP monitoring, but it cannot replace invasive monitoring. Important disadvantages are the requirement for a trained and qualified operator to perform and interpret the measurements and the limited accuracy in estimating absolute ICP values [50, 54, 79, 80].

Near-Infrared Spectroscopy (NIRS)

Near infrared is the name given to the region of the electromagnetic spectrum immediately above the visible region in terms of wavelength. NIRS is an emerging technology that works on the principle of differential absorption of infrared light to detect changes in oxygen and deoxyhemoglobin concentration of blood. NIRS works with wavelengths of 700–1000 nm, where the low absorption allows it to easily pass through skin and bone, resulting in deep tissue penetration that enables it to measure regional changes in cerebral blood oxygen saturation (rSO_2) and cerebral blood volume. Moreover, it can be used to detect changes in CBF and ICP [50, 54, 81–84].

In 1997, Kampfl demonstrated a significant difference in rSO_2 values between normal and elevated ICP in sTBI patients [81], and changes in cerebral oxygenation correlated well with ICP vascular slow waves during CSF infusions and TBI studies [82]. NIRS allows the calculation of certain indices that have been correlated with cerebrovascular pressure reactivity in TBI patients [67]. However, it does not provide an absolute estimate of ICP or facilitate the detection of changes in ICP [50, 54, 84]. This method shows promise, but it cannot currently be used to estimate ICP values [50, 54, 84].

1.3.3 Ancillary Monitoring

1.3.3.1 Cerebral Autoregulation and CBF

Cerebral autoregulation (CA) is defined as the mechanism by which the brain maintains a constant nutrient supply across a breadth of physiologic conditions. CBF is directly proportional to CPP and the fourth power of vascular diameter, and it is indirectly proportional to blood viscosity and cerebral vascular length. CPP is determined by the difference between MAP and ICP [85–87]. The CA curve was first described by Lassen in 1959 [88] as a triphasic curve, and it was suggested that the brain is capable of maintaining a constant perfusion pressure throughout a wide range of mean arterial pressures [85–87]. A systematic review and meta-analysis by de-Lima-Oliveira [86] in 2018 selected 35 studies about the relationship between CA and ICP since the 1980s and observed that there was a clear tendency toward CA impairment with increased ICP [86]. At least four mechanisms are proposed for autoregulation: myogenic (vascular changes), neurogenic (vascular autonomic nerve supply), metabolic (changes in the microenvironment such as pCO_2 and H^+), and endothelial factors (such as nitric oxide) [85]. The assessment of cerebral autoregulation could be static (relationships between CBF and MAP are considered constant) or dynamic (assessment is based on determination of dynamic changes of CBF in response to dynamic changes in MAP) [85].

Cerebral autoregulatory status may also be determined via measuring the cerebrovascular pressure reactivity index (PRx) or the CBF velocity via TCD and near-infrared spectroscopy [13, 54, 85–87]. Increasing CPP, in some cases, may be the only way to increase oxygen delivery to the brain, but this has some costs. Vascular regulation in the traumatized brain is often impaired, causing dissociation between the CBF and the cerebral metabolic demand. Therefore, measuring the CBF may be more important in severely traumatized patients. Thermal diffusion flowmetry and laser Doppler flowmetry are some methods for measuring CBF [85–87].

The concept of the PRx was introduced by Czosnyka [89] in 1997 based on the principle that in MAP elevations there would be cerebral vasoconstriction with a reduction in cerebral blood volume and, consequently, in ICP. PRx reflects the smooth muscle tone of arteries and cerebral arterioles in response to changes in transmural pressure, forming part of the more elaborate physiological phenomenon of CA. The PRx indirectly reflects the CA status and may be utilized to delineate the optimal CPP for a patient [85–87]. In 2000, Luzius Steiner suggested the U-shape relationship between PRx and CPP. He and his colleagues demonstrated that the lowest level in this curve correlated with the CPP level that was associated with the best autoregulation, and this level was termed as the optimal CPP or CPPopt [90]. This was interpreted as the middle point of the upper and lower levels in Lassen's curve. The COGiTATE trial is currently investigating whether therapy based on the targeted value for CPPopt improves outcome [91].

Usually, CA maintains normal CBF when MAP is between 60 and 140 mmHg. CBF of 50–60 mL/100 g/min at a MAP of 80–100 mmHg is normally maintained by vasodilation (when MAP drops to the limit of 60 mmHg) or cerebral vasoconstriction (when MAP rises up to the limit of 150 mmHg), which protects the brain from ischemia or hyperemia despite the physiological fluctuations of CPP. Patients with TBI may have a decrease or loss of CA. In this case, the CBF becomes dependent on the MAP. So if MAP rises, CBF rises too and can cause an increase in brain volume. If MAP drops, CBF also decreases, reducing ICP but possibly causing ischemia and necrosis [84–87].

1.3.3.2 Cerebral Oxygenation

Jugular Venous Oxygen Saturation ($SjvO_2$) and Arterio-Jugular Differences of Oxygen ($AVDO_2$)

Brain oxygenation may be monitored via two invasive modalities: jugular bulb oxygen saturation and $PbtO_2$ by the insertion of a catheter in the brain parenchyma. NIRS is a noninvasive bedside monitoring technique which detects changes in oxygen and deoxyhemoglobin concentration similarly to pulse oximetry [50, 54, 92]. Jugular bulb oximetry ($SjvO_2$) reflects the difference between brain oxygen and brain metabolic rate of oxygen, assuming that arterial oxyhemoglobin saturation, hemoglobin concentration, and the oxygen/hemoglobin dissociation curve remain stable [93, 94]. Myerson [95] first described the percutaneous sampling and analysis of human cerebral venous blood from the jugular bulb in 1927. Gibs [96] observed the arteriovenous difference between oxygen, glucose, and lactate. Moreover, he proposed that cerebral venous blood oxygen saturation measurement allows an estimate of global metabolic demand in relation to oxygen consumption [94]. Catheterizing the dominant internal jugular vein to correctly assess global cerebral oxygenation is recommended for this type of monitoring. The catheter tip should be positioned in the jugular bulb and placement confirmed by lateral skull radiography. $SjvO_2$ provides an indirect measure of CBF. If it is low (<50% for more than 10 min duration), it may reflect hypoperfusion (decreased supply) or an increase in cerebral metabolism (increased demand) [30, 93, 94].

The arteriovenous difference in oxygen supply ($AVDO_2 = CMRO_2/CBF$; $CMRO_2$ = cerebral metabolic rate of oxygen) is the best estimate of the balance between brain metabolism and CBF [97]. When $AVDO_2$ increases, the cerebral metabolic demand is low, and when $AVDO_2$ decreases, this may be suggestive of hyperperfusion or tissue death [89]. $SjvO_2$ levels are correlated with $AVDO_2$ and may be useful in detecting ischemia or hyperemia [93, 94].

However, this method is limited by potential changes in arterial oxygen content, hemodilution, and position of the jugular bulb catheter, as well as by the need for frequent calibration and infrequent complications related to catheter insertion, such as infection, increased ICP, thrombosis, and pneumothorax [93, 94, 98].

Brain Tissue Oxygenation ($PbtO_2$)

Brain hypoxia has been shown to be harmful after a TBI, and it is recognized as a key secondary insult after injury [92, 99, 100]. In recent years, there has been growing evidence that patient outcome is improved after the application of therapy targeted at cerebral tissue oxygen pressure. In this targeted therapy, MAP and percentage of inspired oxygen fraction are often used to maintain this parameter at adequate levels [92, 100].

In 1956, Clark et al. [101] reported the possibility of monitoring oxygen tension in blood and tissue, and in 1993 Meixensberger [102] first demonstrated the concept of $PbtO_2$ monitoring and its potential to assist in management of TBI patients [100, 101]. The use of direct $PbtO_2$ monitors was approved by the US Food and Drug Administration in 2001 [100]. $PbtO_2$ may be measured focally in the brain via either Licox (Integra, USA) or Neurovent (Raumedic, Germany) catheters, both of which have been shown to be safe and to provide accurate data. These devices provide information about the balance between oxygen demand and delivery in an injured brain. They may be affected by changes in capillary perfusion, distance from the capillaries in an edematous brain, and barriers to oxygen diffusion [103].

Recent data suggests that $PbtO_2$ values are directly correlated with patient outcomes. Cerebral hypoxia is an independent predictor of poor prognosis, disconnected from ICP, CPP, and brain imaging changes [100, 104]. $PbtO_2$ monitoring devices appear to discriminate reliably between normal oxygenation, threatened ischemia, and critical ischemia [100]. After elevation of the fraction of inspired O_2, PaO_2 increases to supraphysiological levels, or hyperoxemia. However, the relationship between hypoxemia and outcome in patients with TBI is controversial [85, 100, 104]. The randomized, controlled, multicenter phase III BOOST-3 trial is investigating the outcomes of maintaining a management protocol based on $PbtO_2$ combined with ICP [105]. For now, $PbtO_2$ values should be interpreted in the context of other monitored parameters to establish optimal management in clinical practice [92]. Cerebral hypoxia is a known cause of worse neurological outcome in patients with TBI. It has been observed that a higher frequency of daily episodes of cerebral hypoxia and a longer duration are common in nonsurvivors. Hypoxia is defined as alveolar oxygen pressure (PaO_2) $\leq$ 60 mmHg or O_2 saturation $\leq$ 90% or $PbtO_2 < 20$ mmHg [103–105].

1.3.3.3 Cerebral Microdialysis

Microdialysis consists of inserting an intraparenchymal catheter which allows diffusion of water and soluble substances at the distal end of the catheter across a semipermeable membrane. This permits constant assessment of the biochemical state of the brain tissue and interstitial fluid [106]. This information can help to guide therapy such as MAP parameters, ventilatory rate, and pCO_2 levels, and hyperosmolar therapy as well as the potential need for surgical interventions [106–108]. It could predict secondary damage before detection by clinical manifestations and conventional monitoring [106, 108, 109].

This method was first described in animal studies measuring neurotransmitters by Gaddum (1961) [110] and Myers (1972) [111]. In 1966, Bitto [108, 112] reported a dialysis technique using small volumes of interstitial tissue (e.g., brain), and Delgado (1972) [113] improved it using an electrode in a solution continuously perfused through a dialysis bag, later called a dialytrode. Ungerstedt [114, 115], in the late 1970s and early 1980s, improved the efficiency of microdialysis by enlarging the surface area of the dialysis membrane. The successful use of microdialysis to quantify monoamine levels in neural tissue contributed significantly to the worldwide use of cerebral microdialysis [109].

Microdialysis can reveal the chemical composition of the interstitial fluid. Water and solutes diffuse between the interstitial fluid and perfused solution, which is called the perfusate, and the concentration gradient between these two chambers allows the diffusion of solutes at a constant speed, enabling their measurement in the dialysate. A number of metabolites have been studied and are believed to serve as biomarkers following TBI. The most commonly measured metabolites include glucose, lactate, pyruvate, glycerol, and glutamate [106–109].

Microdialysis has provided important information about TBI pathophysiology and continues to be an important tool as new biochemical markers are being investigated and utilized. However, further studies are necessary to clarify whether interventions based on microdialysis data may improve patient outcomes [106–109].

1.3.4 Multimodal Monitoring

Several parameters can be evaluated at the same time and can be used to establish a patient's prognosis after TBI, detect secondary injuries before irreversible damage occurs, allowing more thorough assessment of patient condition [116–118].

Among the commonly evaluated parameters and techniques are ICP, MAP, central venous oxygen saturation, TCD, ONSD, microdialysis, NIRS, continuous EEG, and other invasive and noninvasive physiologic trends at the bedside [116–118].

The use of a data acquisition and integration device, such as the Moberg CNS monitor, can provide the appropriate display and data synthesis to help clinicians identify significant physiological trends and optimal clinical responses to interventions. By condensing individual monitors and numeric feedback onto a single screen and formatting data into a graphical display, this system can help clinicians increase their understanding and recall of significant patient physiology, thereby improving the quality of patient care [116–118].

1.4 Conclusion

Traditionally, TBI management has focused on treating increased ICP and low CPP. Technological advancement has led to new tools which may provide this information with greater safety. However, research has expanded our knowledge of pathophysiological mechanisms underlying secondary damage to the brain after TBI far beyond these two parameters. Multimodal monitoring holds promise for analyzing a broader set of physiologic parameters to enable more extensive optimization of brain physiology following injury.

Disclosures The authors have nothing to disclose. All the authors declare that there is no financial conflict with the developers or producers of any of the above-mentioned devices.

References

1. Hughes JT. The Edwin Smith Surgical Papyrus: an analysis of the first case reports of spinal cord injuries. Paraplegia. 1988;26(2):71–82. https://doi.org/10.1038/sc.1988.15.
2. Sanchez GM, Burridge AL. Decision making in head injury management in the Edwin Smith Papyrus. Neurosurg Focus. 2007;23(1):E5. https://doi.org/10.3171/foc.2007.23.1.5.
3. Goodrich JT. Cervical spine surgery in the ancient and medieval worlds. Neurosurg Focus. 2007;23(1):E7. https://doi.org/10.3171/foc.2007.23.1.7.
4. Kshettry VR, Mindea SA, Batjer HH. The management of cranial injuries in antiquity and beyond. Neurosurg Focus. 2007;23(1):E8. https://doi.org/10.3171/foc.2007.23.1.8.
5. Zargaran A, Zarshenas MM, Karimi A, Yarmohammadi H, Borhani-Haghighi A. Management of stroke as described by Ibn Sina (Avicenna) in the canon of medicine. Int J Cardiol. 2013;169(4):233–7. Epub 2013 Sep 7. https://doi.org/10.1016/j.ijcard.2013.08.115.
6. Volovici V, Steyerberg EW, Cnossen MC, Haitsma IK, Dirven CMF, Maas AIR, Lingsma HF. Evolution of evidence and guideline recommendations for the medical management of severe traumatic brain injury. J Neurotrauma. 2019;36(22):3183–9. Epub 2019 Jul 31. https://doi.org/10.1089/neu.2019.6474.
7. Missios S. Hippocrates, Galen, and the uses of trepanation in the ancient classical world. Neurosurg Focus. 2007;23(1):E11. https://doi.org/10.3171/foc.2007.23.1.11.
8. Rose FC. The history of head injuries: an overview. J Hist Neurosci. 1997;6(2):154–80. https://doi.org/10.1080/09647049709525700.
9. Talamonti G, D'Aliberti G, Cenzato M. Aulus Cornelius Celsus and the head injuries. World Neurosurg. 2020;133:127–34. Epub 2019 Sep 27. https://doi.org/10.1016/j.wneu.2019.09.119.
10. Padayachy LC, Figaji AA, Bullock MR. Intracranial pressure monitoring for traumatic brain injury in the modern era. Childs Nerv Syst. 2010;26(4):441–52. https://doi.org/10.1007/s00381-009-1034-0.
11. Hawryluk GWJ, Citerio G, Hutchinson P, Kolias A, Meyfroidt G, Robba C, Stocchetti N, Chesnut R. Intracranial pressure: current perspectives on physiology and monitoring. Intensive Care Med. 2022;48(10):1471–81. Epub 2022 Jul 11. https://doi.org/10.1007/s00134-022-06786-y.
12. Sanan A, Haines SJ. Repairing holes in the head: a history of cranioplasty. Neurosurgery. 1997;40(3):588–603. https://doi.org/10.1097/00006123-199703000-00033.
13. Sonig A, Jumah F, Raju B, Patel NV, Gupta G, Nanda A. The historical evolution of intracranial pressure monitoring. World Neurosurg. 2020;138:491–7. Epub 2020 Mar 14. https://doi.org/10.1016/j.wneu.2020.03.028.
14. Niccolò M. Liber introductorius Anatomiæ. Venise: Ed. Francesco Bindoni et Maffeo Pasini; 1536.
15. Cotugno DF. De ischiade nervosa commentaries. Napoli and Bologna: Frates Simonios; 1761.
16. Monro A. Observations on the structure and functions of the nervous system. Lond Med J. 1783;4(2):113–35.
17. Magendie F. Recherches anatomique et physiologique Sur le liquide céphalo-rachidien ou cérebro-spinal. Paris: Méquignon-Marvis fils; 1842.
18. Tubbs RS, Vahedi P, Loukas M, Shoja MM, Cohen-Gadol AA. Hubert von Luschka (1820-1875): his life, discoveries, and contributions to our understanding of the nervous system. J Neurosurg. 2011;114(1):268–72. Epub 2010 Sep 24. https://doi.org/10.3171/2010.8.JNS10683.
19. Retzius MG, Key A. Studien in der Anatomie des Nervensystems und des Bindegewebes. Stockholm: Samson und Wallin; 1875.

20. Goodrich JT. Landmarks in the history of neurosurgery. In: Principles of neurological surgery. Amsterdam: Elsevier; 2018. p. 1–37.
21. Teles RV. Phineas Gage's great legacy. Dement Neuropsychol. 2020;14(4):419–21. PMID: 33354296; PMCID: PMC7735047. https://doi.org/10.1590/1980-57642020dn14-040013.
22. López-Muñoz F, Boya J, Alamo C. Neuron theory, the cornerstone of neuroscience, on the centenary of the Nobel prize award to Santiago Ramón y Cajal. Brain Res Bull. 2006;70(4–6):391–405. Epub 2006 Aug 14. https://doi.org/10.1016/j.brainresbull.2006.07.010.
23. Escalante-Alcalde D, Chimal-Monroy J. Insights into the mechanism of adult neurogenesis - an interview with Arturo Álvarez-Buylla. Int J Dev Biol. 2021;65(1-2-3):153–61. https://doi.org/10.1387/ijdb.200297de.
24. Hawryluk GW, Manley GT. Classification of traumatic brain injury: past, present, and future. Handb Clin Neurol. 2015;127:15–21. https://doi.org/10.1016/B978-0-444-52892-6.00002-7.
25. Stein SC, Georgoff P, Meghan S, Mizra K, Sonnad SS. 150 years of treating severe traumatic brain injury: a systematic review of progress in mortality. J Neurotrauma. 2010;27(7):1343–53. https://doi.org/10.1089/neu.2009.1206.
26. Hawryluk GWJ, Ghajar J. Evolution and Impact of the brain trauma foundation guidelines. Neurosurgery. 2021;89(6):1148–56. https://doi.org/10.1093/neuros/nyab357.
27. Bullock R, Chesnut RM, Clifton G, Ghajar J, Marion DW, Narayan RK, Newell DW, Pitts LH, Rosner MJ, Wilberger JW. Guidelines for the management of severe head injury. Brain trauma foundation. Eur J Emerg Med. 1996 Jun;3(2):109–27. https://doi.org/10.1097/00063110-199606000-00010.
28. The Brain Trauma Foundation. The American Association of Neurological Surgeons. The joint section on Neurotrauma and critical care. Methodology. J Neurotrauma. 2000;17(6-7):561–2. https://doi.org/10.1089/neu.2000.17.561.
29. Brain Trauma Foundation; American Association of Neurological Surgeons; Congress of Neurological Surgeons; Joint Section on Neurotrauma and Critical Care, AANS/CNS, Carney NA. Guidelines for the management of severe traumatic brain injury. Methods. J Neurotrauma. 2007;24 Suppl 1:S3–6. Erratum in: J Neurotrauma. 2008 Mar;25(3):276–8. Carney, Nancy A [added]. https://doi.org/10.1089/neu.2007.9996.
30. Carney N, Totten AM, O'Reilly C, Ullman JS, Hawryluk GW, Bell MJ, Bratton SL, Chesnut R, Harris OA, Kissoon N, Rubiano AM, Shutter L, Tasker RC, Vavilala MS, Wilberger J, Wright DW, Ghajar J. Guidelines for the management of severe traumatic brain injury, fourth edition. Neurosurgery. 2017;80(1):6–15. https://doi.org/10.1227/NEU.0000000000001432.
31. Quincke HI. Verhandlungen des congresses für Innere Medizin. Wiesbaden: Zenther Congress; 1891. p. 321–31.
32. Guillaume J, Janny P. Continuous intracranial manometry; physiopathologic and clinical significance of the method. Presse Med. 1951;59(45):953–5.
33. Wijdicks EFM. Lundberg and his waves. Neurocrit Care. 2019;31(3):546–9. https://doi.org/10.1007/s12028-019-00689-5.
34. Lundberg N. Continuous recording and control of ventricular fluid pressure in neurosurgical practice. Acta Psychiatr Scand Suppl. 1960;36(149):1–193.
35. Lundberg N, Troupp H, Lorin H. Continuous recording of the ventricular-fluid pressure in patients with severe acute traumatic brain injury. A preliminary report. J Neurosurg. 1965;22(6):581–90. https://doi.org/10.3171/jns.1965.22.6.0581.
36. Becker DP, Miller JD, Ward JD, Greenberg RP, Young HF, Sakalas R. The outcome from severe head injury with early diagnosis and intensive management. J Neurosurg. 1977;47(4):491–502. https://doi.org/10.3171/jns.1977.47.4.0491.
37. Miller JD, Becker DP, Ward JD, Sullivan HG, Adams WE, Rosner MJ. Significance of intracranial hypertension in severe head injury. J Neurosurg. 1977;47(4):503–16. https://doi.org/10.3171/jns.1977.47.4.0503.
38. Meyfroidt G, Bouzat P, Casaer MP, Chesnut R, Hamada SR, Helbok R, Hutchinson P, Maas AIR, Manley G, Menon DK, Newcombe VFJ, Oddo M, Robba C, Shutter L, Smith M, Steyerberg EW, Stocchetti N, Taccone FS, Wilson L, Zanier ER, Citerio G. Management

of moderate to severe traumatic brain injury: an update for the intensivist. Intensive Care Med. 2022;48(6):649–66. Epub 2022 may 20. Erratum in: Intensive Care Med 2022 Jul;48(7):989–991. https://doi.org/10.1007/s00134-022-06702-4.
39. Rubiano AM, Griswold DP, Jibaja M, Rabinstein AA, Godoy DA. Management of severe traumatic brain injury in regions with limited resources. Brain Inj. 2021;35(11):1317–25. Epub 2021 Sep 7. https://doi.org/10.1080/02699052.2021.1972149.
40. Schizodimos T, Soulountsi V, Iasonidou C, Kapravelos N. An overview of management of intracranial hypertension in the intensive care unit. J Anesth. 2020;34(5):741–57. Epub 2020 May 21. PMID: 32440802; PMCID: PMC7241587. https://doi.org/10.1007/s00540-020-02795-7.
41. Abraham M, Singhal V. Intracranial pressure monitoring. J Neuroanaesthesiol Crit Care. 2015;2(03):193–203.
42. Vries JK, Becker DP, Young HF. A subarachnoid screw for monitoring intracranial pressure. Technical note. J Neurosurg. 1973;39(3):416–9. https://doi.org/10.3171/jns.1973.39.3.0416.
43. Swann KW, Cosman ER. Modification of the Richmond subarachnoid screw for monitoring intracranial pressure. Technical note. J Neurosurg. 1984;60(5):1102–3. https://doi.org/10.3171/jns.1984.60.5.1102.
44. Ostrup RC, Luerssen TG, Marshall LF, Zornow MH. Continuous monitoring of intracranial pressure with a miniaturized fiberoptic device. J Neurosurg. 1987;67(2):206–9. https://doi.org/10.3171/jns.1987.67.2.0206.
45. Gelabert-González M, Ginesta-Galan V, Sernamito-García R, Allut AG, Bandin-Diéguez J, Rumbo RM. The Camino intracranial pressure device in clinical practice. Assessment in a 1000 cases. Acta Neurochir. 2006;148(4):435–41. Epub 2005 Dec 27. https://doi.org/10.1007/s00701-005-0683-3.
46. Koskinen LO, Olivecrona M. Clinical experience with the intraparenchymal intracranial pressure monitoring Codman MicroSensor system. Neurosurgery. 2005;56(4):693–8; discussion 693-8. https://doi.org/10.1227/01.neu.0000156609.95596.24.
47. Lang JM, Beck J, Zimmermann M, Seifert V, Raabe A. Clinical evaluation of intraparenchymal Spiegelberg pressure sensor. Neurosurgery. 2003;52(6):1455–9; discussion 1459. https://doi.org/10.1227/01.neu.0000065136.70455.6f.
48. Rot S, Dweek M, Gutowski P, Goelz L, Meier U, Lemcke J. Comparative investigation of different telemetric methods for measuring intracranial pressure: a prospective pilot study. Fluids Barriers CNS. 2020;17(1):63. PMID: 33069242; PMCID: PMC7568395. https://doi.org/10.1186/s12987-020-00225-0.
49. Lescot T, Reina V, Le Manach Y, Boroli F, Chauvet D, Boch AL, Puybasset L. In vivo accuracy of two intraparenchymal intracranial pressure monitors. Intensive Care Med. 2011;37(5):875–9. Epub 2011 Feb 26. https://doi.org/10.1007/s00134-011-2182-8.
50. Nag DS, Sahu S, Swain A, Kant S. Intracranial pressure monitoring: gold standard and recent innovations. World J Clin Cases. 2019;7(13):1535–53. PMID: 31367614; PMCID: PMC6658373. https://doi.org/10.12998/wjcc.v7.i13.1535.
51. Evensen KB, Eide PK. Measuring intracranial pressure by invasive, less invasive or non-invasive means: limitations and avenues for improvement. Fluids Barriers CNS. 2020;17(1):34. PMID: 32375853; PMCID: PMC7201553. https://doi.org/10.1186/s12987-020-00195-3.
52. Moraes FM, Silva GS. Noninvasive intracranial pressure monitoring methods: a critical review. Arq Neuropsiquiatr. 2021;79(5):437–46. PMID: 34161530; PMCID: PMC9394557. https://doi.org/10.1590/0004-282X-ANP-2020-0300.
53. Raboel PH, Bartek J Jr, Andresen M, Bellander BM, Romner B. Intracranial pressure monitoring: invasive versus non-invasive methods—a review. Crit Care Res Prac. 2012;2012:950393. Epub 2012 Jun 8. PMID: 22720148; PMCID: PMC3376474. https://doi.org/10.1155/2012/950393.
54. Ballestero MF. Avaliação não invasiva da pressão intracraniana em indivíduos acometidos por traumatismo cranioencefálico grave (Doctoral dissertation, Universidade de São Paulo). 2021.

55. Peters RJ, Hanlo PW, Gooskens RH, Braun KP, Tulleken CA, Willemse J. Non-invasive ICP monitoring in infants: the Rotterdam Teletransducer revisited. Childs Nerv Syst. 1995;11(4):207–13. https://doi.org/10.1007/BF00277655.
56. Vidyasagar D, Raju TN. A simple noninvasive technique of measuring intracranial pressure in the newborn. Pediatrics. 1977;59 Suppl(6 Pt 2):957–61.
57. Hayreh SS. Pathogenesis of oedema of the optic disc (papilloedema). A preliminary report. Br J Ophthalmol. 1964;48(10):522–43. PMID: 14221776; PMCID: PMC506011. https://doi.org/10.1136/bjo.48.10.522.
58. Geeraerts T, Duranteau J, Benhamou D. Ocular sonography in patients with raised intracranial pressure: the papilloedema revisited. Crit Care. 2008;12(3):150. Epub 2008 May 16. PMID: 18495051; PMCID: PMC2481446. https://doi.org/10.1186/cc6893.
59. Khan MN, Shallwani H, Khan MU, Shamim MS. Noninvasive monitoring intracranial pressure—a review of available modalities. Surg Neurol Int. 2017;8:51. PMID: 28480113; PMCID: PMC5402331. https://doi.org/10.4103/sni.sni_403_16.
60. Baurmann M. Über die Entstehung und klinische Bedeutung des Netzhautvenenpulses. Dtsch Ophthalmol Ges. 1925;45:53–9.
61. Firsching R, Müller C, Pauli SU, Voellger B, Röhl FW, Behrens-Baumann W. Noninvasive assessment of intracranial pressure with venous ophthalmodynamometry. Clinical article. J Neurosurg. 2011;115(2):371–4. Epub 2011 Apr 29. https://doi.org/10.3171/2011.3.JNS101275.
62. Reid A, Marchbanks RJ, Burge DM, Martin AM, Bateman DE, Pickard JD, Brightwell AP. The relationship between intracranial pressure and tympanic membrane displacement. Br J Audiol. 1990;24(2):123–9. https://doi.org/10.3109/03005369009077853.
63. Canac N, Jalaleddini K, Thorpe SG, Thibeault CM, Hamilton RB. Review: pathophysiology of intracranial hypertension and noninvasive intracranial pressure monitoring. Fluids Barriers CNS. 2020;17(1):40. PMID: 32576216; PMCID: PMC7310456. https://doi.org/10.1186/s12987-020-00201-8.
64. Rosenberg JB, Shiloh AL, Savel RH, Eisen LA. Non-invasive methods of estimating intracranial pressure. Neurocrit Care. 2011;15(3):599–608. https://doi.org/10.1007/s12028-011-9545-4.
65. Marshall LF, Marshall SB, Klauber MR, van Berkum CM, Eisenberg HM, Jane JA, Luerssen TG, Marmarou A, Foulkes MA. A new classification of head injury based on computerized tomography. J Neurosurg. 1991;75(Supplement):S14–20.
66. Maas AI, Hukkelhoven CW, Marshall LF, Steyerberg EW. Prediction of outcome in traumatic brain injury with computed tomographic characteristics: a comparison between the computed tomographic classification and combinations of computed tomographic predictors. Neurosurgery. 2005;57(6):1173–82; discussion 1173-82. https://doi.org/10.1227/01.neu.0000186013.63046.6b.
67. Raksin PB, Alperin N, Sivaramakrishnan A, Surapaneni S, Lichtor T. Noninvasive intracranial compliance and pressure based on dynamic magnetic resonance imaging of blood flow and cerebrospinal fluid flow: review of principles, implementation, and other noninvasive approaches. Neurosurg Focus. 2003;14(4):e4. https://doi.org/10.3171/foc.2003.14.4.4.
68. Gass A, Barker GJ, Riordan-Eva P, MacManus D, Sanders M, Tofts PS, McDonald WI, Moseley IF, Miller DH. MRI of the optic nerve in benign intracranial hypertension. Neuroradiology. 1996;38(8):769–73. https://doi.org/10.1007/s002340050344.
69. Michaeli D, Rappaport ZH. Tissue resonance analysis; a novel method for noninvasive monitoring of intracranial pressure. Technical note. J Neurosurg. 2002;96(6):1132–7. https://doi.org/10.3171/jns.2002.96.6.1132.
70. Amantini A, Fossi S, Grippo A, Innocenti P, Amadori A, Bucciardini L, Cossu C, Nardini C, Scarpelli S, Roma V, Pinto F. Continuous EEG-SEP monitoring in severe brain injury. Neurophysiol Clin. 2009;39(2):85–93. Epub 2009 Feb 14. https://doi.org/10.1016/j.neucli.2009.01.006.
71. Lescot T, Naccache L, Bonnet MP, Abdennour L, Coriat P, Puybasset L. The relationship of intracranial pressure Lundberg waves to electroencephalograph fluctuations in patients

with severe head trauma. Acta Neurochir. 2005;147(2):125–9; discussion. Epub 2004 Dec 2. https://doi.org/10.1007/s00701-004-0355-8.
72. Chen H, Wang J, Mao S, Dong W, Yang H. A new method of intracranial pressure monitoring by EEG power spectrum analysis. Can J Neurol Sci. 2012;39(4):483–7. https://doi.org/10.1017/s0317167100013998.
73. Marshall LF, Barba D, Toole BM, Bowers SA. The oval pupil: clinical significance and relationship to intracranial hypertension. J Neurosurg. 1983;58(4):566–8. https://doi.org/10.3171/jns.1983.58.4.0566.
74. Taylor WR, Chen JW, Meltzer H, Gennarelli TA, Kelbch C, Knowlton S, Richardson J, Lutch MJ, Farin A, Hults KN, Marshall LF. Quantitative pupillometry, a new technology: normative data and preliminary observations in patients with acute head injury. Technical note. J Neurosurg. 2003;98(1):205–13. https://doi.org/10.3171/jns.2003.98.1.0205.
75. Boev AN, Fountas KN, Karampelas I, Boev C, Machinis TG, Feltes C, Okosun I, Dimopoulos V, Troup C. Quantitative pupillometry: normative data in healthy pediatric volunteers. J Neurosurg. 2005;103(6 Suppl):496–500. https://doi.org/10.3171/ped.2005.103.6.0496.
76. Chen JW, Gombart ZJ, Rogers S, Gardiner SK, Cecil S, Bullock RM. Pupillary reactivity as an early indicator of increased intracranial pressure: the introduction of the neurological pupil index. Surg Neurol Int. 2011;2:82. Epub 2011 Jun 21. PMID: 21748035; PMCID: PMC3130361. https://doi.org/10.4103/2152-7806.82248.
77. Bower MM, Sweidan AJ, Xu JC, Stern-Neze S, Yu W, Groysman LI. Quantitative Pupillometry in the intensive care unit. J Intensive Care Med. 2021;36(4):383–91. Epub 2019 Oct 10. https://doi.org/10.1177/0885066619881124.
78. Aaslid R, Markwalder TM, Nornes H. Noninvasive transcranial Doppler ultrasound recording of flow velocity in basal cerebral arteries. J Neurosurg. 1982;57(6):769–74. https://doi.org/10.3171/jns.1982.57.6.0769.
79. Voulgaris SG, Partheni M, Kaliora H, Haftouras N, Pessach IS, Polyzoidis KS. Early cerebral monitoring using the transcranial Doppler pulsatility index in patients with severe brain trauma. Med Sci Monit. 2005;11(2):CR49–52. PMID: 15668630.
80. Figaji AA, Zwane E, Fieggen AG, Siesjo P, Peter JC. Transcranial Doppler pulsatility index is not a reliable indicator of intracranial pressure in children with severe traumatic brain injury. Surg Neurol. 2009;72(4):389–94. Epub 2009 Jul 15. PMID: 19608224. https://doi.org/10.1016/j.surneu.2009.02.012.
81. Kampfl A, Pfausler B, Denchev D, Jaring HP, Schmutzhard E. Near infrared spectroscopy (NIRS) in patients with severe brain injury and elevated intracranial pressure. A pilot study. Acta Neurochir Suppl. 1997;70:112–4. PMID: 9416295. https://doi.org/10.1007/978-3-7091-6837-0_35.
82. Weerakkody RA, Czosnyka M, Zweifel C, Castellani G, Smielewski P, Brady K, Pickard JD, Czosnyka Z. Near infrared spectroscopy as possible non-invasive monitor of slow vasogenic ICP waves. Acta Neurochir Suppl. 2012;114:181–5. PMID: 22327689. https://doi.org/10.1007/978-3-7091-0956-4_35.
83. Zweifel C, Castellani G, Czosnyka M, Carrera E, Brady KM, Kirkpatrick PJ, Pickard JD, Smielewski P. Continuous assessment of cerebral autoregulation with near-infrared spectroscopy in adults after subarachnoid hemorrhage. Stroke. 2010;41(9):1963–8. Epub 2010 Jul 22. PMID: 20651272. https://doi.org/10.1161/STROKEAHA.109.577320.
84. Kristiansson H, Nissborg E, Bartek J Jr, Andresen M, Reinstrup P, Romner B. Measuring elevated intracranial pressure through noninvasive methods: a review of the literature. J Neurosurg Anesthesiol. 2013;25(4):372–85. PMID: 23715045. https://doi.org/10.1097/ANA.0b013e31829795ce.
85. Armstead WM. Cerebral blood flow autoregulation and dysautoregulation. Anesthesiol Clin. 2016;34(3):465–77. PMID: 27521192; PMCID: PMC4988341. https://doi.org/10.1016/j.anclin.2016.04.002.
86. de Lima-Oliveira M, ASM S, Nogueira RC, de Azevedo DS, Paiva WS, Teixeira MJ, Bor-Seng-Shu E. Intracranial hypertension and cerebral autoregulation: a systematic review and

meta-analysis. World Neurosurg. 2018;113:110–24. Epub 2018 Feb 6. PMID: 29421451. https://doi.org/10.1016/j.wneu.2018.01.194.
87. Tymko MM, Ainslie PN. To regulate, or not to regulate? The devious history of cerebral blood flow control. J Physiol. 2017;595(16):5407–8. Epub 2017 Jul 12. PMID: 28640419; PMCID: PMC5556160. https://doi.org/10.1113/JP274746.
88. Lassen NA. Cerebral blood flow and oxygen consumption in man. Physiol Rev. 1959;39(2):183–238. PMID: 13645234. https://doi.org/10.1152/physrev.1959.39.2.183.
89. Czosnyka M, Smielewski P, Kirkpatrick P, Laing RJ, Menon D, Pickard JD. Continuous assessment of the cerebral vasomotor reactivity in head injury. Neurosurgery. 1997;41(1):11–7; discussion 17–9. PMID: 9218290. https://doi.org/10.1097/00006123-199707000-00005.
90. Steiner LA, Czosnyka M, Piechnik SK, Smielewski P, Chatfield D, Menon DK, Pickard JD. Continuous monitoring of cerebrovascular pressure reactivity allows determination of optimal cerebral perfusion pressure in patients with traumatic brain injury. Crit Care Med. 2002;30(4):733–8. PMID: 11940737. https://doi.org/10.1097/00003246-200204000-00002.
91. Tas J, Beqiri E, van Kaam RC, Czosnyka M, Donnelly J, Haeren RH, van der Horst ICC, Hutchinson PJ, van Kuijk SMJ, Liberti AL, Menon DK, Hoedemaekers CWE, Depreitere B, Smielewski P, Meyfroidt G, Ercole A, Aries MJH. Targeting autoregulation-guided cerebral perfusion pressure after traumatic brain injury (COGiTATE): a feasibility randomized controlled clinical trial. J Neurotrauma. 2021;38(20):2790–800. Epub 2021 Aug 16. PMID: 34407385. https://doi.org/10.1089/neu.2021.0197.
92. Le Roux P, Menon DK, Citerio G, Vespa P, Bader MK, Brophy GM, Diringer MN, Stocchetti N, Videtta W, Armonda R, Badjatia N, Böesel J, Chesnut R, Chou S, Claassen J, Czosnyka M, De Georgia M, Figaji A, Fugate J, Helbok R, Horowitz D, Hutchinson P, Kumar M, McNett M, Miller C, Naidech A, Oddo M, Olson D, O'Phelan K, Provencio JJ, Puppo C, Riker R, Robertson C, Schmidt M, Taccone F, Neurocritical Care Society; European Society of Intensive Care Medicine. Consensus summary statement of the International Multidisciplinary Consensus Conference on Multimodality Monitoring in Neurocritical Care: a statement for healthcare professionals from the Neurocritical Care Society and the European Society of Intensive Care Medicine. Intensive Care Med. 2014;40(9):1189–209. Epub 2014 Aug 20. PMID: 25138226. https://doi.org/10.1007/s00134-014-3369-6.
93. Sinha S, Hudgins E, Schuster J, Balu R. Unraveling the complexities of invasive multimodality neuromonitoring. Neurosurg Focus. 2017;43(5):E4. PMID: 29088949. https://doi.org/10.3171/2017.8.FOCUS17449.
94. Bhardwaj A, Bhagat H, Grover VK. Jugular venous oximetry. J Neuroanaesthesiol Crit Care. 2015;2(03):225–31.
95. Myerson A, Halloran H, Hirsch HL. Technic for obtaining blood from the internal jugular vein and internal carotid artery. Arch Neurol Psychiatry. 1927;17(6):807–8.
96. Gibbs EL, Lennox WG, Nims LF, Gibbs FA. Arterial and cerebral venous blood: arterial-venous differences in man. J Biol Chem. 1942;144(2):325–32.
97. Robertson CS, Contant CF, Gokaslan ZL, Narayan RK, Grossman RG. Cerebral blood flow, arteriovenous oxygen difference, and outcome in head injured patients. J Neurol Neurosurg Psychiatry. 1992;55(7):594–603. PMID: 1640238; PMCID: PMC489173. https://doi.org/10.1136/jnnp.55.7.594.
98. Lewis SB, Myburgh JA, Reilly PL. Detection of cerebral venous desaturation by continuous jugular bulb oximetry following acute neurotrauma. Anaesth Intensive Care. 1995;23(3):307–14. PMID: 7573917. https://doi.org/10.1177/0310057X9502300307.
99. McHugh GS, Engel DC, Butcher I, Steyerberg EW, Lu J, Mushkudiani N, Hernández AV, Marmarou A, Maas AI, Murray GD. Prognostic value of secondary insults in traumatic brain injury: results from the IMPACT study. J Neurotrauma. 2007;24(2):287–93. PMID: 17375993. https://doi.org/10.1089/neu.2006.0031.
100. Maloney-Wilensky E, Le Roux P. The physiology behind direct brain oxygen monitors and practical aspects of their use. Childs Nerv Syst. 2010;26(4):419–30. PMID: 19937246. https://doi.org/10.1007/s00381-009-1037-x.

101. Qlark LC Jr. Monitor and control of blood and tissue oxygen tensions. ASAIO J. 1956;2(1):41–8.
102. Meixensberger J, Dings J, Kuhnigk H, Roosen K. Studies of tissue PO2 in normal and pathological human brain cortex. Acta Neurochir Suppl (Wien). 1993;59:58–63. PMID: 7906079. https://doi.org/10.1007/978-3-7091-9302-0_10.
103. Leach MR, Shutter LA. How much oxygen for the injured brain - can invasive parenchymal catheters help? Curr Opin Crit Care. 2021;27(2):95–102. PMID: 33560016; PMCID: PMC7987136. https://doi.org/10.1097/MCC.0000000000000810.
104. Raj R, Bendel S, Reinikainen M, Kivisaari R, Siironen J, Lång M, Skrifvars M. Hyperoxemia and long-term outcome after traumatic brain injury. Crit Care. 2013;17(4):R177. PMID: 23958227; PMCID: PMC4056982. https://doi.org/10.1186/cc12856.
105. BOOST-3|SIREN [Internet]. https://siren.network/clinical-trials/boost-3. Accessed 10 Oct 2022.
106. Goodman JC, Robertson CS. Microdialysis: is it ready for prime time? Curr Opin Crit Care. 2009;15(2):110–7. PMID: 19578321; PMCID: PMC3593094. https://doi.org/10.1097/MCC.0b013e328325d142.
107. Young B, Kalanuria A, Kumar M, Burke K, Balu R, Amendolia O, McNulty K, Marion B, Beckmann B, Ciocco L, Miller K, Schuele D, Maloney-Wilensky E, Frangos S, Wright D. Cerebral microdialysis. Crit Care Nurs Clin North Am. 2016;28(1):109–24. PMID: 26873764. https://doi.org/10.1016/j.cnc.2015.09.005.
108. Tisdall MM, Smith M. Cerebral microdialysis: research technique or clinical tool. Br J Anaesth. 2006;97(1):18–25. Epub 2006 May 12. PMID: 16698861. https://doi.org/10.1093/bja/ael109.
109. Chefer VI, Thompson AC, Zapata A, Shippenberg TS. Overview of brain microdialysis. Curr Protoc Neurosci. 2009;Chapter 7:Unit7.1. PMID: 19340812; PMCID: PMC2953244. https://doi.org/10.1002/0471142301.ns0701s47.
110. Gaddum JH. Push-pull cannulae. J Physiol. 1961;155:1–2.
111. Myers RD. Methods for perfusing different structures of the brain. In: Methods in psychobiology. New York: Academic Press; 1972. p. 169–211.
112. Bito L, Davson H, Levin E, Murray M, Snider N. The concentrations of free amino acids and other electrolytes in cerebrospinal fluid, in vivo dialysate of brain, and blood plasma of the dog. J Neurochem. 1966;13(11):1057–67. PMID: 5924657. https://doi.org/10.1111/j.1471-4159.1966.tb04265.x.
113. Delgado JM, DeFeudis FV, Roth RH, Ryugo DK, Mitruka BM. Dialytrode for long term intracerebral perfusion in awake monkeys. Arch Int Pharmacodyn Ther. 1972;198(1):9–21. PMID: 4626478.
114. Ungerstedt U, Pycock C. Functional correlates of dopamine neurotransmission. Bull Schweiz Akad Med Wiss. 1974;30(1–3):44–55. PMID: 4371656.
115. Ungerstedt U, Herrera-Marschitz M, Jungnelius U, Stahle L, Tossman U, Zetterström T. Dopamine synaptic mechanisms reflected in studies combining behavioural recordings and brain dialysis. In: Advances in dopamine research. Oxford: Pergamon; 1982. p. 219–31.
116. Foreman B, Lissak IA, Kamireddi N, Moberg D, Rosenthal ES. Challenges and opportunities in multimodal monitoring and data analytics in traumatic brain injury. Curr Neurol Neurosci Rep. 2021;21(3):6. PMID: 33527217; PMCID: PMC7850903. https://doi.org/10.1007/s11910-021-01098-y.
117. Rodriguez A, Smielewski P, Rosenthal E, Moberg D. Medical device connectivity challenges outline the technical requirements and standards for promoting big data research and personalized medicine in neurocritical care. Mil Med. 2018;183(suppl_1):99–104. PMID: 29635618. https://doi.org/10.1093/milmed/usx146.
118. Appavu B, Burrows BT, Nickoles T, Boerwinkle V, Willyerd A, Gunnala V, Mangum T, Marku I, Adelson PD. Implementation of multimodality neurologic monitoring reporting in pediatric traumatic brain injury management. Neurocrit Care. 2021;35(1):3–15. Epub 2021 Mar 31. PMID: 33791948; PMCID: PMC8012079. https://doi.org/10.1007/s12028-021-01190-8.

2 The Importance of Pathways: Trauma Center and Neurocritical Care Unit

Uma Anushka Bagga, Areg Grigorian, Jefferson Chen, Cyrus Dastur, and Jeffry Nahmias

2.1 Introduction

Severe traumatic brain injury (TBI) is a major source of morbidity and mortality, especially in blunt trauma patients. TBI patients incur enormous hospital expenses and can develop multiple complications including pneumonia [1], respiratory failure [2, 3], and venous thromboembolism (VTE) [4, 5]. TBI patients also commonly require prolonged intensive care unit (ICU) treatment, which increases costs even more [1]. Furthermore, the care of these patients is complex and demanding, requiring the integration of skills from numerous medical disciplines (i.e., trauma surgery, critical care, neurosurgery, neurology, physical medicine and rehabilitation, speech

U. A. Bagga
Division of Trauma and Acute Care Surgery, Loma Linda University, Loma Linda, CA, USA

Division of Trauma, Burns and Surgical Critical Care, University of California, Irvine, CA, USA
e-mail: ubagga@llu.edu

A. Grigorian · J. Nahmias (✉)
Division of Trauma, Burns and Surgical Critical Care, University of California, Irvine, CA, USA
e-mail: agrigori@hs.uci.edu

J. Chen
Department of Neurological Surgery, University of California, Irvine, Irvine, CA, USA
e-mail: jeffewc1@hs.uci.edu

C. Dastur
Department of Neurology, University of California, Irvine, Irvine, CA, USA
e-mail: cdastur@hs.uci.edu

E. Brogi et al. (eds.), *Traumatic Brain Injury*, Hot Topics in Acute Care Surgery and Trauma, https://doi.org/10.1007/978-3-031-50117-3_2

language pathology, physical therapy, occupational therapy, etc.) [1]. As such, implementation of a well-designed multidisciplinary clinical pathway is appealing to help ensure high-quality standardized care is maintained despite involvement of multiple specialties and personnel within those specialties.

Clinical pathways are "road maps" that provide a detailed framework for all aspects of patient care during hospitalization [6, 7]. This includes physician and nursing care, pharmacologic therapy, imaging, and laboratory resource utilization. In addition, coordination of rehabilitation with physical, occupational, and speech therapy as well as discharge planning is paramount to the recovery of TBI patients and can be incorporated within a clinical pathway. This enables improved standardization and thus optimal patient care by providing a system that helps minimize fluctuations and/or lapses in evidence-based treatment. In effect the pathway establishes a framework from which further treatment decisions are derived and/or can build upon the scaffold.

Pathways have been demonstrated to improve outcomes [1]. The "technique driven" with standard in cardiac, eye, or orthopedic surgery lend themselves nicely to a clinical pathway approach, but in the complex and unpredictable setting of TBI, which often comes with other traumatic injuries, creating and implementing a standardized pathway requires more detail yet flexibility and frequent modification based on feedback after implementation [8]. An additional key to successful pathway development is input by a multidisciplinary team of physicians, nurses, and members of other services who frequently provide care for the particular patient population the pathway is designed to service [8]. This ensures nuanced clinical aspects of care are appropriately addressed.

In terms of TBI, initial reports on pathway implementation have demonstrated improved length of stay (LOS), ICU LOS, ventilator days, and containment of healthcare expenditures. Also, qualitative pathways have been shown to assist with nursing education and provide channels of communication with patients' families which in turn helps keep family members informed about anticipated therapies, interventions, and potential complications. This helps facilitate increased family engagement as they are privy to the next steps/goals of care.

This chapter will delve deeper into specific aspects of TBI pathways including early enteral feeding, deep vein thrombosis prophylaxis, early tracheostomy placement as well as rehabilitation and referral to post-discharge care.

2.2 Early Tracheostomy

Tracheotomy (often referred to as tracheostomy) is an operative procedure that creates a surgical airway in the cervical trachea. It is performed in patients for many indications including difficulty weaning from a ventilator, airway obstruction, and catastrophic neurologic insult (e.g., TBI) [9]. Tracheostomy also facilitates pulmonary toilet and allows a patient who may require intermittent positive pressure ventilation the opportunity to be liberated from the ventilator for a period of time but then expeditiously reconnect to mechanical ventilation, without risks associated with reintubation. In the general ICU population, multiple studies [10, 11] have been performed with mixed results regarding the impact that a tracheostomy may have on the incidence of ventilator associated pneumonia (VAP), ventilator days, and ICU LOS. However, studies focusing on patients with TBI have demonstrated reduced ventilator days and ICU LOS with early tracheostomy [12, 13].

The definition for early tracheostomy after trauma is variable in the literature, ranging from 2 to 7 days [12–16]. This is distinct from medical ICU populations that historically were recommended to undergo tracheostomy if ventilator liberation failed to occur by 21 days post-intubation and more recently guidelines have suggested within 14 days of intubation [17].

However, a patient intubated for airway protection due to severe TBI is unique in that they have healthy cardiopulmonary systems with uncompromised respiratory mechanics and thus the only indication for mechanical ventilation is their presumed inability to protect their airway from aspiration due to impaired level of consciousness affecting protective reflexes. Therefore, early performance of a tracheostomy enables TBI patients to be liberated from mechanical ventilation early in their hospitalization, thus minimizing ventilator days and the associated complications including VAP, pressure wounds, stress ulcers, and a prolonged ICU LOS [15, 18].

In fact, pathways have enabled this practice to occur in a standardized fashion with tracheostomy placement as early as post-injury day 4 [8]. Furthermore, a meta-analysis of over 5000 patients by Marra et al. which included two randomized controlled trials found that early tracheostomy was associated with reduced ICU LOS, total hospital LOS, and duration of mechanical ventilation [14]. An additional meta-analysis by McCredie et al. similarly noted that early tracheostomy reduced duration of mechanical ventilation and ICU LOS [16]. In addition, they identified a reduced risk of mortality at 6- and 12-month post-tracheostomy [16].

Thus, implementation of a pathway that standardizes indications for early tracheostomy should help preserve ICU resources and minimize complications while potentially improving overall survival from TBI.

2.2.1 Early Physical and Cognitive Rehabilitation

Advances in medical technology and improvements in regional trauma services have increased the number of survivors of TBI, producing social consequences and challenges of an increasing pool of people with cerebral injury. Wider awareness of the scope of the problem and its consequences for society has led to rapid growth in the rehabilitation industry. In fact, three quarters of TBIs that require hospitalization are non-fatal and annually ~80,000 survivors of TBI incur disability or require increased medical care. As such, direct medical costs for TBI treatment are estimated at over $48-billion dollars per year including the costs of rehabilitation [19]. Interestingly, a substantial portion of this cost is related to the need for prolonged inpatient rehabilitation therapy, estimated at $1600 per day [20], with an average LOS of 3–4 months [21].

Physical exercise has remained a mainstay of treatment as it restores the healthy homeostatic regulation of stress and the hypothalamic–pituitary–adrenal axis. Physical activity also attenuates or reverses performance deficits observed in neurocognitive tasks for patients with TBI [22]. In addition, exercise offers a unique non-pharmacologic, non-invasive treatment against vascular risk factors including hypertension, diabetes, cellular inflammation, and aortic rigidity [22]. Exercise also induces direct changes in cerebral vasculature that produce beneficial changes in cerebral blood flow, angiogenesis, and disease improvement [22]. Finally, the improvements induced by physical exercise aid brain plasticity and neurocognitive performance in both healthy individuals and those afflicted by TBI [22].

The duration of physical therapy utilized and complexity of exercises are tailored to the individual TBI patient, considering their state of consciousness, age, and physical status. Moreover, cognitive functions are emphasized and patients are taught to concentrate their attention to a movement being performed [17]. Studies have demonstrated the crucial role of early physical therapy in the recovery of TBI [23], with improved physical function and decreased incidence of ICU acquired weakness compared to patients who do not receive early rehabilitation [24].

Just as important as physical rehabilitation, early cognitive rehabilitation is an important aspect of the recovery following TBI and includes providing therapeutic cognitive activities to improve cognitive functioning and activities of daily living (ADL). The incidence of early cognitive impairment is quite high, even in adults and children with mild TBI [25, 26]. Cognitive rehabilitation also teaches compensation mechanisms to cope with impaired neurologic function [27]. Several studies have shown the beneficial effects of cognitive rehabilitation on planning, organizing, and communicating for TBI patients [27–29]. Recently, a meta-analysis demonstrated that cognitive rehabilitation has positive effects on cognition, especially with respect to problem solving, multitasking, and planning [30]. In addition, patients with TBI receive benefits from a cognitive rehabilitation intervention that targets ADL performance, memory, and self-regulation skills [27, 28].

MacKay et al. showed coma length, rehabilitation stay, and cognitive functioning were significantly better in patients who received formal rehabilitation during their acute trauma admission [31]. A higher proportion of that group (94% vs. 57%) were also discharged home [31]. Similarly Cope and Hall compared 34 TBI patients who had either been referred "early" or "late" to a comprehensive inpatient rehabilitation program. The early group had significant reduction in LOS both in the acute phase and the rehabilitation phase [32]. Another study by Blackerby et al. demonstrated an increase in intensity of rehabilitation for 5–8 h per day decreased LOS [33]. Finally, Aronow et al. demonstrated that rehabilitation can be cost-effective with an average saving of nearly $12,000 per year for TBI patients [34]. Thus, establishing a care pathway for TBI patients that includes early, focused and standardized rehabilitation during acute hospitalization is of paramount importance.

In regard to pathway development, a multicenter trial across Sweden and Iceland studying implementation of a care pathway found that delays in rehabilitation initiation were negatively associated with outcomes for TBI patients. This was measured by the Glasgow outcome scale extended score (GOSE score) performed at 1 year following injury [23]. In addition, a direct clinical pathway including specialized rehabilitation in dedicated units was associated with improved functional independence at 1 year [35].

Thus, rehabilitation should start as early as possible and is best accomplished with a dedicated pathway for TBI. This is likely due to the fact that the recovery curve is steepest in the first 3 months after TBI, and it is therefore important to capitalize on this early phase of recovery to accelerate improvement in function.

2.2.2 Deep Vein Thrombosis (DVT)

VTE is a major and common preventable cause of death worldwide. DVT is especially prevalent among trauma patients with an incidence of up to 60% without prophylaxis and up to 30% with prophylaxis [5, 36, 37].

Major trauma often precipitates Virchow's triad of hypercoagulability, endothelial injury, and venous stasis [38]. Decreased levels of antithrombin III and suppression of fibrinolysis may lead the trauma patient to become hypercoagulable [39]. Also, direct injury to blood vessels can cause endothelial injury worsening the risk of hypercoagulability [39]. Interestingly, TBI patients have an even greater risk of DVT as tissue factor, which is abundant in the brain, is released following TBI, and activates the extrinsic pathway of blood coagulation [40]. In fact, TBI is independently associated with a nearly four times increased risk of DVT formation [41].

Mechanical methods of prophylaxis against DVT have been utilized for many decades and include intermittent pneumatic compression (IPC) devices, graduated compression stockings, and venous foot pumps. IPC devices enhance blood flow in the deep veins of the leg, thereby attempting to prevent venous stasis in an immobilized population (e.g., moderate to severe TBI). Also, IPC devices have been demonstrated to reduce plasminogen activator inhibitor-1, thereby increasing endogenous fibrinolytic activity [42]. Agu et al. demonstrated that mechanical methods reduce postoperative venous thrombosis [43]. A subsequent Cochrane review showed a reduction of VTE by about 50% with the use of graduated compression stockings [44]. However, mechanical pneumatic devices are overall less effective than VTE chemoprophylaxis in preventing VTE. DVT occurs in one-third of moderate to severely brain injured patients [45]. However, only up to 7% of severe TBI patients will develop DVT while on chemoprophylaxis. Historically there has been substantial concern regarding the implementation of chemoprophylaxis as this was thought to put TBI patients at increased risk for intracranial hemorrhage expansion [46]. Currently, there is varied consensus in the literature on the optimal time to initiate DVT chemoprophylaxis in patients who present with intracranial hemorrhage requiring neurosurgical intervention [47]. In addition, there is significant variation across trauma centers [48]. However, initiating VTE chemoprophylaxis 24 h after stable head CT in TBI patients appears to be safe and decreases the rate of DVT formation [46, 49]. In addition, DVT prophylaxis with either subcutaneous low molecular weight heparin (LMWH) or unfractionated heparin (UH) has been shown to be safe with intracranial pressure monitors in place [50, 51], which may be associated with increased risk of VTE [52]. However, LMWH is preferred in TBI patients as it may have a neuroprotective effect mediated by decreased cerebral edema [53].

The exact agent and dosing regimen for a generalized, non-TBI population has been evolving over the past few decades, beginning with a 1996 *New England Journal of Medicine* publication which found that 30 mg of subcutaneous enoxaparin twice daily performed better than 5000 units of subcutaneous heparin twice daily at reducing DVT in moderate to severely injured trauma patients (31% vs. 44%, $p = 0.04$) [54]. Many studies that followed have corroborated this evidence proving the superiority of LMWH compared to UFH in trauma patients with regard to mortality and incidence of pulmonary embolism and DVT [55–57].

Although the results are mixed, recently there has been increased attention to weight-based dosing and adjustment by anti-Xa levels for non-TBI trauma patients. Bellfi et al. demonstrated a correlation between increased dosing of enoxaparin with therapeutic levels of anti-Xa and a reduction in incidence of DVT, however, with a slight increase in risk of hemorrhage for trauma patients [58]. In contrast, a randomized trial by Karcutskie et al. found rates of VTE were not reduced with anti-Xa-guided dosing [59]. Whereas a similar study by Ko et al. found the incidence of DVT was significantly lower in the group who had monitored adjustment of enoxaparin dosing based on Xa levels [60]. However, currently no high-quality studies exist regarding the use of anti-Xa based dosing for TBI patients, although some of the authors of this text are currently pursuing a study on this topic.

In regard to a TBI pathway and VTE prophylaxis, the primary focus of the pathway would be to ensure the optimal time of initiation and dosing of VTE chemoprophylaxis determined by the institution is provided, thereby eliminating provider variation and ensuring the desired standard is achieved. Future research is needed to establish this exact dosing regimen but in the meantime, pathways should incorporate best available evidence coupled with institutional decisions regarding risk and benefit.

2.2.3 Enteral Nutrition

TBI initiates a systemic response characterized by hypermetabolism, hypercatabolism, acute-phase response, decreased immunologic function, hyperglycemia, increased counterregulatory hormones, and serum cytokine levels. Patients with TBI are hypermetabolic for weeks following injury, and only 27% are capable of spontaneously eating sufficient nutritional requirements by discharge [61].

Nutrition can be administered parenterally or enterally via gastric or post-pyloric routes. Early and adequate nutrition is essential. Studies have demonstrated that enteral nutrition is more effective than parenteral nutrition in maintaining the integrity of gastrointestinal mucosa, reducing the incidence of septic morbidity and decreasing the risk of bacterial translocation. Similarly, early small bowel feeding of patients with acute head injury results in a decreased incidence of infections and shorter ICU stay [62].

In fact, early enteral nutrition started within 48 h post-injury has been shown to reduce mortality [63], clinical malnutrition, and prevent bacterial translocation from the gastrointestinal tract, and improve outcomes in severe TBI patients [64].

Furthermore, a study by Hartle et al. found that patients who were not fed within the first 5 days after TBI had significantly increased mortality at 2 weeks, even when controlling for other factors known to affect outcome [65].

However, due to a high incidence of gastroparesis with TBI and/or polytrauma, enteral nutrition support may be difficult. In these cases post-pyloric feeding may be required or if not plausible, then supplemental parenteral nutrition may be necessary until adequate enteral nutrition is achieved.

The incidence of infectious maxillary sinusitis and its relationship to VAP were prospectively studied in critically ill patients who were mechanically ventilated for a period >7 days [66]. Infectious maxillary sinusitis was significantly associated with VAP and its frequency was markedly reduced by inserting endotracheal and gastric tubes via the oral route and not via the nares [66]. The timing of placing a gastrostomy tube is controversial. D'Amelio et al. recommend placing both percutaneous tracheostomy and PEG within 7 days [3] which they found to be associated with a decreased hospital LOS, ICU LOS, and mechanical ventilation without any adverse events [2].

Regardless of the timing for PEG, establishing early feeding access is extremely important in this population and should be addressed in any pathway. When a pathway was established by Spain et al. the target date for placement of PEG was predetermined to be day 4 of hospitalization (with concomitant percutaneous tracheostomy), which allowed some time to see if neurologic status would improve while ensuring that early feeding access was established [1]. Providing early enteral nutrition within 72 h of injury may decrease infection rates and overall complications. Establishing standards of practice and nutrition protocols will assure patients receive optimal nutrition assessment and intervention in a timely manner. This may be best accomplished with a clinical pathway [67].

2.2.4 Neuromonitoring

Methods to measure and monitor brain function have evolved considerably in recent years and now play an important role in the evaluation and management of patients with brain injury [68]. The overall aims of neuromonitoring are to: (1) identify worsening neurological function and secondary cerebral insults that may benefit from specific treatment(s); (2) improve pathophysiological understanding of cerebral disease in critical illness; (3) provide clear physiological data to guide and individualize therapy; (4) assist with prognostication [68]. Elevated intracranial pressure (ICP; >20 mmHg) is associated with increased mortality after acute TBI [69]. The most recent Brain Trauma Foundation guidelines [70] recommend that ICP should be monitored in all salvageable patients with severe TBI (GCS score of 3–8 after resuscitation) and an abnormal head computed tomography (CT) scan. Although non-invasive evaluation of ICP is possible using the transcranial Doppler (TCD)-derived pulsatility index or optic nerve sonography and automated pupillometry which has been shown to be more precise and reproducible than clinical exam [71], the only methods for continuous monitoring of ICP remain invasive.

Intra-ventricular devices have long been considered the "gold standard"; however, intra-parenchymal pressure monitoring provides equivalent pressure measurements. ICP management should also take cerebral perfusion pressure (CPP) into account. Therapies to reduce intracranial hypertension that also may reduce arterial pressure and CPP (for example, barbiturates) require careful titration to preserve adequate cerebral perfusion.

Several techniques can be used to measure brain oxygenation, the most common in the ICU being jugular venous bulb oximetry and direct $PbtO_2$ measurement. Decreases in $PbtO_2$ have been associated with independent chemical markers of brain ischemia in microdialysis studies. Furthermore, the number, duration, and intensity of brain hypoxic episodes ($PbtO_2$ < 15 mmHg) and any $PbtO_2$ values ≤5 mmHg are associated with poor outcome after TBI [72, 73].

Establishing a pathway for the management of elevated ICP based on tiered therapy should help standardize care of severe TBI. General clinical management is considered Tier Zero. Treatment of intracranial hypertension will generally begin at Tier One. Movement to higher tiers reflects increasingly aggressive interventions. Treatments in any given tier are considered equivalent, with selection of one treatment over another based on individual patient characteristics and physician discretion. During any given episode being addressed, multiple items from a single tier can be trialed individually or in combination with the goal of a rapid response. The provider should maintain awareness of the duration of any episode and consider moving to more aggressive interventions in a higher tier quickly if the patient is not responding [74]. In this regard a pathway can help the provider determine which therapies to utilize and when to move on to the next tier of treatments.

2.3 Conclusion

TBI patients represent a challenging population with significant multidisciplinary needs. In addition, they may have varying constellations of concomitant injuries making pathway development to standardize and optimize care challenging. However, TBI patients benefit from early enteral feeding, optimal VTE prophylaxis, early tracheostomy (when appropriate), and intense, multidisciplinary therapy. As such, TBI care pathways have been demonstrated to be helpful in terms of reducing ventilator days, ICU length of stay, morbidity, and improved short-term and longer-term neurologic outcomes. Although labor intensive, TBI pathways may help curtail substantial costs associated with TBI care and lead to improved quality of care and thereby substantially improve the value of care, suggesting a strong return on investment for the development of a TBI pathway.

References

1. Spain DA, et al. Effect of a clinical pathway for severe traumatic brain injury on resource utilization. J Trauma Inj Infect Crit Care. 1998;45:101–5.

2. Moore FA, Haenel JB, Moore EE, Read RA. Percutaneous tracheostomy/gastrostomy in brain-injured patients—a minimally invasive alternative. J Trauma Inj Infect Crit Care. 1992;33:435–9.
3. D'Amelio LF, Hammond JS, Spain DA, Sutyak JP. Tracheostomy and percutaneous endoscopic gastrostomy in the management of the head-injured trauma patient. Am Surg. 1994;60:180–5.
4. Gersin K, et al. The efficacy of sequential compression devices in multiple trauma patients with severe head injury. J Trauma Inj Infect Crit Care. 1994;37:205–8.
5. Geerts WH, Code KI, Jay RM, Chen E, Szalai JP. A prospective study of venous thromboembolism after major trauma. N Engl J Med. 1994;331:1601–6.
6. Forkner J. Clinical pathways: benefits and liabilities. Nurs Manage. 1996;27:35–8.
7. Gadacz TR, Adkins RB, O'Leary JP. General surgical clinical pathways: an introduction. Am Surg. 1997;63:107–10.
8. Vitaz TW, McIlvoy L, Raque GH, Spain DA, Shields CB. Development and implementation of a clinical pathway for spinal cord injuries. J Spinal Disord. 2001;14:271–6.
9. Fernandez-Bussy S, et al. Tracheostomy tube placement. J Bronchol Interv Pulmonol. 2015;22:357–64.
10. Sugerman HJ, et al. Multicenter, randomized, prospective trial of early tracheostomy. J Trauma Inj Infect Crit Care. 1997;43:741–7.
11. Livingston DH. Prevention of ventilator-associated pneumonia. Am J Surg. 2000;179:12–7.
12. Rodriguez JL, et al. Early tracheostomy for primary airway management in the surgical critical care setting. Br J Surg. 1990;77:1406–10.
13. Arabi Y, Haddad S, Shirawi N, Shimemeri AA. Early tracheostomy in intensive care trauma patients improves resource utilization: a cohort study and literature review. Crit Care. 2004;8:R347.
14. Marra A, et al. Early vs. late tracheostomy in patients with traumatic brain injury: systematic review and meta-analysis. J Clin Med. 2021;10:3319.
15. Möller MG, et al. Early tracheostomy versus late tracheostomy in the surgical intensive care unit. Am J Surg. 2005;189:293–6.
16. McCredie VA, et al. Effect of early versus late tracheostomy or prolonged intubation in critically ill patients with acute brain injury: a systematic review and meta-analysis. Neurocrit Care. 2017;26:14–25.
17. Durbin CG. Tracheostomy: why, when, and how? Respir Care. 2010;55:1056–68.
18. de Franca SA, Tavares WM, Salinet ASM, Paiva WS, Teixeira MJ. Early tracheostomy in severe traumatic brain injury patients: a meta-analysis and comparison with late tracheostomy. Crit Care Med. 2020;48:e325–31.
19. Chestnut R, et al. Rehabilitation for traumatic brain injury: summary. AHRQ Evidence Report Summaries.
20. Mayer NH, Pelensky J, Whyte J, Fidler-Sheppard R. Characterization and correlates of medical and rehabilitation charges for traumatic brain injury during acute rehabilitation hospitalization. Arch Phys Med Rehabil. 2003;84:242–8.
21. Barnes MP. Rehabilitation after traumatic brain injury. Br Med Bull. 1999;55:927–43.
22. Archer T. Influence of physical exercise on traumatic brain injury deficits: scaffolding effect. Neurotox Res. 2012;21:418–34.
23. Godbolt AK, et al. Associations between care pathways and outcome 1 year after severe traumatic brain injury. J Head Trauma Rehabil. 2015;30:E41–51.
24. Fuke R, et al. Early rehabilitation to prevent postintensive care syndrome in patients with critical illness: a systematic review and meta-analysis. BMJ Open. 2018;8:e019998.
25. Keys ME, et al. Early cognitive impairment is common in pediatric patients following mild traumatic brain injury. J Trauma Acute Care. 2021;91:861–6.
26. Delaplain PT, et al. Early cognitive impairment is common after intracranial hemorrhage with mild traumatic brain injury. J Trauma Acute Care. 2020;89:215–21.
27. Park HY, Maitra K, Martinez KM. The effect of occupation-based cognitive rehabilitation for traumatic brain injury: a meta-analysis of randomized controlled trials. Occup Ther Int. 2015;22:104–16.

28. Goverover Y, Johnston MV, Toglia J, DeLuca J. Treatment to improve self-awareness in persons with acquired brain injury. Brain Inj. 2007;21:913–23.
29. Salazar AM, et al. Cognitive rehabilitation for traumatic brain injury: a randomized trial. JAMA. 2000;283:3075–81.
30. Kennedy MRT, et al. Intervention for executive functions after traumatic brain injury: a systematic review, meta-analysis and clinical recommendations. Neuropsychol Rehabil. 2008;18:257–99.
31. Mackay LE, Bernstein BA, Chapman PE, Morgan AS, Milazzo LS. Early intervention in severe head injury: long-term benefits of a formalized program. Arch Phys Med Rehabil. 1992;73:635–41.
32. Cope DN, Hall K. Head injury rehabilitation: benefit of early intervention. Arch Phys Med Rehabil. 1982;63:433–7.
33. Blackerby WF. Intensity of rehabilitation and length of stay. Brain Inj. 1990;4:167–73.
34. Aronow HU. Rehabilitation effectiveness with severe brain injury: translating research into policy. J Head Trauma Rehabil. 1987;2:24–36.
35. Sveen U, et al. Rehabilitation pathways and functional independence one year after severe traumatic brain injury. Eur J Phys Rehabil Med. 2016;52:650–61.
36. Nielson S Jr, et al. Early detection of deep venous thrombosis in trauma patients. Cureus. 2020;12:e9370.
37. Meissner MH, Chandler WL, Elliott JS. Venous thromboembolism in trauma: a local manifestation of systemic hypercoagulability? J Trauma Inj Infect Crit Care. 2003;54:224–31.
38. Kitagawa K, Sakoda S. Mechanism underlying thrombus formation in cerebral infarction. Rinsho Shinkeigaku. 2009;49:798–800.
39. Hak DJ. Prevention of venous thromboembolism in trauma and long bone fractures. Curr Opin Pulm Med. 2001;7:338–43.
40. Sase T, et al. Tissue factor messenger RNA levels in leukocytes compared with tissue factor antigens in plasma from patients in hypercoagulable state caused by various diseases. Thromb Haemost. 2004;92:132–9.
41. Reiff DA, et al. Traumatic brain injury is associated with the development of deep vein thrombosis independent of pharmacological prophylaxis. J Trauma Inj Infect Crit Care. 2009;66:1436–40.
42. Roberts VC, Sabri S, Beeley AH, Cotton LT. The effect of intermittently applied external pressure on the haemodynamics of the lower limb in man. Br J Surg. 1972;59:223–6.
43. Agu O, Hamilton G, Baker D. Graduated compression stockings in the prevention of venous thromboembolism. Br J Surg. 1999;86:992–1004.
44. Amaragiri SV, Lees T. Elastic compression stockings for prevention of deep vein thrombosis. Cochrane Database Syst Rev. 2000(3):CD001484. https://doi.org/10.1002/14651858.cd001484.
45. Ekeh AP, Dominguez KM, Markert RJ, McCarthy MC. Incidence and risk factors for deep venous thrombosis after moderate and severe brain injury. J Trauma Inj Infect Crit Care. 2010;68:912–5.
46. Scudday T, et al. Safety and efficacy of prophylactic anticoagulation in patients with traumatic brain injury. J Am Coll Surg. 2011;213:148–53.
47. Farr S, et al. Risks, benefits, and the optimal time to resume deep vein thrombosis prophylaxis in patients with intracranial hemorrhage. Cureus. 2019;11:e5827.
48. Yeates EO, et al. Chemoprophylaxis and venous thromboembolism in traumatic brain injury at different trauma centers. Am Surg. 2020;86:362–8.
49. Farooqui A, Hiser B, Barnes SL, Litofsky NS. Safety and efficacy of early thromboembolism chemoprophylaxis after intracranial hemorrhage from traumatic brain injury: clinical article. J Neurosurg. 2013;119:1576–82.
50. Dengler BA, et al. Safety of chemical DVT prophylaxis in severe traumatic brain injury with invasive monitoring devices. Neurocrit Care. 2016;25:215–23.

51. Chi G, Lee JJ, Sheng S, Marszalek J, Chuang ML. Systematic review and meta-analysis of thromboprophylaxis with heparins following intracerebral hemorrhage. Thromb Haemost. 2022;122:1159–68.
52. Allen A, et al. Intracranial pressure monitors associated with increased venous thromboembolism in severe traumatic brain injury. Eur J Trauma Emerg Surg. 2021;47:1483–90.
53. Li S, et al. Does enoxaparin interfere with HMGB1 signaling after TBI, a potential mechanism for reduced cerebral edema and neurologic recovery. J Trauma Acute Care. 2016;80:381–9.
54. Geerts WH, et al. A comparison of low-dose heparin with low-molecular-weight heparin as prophylaxis against venous thromboembolism after major trauma. N Engl J Med. 1996;335:701–7.
55. Byrne JP, et al. Effectiveness of low-molecular-weight heparin versus unfractionated heparin to prevent pulmonary embolism following major trauma. J Trauma Acute Care. 2017;82:252–62.
56. Tran A, et al. Efficacy and safety of low molecular weight heparin versus unfractionated heparin for prevention of venous thromboembolism in trauma patients. Ann Surg. 2022;275:19–28.
57. Jacobs BN, et al. Unfractionated heparin versus low-molecular-weight heparin for venous thromboembolism prophylaxis in trauma. J Trauma Acute Care. 2017;83:151–8.
58. Bellfi LT, et al. Impact of increased enoxaparin dosing on anti-Xa levels for venous thromboembolism prophylaxis in trauma patients. Am Surg. 2022;88:2158–62.
59. Karcutskie CA, et al. Association of anti–factor Xa–guided dosing of enoxaparin with venous thromboembolism after trauma. JAMA Surg. 2017;153:144.
60. Ko A, et al. Association between Enoxaparin dosage adjusted by anti–factor Xa trough level and clinically evident venous thromboembolism after trauma. JAMA Surg. 2016;151:1006.
61. Borzotta AP, et al. Enteral versus parenteral nutrition after severe closed head injury. J Trauma Inj Infect Crit Care. 1994;37:459–68.
62. Roberts PR. Nutrition in the head-injured patient. New Horiz. 1995;3:506–17.
63. Doig GS, Heighes PT, Simpson F, Sweetman EA. Early enteral nutrition reduces mortality in trauma patients requiring intensive care: a meta-analysis of randomised controlled trials. Injury. 2011;42:50–6.
64. Chiang Y-H, et al. Early enteral nutrition and clinical outcomes of severe traumatic brain injury patients in acute stage: a multi-center cohort study. J Neurotrauma. 2012;29:75–80.
65. Härtl R, Gerber LM, Ni Q, Ghajar J. Effect of early nutrition on deaths due to severe traumatic brain injury. J Neurosurg. 2008;109:50–6.
66. Rouby JJ, et al. Risk factors and clinical relevance of nosocomial maxillary sinusitis in the critically ill. Am J Resp Crit Care. 1994;150:776–83.
67. Vizzini A, Aranda-Michel J. Nutritional support in head injury. Nutrition. 2011;27:129–32.
68. Stocchetti N, et al. Clinical review: neuromonitoring—an update. Crit Care. 2013;17:201.
69. Marmarou A, et al. Impact of ICP instability and hypotension on outcome in patients with severe head trauma. J Neurosurg. 1991;75:S59–66.
70. Bratton SL, et al. Guidelines for the management of severe traumatic brain injury. VI. Indications for intracranial pressure monitoring. J Neurotrauma. 2007;24(Suppl 1):S37–44.
71. Phillips SS, Mueller CM, Nogueira RG, Khalifa YM. A systematic review assessing the current state of automated pupillometry in the NeuroICU. Neurocrit Care. 2019;31:142–61.
72. Dings J, Meixensberger J, Jäger A, Roosen K. Clinical experience with 118 brain tissue oxygen partial pressure catheter probes. Neurosurgery. 1998;43:1082–94.
73. van den Brink WA, et al. Brain oxygen tension in severe head injury. Neurosurgery. 2000;46:868–78.
74. Hawryluk GWJ, et al. A management algorithm for patients with intracranial pressure monitoring: the Seattle international severe traumatic brain injury consensus conference (SIBICC). Intensive Care Med. 2019;45:1783–94.

3 The Central Role of Specialized Neurocritical Care Teams: Standards of Neurologic Critical Care Units

Amanda Hambrecht and Marko Bukur

3.1 Introduction

Intensive care units (ICUs) have evolved over the past 70 years, transforming into a distinct medical subspecialty that has become an integral part of the healthcare system. The earliest ICU model is credited to Florence Nightingale during the Crimean War, when she established nursing-run units to care for the most critically wounded [1]. Over the next century, the concept of an ICU was adapted by hospital systems and developed internationally and throughout the USA. Intensive care functions as a clinical specialty and care delivery system, providing comprehensive and specialized nursing and medical care to the most critically ill patients, often with multiple organ insufficiency. Intensive care medicine is defined by the manner in which the ICU is integrated into the hospital system, the actual care provided to patients and their families, and the clinical outcomes achieved [2]. In the early 2000s, there were approximately four million ICU admissions each year in the USA, resulting in over $80 billion in healthcare costs [3].

3.2 Organization of Intensive Care Units

With the increasing prevalence of ICUs in hospitals around the world, multidisciplinary organizations have been created in an attempt to standardize intensive care medicine. Working with The World Federation of Societies of Intensive and Critical

A. Hambrecht
Department of Trauma and Acute Care Surgery, Los Angeles County Hospital, University of Southern California, Los Angeles, Los Angeles, CA, USA

M. Bukur (✉)
Division of Acute Care Surgery, Department of Surgery, New York University Grossman School of Medicine, Health + Hospitals/Bellevue Hospital, New York, NY, USA
e-mail: marko.bukur@nyulangone.org

E. Brogi et al. (eds.), *Traumatic Brain Injury*, Hot Topics in Acute Care Surgery and Trauma, https://doi.org/10.1007/978-3-031-50117-3_3

Care Medicine, a professional society with global clinician representation, Marshall and colleagues developed an outline to distinguish intensive care from routine clinical care [1]. The discrete space for an ICU within a hospital or healthcare center allows for the concentration of clinical expertise and support technologies to maximally benefit patients. Rooms should accommodate a myriad of support and monitoring devices, capable of performing invasive and noninvasive continuous monitoring. The ideal team to provide such critical care services should include nursing and medical staff with advanced training in intensive care medicine. In order to provide the highest quality care, intensivists must be dedicated to continuous quality improvement, with persistent efforts to improve patient care and implement evidence-based practices.

3.3 Rationale for the Development of Neurocritical Care Units

Over time, the field of ICU medicine has become further defined, with intensivists receiving specific and targeted training in different areas of medicine. Studies have shown that lower levels of diagnostic diversity within an ICU are associated with decreased mortality [4]. One such area is neurocritical care, a specialty focusing on the care of patients with neurological illnesses, ranging from epilepsy and cerebrovascular accidents to traumatic brain injury. An observational, international study from nearly 50 countries identified dedicated neurocritical care units (NCCU) in two-thirds of countries around the world, with over 80% in North America [5]. The ideal goal of an NCCU is to provide balanced care to neurologically injured patients, with interventions highly focused on neuroprotection and preventing secondary brain injury while addressing and treating the non-neurologic organ dysfunction often seen in the critically ill. Care by each member of the team has a neurologic focus with special attention paid to the neurologic consequences of systemic organ dysfunctions. These NCCUs play a critical role in delivering specialized care in trauma facilities. In hospitals with both neurocritical and surgical intensive care units, patients with isolated head trauma or those with minor polytrauma and major head injuries tend to be admitted to the neurological ICU. Studies have found traumatic brain injury patients admitted to a neurointensivist run ICUs had lower ICU- and in-hospital mortality, as well as improved outcomes [6]. A secondary analysis from Lombardo and colleagues evaluated nearly 2500 patients admitted to intensive care units in 11 level I trauma centers across the USA [7]. Patients were categorized as isolated TBI with a head abbreviated injury scale (AIS) score ≥ 2 with other regions <2, or polytrauma with a head injury as well as AIS ≥ 3 in the chest, abdomen, pelvis, or long bones. Patients were admitted to NCCU, trauma ICU (TICU), or general ICU (Med/Surg), although not all centers had all three types of ICUs available. They found that among all patients with TBI and increasing injury severity scores, admission to a specialty ICU, such as NCCU or TICU, was protective of in-hospital mortality compared to a general ICU. This survival benefit was also seen in the polytrauma cohort with TBI admitted to specialty ICUs. A large cohort study from the UK additionally found that management in an NCCU may be cost-effective compared to a general critical care unit and recommend that all patients with severe TBI be considered for transfer to a neurological intensive care unit, regardless of their need for surgery [8].

3.4 Benefits of Neurocritical Care Units

An admission path for TBI patients to neurocritical care units has been associated with lower mortality, higher chance of functional recovery, and increased likelihood of being discharged home [9, 10]. Higher hospital volume has also been associated with improved outcomes in multiple neurological diagnoses, including traumatic brain injury [11, 12]. This is posited to be due to greater clinician experience within a higher volume unit, emphasizing and adhering to protocols designed to prevent secondary brain injury. A decade-long population-based study of more than 4000 neurocritical care patients found decreased mortality over time and an increase in the number of patients being discharged home after the creation of a neurocritical care unit, within which these patients could be clustered. The success of these units was partly attributed to the subsequent implementation of traumatic brain injury protocols [13]. A retrospective study of 123 traumatic brain injury patients by Pineda and colleagues found stronger adherence to evidence-based protocols after the implementation of neurocritical care programs, with more intensive therapy and intracranial pressure monitoring for intracranial hypertension, and ultimately, an increase in the number of patients being discharged home [14]. And while the cause–effect relationship of NCCUs, care from neurointensivists, and patient outcomes still need to be fully established and defined, studies have found better outcomes, improved communication among consulting specialties [11], and increased compliance to Brain Trauma Foundation guidelines in patients with traumatic brain injury cared for in a neurocritical care unit [15–17]. Adherence to Brain Trauma Foundation guidelines has been associated with significant reduction in ICU length of stay, hospital length of stay, and hospital charges [15]. Institutional adoption of these protocols has allowed for the standardization of care, significantly improving survival outcomes after traumatic brain injury [18–20].

3.5 Neurocritical Care Unit Requirements

Formal training in neurocritical care has resulted in highly trained subspecialized teams with expertise in managing critically ill patients with neurologic diseases. Studies of these NCC teams have shown improved patient outcomes [21]. Founded in 2002, the Neurocritical Care Society (NCS) is a nonprofit, international organization dedicated to improving outcomes for patients with life-threatening neurological illnesses. It is supported by the Society of Critical Care Medicine (SCCM) and accepted by the United Council of Neurological Subspecialties, an organization committed to establishing training standards for neurological subspeciality fellowships.

In 2018, NCS guidelines summarized the standards for neurologic critical care units [21]. The three tiers of NCCUs range from level I units that can care for complex neurological emergencies, often requiring advanced interventions, to level II units that can manage acutely ill but stable patients, and finally level III units that can stabilize emergent patients prior to transferring to a higher level of care. The majority of NCCUs in trauma centers are considered level I, able to provide the most comprehensive neurocritical care. Neurointensivist-led teams have been associated with decreased mortality, improved functional outcomes, and improved resource utilization [21]. A neurointensivist or appropriate in-house provider is recommended to be on-site and available at bedside within minutes, 24 h a day, 7 days a week. Nursing expertise in neurocritical care is also important for good patient outcomes. It is recommended that nursing educational programs include training on interventions specific to neurocritical care, including monitoring, procedures, and devices. The Emergency Neurologic Life Support curriculum offers early management strategies for multiple neurocritical care diagnoses, highlighting the key priorities in treatment plans. The neurocritical care unit itself should be able to evaluate, diagnose, and treat a variety of neurological diagnoses. Essential equipment includes ventilators with end-tidal carbon dioxide monitors, arterial and central venous access monitors, hemodynamic and intracranial monitoring equipment, transcranial Doppler, electroencephalogram, and external ventricular drainage systems. Radiology services including computed tomography, ultrasound, magnetic resonance imaging, and transthoracic echocardiogram should be available 24 h a day. Neurocritical care unit specific medications should be immediately accessible including analgesics, sedatives, osmotic agents such as mannitol and 23.4% hypertonic saline, antiepileptic agents, and antihypertensive medications.

The unit should have a dedicated medical director with formal neurocritical care training who leads regular leadership meetings to evaluate quality and safety and monitor morbidity and mortality. High-quality care requires safe care that minimizes risks and optimizes benefits and needs regular review to assess outcomes and performance measures. Medical subspecialists from multiple services should be readily available, including but not limited to, general surgery, vascular surgery, cardiothoracic surgery, cardiology, nephrology, pulmonology, and gastroenterology. A critically ill patient may have multiorgan dysfunction or develop hospital-associated complications requiring consultation with several ancillary care teams. Effective and clear communication among consulting services are critical for safe and optimal patient care.

A multidisciplinary care team is recommended, with medical and nursing staff having specialized training in neurocritical care. The team can include members from respiratory therapy, pharmacy, physiatry, nutrition, speech and language pathology, social workers, and spiritual leaders. Improved patient outcomes and cost-effective care have been associated with respiratory therapy-driven weaning protocols, tracheostomy management, and oxygen titration strategies [21].

Pharmacists are considered essential members of neurocritical care teams. They have been shown to reduce medication costs, decrease adverse drug reactions, improve morbidity and mortality, and decrease both the ICU and hospital length of stays [21, 22]. The Joint Commission and Society of Critical Care Medicine recommend integrating a dedicated pharmacist into the ICU team [21]. Physical, occupational, and speech and language therapy should be available 7 days a week. Daily physical therapy improves functional status by the time of discharge, reduces the number of intubated days and improves rates ICU delirium [22]. Most importantly, care provided by each member of the multidisciplinary team should have a neurologic focus with consideration given to the intracranial ramifications of treatment plan decisions or modifications.

3.6 Conclusion

Caring for a critically ill patient is a complex and complicated endeavor. Intensive care medicine necessitates a comprehensive care plan that focuses on each organ system with intense detail. Subspecialized intensive care medicine, such as neurocritical care, shifts the focus of that care plan toward the neurologic organ system. Within a trauma facility, neurocritical care units should be able to provide care for a multitude of neurological diagnoses, including neurological emergencies. All team members in that unit frame their care plans with a neurologic focus, recognizing the complex relationship between neurologic injury and the rest of the body. As such, these multidisciplinary care teams provide the epitome of individualized patient care.

References

1. Marshall JC, Bosco L, Adhikari NK, Connolly B, Diaz JV, Dorman T, et al. What is an intensive care unit? A report of the task force of the World Federation of Societies of Intensive and Critical Care Medicine. J Crit Care. 2017;37:270–6.
2. Curtis JR, Cook DJ, Wall RJ, Angus DC, Bion J, Kacmarek R, et al. Intensive care unit quality improvement: a "how-to" guide for the interdisciplinary team. Crit Care Med. 2006;34:211–8.
3. Halpern NA, Pastores SM. Critical care medicine in the United States 2000-2005: an analysis of bed numbers, occupancy rates, payer mix, and costs. Crit Care Med. 2010;38(1):65–71.
4. Lott JP, Iwashyna TJ, Christie JD, Asch DA, Kramer AA, Kahn JM. Critical illness outcomes in specialty versus general intensive care units. Am J Respir Crit Care Med. 2009;179:676–83.
5. Suarez JI, Martin RH, Bauza C, Georgiadis A, Venkatasubba Rao CP, Calvillo E, et al. Worldwide Organization of Neurocritical Care: results from the PRINCE study part 1. Neurocrit Care. 2020;32(1):172–9.
6. Varelas PN, Eastwood D, Yun HJ, Spanaki MV, Hacein Bey L, Kessaris C, et al. Impact of a neurointensivist on outcomes in patients with head trauma treated in a neurosciences intensive care unit. J Neurosurg. 2006;104:713–9.
7. Lombardo S, Scalea T, Sperry J, Coimbra R, Vercruysse G, Enniss T, et al. Neuro, trauma, or med/surg intensive care unit: does it matter where multiple injuries patients with traumatic brain injury are admitted? Secondary analysis of the American Association for the Surgery of Trauma multi-institutional trials committee decompressive craniectomy study. J Trauma Acute Care Surg. 2017;82(3):489–96.

8. Harrison DA, Prabhu G, Grieve R, Harvey SE, Sadique MZ, Gomes M, et al. Risk adjustment in neurocritical care (RAIN)—prospective validation of risk prediction models for adult patients with acute traumatic brain injury to use to evaluate the optimum location and comparative costs of neurocritical care: a cohort study. Health Technol Assess. 2013;17(23):vii–viii.
9. Kramer AH, Zygun DA. Neurocritical care: why does it make a difference? Curr Opin Crit Care. 2014;20(2):174–81.
10. Samuels O, Webb A, Culler S, Martin K, Barrow D. Impact of a dedicated neurocritical care team in treating patients with aneurismal subarachnoid hemorrhage. Neurocrit Care. 2011;14(3):334–40.
11. Mauritz W, Steitzer H, Bauer P, Dolanski-Aghamanoukjan L, Metnitz P. Monitoring of intracranial pressure in patients with severe traumatic brain injury: an Austrian prospective multicenter study. Intensive Care Med. 2008;34:1208–15.
12. Shi HY, Hwang SL, Lee KT, Lin CL. Temporal trends and volume-outcome associations after traumatic brain injury: a 12-year study in Taiwan. J Neurosurg. 2013;118:732–8.
13. Kramer AH, Zygun DA, Doig CJ, Zuege DJ. Incidence of neurologic death among patients with brain injury: a cohort study in a Canadian Health Region. CMAJ. 2013;185:E838–45.
14. Pineda JA, Leonard JR, Mazotas IG, Noetzel M, Limbrick DD, Keller MS, et al. Effect of implementation of a paediatric neurocritical care programme on outcomes after severe traumatic brain injury: a retrospective cohort study. Lancet Neurol. 2013;12:45–52.
15. Fakhry SM, Trask AL, Waller MA, Watts DD. Management of brain-injured patients by an evidence-based medicine protocol improves outcomes and decreases hospital charges. J Trauma. 2004;56:492–9.
16. Talving P, Karamanos E, Teixeria PG, Skiada D, Lam L, Belzberg H, et al. Intracranial pressure monitoring in severe head injury: compliance with brain trauma foundation guidelines and effect on outcomes. J Neurosurg. 2013;119:1248–54.
17. Palmer S, Bader MK, Qureshi A, Palmer J, Shaver T, Borzatta M, Stalcup C. The impact of outcomes in a community hospital setting using the AANS traumatic brain injury guidelines. J Trauma. 2001;50:657–754.
18. Patel HC, Menon DK, Tebbs S, Hawker R, Hutchinson PJ, Kirkpatrick PJ. Specialist neurocritical care and outcome from head injury. Intensive Care Med. 2002;28:547–53.
19. Elf K, Nilsson P, Enblad P. Outcome after traumatic brain injury improved by an organized secondary insult program and standardized neurointensive care. Crit Care Med. 2002;30:2129–34.
20. Kurtz P, Fitts V, Sumer Z, Jalon H, Cooke J, Kvetan V, et al. How does care differ for neurological patients admitted to a neurocritical care unit versus a general ICU? Neurocrit Care. 2011;15:477–80.
21. Moheet AM, Livesay SL, Abdelhak T, Bleck TP, Human T, Karanjia N, et al. Standards for neurologic critical care units: a statement for healthcare professionals from the Neurocritical Care Society. Neurocrit Care. 2018;29:145–60.
22. Schwieckert WD, Pohlman MC, Pohlman AS, Nigos C, Pawlik AJ, Esbrook CL, et al. Early physical and occupational therapy in mechanically ventilated, critically ill patients: a randomized controlled trial. Lancet. 2009;373:1874–82.

4 The Central Role of a Specialized Neurocritical Care Team: Nursing Perspective in Neurocritical Care Practice

Azeem A. Rehman, Shanna Morgan,
and Nicholas J. Brandmeir

4.1 Introduction

The successful medical care of patients in the neurocritical care unit is a complex and specialized undertaking. Components of the critical care team are varied and include physicians, physician extenders, nurses, pharmacists, dieticians, physical, occupational, and speech therapists, social workers, and many others. The team members most closely focused on the continuous monitoring, assessment, and treatment of patients are the bedside nurses. The bedside nurse interacts with all members of the treatment team as well as patients and families and provides specialized skills and knowledge necessary for the optimal performance of the entire team. A simplified schematic of some of the clinical relationships involved in bedside nursing in the neurocritical care unit is provided in Fig. 4.1. The goal of this chapter is to describe the contributions of the bedside nurse as well as to provide an outline of optimal organization and utilization of these vital professionals.

A. A. Rehman · N. J. Brandmeir (✉)
Department of Neurosurgery, Rockefeller Neuroscience Institute, West Virginia University, Morgantown, WV, USA
e-mail: Azeem.Rehman@hsc.wvu.edu; Nicholas.Brandmeir@hsc.wvu.edu

S. Morgan
Neuroscience Critical Care Unit, Rockefeller Neuroscience Institute, West Virginia University, Morgantown, WV, USA
e-mail: swatson6@wvumedicine.org

E. Brogi et al. (eds.), *Traumatic Brain Injury*, Hot Topics in Acute Care Surgery and Trauma, https://doi.org/10.1007/978-3-031-50117-3_4

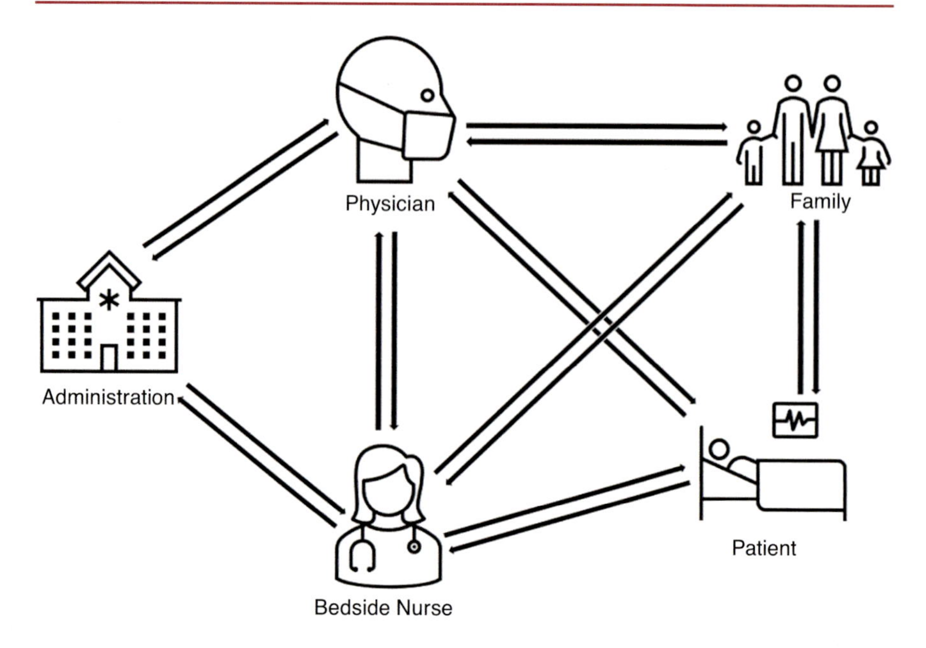

Fig. 4.1 Clinical relationships of the bedside nurse. Greatly simplified schematic of the relationships impacting the bedside nurse and the patient in the neurocritical care unit

4.2 Staffing

Despite the widespread availability of highly specialized teams, neurocritical care is still rigorous and unpredictable, primarily due to patient pathology and the frequent need for advanced intervention in a short period of time. The Neurocritical Care Society published a statement to provide an organizational framework for the development and maintenance of neurocritical care units. This document recommends a nurse-to-patient ratio of 2:1, with additional criteria detailing when a 1:1 ratio is appropriate [1]. The nursing ratio directly impacts patient outcomes. For instance, Neuraz et al. demonstrated that in critically ill patients, a significant increase in mortality occurred when the patient-to-nurse ratio was greater than 1:2.5 [2]. A separate study found that higher nursing staffing results in a decrease in adverse events and length of stay [3].

With that said, staffing is more than just a number. There is no set process to determine appropriate staffing; workflow must be adjusted to ensure that a nurse is not performing 15 hours of work during a 12-hour shift. Neurocritical care patients are unique, requiring frequent neurologic assessments and constant transportation out of the intensive care unit for diagnostic testing. Often, these evaluations are random in terms of their occurrences and are time-sensitive. While a diagnostic test is being performed, a nurse must leave his/her other patient for an extended period, requiring another nurse to add an additional patient to his/her assignment. In surgical patients, Aiken et al. found that a 7% increase in death occurs when an additional patient is added to a nursing assignment [4]. To address this issue, the addition of a circulating nursing position, one who does not have a patient assignment, can help mitigate these challenges. To some degree, the workload needs to be quantified for neurocritical care nurses to justify additional staffing needs to not only improve patient outcomes but also to prevent burnout and promote retention.

4.3 Education

Neurocritical care represents a subspeciality within intensive care practice that requires unique nursing skill sets. As such, standardized certification and educational curricula tailored to these needs are necessary. In addition to Advanced Cardiac Life Support (ACLS) and Basic Life Support (BLS), neurocritical care nurses should also undergo Emergency Neurological Life Support (ENLS) training or equivalent certification. ENLS is designed to provide all healthcare professionals with a set of protocols and strategies to manage a variety of neurological emergencies. Research suggests that a specialty certification process that provides knowledge for nurses leads to improved patient outcomes [5].

In addition, nursing subspeciality certification is frequently used as an indicator for quality of care by hospital systems and external regulatory bodies. Beyond certification, neurocritical care nurses should participate in educational activities at the institutional and national levels. These endeavors should include formalized continuing education credits. The Neurocritical Care Society recommends an annual goal of 8 h for all members of the neurocritical care team, with CORE members (such as a nurse manager) encouraged to have 32 h yearly.

4.4 Clinical Care

Patients in the neurocritical care unit require highly sophisticated monitoring of neurologic functions and physiologic parameters in order to prevent and mitigate secondary neurologic injury. To accomplish these goals, neurocritical care nurses focus on neuroprotection by administering interventions targeted at such parameters as blood pressure, brain tissue oxygenation, and cerebral perfusion pressure. The neurocritical care nurse is responsible for integrating a variety of clinical data—brain tissue oxygenation, electroencephalography, intracranial pressure monitoring, vital signs, and others—and linking this information to a patient's chart. Frequently, the bedside nurse is the first to appreciate fluctuations in these values. Beyond just identifying variations, the nurse often correlates these changes to the clinical assessment of the patient and intervenes accordingly. In this role, the bedside nurse benefits from increased training not only in identification of changes in neurologic and vital signs but also in recognition of normal variations in physical exam and vital signs, such as intracranial pressure excursions with coughing or straining, and normal pupillary asymmetry. Adjunctive technology can facilitate these processes by providing objective measures, as in quantitative pupillometry, or by allowing time-linked reporting of various physiologic events, such as with the Moberg device (Moberg Research Inc., Ambler, PA, USA). This type of specialized training and technology can improve the ability of the nurse to ensure optimal and timely care by providing both sensitive and specific reports to the physician caring for the patient.

As an example, the utility of nurses in interpreting bedside electroencephalography to allow for earlier seizure identification has been evaluated [6]. Kang et al. conducted a prospective study demonstrating that neurocritical care nurses exhibited a high sensitivity (85.1%) and specificity (89.8%) for interpreting real-time quantitative electroencephalography to detect recurrent non-convulsive seizures. This study supports the role of nurses as important frontline screeners to alert the neurophysiologist to review the encephalographic data.

Nurses should also be involved in creating standardized processes of care, including formal guidelines, care pathways, and checklists. One such example involves documentation of a secondary insult as a checklist item after every shift to ensure the event will be relayed to the next shift as well as to the clinical rounding team [7]. Ultimately, the goal is to maximize efforts to prevent secondary insults by highlighting some of the major issues during the prior shift. To further promote safety, the use of technology for computerized order entry, barcode medication administration, and standardized communication pathways should be adopted. Nurses can also provide insight into barriers to providing care, particularly when introducing new technology or guidelines.

All practice and policies related to bedside nursing in the neurocritical care unit should be focused on allowing the bedside nurse time and energy to provide care to his/her patients. To this end, policies and practices that increase the need for nurses to chart or interact with computers/screens should be carefully evaluated and countered with technology if at all possible. If this is not feasible, the value of the charting should be carefully weighed against the decrease in bedside care that it inevitably will cause.

4.5 End-of-Life Care

End-of-life care can be defined as the care and support a patient and his/her family receive once the decision to withdraw or withhold treatment has been made [8]. In the neurocritical care setting, most deaths occur after withdrawal of life-sustaining measures. As such, end-of-life care is an essential component of neurocritical care. The practice pattern in the USA involves a shared decision-making process involving the treatment team and the patient's family. Frequently, mortality and long-term disability are challenging to prognosticate. Given that the neurocritical care nurse spends the most time at bedside, he/she can provide valuable insight into the family perspective. Thus, nursing involvement in the transition to end-of-life care is essential. Moreover, when the decision to withdraw life-sustaining measures occurs, nurses must continue to support the patient and family, including the time after the patient passes away. Often, the level of satisfaction a family has with end-of-life care is directly linked to communication.

Nursing communication with families is particularly important in the neurocritical care setting given that patients frequently have an altered sensorium. This situation can be challenging for a nurse who strives to uphold the personal rights of a patient while still providing the family with enough information to be informed and make medical decisions. Equally important is nursing collaboration with physicians during end-of-life care. Nurses in the neurocritical care unit rarely have the opportunity to interact with patients after their recovery from their critical illness. This can give nursing staff an overly pessimistic view of long-term outcomes of patients with neurological injuries. Specific education and, wherever possible, interaction with former and now-recovered patients should be encouraged to allow bedside nurses to observe the ultimate value of their care in allowing patients to return to functional lives.

In a pilot study evaluating end-of-life care, nurses reported lower perception of collaboration, higher moral distress, and less satisfaction with quality of care when compared to physicians. Regarding moral distress, nurses report feeling pressure to continue futile aggressive treatment. Additionally, more collaboration with physicians was linked to greater satisfaction with the quality of care [9]. It is critical that nurses understand the benefits and outcomes associated with aggressive care in the neurocritical care unit so that they are able to provide optimal care to patients while avoiding the hazards described above. We also advocate for early discussion with patients' families regarding their willingness to proceed with prolonged aggressive measures. Often these conversations can avoid the scenario of eventual withdrawal of life-sustaining support only after a long period of aggressive, intensive care that was always felt to have little chance of producing a good outcome.

Nursing collaboration with physicians is important to provide transparency and consistency in decision-making. Nurses can also provide insight into the clinical and psychological condition of the patient. Signals shown by the patient's family are often seen only by the nurse. The relationship that a nurse develops with both a patient and the family can result in emotional distress. Emotional support systems must be available to nurses.

4.6 Research

Nurses must also play an active role in research projects related to neurocritical care. Often nurses are the primary collectors of data that is used for outcome analysis in neurocritical care studies. This is especially true in retrospective studies that rely on data already contained in the patient's chart. This highlights the importance of routine and prospective standardization of nursing assessments throughout the unit to allow both research and quality improvement through analysis of data. Traditionally, nursing research was primarily non-experimental. Several scoring scales related to sedation, pain control, and arousal are utilized in the intensive care unit. Nurses are in a central position to discuss incorporation of such scales from a practical perspective. In addition to standard data collection and qualitative observations, nurses can intervene to improve patient care. For instance, in a nursing-directed study, the nurses in a neurocritical care unit implemented a "Quiet Time" protocol to minimize external environmental stimuli, resulting in a greater duration of sleep for patients [10]. This study highlights the importance of nurses directing research not only to identify nursing activities that can be adjusted to improve patient care but also to comment on the feasibility of incorporating such changes. Ultimately, a model of nursing research that embraces quantitative analysis to evaluate nursing interventions will allow the continued refinement and improvement of nursing practice in the neurocritical care unit.

4.7 Leadership

Nursing leadership is important to enhance recruitment and retention of specialist nurses. Moreover, nursing leadership will set the standards of practice in the neurocritical care unit and oversee the educational agenda for the staff nurses who work there. Nursing leadership typically involves a nurse manager, a nurse educator, and several experienced bedside nurses with additional education who serve as charge nurses for different shifts. Administrative and leadership functions are supplemented by the creation of nurse-centered, unit-specific committees to focus on the evaluation of practice and policies that affect the patients and nurses. This ensures that all policies are assessed by the nurses responsible for following them and makes certain that the policies not only improve job satisfaction and patient care but also maintain judicious use of time and financial resources.

Nurse leadership also creates a dedicated, consistent contact point for physician leadership. Together, this relationship allows nursing staff to propagate shared goals and initiatives and to receive feedback on new or old practices and how they impact patient care and nurse job satisfaction. Closing this feedback loop is essential to prevent the accumulation of counterproductive policies.

4.8 Conclusion

Nursing practice and care are central to the treatment of critically ill patients with neurologic injuries. Moreover, organization and maintenance of a specialized nursing staff are essential if a hospital is to achieve its missions, including education, research, and patient care. This is only possible with close collaboration and mutual support between the nursing and medical staffs, which can amplify each of their unique strengths.

References

1. Moheet AM, Livesay SL, Abdelhak T, Bleck TP, Human T, Karanjia N, et al. Standards for neurologic critical care units: a statement for healthcare professionals from the Neurocritical Care Society. Neurocrit Care. 2018;29(2):145–60. http://www.ncbi.nlm.nih.gov/pubmed/30251072.
2. Neuraz A, Guérin C, Payet C, Polazzi S, Aubrun F, Dailler F, et al. Patient mortality is associated with staff resources and workload in the ICU: a multicenter observational study. Crit Care Med. 2015;43(8):1587–94. http://www.ncbi.nlm.nih.gov/pubmed/25867907.
3. Frith KH, Anderson EF, Caspers B, Tseng F, Sanford K, Hoyt NG, et al. Effects of nurse staffing on hospital-acquired conditions and length of stay in community hospitals. Qual Manag Health Care. 2010;19(2):147–55. http://www.ncbi.nlm.nih.gov/pubmed/20351541.
4. Aiken LH, Clarke SP, Sloane DM, Sochalski J, Silber JH. Hospital nurse staffing and patient mortality, nurse burnout, and job dissatisfaction. JAMA. 2002;288(16):1987–93. http://www.ncbi.nlm.nih.gov/pubmed/12387650.
5. Fleischman RK, Meyer L, Watson C. Best practices in creating a culture of certification. AACN Adv Crit Care. 2011;22(1):33–49. http://www.ncbi.nlm.nih.gov/pubmed/21297390.
6. Kaleem S, Kang JH, Sahgal A, Hernandez CE, Sinha SR, Swisher CB. Electrographic seizure detection by neuroscience intensive care unit nurses via bedside real-time quantitative EEG. Neurol Clin Pract. 2021;11(5):420–8. http://www.ncbi.nlm.nih.gov/pubmed/34840869.
7. Nyholm L, Lewén A, Fröjd C, Howells T, Nilsson P, Enblad P. The use of nurse checklists in a bedside computer-based information system to focus on avoiding secondary insults in neurointensive care. ISRN Neurol. 2012;2012:903954. http://www.ncbi.nlm.nih.gov/pubmed/22844615.
8. Latour JM, Fulbrook P, Albarran JW. EfCCNa survey: European intensive care nurses' attitudes and beliefs towards end-of-life care. Nurs Crit Care. 2009;14(3):110–21. http://www.ncbi.nlm.nih.gov/pubmed/19366408.
9. Hamric AB, Blackhall LJ. Nurse-physician perspectives on the care of dying patients in intensive care units: collaboration, moral distress, and ethical climate. Crit Care Med. 2007;35(2):422–9. http://www.ncbi.nlm.nih.gov/pubmed/17205001.
10. Olson DM, Borel CO, Laskowitz DT, Moore DT, McConnell ES. Quiet time: a nursing intervention to promote sleep in neurocritical care units. Am J Crit Care. 2001;10(2):74–8. http://www.ncbi.nlm.nih.gov/pubmed/11244674.

Part II

Diagnosis and Neuromonitoring

Clinical Evaluation: Neurological Examination and Standardized Scales

5

Andrea Viscone, Davide Corbella, and Matteo Giuseppe Felice Vascello

5.1 Neurological Evaluation in Trauma

5.1.1 Introduction

The Advanced Trauma Life Support (ATLS) protocol mandates an evaluation of the neurological functions after assessing and stabilizing airways, breath, and circulatory function [1]. The neurological physical examination identifies the involvement of the central nervous system (CNS) in the damage. It directs fundamental choices like the destination of the patient from the territory, diagnostic paths, immediate treatments, and shade lights on patient's prognosis. The physical examination of the neurological functions has scores aimed at standardizing communications between the healthcare providers to detect the deteriorating patient most efficiently. Every phase of the neurocritical patients (i.e., crash scene, emergency department (ED), neurocritical care unit (NCCU)) has its specific objective and pitfalls. Consequently, every phase will focus on exploring different signs and symptoms. We will first present an evaluation scheme focusing on the various treatment phases. The final part of this chapter will focus on the confused, traumatized patient highlighting the possible physiology, quantification, and identification.

A. Viscone · D. Corbella (✉)
NeuroTrauma Intensive Care Unit, Department of Anesthesia, Emergency and Critical Care, Azienda Socio Sanitaria Territoriale Papa Giovanni XXIII, Bergamo, Italy
e-mail: aviscone@asst-pg23.it; dcorbella@asst-pg23.it

M. G. F. Vascello
Clinical Psychology Unit, Physical Medicine and Rehabilitation Unit, Department of Mental Health, Azienda Socio Sanitaria Territoriale Papa Giovanni XXIII, Bergamo, Italy
e-mail: mvascello@asst-pg23.it

E. Brogi et al. (eds.), *Traumatic Brain Injury*, Hot Topics in Acute Care Surgery and Trauma, https://doi.org/10.1007/978-3-031-50117-3_5

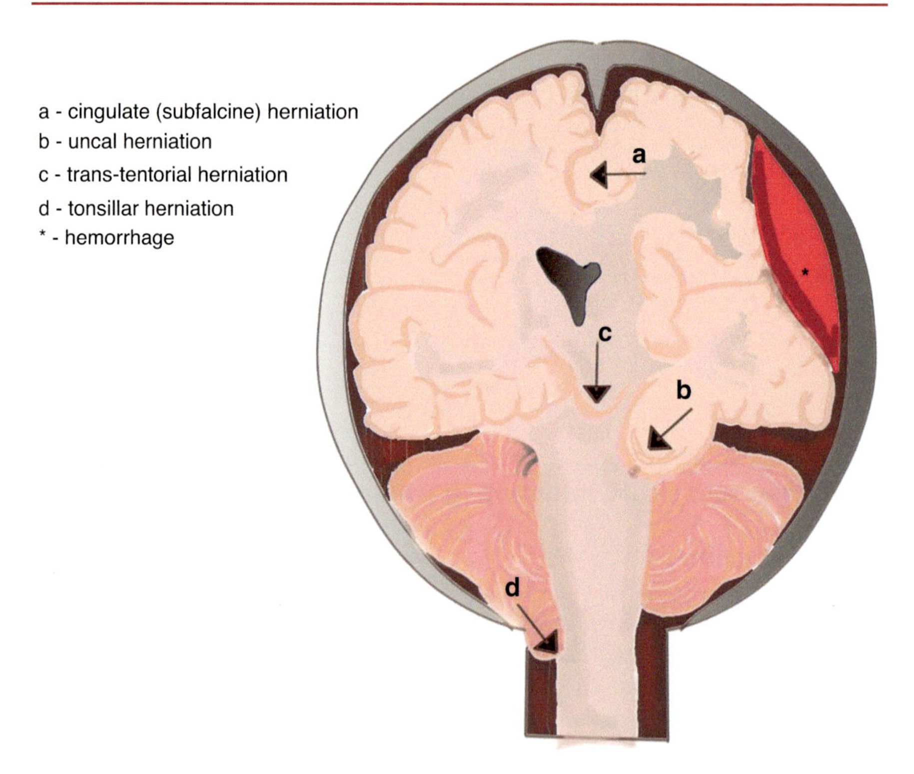

Fig. 5.1 Example of primary damage in TBI. Cerebral herniation types

5.1.2 Traumatic Brain Injury

Traumatic brain injury (TBI) is usually characterized by primary damage, linked to the direct traumatic harmful effect on both cerebral parenchyma and skull and secondary damage due to the development of high intracranial pressure (see Monroe-Kelly doctrine), to the localized mass effect, to events of ischemia or hypoxia and cerebral oedema (Fig. 5.1). A more subtle form of primary damage is the diffuse axonal injury (DAI): shearing of axons that happens when the brain is injured as it shifts and rotates inside the skull. TBI could present with different clinical scenarios, from confusion/dysphoric state to conscience deficit to coma or peripheral deficit.

5.2 Crash Scene

5.2.1 Objectives

On the crash scene, the main objective is to assess and obtain a secure airway and stable vital functions, as per ATLS protocol. If the neurologic evaluation highlights a CNS trauma, perfusion and oxygenation targets must grant an adequate oxygen supply to the brain (mean arterial pressure > 90 mmHg and SpO_2 > 90%) [2, 3]. The ventilation strategy should be protective and avoid hypo- and hyperventilation unless imminent cerebral herniation is suspected. For intubation maneuvers, adequate sedation and neuromuscular block are mandatory, as continuous sedation after. The physical exam can raise the suspicion of a neurosurgical emergency. It should trigger specific drug treatment (e.g., hypertonic saline or mannitol infusion and transient hyperventilation) and the dispatchment to a neurosurgical-capable hospital.

5.2.2 Pitfalls

On the scene, it is frequent to over- or underrate the trauma severity. Multiple confounders make neurological assessment unreliable: drugs or alcohol assumption, metabolic causes such as hypo- or hyperglycemia, shock, hypotension or hypoxia, and post-critical period. Healthcare providers should pay attention to the context in which they examine the patient and the dynamic of the event. They must repeat the neurological examination at the scene and during hospital transportation: brain lesions are evolutive, and the patient could worsen abruptly. Distracting lesions (e.g., amputations) constitute a significant pitfall. They could bring to a careless neurological evaluation or mask a worsening in conscience status (or could mask it as a consequence of hypovolemic or hemorrhagic shock). It is essential to check for consistency between the trauma dynamic and patient's clinical severity (e.g., an unconscious patient following a very low-energy trauma could suggest that the neurological alteration could be the cause and not the consequence of the traumatic event).

5.2.3 Clinical Examination and Scores

Conscience evaluation in TBI patients could inform about the damage suffered. DAI, obstructive hydrocephalus, and cerebral hemorrhage compressing brain parenchyma are all causes of conscience alterations and coma. A simple way to evaluate neurological functions is with the Glasgow Coma Scale (GCS, Table 5.1), a widely diffuse and validated grading score for traumatic patients [4]. It explores three items—eye-opening, verbal, and motor response—scoring each according to

Table 5.1 Glasgow Coma Scale

Score	Eye-opening response	Verbal response	Motor response
6			Obeys command
5		Oriented to time/place/person	Moves to localize pain
4	Spontaneously	Confused	Withdraw from pain
3	To speech	Inappropriate words	Abnormal flexion
2	To pain	Incomprehensible sounds	Abnormal extension
1	No response	No response	No response

Table 5.2 Full Outline of Unresponsiveness Score

Score	Eye response	Motor response	Brainstem reflexes	Respiration pattern
4	Open, tracking, blinking to command	Thumbs-up, fist, or peace sign	Pupil and corneal reflexes present	Not intubated, regular pattern
3	Open but not tracking	Localizing to pain	One pupil wide and fixed	Not intubated, Cheyne–Stokes pattern
2	Closed but open to loud voice	Flexion response to pain	Pupil or corneal reflex absent	Not intubated, irregular breathing
1	Closed but open to pain	Extension response to pain	Pupil and corneal reflexes absent	Breaths above ventilatory rate
0	No response	No response/ myoclonus status	Absent pupil, corneal and cough reflexes	Breaths at ventilator rate/apnea

patient's best performance. The motor evaluation must consider the best response in a side unaffected by motor pathway lesion (i.e., eye closing after command in a tetraplegic patient). A verbal response is not testable (NT) in intubated patients. Health care providers can report GCS as the sum of the three items or each item points separated. Both ways are correct and depend on the information we want to provide. For example, TBI is classified as severe if GCS is less than 9, mild between 9 and 13, and moderate if higher than 13. A decrease of two GCS points is a significant worsening that needs action. Motor response score in GCS for TBI patients correlates with the outcome and should always be reported unbundled. The GCS-Pupils Score (GCS-P) [5] integrates pupils' reactivity to light (if absent, it could mean brainstem damage) with the Pupils Reactivity Score (PRS). To obtain GCS-P, we should subtract PRS from GCS score: e.g., if a patient has a GCS score of 9 and a PRS of 2, GCS-P will be GCS – PRS = 9–2 = 7.

The GCS has two primary limits: it is not testable in intubated patients and does not explore brainstem reflexes. The Full Outline of Unresponsiveness Score (FOUR, Table 5.2) [6] tries to overcome these limitations and shows an excellent correlation to mortality in severely traumatized patients. FOUR explore four items: eye-opening and motor response (but only for upper extremities) like GCS plus brainstem reflexes—as a response to light and corneal reflex—and respiratory pattern. It ranges from 0 in an unconscious apneic patient with no brainstem reflexes to 16 in a normal awake patient. The first clinical evaluation can easily miss signs and symptoms of a basicranium fracture. Those lesions could cause a dura mater tearing due to the contiguity between the dura mater and bone. Basicranium fracture and most dura mater lesions could be suspected from the trauma dynamic (e.g., direct trauma or the indirect distribution force of a precipitation trauma with landing on feet).

Providers must actively look for signs of basilar skull fracture:

- Evidence of depressed skull fracture at palpation;
- Rhinorrhoea: leak of CSF from the nose, likely after basilar skull fracture in the anterior portion;
- Otorrhea: leak of CSF from the ear, as in the event of a basilar skull fracture in the middle portion;

- Hemotympanum: the presence of blood in the middle ear, visible with an otoscope as blood trapped behind the eardrum;
- Battle's sign: bruising over the mastoid process or in the retro-auricular region;
- Raccoon sign: unilateral or bilateral progressive periorbital ecchymosis associated with oedema.

Recognizing those signs on the scene prompts the transport to a hospital with a neurosurgery ward because a basilar skull fracture is a potential neurosurgical emergency.

A TBI patient must be treated as a spine injury until proven otherwise due to the high rate of co-presence of TBI and spine injury [2]. Traumatic spine injury could be seen as a vertebral fracture, a ligamentous lesion, or a medullary damage. A medullary lesion manifests as a tearing (e.g., a vertebral fracture with fragments lacerating the nervous fibers) or a contusion (e.g., for a peridural hematoma or local oedema). Chances are higher if the medullary canal is stenotic. Several devices are designed to immobilize the spine: cervical collar, spinal board, and KED. Symptoms, their severity, and their localization in case of a medullary lesion will change accordingly to the level involved. As a general rule, the more severe lesions are more cranial; the most serious are above C5 level, as they will determine respiratory palsy. At the crash scene, healthcare providers should check for pain at the spine level (spontaneous or after palpation), sensory or motor impairment, and early signs of a medullary lesion like priapism (persistent and painful erection).

5.3 Emergency Department

5.3.1 Objectives

Once in the ED, the ED physician should undertake a thorough neurologic exam to localize a CNS lesion. We will need a "top" down" neurologic examination, which includes language, executive function, brainstem reflexes, tone, strength, coordination, sensation, and reflexes (tendon, cutaneous, grasp, plantar, and coordinated, nocifensive motor responses). The providers need to customize the exam accordingly to the actual presentation of the patient. There is no point in testing an executive function in a deeply sedated or hypotensive hypoxic patient. Providers must periodically repeat the neurological examination due to the TBI evolutive nature and be ready for a mixed neurologic picture, as trauma can affect CNS areas far from each other. Physical exam, past medical history, and crash mechanism lead to the choices for secondary diagnostic exams (CT scan, EEG, transcranial color Doppler, MRI) and hereafter medical vs. surgical treatment. The clinical exam should raise suspicion and lead to diagnostic exams for spinal and vascular injuries.

5.3.2 Pitfalls

Cardiac and respiratory instability profoundly affect the neurologic clinical exam and should be addressed before performing any evaluation.

Sedative, analgesic, and neuromuscular blocking agents can profoundly affect the neurologic exam, and their administration must be kept in mind while evaluating a traumatized patient. Even analgesic drugs could impact neurological evaluation; generally speaking, we should maintain an adequate sedative and analgesic plan for the patients trying to minimize the conscience alteration. The ED physician should perform a sedation holiday before performing a clinical exam; if unfeasible or unsafe, he should at least regularly check for pupil dimension and reactivity to light.

5.3.3 Clinical Examination and Scores

In the setting of ED, we should, at least, maintain a regular neurological evaluation with GCS or FOUR to intercept clinical worsening. The clinical worsening can be defined by a decrease of two points in a GCS or FOUR scale or the occurrence, or worsening, of neurological signs, and should prompt action to determine the cause. In the awake and oriented patient, we could perform the classical neurologic examination by "the systems," i.e., hemisphere considering separate lobes, cerebellum, brainstem, and spinal cord. The main point is to orient the macrolocalization of the lesion and rule out the occurrence of a new lesion in an unaffected area. Cerebral hemispheric lesions show disturbances in multitasking and switching, reasoning, abnormality of perception, memory disturbances, weakness, visual field defects and, eventually, abnormal levels of consciousness. Brainstem lesions produce a cranial nerve deficit, with or without hemiparesis, impairment of motor eyes and visual impairment. Cerebellar lesions bring gait and coordination disorders. Romberg's test could assess coordination: in case of a cerebellar lesion, the patient will tend to lateropulsion; in proprioceptive impairment, the patient will not stand with eyes closed. Another possibility is the finger-to-nose test: the patient should reach the nose tip with both indexes alternatively and rapidly; failure in this test could mean dysmetria secondary to cerebellar damage.

The ED physician must rule out the need for endotracheal intubation. The main reasons to perform endotracheal intubation in ED are GCS < 9, lack of spontaneous airway protection, airway obstruction, persistent hypoxemia despite non-invasive oxygen therapy, respiratory failure, need for sedation in an agitated patient, need for sedation, and airway protection for patient transport.

5.3.4 Spinal Injury

In the USA, 3.5% of all patients accepted in the ED for trauma are evaluated for a cervical spine lesion; of those, only 2% present one [7, 8]. Despite the rarity of C-spine lesions, providers must actively look for them to prevent further damage in these highly disabling lesions. At the same time, we should avoid futile radiological exams in low-risk patients. The authors proposed two evaluation systems to stratify the probability that a c-spine lesion is present:

Nexus Criteria [9]: it considers five criteria: focal neurologic deficit, pain at the palpation on neck midline, a story of drug abuse, normal conscious state, and absence of distracting lesions. If those criteria are unmet, then the patient does not need a radiologic evaluation of the C-spine.

Canadian C-Spine Rule [10]: more sensible than NEXUS criteria, validated for patients older than 16. It is a flowchart that evaluates imaging indications. It comprises high-risk criteria (age ≥ 65 years, dangerous mechanism of trauma, and paresthesia at the extremities), low-risk criteria, and, if those are unmet, patient's ability to rotate the head.

However, both scales give no clues on which radiologic exam performs.

Medullary damage could be complete or incomplete. A complete lesion shows bilateral flaccid paralysis of muscles below the lesion level, associated with hypo-anesthesia and dysautonomia in the same region, hemodynamic instability if lesion's level is high, and loss of sphincteric control. Flaccid paralysis will become spastic with tendons hyperreflexia after days from the primary injury. On the contrary, incomplete medullary lesions show sensory or motor deficits, mono- or bilateral depending on the lesion sites, possible sphincteric alterations, and tendons' hyper-reflexia. Those findings could be temporary (in case of contusion or concussion) or permanent. We identify several medullary syndromes by their site of damage and the symptoms below the lesion level. The American Spinal Injury Association reports a thorough evaluation of spine symptoms and function and its classification [11] (Fig. 5.2).

The medulla midsection causes Brown-Sequard syndrome. The patient shows ipsilateral spastic paralysis, loss of epicritic sensibility, and loss of contralateral thermic and pain sensibility. A direct lesion of the anterior portion of the medulla and anterior spinal artery section can cause the anterior medullary syndrome. It shows loss of bilateral motor and pain sensibility; the posterior pathways are intact, so vibration and proprioception are unremarkable. Hyperextension trauma in a

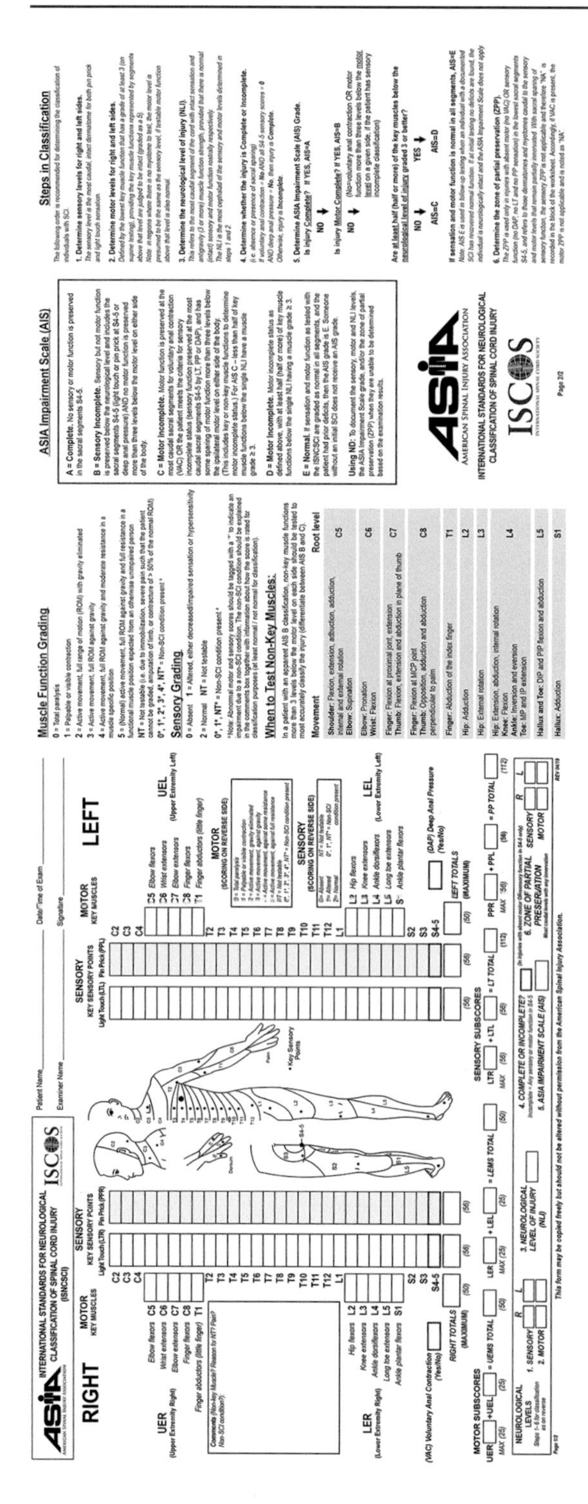

Fig. 5.2 International Standards for Neurological Classification of Spinal Cord Injury from the American Spinal Injury Association (2019) [11]

patient with cervical spinal canal stenosis can lead to central medullary syndrome. Motor function is compromised with worse symptoms in the upper than lower extremities. Depending on the involvement of the posterior or spinothalamic tract, we could observe a loss of superficial tactile and proprioceptive sensibility or a loss of thermic, pain and deep tactile sensibility. Medullary hemorrhage can prompt inferior motoneuron symptoms such as weakness, muscular atrophy, fasciculation, and tendons' hyporeflexia on the upper extremities. Compression to the terminal nerve roots below the L2 level can cause a cauda equina syndrome characterized by acute loss of lumbar plexus function, a structure which grants sensory and motor innervation to the low abdomen and lower extremities. Depending on the syndrome severity, we could observe lumbar back pain irradiated to the leg with hyposthenia and hypoesthesia, bladder dysfunction, sphincteric dysfunction, or saddle anesthesia.

5.3.4.1 Clinical Examination and Spinal Injury Score

Sensitive symptoms' level identifies the medullary lesion level. The cutaneous surface should be evaluated at the four extremities, torso, and abdomen. Sensory exams include light touch sensation (brush), pain sensation (pinprick), and position sense (evaluated by asking the patient, with his eyes closed, to identify passive change of position of fingers). Thermal sense is not tested in the ED. We could identify several sensitive alterations:

- anesthesia: complete loss of sensitivity below the lesion's level;
- hypoesthesia: reduction of sensitivity in its various components;
- allodynia: painful sensation triggered by a stimulus that typically would not be painful, usually not linked to medullary compression;
- hyperalgesia: pathological accentuation of the perception of a painful trigger, usually found in neuritis or thalamic syndromes, not linked to the medullary lesion.

5.3.5 Motor Symptoms

We should test muscle tone at all the extremities, with a scoring system ranging from 0 (no muscle contraction) to 5 (normal strength) [12], as in Table 5.3. We could assess alteration as plegia, paralysis, or hyposthenia.

Table 5.3 Royal Medical Research Council Strength Grading Scale

Grade	Strength
0	No contraction
1	Flicker or trace of contraction
2	Active movement with gravity eliminated
3	Active movement against gravity
4	Active movement against resistance
5	Normal strength

Table 5.4 Scale for tendon reflex assessment

Score	Description
0	Absent
1+	Low response
2+	Normal response
3+	Brisk response
4+	Exhaustible response
5+	Continuous clonus

5.3.6 Tendons' Reflexes Evaluation

The deep reflexes test evaluates sensitive and motor fibers at a certain spine level. With a neurology hammer, we trigger muscle contraction that is usually immediate and symmetrical. Pathological responses can be augmented (hyperreflexia), reduced (hyporeflexia), or absent (areflexia); we could alternatively use the score reported in Table 5.4 [13]. We usually test:

- bicipital reflex (C5-C6): examiner should maintain patient's elbow at 90° keeping his thumb on the bicipital tendon: a hammer strike on the thumb should provoke a mild elbow flexion;
- tricipital reflex (C7): examiner should maintain patient's elbow at 90°, striking the tricipital tendon (located just in proximity of elbow bone prominence); we should obtain a forearm extension;
- patellar reflex (L2–L3–L4): the patient is sitting, his lower extremities relaxed and not touching the floor: a hit on the patellar tendon should provoke a mild extension of the knee;
- Achilles tendon reflex (S1): the examiner should grab patient's foot; the leg must be relaxed; a hammer strike on the Achilles tendon should provoke a mild plantar flexion.

5.3.7 Vascular Injuries

Vascular lesions are often concomitant [14] with traumatic brain injuries and should be addressed in the ED or as soon as the suspicion arises. Traumatic damage of neck and intracranial arteries should be ruled out by a CTA when one of these signs is present: facial fractures (Le Fort II and III), basicranium fractures involving the carotid canal, DAI and GCS score ≤5, evidence of neck lesions, cervical spine fractures involving C1, C2, or C3 or cervical spine fractures involving transverses foramen, cervical dislocation, and fracture of clavicula and the first three ribs. A carotid-cavernous fistula is usually a late event after a TBI and sometimes even after a minor one. Bulging eyes, chemosis, bruit (i.e., a blowing sound in the vessel that can be heard with a stethoscope), and a deteriorating vision suggest the need to perform a CTA to rule out a carotid-cavernous fistula.

5.4 Neurocritical Care Unit

5.4.1 Objective

In the ICU, the main focus is the treatment of the primary damage and prevention, early recognition and prompt treatment of the secondary damage. Accordingly to this targets, the aims of the neurologic examination are: (1) look for new neurological signs that can herald new lesions or evolutions of the primary damage (see Fig. 5.4 for a quick reference of clinical signs heralding neuroworsening); (2) define the trajectory of the neurologic lesions, for example, stable hemiplegia or recovery from that; (3) address the clinical need of a tracheostomy or gastric feeding tube; (4) try to formulate a prognosis to counsel the family or the patient. TBI is a polyhedric entity that shows multiple injuries simultaneously like ischemia, cerebral hypoxia, cerebral oedema, reduction in cerebral blood flow, rise in ICP, and mass effect. Those hits are present and evolve; a thorough neurologic clinical exam is the gold standard to detect their evolution.

5.4.2 Pitfalls

The critical care patient is often intubated, under sedation, and on several drugs that may impact the clinical evaluation and whose pharmacokinetic and dynamic can be quite unpredictable. Moreover, other circumstances hamper the value of a neurological exam, like hypoxia, circulatory failure, rise in blood urea, hypercarbia, or sepsis. Neurological evaluation should be performed, if possible, after sedative withdrawal in a patient without confounding factors (see Fig. 5.3). We should always be aware that a neurological worsening can arise from non-neurological causes, although we must first rule out a neurological cause. Many ICU patients cannot have their sedation suspended and show confounding factors. The lack of the possibility to perform a sound clinical exam is the main reason for fostering the clinic with other tools in a multimodal manner [15] (i.e., cEEG, TCCD, pupillometry, PtO2, ICP monitoring, near infrared spectroscopy).

5.4.3 Clinical Examination and Scores

Scales like the GCS or the FOUR have a role in monitoring patient's consciousness but cannot substitute a clinical exam. A previously intact patient can develop a left hemiplegia and still be a GCS15! Despite the presence of sedation, organ failures, and systemic inflammation, the intensivist should try to perform a complete "top down" neurologic evaluation. A neurologic clinical exam in ICU should, at least, explore consciousness, language function, cranial nerves, gaze, relevant reflexes and motor function; moreover, it should answer relevant questions like the need for a tracheostomy or feeding tube. Pain, agitation, and sedation will be the focus of other chapters.

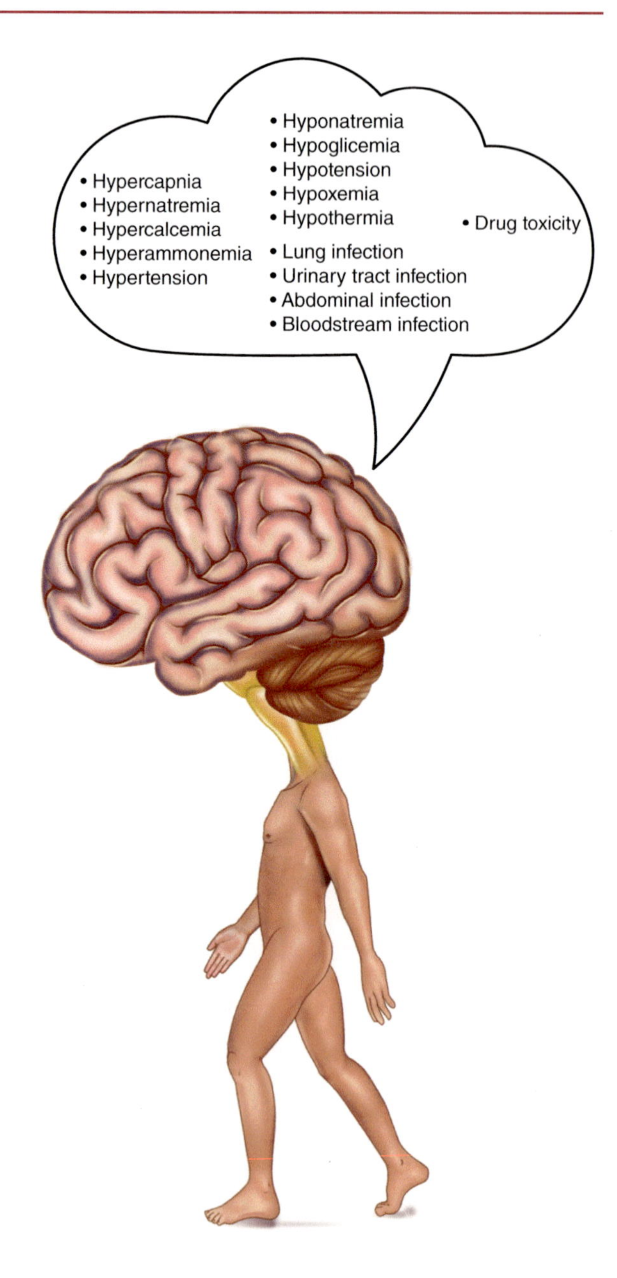

Fig. 5.3 Systemic causes of neurological impairment

5.4.3.1 Language

A thorough assessment of language and speech is rarely possible in ICU. However, we should try to classify aphasia correctly by replying to three simple questions the speech fluent? Can the patient comprehend a spoken message? Is the patient able to repeat words or phrases? Defining the type of aphasia helps formulate a prognosis upon language function, as most aphasias ameliorate over time and help localize a lesion.

5.4.3.2 Cranial Nerves

The integrity of cranial nerves (CN) and their pathways is an easy way to map in time and space lesions of the CNS. If feasible and reliable, we should systematically assess all of them.

Olfactory nerve (I CN): it is not relevant in the patient's evaluation, but a lack of smell sense suggests a telencephalic lesion.

Optic nerve (II CN): in an awake patient, we could test visual field deficits and pupils' response to light. This nerve is involved, together with III CN, in pupils' contraction as a response to light: an optic nerve lesion means the loss of both direct and consensual reflex on the lesion side; both will be maintained contralaterally. Consensual reflex is pupil's response contralaterally to a light trigger. Alteration in the visual field would be secondary to a chiasmatic or optic radiation lesion (Fig. 5.5), but we should not see an alteration of pupillary light reflex. Ultra-sound scan of nerve's sheet can raise the suspicion of a risen ICP. The ICU physician should perform an ophthalmoscopy at least to rule out a pale, swollen retina disk and the presence of a retinal or vitreous hemorrhage.

Oculomotor nerve (III CN), trochlear nerve (IV CN), and abducens nerve (VI CN): they control gaze and response to light and are involved in many reflexes. III CN controls pupils' response to light, and a direct lesion brings to loss of direct light reflex on the damaged side and loss of consensual reflex contralaterally. It controls eye movement upward and toward the nose. IV CN enables eyes' downward rotation and movements away from the nose through the superior oblique muscle. VI CN is responsible for eye movement away from the nose. Their direct lesion can lead to consequent impairment of eye movement.

The trigeminal nerve (V CN) is the face main sensory nerve. Its integrity involves corneal reflex (bilateral blink reflex after corneal stimulation with saline or a light touch with a gauze) and sensory sensation.

The facial nerve (VII CN): the main motor cranial nerve. It is involved in corneal and blinking reflex through its innervation on the orbicularis oculi muscle.

Vestibulocochlear or auditory vestibular nerve (VIII CN): its vestibular components play a role in the oculocephalic reflex. Acoustic blinking reflex explores VIII CN auditory components in an unresponsive patient that is otherwise difficult to explore. Dizziness and nystagmus are the most frequent symptoms of vestibular fibers injury, and tinnitus and hypoacusis for the cochlear components.

The glossopharyngeal nerve (IX CN) controls the swallow and cough reflex with the vagus nerve.

The vagus nerve (X CN) is exceptionally complex, running through the chest and toward the abdomen; we need to test swallow and carinal reflex. A stimulation of the hypopharynx should trigger a swallow or a gag reflex, while a direct stimulation of the carina should trigger a diaphragmatic movement or a cough.

The accessory nerve (XI CN) is tested by asking the patient to lift the shoulders against resistance.

The hypoglossal nerve (XII CN) is a motor nerve that controls tongue muscles. Its injury impairs swallowing and speech. We can evaluate XII CN by asking the patient to protrude the tongue that would be deviated toward the affected side.

5.4.3.3 Resting Eye Position and Gaze

Abnormalities in resting eye position are often pathologic. A horizontal-conjugate deviation indicates a hemispheric injury, a downward eye deviation suggests an injury in the thalamus or posterior midbrain, an upward deviation usually indicates a bilateral hemispheric lesion, and a skew deviation in a comatose patient is often associated with a basilary stroke. Visual tracking is a complex reflex that needs input from the visual cortex. Failure to horizontal visual tracking can be associated with lesions of the oculomotor (mesencephalon) and abducens nucleus (pons), whereas failure in vertical tracking suggests lesions in the periaqueductal gray matter of the mesencephalon (oculomotor and trochlear nuclei).

5.4.3.4 Relevant Reflexes

The blinking reflex is blinking in response to a menace like a loud sound or a rapid-approaching hand to the open eye. Whereas a visual stimulus needs an intact cortex, the acoustic one is only through the brainstem and does not need any cortical input and it helps in discriminating the level of a new CNS lesion.

Pupillary diameter and pupillary light reflex need an intact optic tract, Edinger Westphal nucleus, and CN III to elicit a pupillary contraction to light. Abnormalities, and their most likely reasons, can be: a fixed pupil is often due to a lesion in the tectum or pretectum with involvement of the posterior commissure; stretching or compressing the oculomotor nerve or the midbrain oculomotor complex results in a dilated pupil where a lesion in the descending sympathetic tracts results in a pupil fixed in mid-position; finally, pinpoint pupils are seen in pontine lesions, but light reflex is intact.

The oculovestibular reflex is elicited in comatose patients injecting cold water into the ear canals; in the physiologic response, both eyes should slowly move toward the cold stimulus. This reflex explores the cranial nerves III, IV, VI, and VIII, and its failure is related to a brainstem injury. If both eyes fail to move, it indicates a midbrain lesion. If only an eye fails to move, it indicates a same-side CN VI palsy or an opposite-side internuclear ophthalmoplegia. Doll's eyes or oculocephalic reflex is elicited by moving passively from right-to-left the head with the eyes open; if the reflex is intact, the eyes move left-to-right, and the gaze is fixed.

The absence of carinal reflex, pupillary light reflex, corneal reflex, and oculovestibular reflex is a sign of loss of brainstem function. The law in several countries requires their concomitant presence to declare death by neurological criteria.

Babinski reflex is a plantar reflex elicited by firmly stroking the sole of patient's foot with a pointed stick and is a frequent cause of enthusiasm in residents. The abnormal response is the hallux dorsiflexion and is associated with any condition that depresses the forebrain (i.e., acute brain injury or general anesthesia).

5.4.3.5 Motor Function

The assessment of motor function classically goes through these six items: (1) tone and position; (2) spontaneous movements; (3) evoked movements; (4) strength; (5) symmetry; and (6) a motor response. As a minimum standard, we should rate motor response after a painful stimulus into no response, extension, abnormal flexion, withdrawal, localization, and execution after a verbal command. This progression of symptoms correlates with lesser severity and extension of the brain damage. In ICU, we should be able to track the presence and onset of abnormal movements, like jerk movements or generalized myoclonus, and we should rate strength and symmetry as they are essential in spinal patients, progression, or recovery, from a CNS lesion.

5.4.4 Neuroworsening

Critical neuroworsening is a broad definition that list a series of signs and symptoms that depicts a specific situation of critical deterioration requiring emergent evaluation and management. Critical neuroworsening [16] was first proposed in the late 1990s as an early endpoint to demonstrate the efficacy of a drug or intervention in TBI. Seattle International Severe Traumatic Brain Injury Consensus Conference [17, 18] proposed the last lists of symptoms to define critical neuroworsening (i.e., a spontaneous decrease in the GCS motor score of ≥1, a decrease in pupillary reactivity, a new pupillary asymmetry or mydriasis, a new focal motor deficit, herniation syndrome). Despite the fact that not every neuroworsening is critical we believe that every neuroworsening should be addressed. A list of sensitive localizing and non-localizing signs and symptoms is provided in Fig. 5.4. A clinical exam can be difficult in the ICU environments where multiple confounding factors are present. However, we should try "to exam" as much as possible paying special attention to consciousness and its fluctuances, brainstem, reflexes, and motor responses.

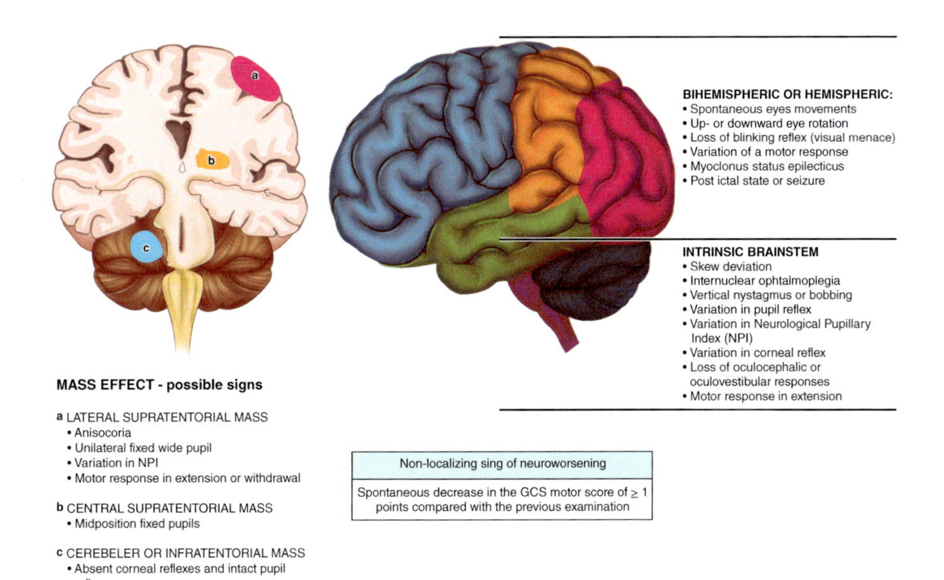

Fig. 5.4 Localizing and not localizing signs and symptoms

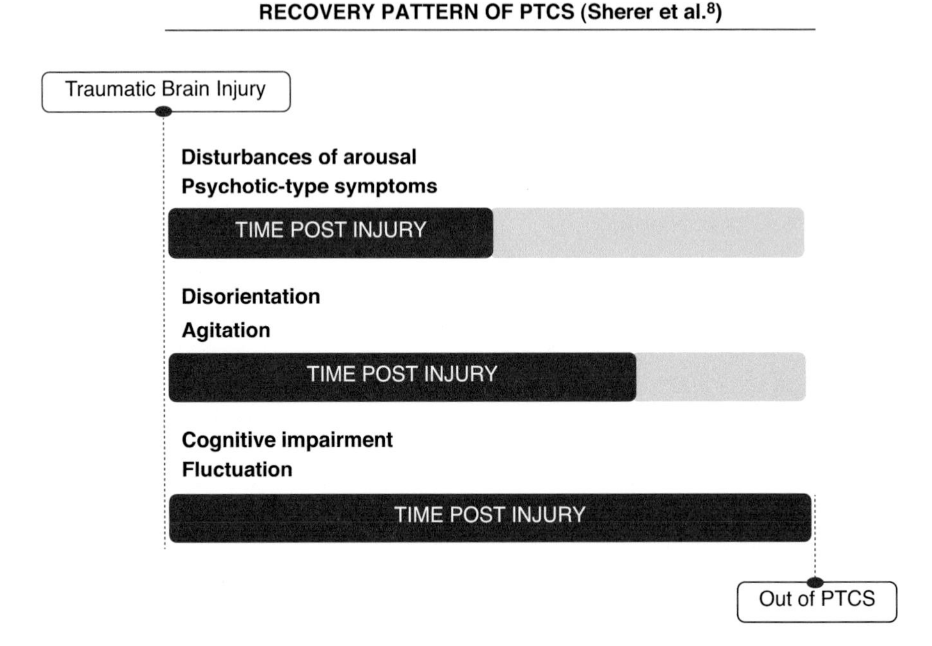

Fig. 5.5 Recovery pattern of PTCs (Sherer et al. [25]). This picture shows the recovery pattern of 7 key symptoms of Post-Traumatic Confusional State (PTCS): nighttime sleep disturbance and decreased daytime arousal (disturbances of arousal), psychotic-type symptoms, disorientation, agitation, cognitive impairment and fluctuation

5.4.5 Confusional State Following TBI

The majority of severe TBI undergo a period during which they recover responsiveness but are confused [19]. In mild to moderate TBI, the unconsciousness period and consequent confusion are generally much shorter; in some cases (e.g., concussion), the former can be absent and the latter so brief that it is tough to detect [20].

This confusion is commonly termed post-traumatic amnesia, post-traumatic confusional state, or *delirium*. Historically, the neurosurgery and rehabilitation literature defined *post-traumatic amnesia* (PTA) as the early phase of recovery after TBI characterized by a confusional state. The term PTA suggests that memory disturbance is the hallmark of patients' symptomatology in this state. PTA is a clinical condition of generalized cognitive disturbance characterized by disorientation, inability to store and retrieve new memories (anterograde amnesia), recall events preceding the brain injury (retrograde amnesia), and sometimes agitation and delusions. The term "post-traumatic amnesia" was first used by Symonds [21]; its duration includes the period of coma and is calculated from the time of injury until the return of the capacity to acquire and retrieve new memories [22].

Some authors stated that PTA is a complex condition that involves working memory and speed information processing deficits in addition to orientation and memory disorders [23].

Stuss et al. [24] studied patients with PTA and found that the performance on attentional tasks improved before the return to orientation. They concluded that attentional disturbance is a crucial aspect of confusion after TBI and suggested using *post-traumatic confusional state* (PTCS) instead of PTA. Sherer et al. [25] identified seven key symptoms of PTCS in the post-acute phase of TBI recovery. These are disorientation, cognitive impairment (memory and attentional/executive control), fluctuation in symptoms presentation, agitation, nighttime sleep disturbance, decreased daytime arousal, and psychotic-type symptoms.

Sherer et al. [26] further investigated the pattern of early recovery of PTCS symptomatology, showing that it was characterized first by the resolution of disturbances of arousal (nighttime sleep disturbance and decreased daytime arousal) and psychotic-type symptoms, and then by the resolution of disorientation and agitation. Cognitive impairment and fluctuation of symptoms presentation were the most long-lasting symptoms (see Fig. 5.5). Finally, there is increasing evidence of the neuroanatomical substrates of PTCS/PTA, provided by neuroimaging studies [27–29].

Many standardized scales have been developed for measuring the duration of PTA. The first instrument was the Galveston Orientation and Amnesia Test (GOAT), developed by Levin et al. [30]. Other PTA scales are the Oxford PTA Scale [31], the Westmead PTA Scale (WPTAS) [32], the revised-WPTAS [33]. Recently, Sherer et al. [25] proposed the Confusion Assessment Protocol (CAP), which extends the assessment by incorporating elements associated with the more comprehensive construct of PTCS.

PTA duration is significantly related to short-, medium-, and long-term outcomes in mild to severe TBI, measured by global outcome measures, such as Glasgow Outcome Scale (GOS), Glasgow Outcome Scale Extended (GOS-E), or Disability Rating Scale [34–38], or by more specific domains as community integration [39, 40], cognitive and behavioral dysfunction [38, 41–43], psychosocial dysfunction [44–46], independent living [34, 47], and occupational status [34, 37, 48, 49]. Furthermore, some studies have shown that PTA duration is a better predictor of psychosocial, cognitive, and functional outcomes than other acute severity indexes, such as the GCS, time to follow commands (TFC), and the loss of consciousness (LOC) duration [34, 37, 39, 40, 42, 49, 50]. Recently, some authors have shown that PTCS and its severity also predict TBI outcomes, such as the functional status at rehabilitation discharge and the return to employment [25, 51, 52].

The psychiatric literature generally refers to this period of confusion after TBI as d*elirium*, and this term is commonly used in the ICU clinical practice [53]. The Diagnostic and Statistical Manual of Mental Disorders, Fifth Edition (DSM-5) defines delirium as a reduced ability to direct, focus, sustain, and shift attention and reduced awareness of the environment. The disturbance develops over a short period (usually hours to a few days), represents an acute change from baseline attention and awareness, and tends to fluctuate in severity during the day. It is often associated with additional disturbances in cognition (e.g., memory deficit, disorientation, language, visuospatial ability, or perceptual disturbances) [54].

Based on arousal level, delirium shows three psychomotor subtypes: hyperactive (hyperarousal, agitation), hypoactive (hypoarousal, slowness, lethargy), and mixed (includes the features of both previous subtypes) [55].

The DSM-5 criteria provide the standard reference for diagnosing delirium. However, these criteria are difficult to apply in the ICU context. For this reason, several tools have been developed to screen delirium in ICU patients. In particular, two instruments have been validated and widely employed: the Confusion Assessment Method for the Intensive Care Unit (CAM-ICU) [56] and the Intensive Care Delirium Screening Checklist (ICDSC) [57]. These instruments have been recommended by the Society of Critical Care Medicine Clinical Practice Guidelines on Pain, Agitation, and Delirium [58, 59].

Recently, some authors applied these instruments to TBI in the neuro-ICU context [60, 61] and provided evidence that delirium is associated with worse outcomes, such as a long stay in ICU [60], functional and cognitive impairment [62–64].

For a more detailed discussion on ICU delirium, see Chap. 14.

Ultimately, the scientific literature termed the acute confusion after TBI mainly PTCS/PTA (rehabilitation context) or delirium (NCCU context). Acute confusion can commonly occur immediately after TBI or after an emergency from a coma (severe TBI). It is part of TBI neuropathology [27–29] and represents an index of recovery from the acute stage [65, 66]. Since its severity and duration are excellent predictors of long-term outcomes of TBI [67], it could be useful to create instruments for its detection in NCCU and the subsequent rehabilitative contexts.

References

1. American College of Surgeons, Committee on Trauma. Advanced Trauma Life Support® Student Course Manual. 10th ed; 2018.
2. Carney N, Totten AM, O'Reilly C, Ullman JS, Hawryluk GWJ, Bell MJ, et al. Guidelines for the management of severe traumatic brain injury, fourth edition. Neurosurgery. 2017;80:6–15.
3. Kochanek PM, Carney N, Adelson PD, Ashwal S, Bell MJ, Bratton S, et al. Guidelines for the acute medical management of severe traumatic brain injury in infants, children, and adolescents—second edition. Pediatr Crit Care Med. 2012;13(Suppl 1):S1–82.
4. Teasdale G, Jennett B. Assessment of coma and impaired consciousness. A practical scale. Lancet. 1974;2:81–4.
5. Brennan PM, Murray GD, Teasdale GM. Simplifying the use of prognostic information in traumatic brain injury. Part 1: the GCS-pupils score: an extended index of clinical severity. J Neurosurg. 2018;128:1612–20.
6. Wijdicks EFM, Bamlet WR, Maramattom BV, Manno EM, McClelland RL. Validation of a new coma scale: the FOUR score. Ann Neurol. 2005;58:585–93.
7. Brown CVR, Antevil JL, Sise MJ, Sack DI. Spiral computed tomography for the diagnosis of cervical, thoracic, and lumbar spine fractures: its time has come. J Trauma. 2005;58:890–5; discussion 895–896.
8. Como JJ, Diaz JJ, Dunham CM, Chiu WC, Duane TM, Capella JM, et al. Practice management guidelines for identification of cervical spine injuries following trauma: update from the eastern association for the surgery of trauma practice management guidelines committee. J Trauma. 2009;67:651–9.
9. Hoffman JR, Mower WR, Wolfson AB, Todd KH, Zucker MI. Validity of a set of clinical criteria to rule out injury to the cervical spine in patients with blunt trauma. National Emergency X-Radiography Utilization Study Group. N Engl J Med. 2000;343:94–9.
10. Stiell IG, Wells GA, Vandemheen KL, Clement CM, Lesiuk H, De Maio VJ, et al. The Canadian C-spine rule for radiography in alert and stable trauma patients. JAMA. 2001;286:1841–8.

11. Kalsi-Ryan S. International standards for neurological classification of spinal cord injury (ISNCSCI) *. In: Vaccaro AR, Fisher CG, Wilson JR, editors. 50 Landmark Papers [Internet]. 1st ed. Boca Raton, FL: CRC; 2018. p. 83–6. https://doi.org/10.1201/9781315154053-16.
12. Aids to the examination of the peripheral nervous system [Internet]. 2016. https://www.ukri.org/publications/aids-to-the-examination-of-the-peripheral-nervous-system/.
13. Walker HK. Deep tendon reflexes. In: Walker HK, Hall WD, Hurst JW, editors. Clinical methods: the history, physical, and laboratory examinations [internet]. 3rd ed. Boston: Butterworths; 1990. http://www.ncbi.nlm.nih.gov/books/NBK396/.
14. Esnault P, Cardinale M, Boret H, D'Aranda E, Montcriol A, Bordes J, et al. Blunt cerebrovascular injuries in severe traumatic brain injury: incidence, risk factors, and evolution. J Neurosurg. 2017;127:16–22.
15. Le Roux P, Menon DK, Citerio G, Vespa P, Bader MK, Brophy GM, et al. Consensus summary statement of the international multidisciplinary consensus conference on multimodality monitoring in neurocritical care: a statement for healthcare professionals from the Neurocritical Care Society and the European Society of Intensive Care Medicine. Intensive Care Med. 2014;40:1189–209.
16. Morris GF, Juul N, Marshall SB, Benedict B, Marshall LF. Neurological deterioration as a potential alternative endpoint in human clinical trials of experimental pharmacological agents for treatment of severe traumatic brain injuries. Executive Committee of the International Selfotel Trial. Neurosurgery. 1998;43:1369–72; discussion 1372–1374.
17. Chesnut R, Aguilera S, Buki A, Bulger E, Citerio G, Cooper DJ, et al. A management algorithm for adult patients with both brain oxygen and intracranial pressure monitoring: the Seattle International Severe Traumatic Brain Injury Consensus Conference (SIBICC). Intensive Care Med. 2020;46:919–29.
18. Hawryluk GWJ, Aguilera S, Buki A, Bulger E, Citerio G, Cooper DJ, et al. A management algorithm for patients with intracranial pressure monitoring: the Seattle International Severe Traumatic Brain Injury Consensus Conference (SIBICC). Intensive Care Med. 2019;45:1783. https://doi.org/10.1007/s00134-019-05805-9.
19. Giacino JT, Fins JJ, Laureys S, Schiff ND. Disorders of consciousness after acquired brain injury: the state of the science. Nat Rev Neurol. 2014;10:99–114.
20. Povlishock JT, Katz DI. Update of neuropathology and neurological recovery after traumatic brain injury. J Head Trauma Rehabil. 2005;20:76–94.
21. Symonds CP. Concussion and contusion of the brain and their sequelae. In: Brock S, editor. Injuries of the skull, brain and spinal cord: neuro-psychiatric, surgical, and medico-legal aspects. London: Bailliere, Tindall and Cox. p. 69–111.
22. Russell WR, Nathan PW. Traumatic amnesia. Brain. 1946;69:280–300.
23. Wilson BA, Evans JJ, Emslie H, Balleny H, Watson PC, Baddeley AD. Measuring recovery from post traumatic amnesia. Brain Inj. 1999;13:505–20.
24. Stuss DT, Binns MA, Carruth FG, Levine B, Brandys CE, Moulton RJ, et al. The acute period of recovery from traumatic brain injury: posttraumatic amnesia or posttraumatic confusional state? J Neurosurg. 1999;90:635–43.
25. Sherer M, Nakase-Thompson R, Yablon SA, Gontkovsky ST. Multidimensional assessment of acute confusion after traumatic brain injury. Arch Phys Med Rehabil. 2005;86:896–904.
26. Sherer M, Yablon SA, Nakase-Richardson R. Patterns of recovery of posttraumatic confusional state in neurorehabilitation admissions after traumatic brain injury. Arch Phys Med Rehabil. 2009;90:1749–54.
27. De Simoni S, Grover PJ, Jenkins PO, Honeyfield L, Quest RA, Ross E, et al. Disconnection between the default mode network and medial temporal lobes in post-traumatic amnesia. Brain. 2016;139:3137–50.
28. Cho MJ, Jang SH. Relationship between post-traumatic amnesia and white matter integrity in traumatic brain injury using tract-based spatial statistics. Sci Rep. 2021;11:6898.
29. Osmanlıoğlu Y, Parker D, Alappatt JA, Gugger JJ, Diaz-Arrastia RR, Whyte J, et al. Connectomic assessment of injury burden and longitudinal structural network alterations in moderate-to-severe traumatic brain injury. Hum Brain Mapp. 2022;43:3944–57.

30. Levin HS, O'Donnell VM, Grossman RG. The Galveston orientation and amnesia test. A practical scale to assess cognition after head injury. J Nerv Ment Dis. 1979;167:675–84.
31. Fortuny LA, Briggs M, Newcombe F, Ratcliff G, Thomas C. Measuring the duration of post traumatic amnesia. J Neurol Neurosurg Psychiatry. 1980;43:377–9.
32. Shores EA, Marosszeky JE, Sandanam J, Batchelor J. Preliminary validation of a clinical scale for measuring the duration of post-traumatic amnesia. Med J Aust. 1986;144:569–72.
33. Ponsford J, Willmott C, Rothwell A, Kelly A-M, Nelms R, Ng KT. Use of the Westmead PTA scale to monitor recovery of memory after mild head injury. Brain Inj. 2004;18:603–14.
34. Brown AW, Malec JF, McClelland RL, Diehl NN, Englander J, Cifu DX. Clinical elements that predict outcome after traumatic brain injury: a prospective multicenter recursive partitioning (decision-tree) analysis. J Neurotrauma. 2005;22:1040–51.
35. Ponsford J, Draper K, Schönberger M. Functional outcome 10 years after traumatic brain injury: its relationship with demographic, injury severity, and cognitive and emotional status. J Int Neuropsychol Soc. 2008;14:233–42.
36. Walker WC, Ketchum JM, Marwitz JH, Chen T, Hammond F, Sherer M, et al. A multicentre study on the clinical utility of post-traumatic amnesia duration in predicting global outcome after moderate-severe traumatic brain injury. J Neurol Neurosurg Psychiatry. 2010;81:87–9.
37. Walker WC, Stromberg KA, Marwitz JH, Sima AP, Agyemang AA, Graham KM, et al. Predicting long-term global outcome after traumatic brain injury: development of a practical prognostic tool using the traumatic brain injury model systems National Database. J Neurotrauma. 2018;35:1587–95.
38. Hart T, Novack TA, Temkin N, Barber J, Dikmen SS, Diaz-Arrastia R, et al. Duration of posttraumatic amnesia predicts neuropsychological and global outcome in complicated mild traumatic brain injury. J Head Trauma Rehabil. 2016;31:E1–9.
39. Doig E, Fleming J, Tooth L. Patterns of community integration 2-5 years post-discharge from brain injury rehabilitation. Brain Inj. 2001;15:747–62.
40. Fleming J, Tooth L, Hassell M, Chan W. Prediction of community integration and vocational outcome 2-5 years after traumatic brain injury rehabilitation in Australia. Brain Inj. 1999;13:417–31.
41. de Guise E, LeBlanc J, Feyz M, Lamoureux J, Greffou S. Prediction of behavioural and cognitive deficits in patients with traumatic brain injury at an acute rehabilitation setting. Brain Inj. 2017;31:1061–8.
42. Haslam C, Batchelor J, Fearnside MR, Haslam SA, Hawkins S, Kenway E. Post-coma disturbance and post-traumatic amnesia as nonlinear predictors of cognitive outcome following severe closed head injury: findings from the Westmead head injury project. Brain Inj. 1994;8:519–28.
43. van der Naalt J, van Zomeren AH, Sluiter WJ, Minderhoud JM. Acute behavioural disturbances related to imaging studies and outcome in mild-to-moderate head injury. Brain Inj. 2000;14:781–8.
44. Wood RL, Rutterford NA. Demographic and cognitive predictors of long-term psychosocial outcome following traumatic brain injury. J Int Neuropsychol Soc. 2006;12:350–8.
45. Draper K, Ponsford J, Schönberger M. Psychosocial and emotional outcomes 10 years following traumatic brain injury. J Head Trauma Rehabil. 2007;22:278–87.
46. Tate RL, Broe GA, Cameron ID, Hodgkinson AE, Soo CA. Pre-injury, injury and early post-injury predictors of long-term functional and psychosocial recovery after severe traumatic brain injury. Brain Impairment. 2005;6:75–89.
47. Eastvold AD, Walker WC, Curtiss G, Schwab K, Vanderploeg RD. The differential contributions of posttraumatic amnesia duration and time since injury in prediction of functional outcomes following moderate-to-severe traumatic brain injury. J Head Trauma Rehabil. 2013;28:48–58.
48. van der Naalt J, van Zomeren AH, Sluiter WJ, Minderhoud JM. One year outcome in mild to moderate head injury: the predictive value of acute injury characteristics related to complaints and return to work. J Neurol Neurosurg Psychiatry. 1999;66:207–13.

49. Sherer M, Sander AM, Nick TG, High WM, Malec JF, Rosenthal M. Early cognitive status and productivity outcome after traumatic brain injury: findings from the TBI model systems. Arch Phys Med Rehabil. 2002;83:183–92.
50. Perrin PB, Niemeier JP, Mougeot J-L, Vannoy CH, Hirsch MA, Watts JA, et al. Measures of injury severity and prediction of acute traumatic brain injury outcomes. J Head Trauma Rehabil. 2015;30:136–42.
51. Sherer M, Yablon SA, Nakase-Richardson R, Nick TG. Effect of severity of post-traumatic confusion and its constituent symptoms on outcome after traumatic brain injury. Arch Phys Med Rehabil. 2008;89:42–7.
52. Nakase-Richardson R, Yablon SA, Sherer M. Prospective comparison of acute confusion severity with duration of post-traumatic amnesia in predicting employment outcome after traumatic brain injury. J Neurol Neurosurg Psychiatry. 2007;78:872–6.
53. Ganau M, Lavinio A, Prisco L. Delirium and agitation in traumatic brain injury patients: an update on pathological hypotheses and treatment options. Minerva Anestesiol. 2018;84:632–40.
54. American Psychiatric Association. Diagnostic and statistical manual of mental disorders. 5th ed; 2023. https://doi.org/10.1176/appi.books.9780890425596.
55. Meagher D. Motor subtypes of delirium: past, present and future. Int Rev Psychiatry. 2009;21:59–73.
56. Ely EW, Margolin R, Francis J, May L, Truman B, Dittus R, et al. Evaluation of delirium in critically ill patients: validation of the confusion assessment method for the intensive care unit (CAM-ICU). Crit Care Med. 2001;29:1370–9.
57. Bergeron N, Dubois MJ, Dumont M, Dial S, Skrobik Y. Intensive care delirium screening checklist: evaluation of a new screening tool. Intensive Care Med. 2001;27:859–64.
58. Barr J, Fraser GL, Puntillo K, Ely EW, Gélinas C, Dasta JF, et al. Clinical practice guidelines for the management of pain, agitation, and delirium in adult patients in the intensive care unit. Crit Care Med. 2013;41:263–306.
59. Devlin JW, Skrobik Y, Gélinas C, Needham DM, Slooter AJC, Pandharipande PP, et al. Clinical practice guidelines for the prevention and management of pain, agitation/sedation, delirium, immobility, and sleep disruption in adult patients in the ICU. Crit Care Med. 2018;46:e825–73.
60. Duceppe M-A, Williamson DR, Elliott A, Para M, Poirier M-C, Delisle M-S, et al. Modifiable risk factors for delirium in critically ill trauma patients: a multicenter prospective study. J Intensive Care Med. 2019;34:330–6.
61. Frenette AJ, Bebawi ER, Deslauriers LC, Tessier A-AL, Perreault MM, Delisle M-S, et al. Validation and comparison of CAM-ICU and ICDSC in mild and moderate traumatic brain injury patients. Intensive Care Med. 2016;42:122–3.
62. Robinson D, Thompson S, Bauerschmidt A, Melmed K, Couch C, Park S, et al. Dispersion in scores on the Richmond agitation and sedation scale as a measure of delirium in patients with subdural hematomas. Neurocrit Care. 2019;30:626–34.
63. Nekrosius D, Kaminskaite M, Jokubka R, Pranckeviciene A, Lideikis K, Tamasauskas A, et al. Association of COMT Val158Met polymorphism with delirium risk and outcomes after traumatic brain injury. J Neuropsychiatry Clin Neurosci. 2019;31:298–305.
64. Ishida T, Inoue T, Inoue T, Saito A, Suzuki S, Uenohara H, et al. Functional outcome in patients with chronic subdural hematoma: postoperative delirium and operative procedure. Neurol Med Chir (Tokyo). 2022;62:171–6.
65. Ponsford J, Carrier S, Hicks A, McKay A. Assessment and management of patients in the acute stages of recovery after traumatic brain injury in adults: a worldwide survey. J Neurotrauma. 2021;38:1060–7.
66. Wang Z, Winans NJ, Zhao Z, Cosgrove ME, Gammel T, Saadon JR, et al. Agitation following severe traumatic brain injury is a clinical sign of recovery of consciousness. Front Surg. 2021;8:627008.
67. Sherer M, Katz DI, Bodien YG, Arciniegas DB, Block C, Blum S, et al. Post-traumatic confusional state: a case definition and diagnostic criteria. Arch Phys Med Rehabil. 2020;101:2041–50.

6 Neuroradiological Imaging for Traumatic Brain Injury

Hansen Deng, John K. Yue, and David O. Okonkwo

6.1 Introduction to Neuroimaging

Radiological imaging of the patient with traumatic brain injury (TBI) is a critical component of saving lives and directing clinical care. The initial evaluation of the trauma patient includes the rapid detection of intracranial mass lesions requiring neurosurgical intervention as well as assessment of the need for invasive neuromonitoring. Neuroimaging for TBI also provides key insights to parse out the heterogeneous manifestations of the injury and the overall burden of injury.

For these reasons, the heterogeneity of TBI presentation is a barrier to precise diagnosis of intracranial injuries and prognostication of long-term functional outcomes. Regardless of current limitations in care delivery and the emerging role of blood biomarkers to potentially fill these knowledge gaps, the early standard of management of patients with suspected TBI in the emergency department is similar across health care systems. Standardized protocols include (1) initial stabilization and resuscitation, (2) acquiring an accurate neurological examination, and (3) neuroimaging to assist with clinical decision-making. Neuroimaging remains an essential component of guiding management in the TBI patient population.

H. Deng · D. O. Okonkwo (✉)
Department of Neurological Surgery, University of Pittsburgh Medical Center, Pittsburgh, PA, USA
e-mail: okonkwodo@upmc.edu

J. K. Yue
Department of Neurological Surgery, University of California, San Francisco, San Francisco, CA, USA

E. Brogi et al. (eds.), *Traumatic Brain Injury*, Hot Topics in Acute Care Surgery and Trauma, https://doi.org/10.1007/978-3-031-50117-3_6

6.2 Computed Tomography as the Workhorse

The introduction of computed tomography (CT) into routine clinical care in the mid 1970s heralded the dawn of modern management of TBI. A head CT scan is now a near-universal imaging modality for the patient who presents with a history of trauma and obvious or suspected TBI. Neuroimaging is pursued after the initial evaluation and stabilization of the trauma patient and rapid clinical assessment of neurologic status, including a Glasgow Coma Scale (GCS) score.

In patients with GCS scores 13–15, the National Emergency X-Radiography Utilization Study II (NEXUS-II), Canadian Head CT Rule, and the New Orleans Criteria are widely used to determine the need for a non-contrast CT of the head [1–3]. In patients with more significant TBI (GCS scores 3–13), a head CT is a class I recommendation according to the American College of Radiology [4]. Because of CT's speed and wide accessibility across medical institutions, it remains the gold standard for localization of traumatic intracranial pathologies that may need emergent neurosurgical intervention (Fig. 6.1). Current technology for brain imaging allows for multi-slice spiral scans of up to 320 slices, although CT sequences between 32 to 64 slices, frequently in 2.5-mm or 5-mm thickness with multiplanar reconstructions in sagittal and coronal reformats, are preferred at most trauma centers.

Head CT is most commonly performed as a non-contrast study to detect fractures, pneumocephalus, herniation, epidural hematoma (EDH), subdural hematoma (SDH), subarachnoid hemorrhage, intraventricular hemorrhage, and parenchymal contusions. The addition of a contrast-enhanced phase is performed for specific

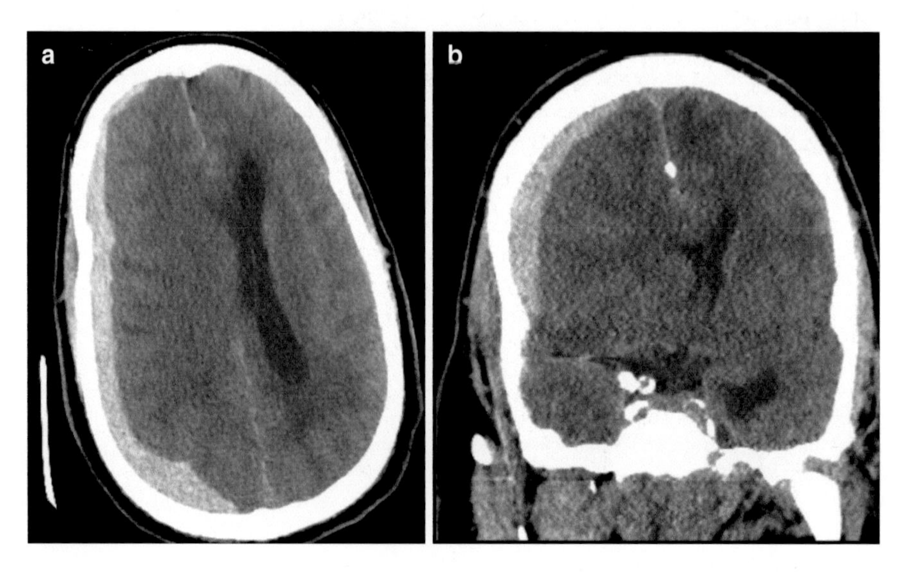

Fig. 6.1 (**a**) Axial noncontrast head CT showing acute right SDH with midline shift. (**b**) Coronal image demonstrating rightward displacement of the uncus with impending herniation

indications. In patients who potentially had contrasted imaging of the chest or abdomen as part of a polytrauma work-up, dual energy CT, also known as spectral CT, can be considered. Dual energy CT uses two separate X-ray photon energy spectra, whereas conventional single energy CT produces a single image set. This allows reconstruction of iodine concentration maps to discern the attenuation properties of blood products, which are at different energy levels from that of iodine contrast. The plasma half-life of intravenously administered iodinated contrast medium is approximately 2–4 h, with nearly 100% clearance from the bloodstream within 24 h.

The advantages of CT over magnetic resonance imaging (MRI) include enhanced detection of calvarial and skull base fractures. Particularly in patients with penetrating TBI and metallic foreign bodies, CT can provide a rapid evaluation without any delay caused by safety screening measures (Fig. 6.2) Patients with a positive initial head CT scan usually undergo neurosurgical evaluation and often receive repeat imaging 4–6 h after the first scan in order to verify stability of the bleed. The Brain Injury Guidelines (BIG) provide an algorithm for triage by stratifying patients based on the size of the traumatic pathology, which is a departure from standard of practice and would need external validation at other institutions and, importantly, understanding of its specificity [5, 6].

After discharge, a repeat head CT is often obtained 4 weeks post-trauma as part of routine follow-up. Different pathophysiological processes appear to dictate the temporal formation of chronic SDH, including radiographic evidence of an evolved acute SDH versus a subdural hygroma on baseline imaging [7] (Fig. 6.3).

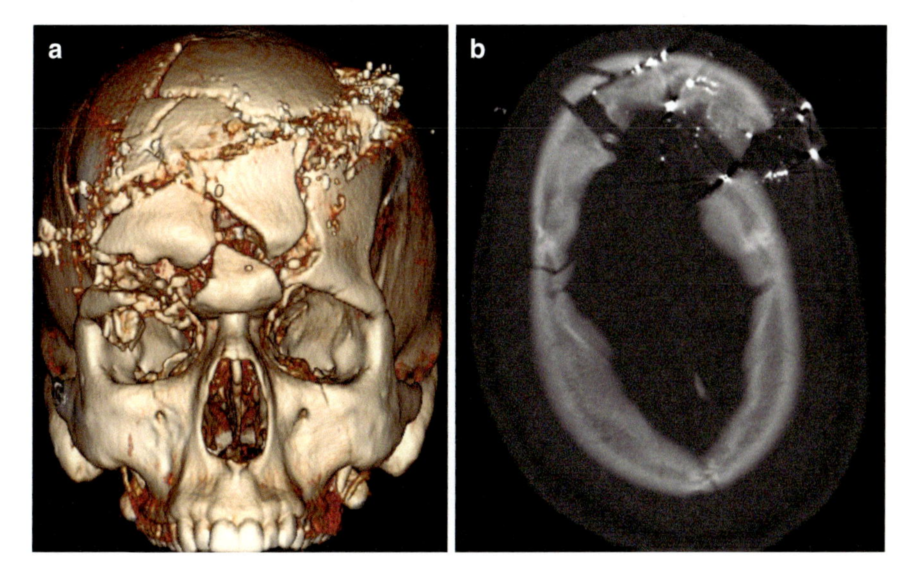

Fig. 6.2 (**a**) Reconstructed head CT showing severe craniofacial injury from gunshot wound. (**b**) Axial view in bone windows revealing multiple comminuted calvarial fractures and bullet fragments

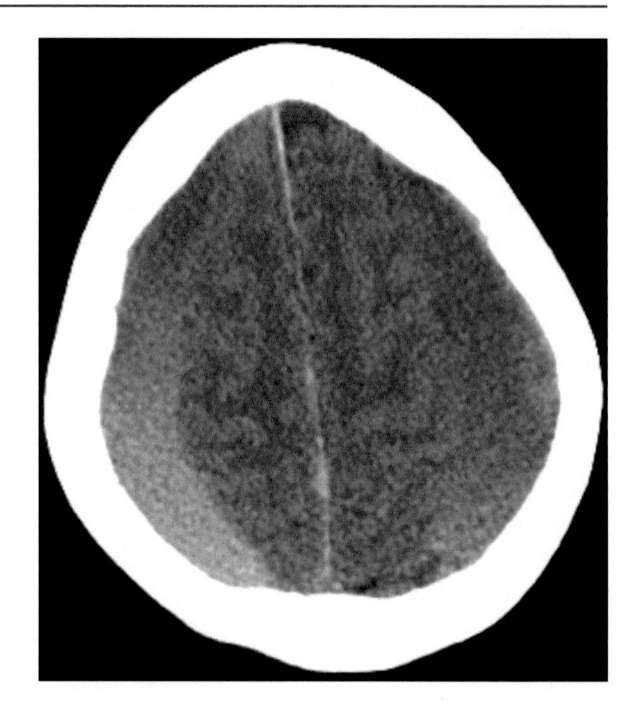

Fig. 6.3 Axial head CT showing bilateral convexity SDHs of mixed densities, with acute components visible more on the right than the left

6.3 CT Angiography and Blunt Cerebrovascular Injury Screening

In patients who have sustained high-velocity trauma, fractures commonly occur in proximity to key vascular structures, potentially necessitating additional work-up. CT can identify fractures that extend through the petrous carotid canal or jugular foramen or cross structures such as the superior sagittal sinus or transverse or sigmoid sinus. On a case-by-case basis, further contrast-enhanced examination with an acquisition delay in the arterial phase for CT angiography (CTA) or the venous phase for CT venography (CTV) can provide accurate depictions of cerebrovascular anatomy and patency (Fig. 6.4). The Denver criteria are widely utilized to identify trauma patients with specific signs, symptoms, or high-energy traumatic injuries that are often associated with blunt cerebrovascular injury and thus may require further evaluation with CTA imaging [8].

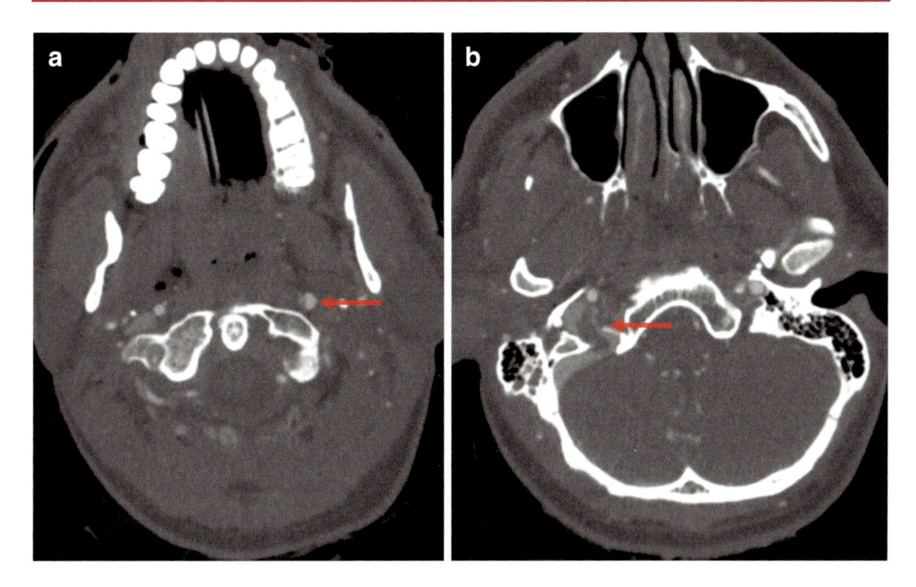

Fig. 6.4 (**a**) Axial view of CTA of the neck showing a cervical internal carotid artery dissection with vessel flap (arrow). (**b**) Axial view of CTV of the brain revealing a nonocclusive thrombus located in the right jugular bulb and extending into the sigmoid sinus (arrow)

6.4 Magnetic Resonance Imaging as an Important Adjunctive Modality

In current diagnostic paradigms, GCS score and CT findings in combination with clinical and laboratory data form the basis of initial TBI diagnosis and management. Magnetic resonance imaging (MRI) has higher sensitivity than CT to detect EDH, SDH, nonhemorrhagic cortical contusions, brainstem injuries, and diffuse axonal injury (DAI), especially as the composition of traumatic blood products changes over time. However, the limitations of MRI include longer imaging time, limited accessibility, higher cost, and the need to screen for metallic foreign objects, particularly in penetrating trauma.

Emerging evidence has highlighted the clinical and prognostic implications of MR findings of TBI, particularly in the setting of a normal head CT. As such, MRI can be an important adjunct for TBI patients with ongoing signs and symptoms despite a normal head CT [9, 10]. In patients with more severe TBI, MRI can be performed in the subacute period within a week of the initial trauma (Fig. 6.5). In the acute period after moderate to severe TBI, the physiologic capacity of the patient to tolerate MRI should be carefully assessed to reduce the risk of worsening secondary brain injury. Multidisciplinary discussion among the neurointensivists, neurosurgeons, and trauma team can establish patient readiness for MRI. Intracranial hypertension, presence of multimodality monitoring—which may not be

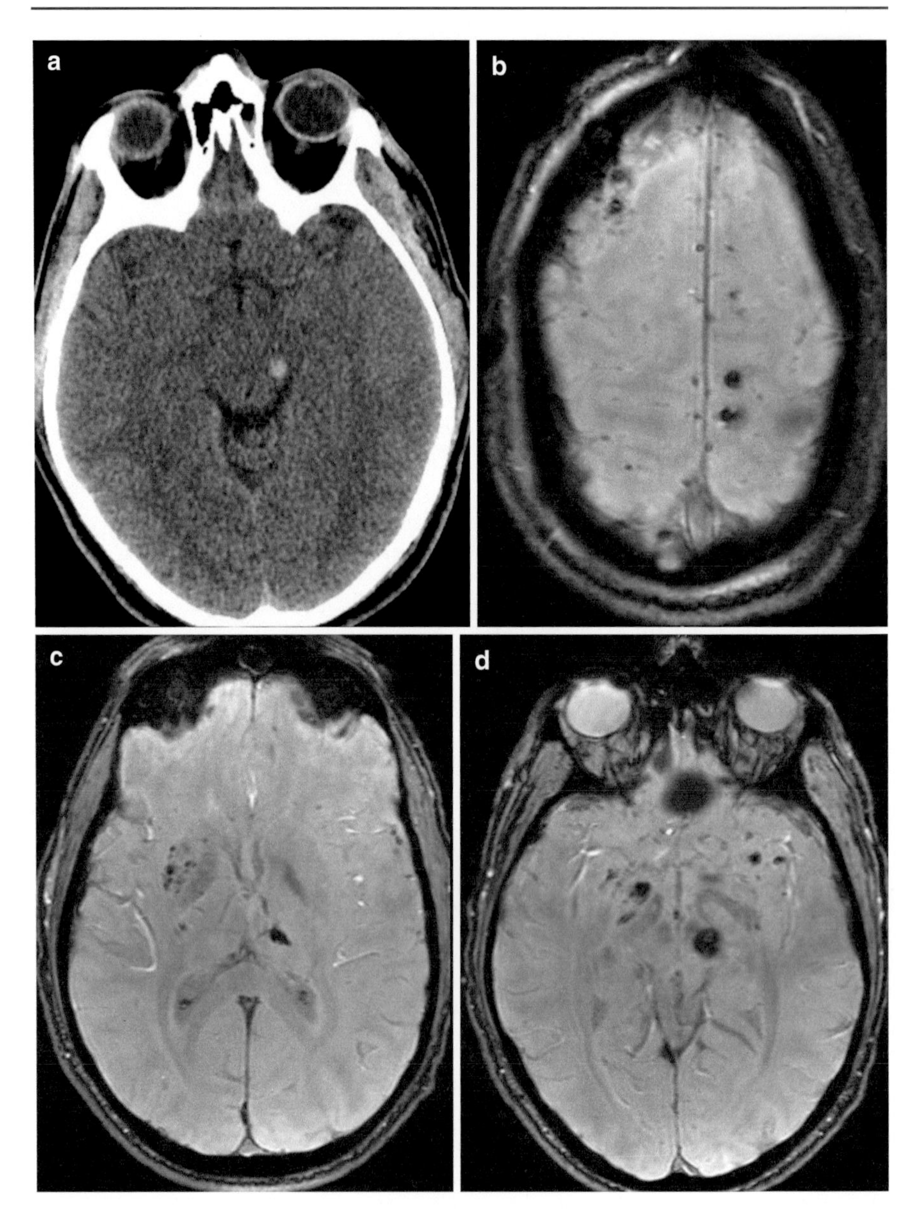

Fig. 6.5 (**a**) Axial head CT head showing punctate hemorrhages in the midbrain concerning for DAI. (**b**) Susceptibility-weighted MRI sequence showing bilateral DAI in grey-white matter junction, as well as (**c**) involving the right lentiform nucleus and internal capsule and (**d**) the left midbrain

MRI-compatible—and signs of hemodynamic or cardiopulmonary instability should be addressed definitively prior to MRI. In patients with resolving intracranial hypertension, laying the patient flat can first be performed by the clinician as a simple bedside evaluation of MRI tolerance, especially while an external ventricular drain (EVD) and/or multimodality monitoring are available to obtain intracranial physiologic data.

Administration of contrast with MRI is not routinely performed in the TBI patient population. The sequences for non-enhanced brain MRI may include T1-weighted and T2-weighted sequences, diffusion-weighted imaging (DWI), susceptibility-weighted imaging (SWI), and fat-suppressed fluid-attenuated inversion-recovery (FLAIR). In terms of detecting intracranial hemorrhage, SWI possesses higher sensitivity than gradient-recalled-echo (GRE) imaging. Similar to CT venography, MRI venography can be helpful in cases where a fracture traverses a dural venous sinus. DWI may be important in the detection of DAI in patients who sustained high-velocity injuries with significant rotational force. Detection of DAI burden can guide prognostication and clinical decision-making in patients with delayed recovery of consciousness [11].

6.5 Advanced Applications of MRI to Aid Prognostication

Diffusion tensor imaging (DTI) quantifies the parameters of water diffusion in brain tissue, and postprocessing techniques allow for the identification of specific axonal tracts and trauma-induced disruptions to their integrity. In the mild TBI patient population, reductions in anisotropy correlating with white matter injury have been linked to functional outcomes at 3 and 6 months post-injury [12]. Due to the considerable heterogeneity in sample characteristics and technical aspects of imaging analysis, larger longitudinal studies using standardized data acquisition techniques and post-processing parameters are still needed for DTI to become a useful tool in TBI care.

MR Spectroscopy (MRS) is commonly utilized to aid in the diagnosis of brain neoplasms and demyelinating diseases, but more recently it has been applied in the setting of TBI. MRS can analyze specific biochemical metabolites in order to differentiate their concentrations in tissue. Common biomarkers include choline, N-acetylaspartate, myo-inositol, glutamate, and lipids [13]. Applications of MRS include evaluating the burden of DAI-associated microhemorrhages. It may also have the potential to correlate metabolic biomarkers with neurological outcomes, although such findings remain exploratory in nature and in need of normative data prior to clinical adoption.

6.6 Special Neuroimaging Modalities

Traumatic brain injury can be exacerbated by secondary injuries, particularly cerebral ischemia, which cannot be readily detected using conventional CT. A specialized version of contrast-enhanced study, CT perfusion scanning, can identify regional changes in cerebral blood flow after neurotrauma. CT perfusion studies are commonly used in patients with acute stroke, aneurysmal subarachnoid hemorrhage, and other cerebrovascular disorders. These studies obtain dynamic sequential CT slices with cine mode following intravenous administration of a 40-mL dose of nonionic iodinated contrast material. They provide quantitative assessment of brain perfusion within 5 min of postprocessing. Perfusion CT data can provide prognostic information regarding functional outcomes after TBI. Findings of normal brain perfusion or hyperemia can be associated with favorable recovery, whereas oligemia can be suggestive of unfavorable outcomes due to prolonged loss of autoregulation and intracranial hypertension after severe TBI [14].

Advanced applications in nuclear medicine imaging can now reliably reveal metabolic and functional alterations in specific regions of the injured brain, which may have additional prognostic value as part of creating an individualized recovery trajectory and rehabilitative plan. Single Photon Emission Computed Tomography (SPECT) provides quantitative analysis of cerebral blood flow, with technetium-labeled hexamethylpropyleneamine oxide (99Tc-HMPAO) being the most commonly used tracer. Particularly in patients with mild TBI and persistent neurological or psychiatric symptoms, SPECT is able to provide lesion localization that is not detectable on CT or MRI [15].

6.7 Considerations in Penetrating Traumatic Brain Injury

Penetrating cerebrovascular injury (PCVI) may result in such vascular pathologies as traumatic pseudoaneurysms, direct arterial injury, venous sinus stenosis or occlusion, and dural arteriovenous fistulas. These conditions are associated with high risks of secondary injury and require close vascular follow-up, which can be conducted with neuroimaging modalities like CTA and digital subtraction angiography (DSA). The diagnostic yield of CTA appears to be better in cervical spine injuries associated with penetrating neck trauma than in the diagnosis of penetrating intracranial arterial injuries [16, 17]. Once patients have been stabilized from their acute injuries, DSA should be considered in patients with penetrating neurotrauma, particularly when there is a possibility that urgent endovascular management and therapeutic intervention may be needed (Fig. 6.6).

Vasospasm following TBI may dramatically affect neurological outcomes. It can occur in a delayed manner with or without initial CT findings of traumatic subarachnoid hemorrhage. Serial transcranial Doppler ultrasonography protocols have been employed for vasospasm surveillance. If concern arises for clinical vasospasm requiring prompt treatment, CTA of the neck and head can be rapidly obtained. Subsequently, DSA could be performed for real-time detection and treatment of suspected vasospasm.

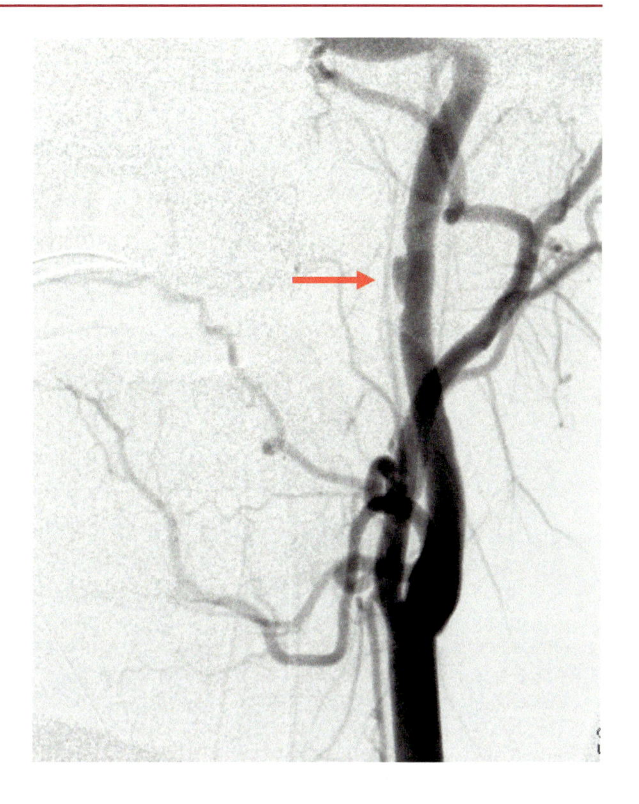

Fig. 6.6 Selective DSA of the left common carotid artery showing a dissection of the cervical segment of the internal carotid artery and an associated traumatic pseudoaneurysm (arrow)

6.8 On the Horizon: Non-invasive Modalities for Neuroimaging (NIRS)

Instead of gamma-emitting radioisotope tracers, positron emission tomography (PET) imaging uses [18F]fluorodeoxyglucose (FDG), a positron-emitting isotope attached to deoxyglucose that accumulates in brain tissue in proportion to glucose uptake and phosphorylation. FDG-PET has the capability to measure alterations in cerebral glucose metabolism after TBI [14]. Brain injury can be followed by a period of sustained hypometabolism that may be identified through decreased FDG uptake, which can last for days to months and be associated with cellular and functional alterations. Although clinical studies performed to date have generally been underpowered, there seem to be emerging patterns of metabolic changes that are reflective of secondary pathophysiology. These include an apparent increase in glucose utilization after TBI, followed by sustained hypometabolism during the subacute and chronic phases post-injury in specific regions of the brain in the frontal and temporal lobes [18]. The cost and difficulty of PET scanning have so far limited its use in the TBI population.

References

1. Haydel MJ, Preston CA, Mills TJ, Luber S, Blaudeau E, DeBlieux PM. Indications for computed tomography in patients with minor head injury. N Engl J Med. 2000;343(2):100–5.
2. Stiell IG, Wells GA, Vandemheen K, et al. The Canadian CT head rule for patients with minor head injury. Lancet. 2001;357(9266):1391–6.
3. Mower WR, Hoffman JR, Herbert M, et al. Developing a decision instrument to guide computed tomographic imaging of blunt head injury patients. J Trauma. 2005;59(4):954–9.
4. Wintermark M, Sanelli PC, Anzai Y, et al. Imaging evidence and recommendations for traumatic brain injury: conventional neuroimaging techniques. J Am Coll Radiol. 2015;12(2):e1–e14.
5. Khan AD, Elseth AJ, Brosius JA, et al. Multicenter assessment of the brain injury guidelines and a proposal of guideline modifications. Trauma Surg Acute Care Open. 2020;5(1):e000483.
6. Joseph B, Obaid O, Dultz L, et al. Validating the brain injury guidelines: results of an American Association for the Surgery of Trauma prospective multi-institutional trial. J Trauma Acute Care Surg. 2022;93(2):157–65.
7. Edlmann E, Whitfield PC, Kolias A, Hutchinson PJ. Pathogenesis of chronic subdural hematoma: a cohort evidencing de novo and transformational origins. J Neurotrauma. 2021;38(18):2580–9.
8. Biffl WL, Moore EE, Offner PJ, et al. Optimizing screening for blunt cerebrovascular injuries. Am J Surg. 1999;178(6):517–22.
9. Yue JK, Yuh EL, Korley FK, et al. Association between plasma GFAP concentrations and MRI abnormalities in patients with CT-negative traumatic brain injury in the TRACK-TBI cohort: a prospective multicentre study. Lancet Neurol. 2019;18(10):953–61.
10. Schweitzer AD, Niogi SN, Whitlow CT, Tsiouris AJ. Traumatic brain injury: imaging patterns and complications. Radiographics. 2019;39(6):1571–95.
11. Deng H, Nwachuku EL, Wilkins TE, et al. Time to follow commands in severe traumatic brain injury survivors with favorable recovery at 2 years. Neurosurgery. 2022;91(4):633–40.
12. Yuh EL, Cooper SR, Mukherjee P, et al. Diffusion tensor imaging for outcome prediction in mild traumatic brain injury: a TRACK-TBI study. J Neurotrauma. 2014;31(17):1457–77.
13. Marino S, Ciurleo R, Bramanti P, Federico A, De Stefano N. 1H-MR spectroscopy in traumatic brain injury. Neurocrit Care. 2011;14(1):127–33.
14. Wintermark M, van Melle G, Schnyder P, et al. Admission perfusion CT: prognostic value in patients with severe head trauma. Radiology. 2004;232(1):211–20.
15. Raji CA, Tarzwell R, Pavel D, et al. Clinical utility of SPECT neuroimaging in the diagnosis and treatment of traumatic brain injury: a systematic review. PLoS One. 2014;9(3):e91088.
16. Ares WJ, Jankowitz BT, Tonetti DA, Gross BA, Grandhi R. A comparison of digital subtraction angiography and computed tomography angiography for the diagnosis of penetrating cerebrovascular injury. Neurosurg Focus. 2019;47(5):E16.
17. Hawryluk GWJ, Selph S, Lumba-Brown A, et al. Rationale and methods for updated guidelines for the management of penetrating traumatic brain injury. Neurotrauma Rep. 2022;3(1):240–7.
18. Byrnes KR, Wilson CM, Brabazon F, et al. FDG-PET imaging in mild traumatic brain injury: a critical review. Front Neuroenerg. 2014;5:13.

7 Interactions Between Volumes, Flows and Pressures in the Brain: Intracranial Pressure, Cerebral Perfusion Pressure, Cerebral Autoregulation and the Concept of Compensatory Reserve

Agnieszka Zakrzewska, Adam Pelah, and Marek Czosnyka

Primary brain injury occurs as an immediate result of a trauma insult. Secondary brain injury develops in the following hours or days, as a cascade of pathophysiological events subsequent to the primary injury [1]. While the extent of the initial injury to the brain is beyond the medical approach, the secondary injury has become a target for modern diagnostic and treatment procedures in severely head-injured patients. Nonetheless the Marshall computed tomography classification grade, whether a patient undergoes a preceding head surgery or is directly admitted to the intensive care settings, all therapeutical means are aimed at preventing progress of the secondary brain injury. Thus, a real-time registration of physiological parameters which reflect functioning and metabolism of the brain is an asset in neurocritical care.

Extracranial physiological factors which may induce expansion of the secondary damage of the brain are hypoxia, hypotension, hyper- or hypocarbia, hyper- or hypoglycaemia, hyperthermia, hyponatremia, anaemia, disturbed viscosity or coagulation disorders. Intracranial factors may include intracranial hypertension, decrease in cerebral perfusion pressure, ischemia, vasospasm, seizures, spreading depolarisations, oedema, or brain herniation.

A. Zakrzewska · A. Pelah · M. Czosnyka (✉)
Brain Physics Laboratory, Division of Neurosurgery, Department of Clinical Neurosciences, Cambridge University Hospitals, Cambridge, UK
e-mail: apz21@cam.ac.uk; ap2238@cam.ac.uk; mc141@medschl.cam.ac.uk

E. Brogi et al. (eds.), *Traumatic Brain Injury*, Hot Topics in Acute Care Surgery and Trauma, https://doi.org/10.1007/978-3-031-50117-3_7

7.1 Intracranial Pressure

Historically, intracranial pressure (ICP) is defined as a pressure exerted against a needle introduced into the cerebrospinal fluid (CSF) space in order to prevent the fluid escape.

Although intraparenchymal sensors are most commonly used to measure ICP, measurement of the CSF pressure via intraventricular catheter and external ventricular drainage system remains a golden standard of ICP monitoring.

The thresholds of normal ICP are not precisely defined and depend on age or body position and vary between individuals. The normal ICP range in adults and youth is below 10–15 mmHg [2]. It ranges from 3 to 7 mmHg in young children, from 1 to 6 mmHg in term infants, and can be negative in newborns or in adults and children in the vertical position [3–5].

ICP monitoring is recommended for all salvageable patients after TBI with post-resuscitation Glasgow Coma Scale (GCS) score between 3 and 8, and an abnormal CT scan, and for those with a normal CT scan after severe TBI who meet 2 or more of the following criteria: age above 40 years, uni- or bilateral motor posturing, or systolic blood pressure below 90 mmHg [6].

ICP above 22 mmHg is associated with elevated mortality following head injury and is a target for clinical management [6, 7]. Intracranial hypertension following TBI may be caused by mass lesion, oedema, vasodilation, hyperaemia, reduced venous outflow or acute hydrocephalus.

7.1.1 Intracranial Compliance and Compensatory Reserve

The Monroe-Kellie doctrine describes relationships between volumes and pressures in the intracranial space. The hypothesis states that the total volume of the intracranial compartment is constant. In normal conditions, the brain and the interstitial fluid constitute about 75% of the cranial volume, while blood and cerebrospinal fluid (CSF) constitute approximately 12% of the volume each. According to the doctrine, the increase in volume of one of these constituents induces a decrease in volume of another [8, 9]. Different components of the volume produce different components of the pressure. Volume exchange can induce changes in pressure. Mechanisms of increase of the intracranial volume include increase in CSF, increase in cerebral blood volume (CBV), vasogenic, neurotoxic and ischemic oedema [10] (Figs. 7.1 and 7.3c).

The ability of the intracranial compartment to accommodate an increase in volume without a significant increase in pressure is determined by the intracranial compliance (ICC). It was tested in the past by a manoeuvre of injecting an additional fluid in the CSF compartment. ICC can be expressed as change in volume per change in pressure, ICC = $\Delta V/\Delta P$ (ΔV—change in volume, ΔP—change in pressure). However, due to the non-linear exponential shape of the pressure volume

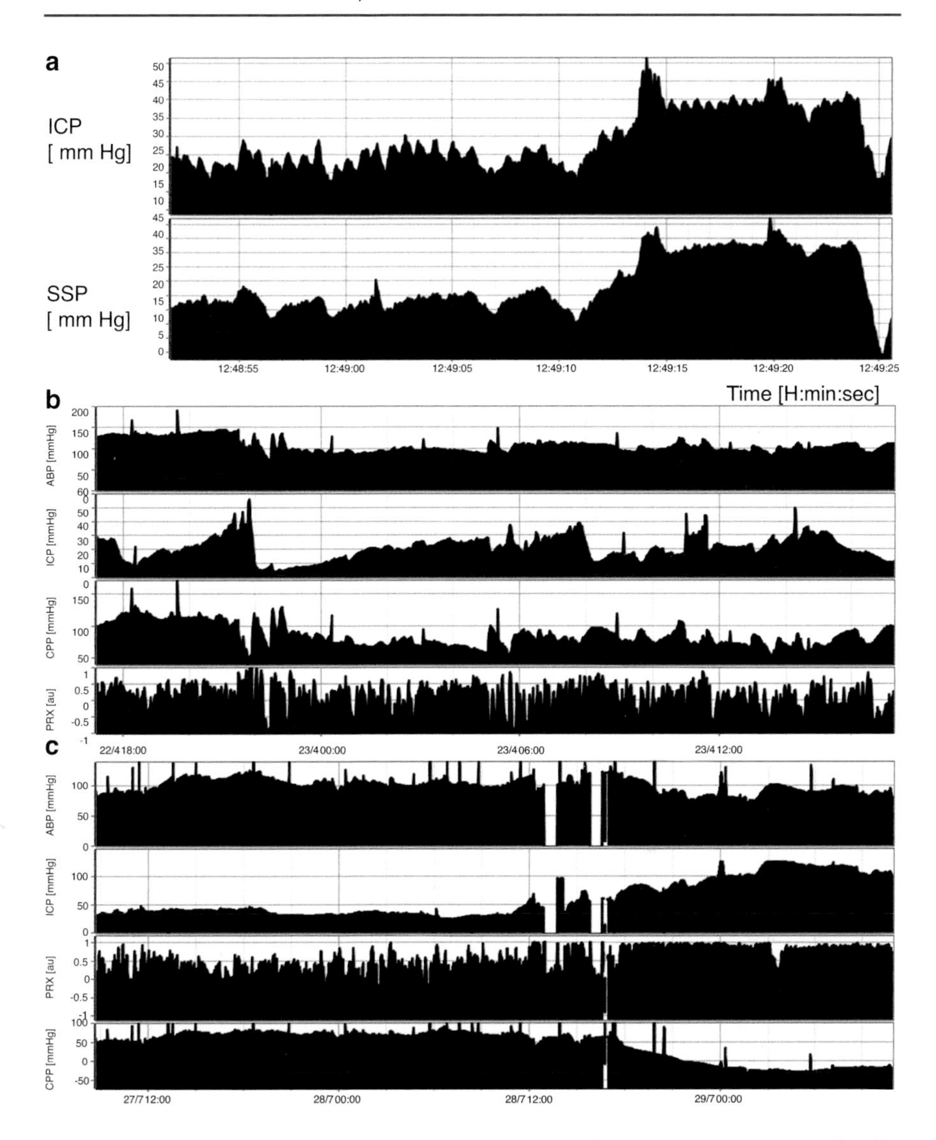

Fig. 7.1 Examples of ICP waveforms reflecting changes of different volume components listed in Monro-Kellie doctrine. *ABP* arterial blood pressure, *ICP* intracranial pressure, *CPP* cerebral perfusion pressure, *PRx* pressure reactivity index, *SSP* sagittal sinus pressure. (**a**) ICP and direct sagittal sinus pressure (SSP) monitored in patient with idiopathic intracranial hypertension during brief neck compression (Queckenstedt test). Obstruction of venous outflow produces immediate increase in ICP. (**b**) One of mechanisms of increase of the intracranial volume is an augmentation of CSF volume. An example of unstable ICP in patient after TBI (15 h after admission) with computed tomography picture consistent with acute hydrocephalus. (**c**) Gradual rise in ICP (over 2 days) leading to decrease in CPP virtually to 0 mmHg. This is accompanied by deterioration in PRx. Nature of refractory intracranial hypertension is often related to fast advancing brain oedema

curve, compliance is dependent on ICP and decreases when ICP increases. A measure of compliance invariant on ICP is described by the pressure-volume index (PVI), where PVI = $\Delta V/\log Pi/Po$ (ΔV—change in volume, *Po*—initial pressure, *Pi*—pressure increased by a volume change) [11]. The opposite ratio of pressure change to volume change defines the elastance index [12]. The volume-pressure response (VPR) is a measure of the intracranial elastance [13, 14].

The intracranial pressure interferes with the cerebral compliance. When an extra volume is introduced into the cranial cavity, the ICP initially rises linearly, independently of the cerebral compliance, until the lower breakpoint (Fig. 7.2). This is the phase of a good compensatory reserve. Further addition of volume, above the lower

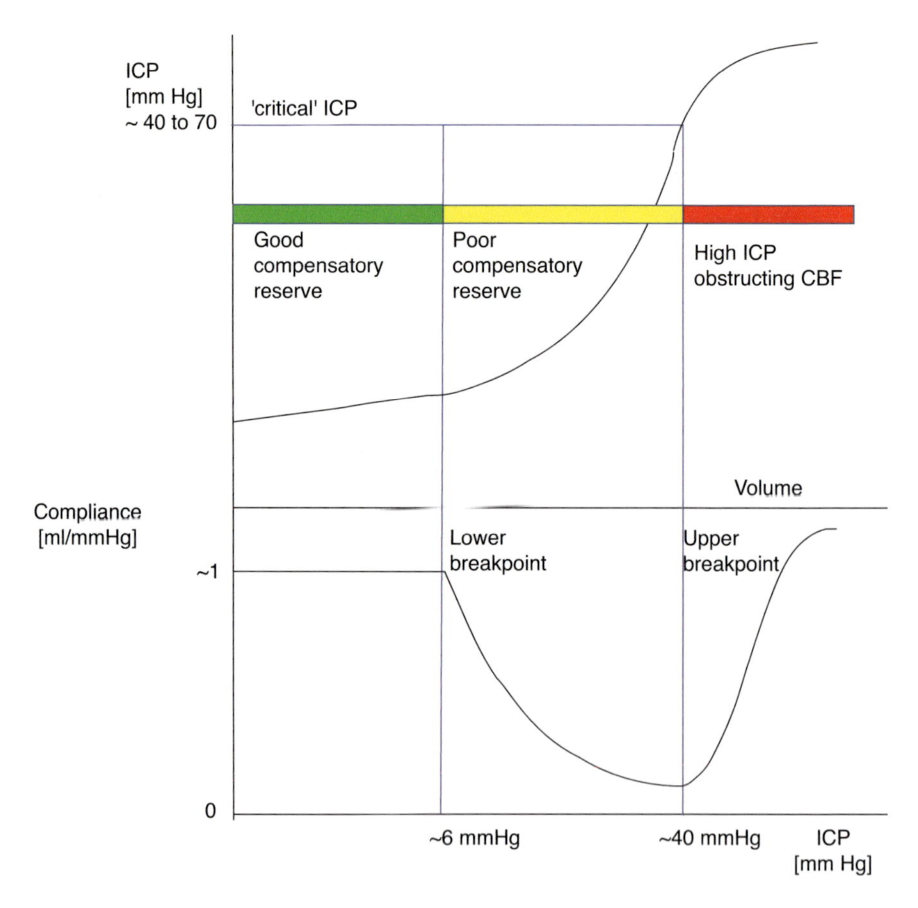

Fig. 7.2 General shape of the pressure-volume curve (upper panel) and related brain compliance (lower panel). There are three distinct zones. ICP first increases linearly with extra volume-zone of good compensatory reserve. Upon further volume load, the curve becomes exponential, indicating poor compensatory reserve. Past this zone, with further volume load, ICP is critically high, leading to arterial bed compression, decreased blood flow, and a high risk of brain ischaemia

breakpoint, is reflected in the exponential rise in ICP and decline of the compliance. This is the phase of a poor compensatory reserve. When the ICP values become very high, above the critical, upper breakpoint, the pressure-volume curve deflects to the right and the compliance increases. In this phase the compression of the arterial bed starts, blood flow through the brain decreases with a high risk of developing ischemia. The breakpoints are individual and may be affected by the cerebral perfusion pressure, partial pressure of carbon dioxide (PaCO2) or anaesthetic drugs and the level of sedation [15, 16].

7.1.2 Intracranial Pressure Transients and Waveform

The normal ICP waveform is composed of repetitive waves related to rapid changes in arterial blood pressure (ABP) (pulse waveform), superimposed on slower respiratory waves. Other cyclic, more or less pathological, waves are slow vasogenic waves that were described by Lundberg as B and C waves [17].

Non-repetitive transients of changing ICP in various pathophysiological conditions may present various patterns: low and stable, elevated and stable, A (plateau) waves, waves related to increase in cerebral blood flow (CBF), refractory intracranial hypertension, etc. [18]. Figure 7.3 presents some examples of various ICP waveforms.

Plateau waves are a particular type of waves characterised by ICP elevation above 40 mmHg, with ICP increase of greater than or equal to 15 mmHg and cerebral perfusion pressure (CPP) decreases of greater than or equal to 10 mmHg [19]. A waves may reflect increase in arterial CBV (Fig. 7.3c). They last approximately 15–20 min, usually resolve spontaneously and are accompanied by decrease in CBF and partial pressure of brain tissue oxygen (PtO_2) [20].

A special subtype of the vasogenic waveform components are slow waves, classified historically by Lundberg as B waves [21]. All components of periodicity from 20 s to 3 min can be classified as slow waves. The power of slow waves is thought to be an independent predictor of outcome from TBI. The low magnitude of slow waves correlates with fatal outcome [7, 18, 22]. Slow waves, due to their peculiar frequency, carry information about cerebrovascular reactivity.

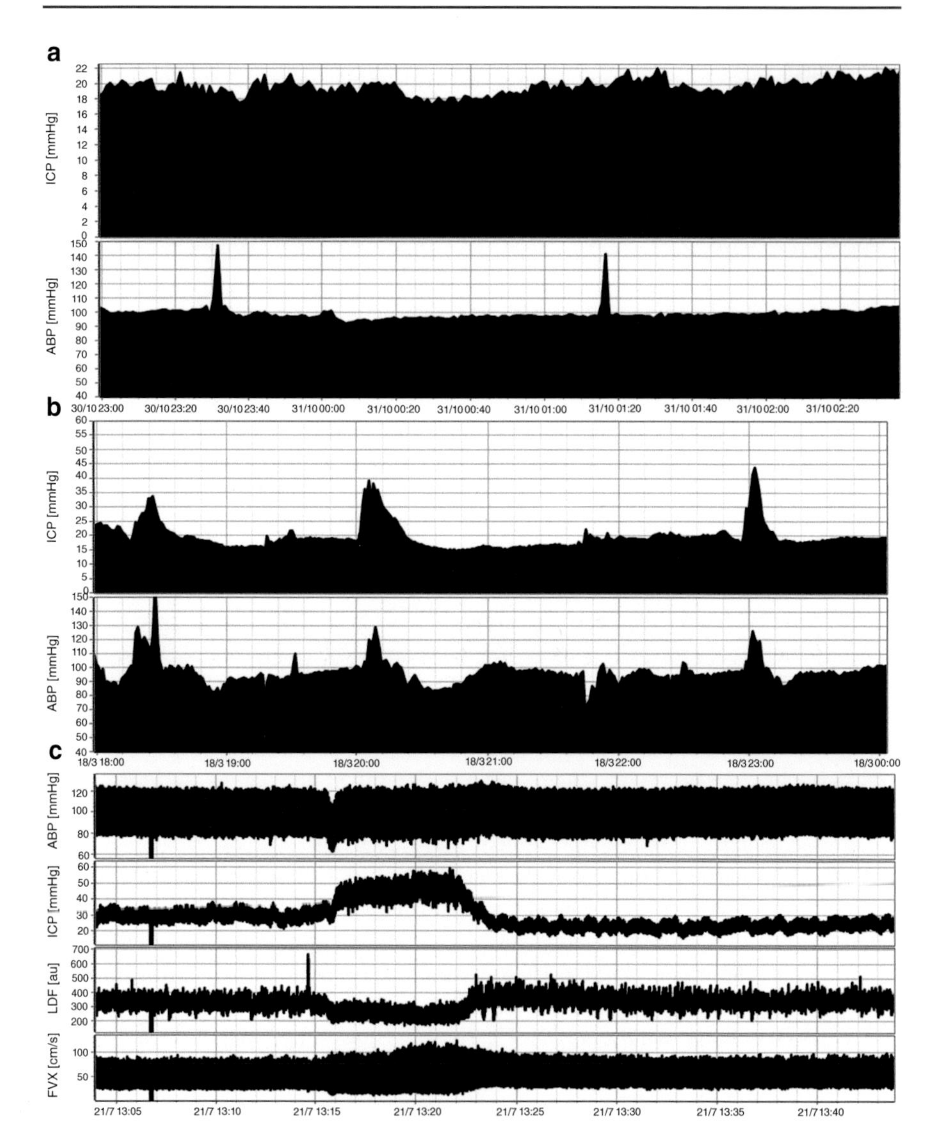

Fig. 7.3 Examples of selected patterns of ICP waveform. *ABP* - arterial blood pressure, *ICP* intracranial pressure, *CPP* cerebral perfusion pressure, *LDF* laser doppler flowmetry, *FVx* maximal blood flow velocity in MCA, *CBF* cerebral blood flow, *CBV* cerebral blood volume, *CBFV* cerebral blood flow velocity. (**a**) Stable and moderately increased ICP (mean 20 mmHg). (**b**) Changes in ICP caused by spike-like increases in blood pressure (ABP). If variations of ABP are fast and deep, no matter what the state of cerebrovascular reactivity is, ICP follows changes in ABP. (**c**) Plateau wave of ICP—an example of active rise in arterial blood volume. Cortical blood flow was monitored using LDF. FVx was monitored using Transcranial Doppler. During plateau waves CBF decreases as a consequence of decrease in CPP. (**d**) 'Metabolic' waves of ICP. They are caused by increase in CBV, associated with an increase in CBF. CBF was monitored using transcranial doppler. (**e**) B waves of ICP. The same direction of changes of ICP and blood flow velocity which is similar to 'metabolic waves' (Figure (**d**)), but B waves are much faster (20 s to 3 min period). They carry information about autoregulation of CBF

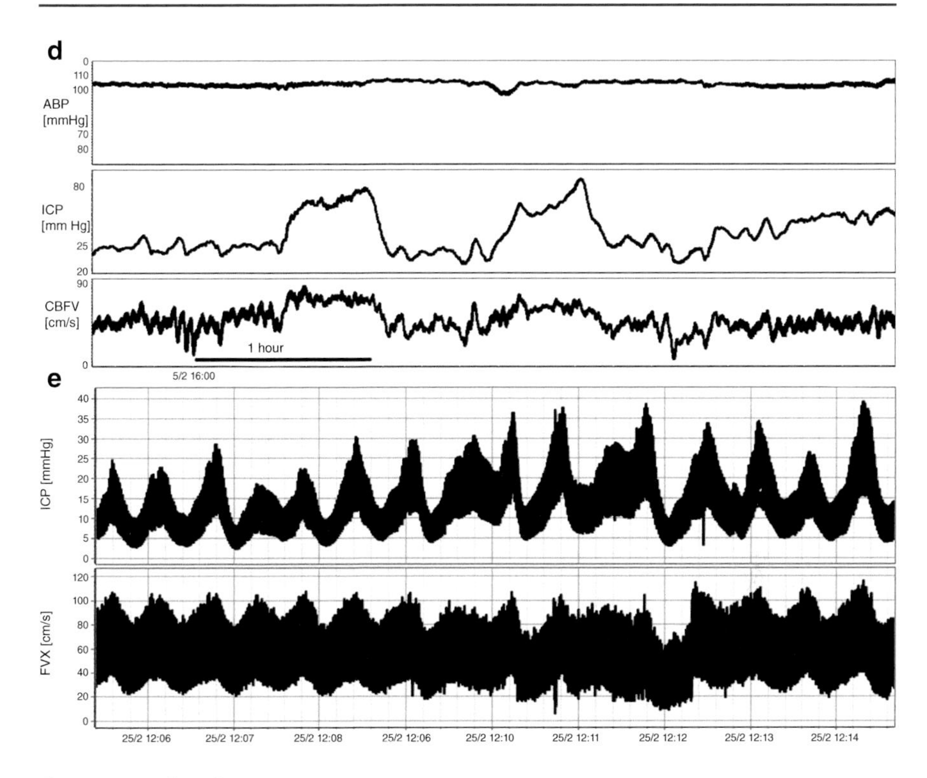

Fig. 7.3 (continued)

7.1.3 Intracranial Pressure Pulse Waveform

Visual inspection of intracranial pressure pulse waveform usually reveals three peaks: P1—percussion wave, P2—tidal wave, P3—dicrotic wave (Fig. 7.4). Morphology of ICP waveform is important because P1/P2 relation indirectly describes brain compliance. In normal physiological conditions P1 exceeds P2 and P2 exceeds P3, indicating good intracranial compliance [23].

An increase in ICP (an exception is an increase caused by obstruction of venous outflow) is accompanied by a change of shape of its waveform, with a disproportionate rise in the P2 and P3 peaks and depletion of the intracranial compliance (Fig. 7.4). Detection of these changes in pulse wave's shape can be of clinical significance above the ICP value itself. Intracranial compliance is considered to be an earlier and more sensitive indicator of life-threatening intracranial hypertension leading to rapid neurological deterioration [24].

The ICP pulse waveform has several harmonic components, of which the fundamental component (1st harmonic) has a frequency equal to the heart rate. Apart from classification of the pulse waveform based on visual inspection, it is possible to calculate its derivatives while recording the ICP signal at the bedside.

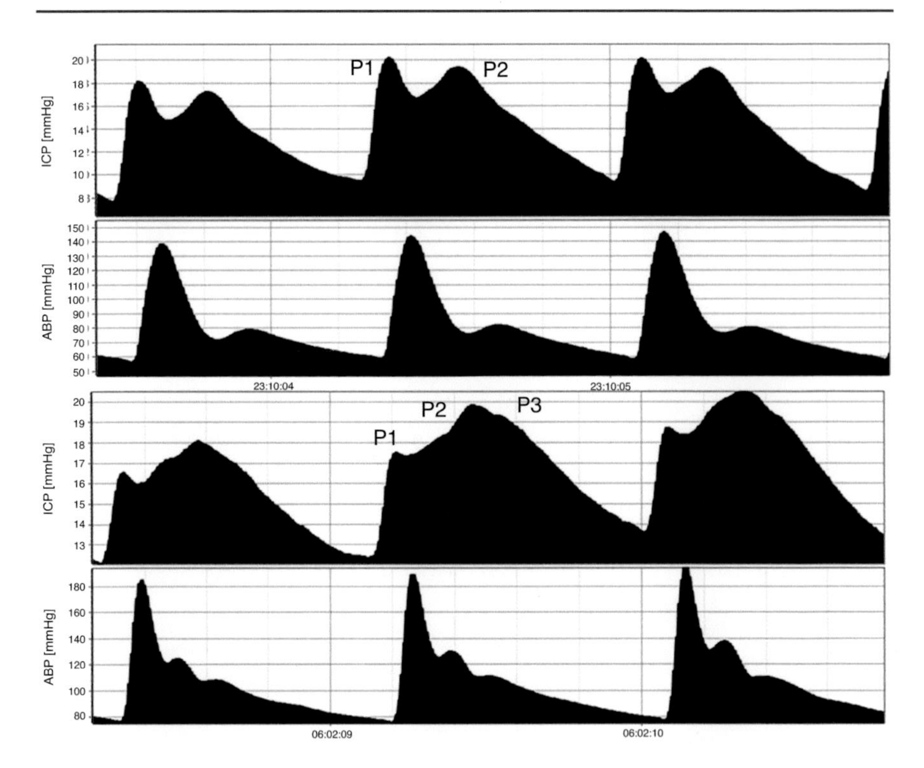

Fig. 7.4 Illustrations of P1/P2 in patient with intracranial hypertension who eventually died due to brain stem herniation. Upper graph shows early recording with good compliance, P1 > P2; P3 is invisible. Lower graph demonstrates deteriorating compliance (closer to event of terminal rise in ICP), P1< P2 and P3 (hardly visible on trailing edge of dominant P2). Note that the level of mean ICP in both cases were similar

One useful index is the high frequency centroid (HFC), a power-weighted average frequency within 4–15 Hz band of the ICP power density spectrum [25].

Another modality in the analysis of the ICP waveform is the higher harmonics centroid (HHC). The HHC can be defined as the centre of mass of ICP waveform harmonics from 2nd to 10th expressed as consecutive integers, where mass corresponds to amplitude of these harmonics [19].

The HFC and HHC correlate well with ICP, and they decrease during slow but deep rises in ICP. Their decline can be a warning sign of escalating intracranial hypertension. The advantage of ICP monitoring supplemented by this computerised analysis is rapid and continuous detection, as well as independence of zero drift which often affects ICP recordings [19] (Fig. 7.5).

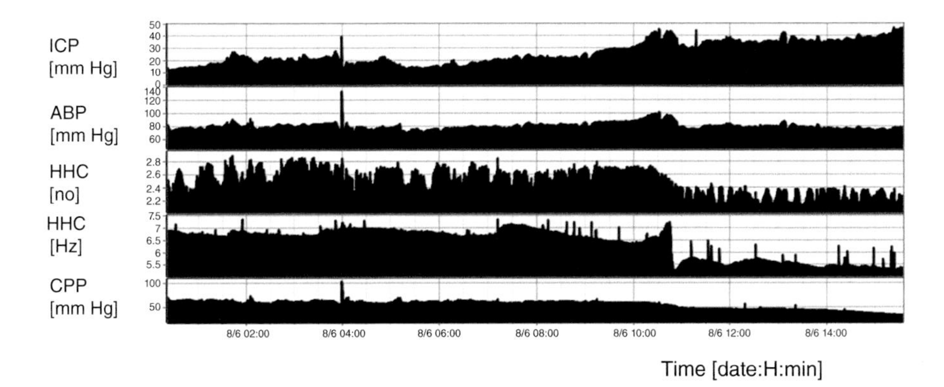

Fig. 7.5 Example of decrease in higher harmonic centroid (HHC) and higher frequency centroid (HFC) of intracranial pressure pulse waveform in patient with gradual increase in ICP

7.2 Cerebral Metabolism and Autoregulation of Cerebral Blood Flow

The brain depends on the supply of oxygen and glucose. Disturbances of both the delivery and the turnover of substrates can play role in the progress of the secondary brain injury. Thus, a physiological entity which is crucial for brain function is cerebral blood flow (CBF), which is regulated by the brain in order to maintain an adequate supply of substrates. CBF depends on the cerebral metabolic rate of oxygen ($CMRO_2$) mainly and the cerebral metabolic rate of glucose (CMRG), so on increasing or decreasing metabolic demands. A normal $CMRO_2$ value in adults is approximately 3.3 mg/100 g/1 min and the CMRG is 5.5 mg/100 g/1 min [26, 27].

As the brain metabolism is mainly aerobic, the $CMRO_2$ is considered its measure. The Fick equation relates cerebral blood flow with metabolism: $CMRO_2 = CBF \times AVDO_2$ (arteriovenous difference of oxygen) [28]. $AVDO_2$ is obtained from the difference between arterial and jugular blood content [29, 30]. It is maintained relatively constant by the brain while regional CBF changes to meet the augmented or reduced metabolic demand.

Normal mixed sub- and cortical CBF ranges within 55–60 ml/100 g/min. CBF greater than 60 ml/100 g/min is a stage of hyperaemia when CBF exceeds cerebral metabolic demand. Cerebral ischemia is a state when CBF is insufficient to match the metabolic demands of the brain. It is one of the mechanisms of the expansion of the secondary brain injury after head trauma, when the brain becomes more vulnerable. 18 ml/100 g/min is considered a critical threshold of CBF [31]. The brain initially buffers decreasing CBF to prevent ischemia by increasing oxygen extraction from the blood. Further decline in CBF results in reduction of the synaptic activity of neurons. A prolonged, critical decrease of CBF below 10 ml/100 g/min causes alternations in active transport through the membrane, cell swelling and eventually cell death.

Cerebral autoregulation is the ability to control CBF by adjustment in vessel calibre [32]. CBF can rise as a result of vasodilation and decrease as a result of vasoconstriction of arterial vasculature. It is regulated by a few different physiological mechanisms, including neurogenic, metabolic, myogenic or chemical, of which myogenic pressure autoregulation is the most referred to type in scientific papers. The vascular endothelium has been also reported as a key mediator in these processes. However, not all mechanisms are well studied, thus the whole picture of interactions, how the regional CBF is coupled with the regional functional activity, metabolism, perfusion pressure or blood viscosity, is not entirely clear.

7.2.1 Cerebral Perfusion Pressure

It is challenging to count CBF in the clinical settings and complicated to monitor it in continuous, real-time mode. However, CBF is associated with CPP, which can be measured in critical care setting based on the ICP monitoring. CPP can be quantitated as the difference between mean arterial pressure (MAP) and ICP, as CPP = MAP − ICP. MAP is assumed to be the mean carotid pressure (MCP) in fact, with the transducer zeroing at the level of the foramen of Monroe [33, 34].

7.2.2 Pressure Autoregulation

Pressure autoregulation is an ability of changing the vessels tone, namely cerebrovascular resistance (CVR) in response to changes in CPP, in order to maintain the CBF relatively stable. The diameter of venules remains constant in general. Arterioles of a diameter from 30 to 300 μm are considered cerebral resistance vessels which ensure this autoregulation of the blood flow [32, 35]. The CVR can be expressed as CVR = CPP/CBF [36]. The pressure autoregulation is the most quoted type of cerebral autoregulation.

Autoregulation is impaired outside its limits of CPP, below 40 mmHg and above 150 mmHg in normal condition. These limits can be altered following severe brain injury. Below the lower limit of autoregulation, after maximal dilation, the diameter of cerebral arterioles starts to passively decrease with declining CPP, resulting in critical decrease in CBF. This gradual decrease is further accelerated by closing of cerebral arterioles caused by critical closing phenomenon, on average at CPP around 20 mmHg. Above the upper limit of autoregulation, when cerebral arterioles cannot constrict further, their diameter starts to passively augment, resulting in increase in CBF [37] (Fig. 7.6).

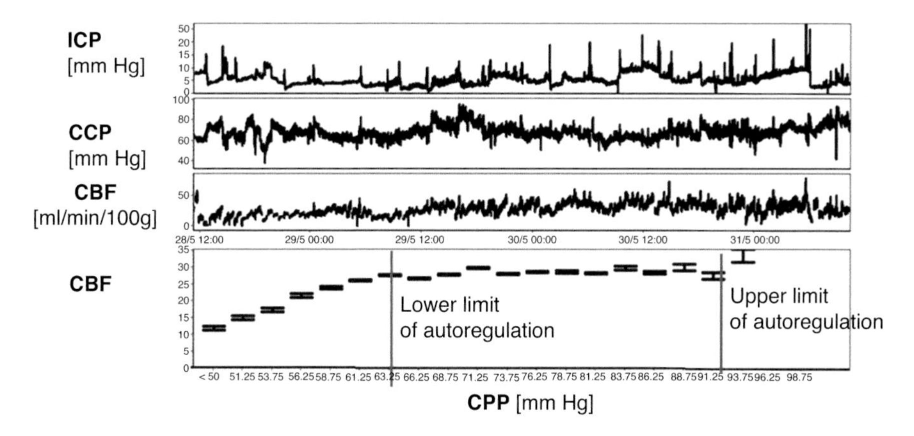

Fig. 7.6 Pressure autoregulation CBF/CPP curve, known as Lassen curve. 4-day recording of intracranial pressure (ICP) and cerebral blood flow (CBF), via a thermal dilution probe, shows good CBF autoregulation range between its lower (~60 mmHg) and upper (~92 mmHg) limits

7.2.3 Blood Viscosity and Cerebral Blood Flow Coupling

CBF also depends on the viscosity of the blood. Blood viscosity is determined by the haematocrit, mechanical properties of red blood cells, as well as plasma proteins.

The relationship between blood flow and perfusion pressure, radius and length of vessel, and blood viscosity can be described according to the Poiseuille's law of fluid dynamics. Poiseuille's equation for the cerebral circulation can be expressed as follows: $CBF = k\ (CPPd^4)/8lv$, where k is constant, d is a diameter of a vessel, l is length of a vessel and v is viscosity. Based on the above equation, $CVR = 8lv/d^4$, thus greater viscosity generates greater vascular resistance. CBF is kept relatively constant thanks to its coupling with the viscosity, which involves the mechanism of adjusting the vessel diameter. With augmenting viscosity, the vessel diameter increases reducing CVR and maintaining CBF unchanged [28].

7.2.4 Cerebral Blood Volume

While CBF is determined by CPP, vascular diameter and blood viscosity, the diameter of the vascular bed is the only determinator of the CBV. Decrease in the diameter of the vasculature causes decrease in CBV and vice versa. CBV has a major influence on ICP.

CBV can be defined by the product: CBV = CB F MTT, where MTT is a mean transit time of the blood through cerebral blood vessels. Most of CBV is contained within vessels of diameter between 30 and 300 μm [28]. CBV accounts for 130–150 ml approximately but can be actively regulated by vasomotor processes.

7.2.5 Carbon Dioxide Reactivity

CBF and CBV are also dependent on fluctuations of the partial pressure of the carbon dioxide in arterial blood ($PaCO_2$). An increase or decrease of $PaCO_2$ by 1 mmHg induces a 2–3% increase or decrease in CBF. Unlike the autoregulation response where $AVDO_2$ is maintained relatively constant, CO_2 reactivity generates changes in $AVDO_2$ in order to compensate for variations in CBF [28].

Hypoventilation and elevated $PaCO_2$ causes vasodilation and a rise in CBF and ICP which in turn reduces CPP. Vice versa, hyperventilation diminishes CBF and ICP via vasoconstriction. Therefore, both sequelae that follow hypercarbia and hypocarbia can lead to ischemia in some areas of the brain if not managed appropriately [22]. Thus, prolonged, prophylactic hyperventilation with $PaCO_2 \leq 25$ mmHg is not recommended. Short term hyperventilation as a vasoconstrictory stimulus can stabilise ICP during prolonged plateau waves. Although hyperventilation is recommended as a temporal treatment of intracranial hypertension, it should be avoided during the first 24 h after TBI when CBF is critically reduced [14]. If hyperventilation is implemented, $AVDO_2$ measurement by jugular venous oximetry or PtO_2 is recommended [38–40].

Unlike pressure autoregulation, CO_2 reactivity is often present after acute brain injury. This phenomenon is sometimes referred to as dissociation of CO_2 reactivity and pressure autoregulation [41]. When it is absent, with the failure of both mechanisms, the prognosis for outcome is fatal [42].

7.2.6 Pressure Reactivity After Traumatic Brain Injury

Cerebral autoregulation and cerebrovascular reactivity are impaired following severe TBI. The cerebrovascular reactivity is usually not affected globally but is rather disturbed in certain regions of the injured brain.

The pressure reactivity is described by a relationship between arterial blood pressure and intracranial pressure and can be detected in patients under monitoring in clinical settings. It is one of the mechanisms of cerebral autoregulation which helps to maintain an almost constant CBF in healthy conditions.

Pressure reactivity index (PRx) was introduced as a tool in monitoring cerebral autoregulation in patients with acute brain injury in critical care. It is calculated in an online, continuous way, as a Pearson correlation coefficient between averaged ABP and ICP. Their average values are calculated every 10 seconds and the correlation of 30 consecutive values is taken to obtain the PRx [43] (Fig. 7.7).

The distribution of PRx in different outcome groups revealed that pressure reactivity is significantly worse in patients with fatal outcome. The mortality indicated a threshold rise from 20% to 70% when averaged PRx increased above 0.3 [44]. The threshold for differentiating between favourable and unfavourable outcome after TBI was identified as PRx of 0.05. PRx averaged value below 0.05 predicts favourable

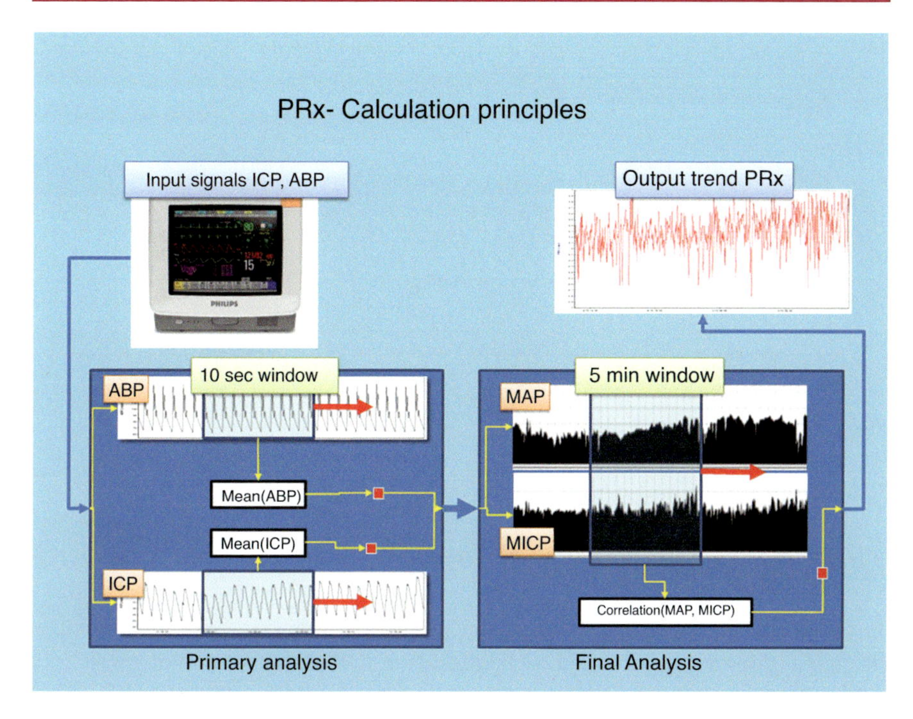

Fig. 7.7 The schematic diagram illustrating calculation of PRx. High frequency sampled ABP and ICP signals are transferred from bedside monitors to computer's memory. 10 second averages are then calculated and transferred to second buffer with sampling frequency of 10 s. Subsequent 30 samples of mean ICP and ABP are taken for calculation of PRx-correlation coefficient between mean ABP and ICP. Calculated PRx is 'noisy'. In most cases it should be time averaged (over a 30-minute period) to judge about the state of cerebrovascular reactivity. Higher PRx indicates worse reactivity, with a value >0.3 associated with autoregulatory failure and increased incidence of mortality (>60%). Value of PRx <0.05 correlates with an excellent reactivity and favourable outcome

outcome following severe head injury [7]. The autoregulation failure with elevated PRx is also associated with higher incidence of the intracranial hypertension.

7.2.7 CPP-oriented Therapy

PRx can be used as an indicator of optimal CPP (CPPopt). The relationship between CPP and PRx over a longer period of several hours shows a U-shape curve indicating a minimal best reactivity at CPPopt (Fig. 7.7). It was demonstrated that CPP between 70 and 90 mmHg ensures preserved pressure reactivity and thus, autoregulation [45]. The difference between observed CPP and CPPopt is strongly correlated with outcome from TBI. The rate of favourable outcome reaches the highest probability value when CPP follows the optimal CPP [46] (Fig. 7.8).

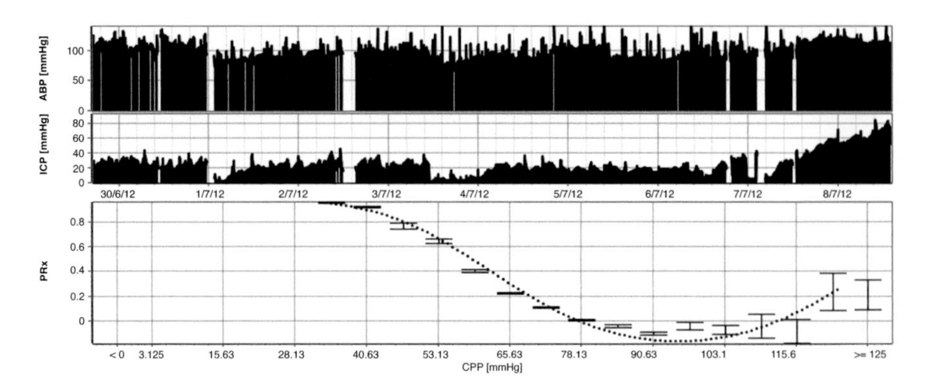

Fig. 7.8 U shape curve constructed by plotting PRx against CPP in patient who died from refractory intracranial hypertension. The curve shows optimal CPP around 90 mmHg

7.2.8 RAP Index

In the ICP monitoring, RAP index is a moving correlation coefficient between mean ICP (10-s average) and pulse amplitude of ICP (AMP), measured every 3 or 5 minutes. It is a reliable measure of compensatory reserve and intracranial compliance. A RAP coefficient close to 0 indicates a good pressure–volume compensatory reserve, when change in volume causes minor or no change in pressure. When RAP increases to +1 the compensatory reserve is low, and any addition of volume generates elevation of ICP. Negative RAP indicates terminal vascular insufficiency when the arterioles collapse [47]. Low average RAP index combined with elevated ICP (>20 mmHg) is associated with unfavourable outcome after TBI [48] (Fig. 7.9).

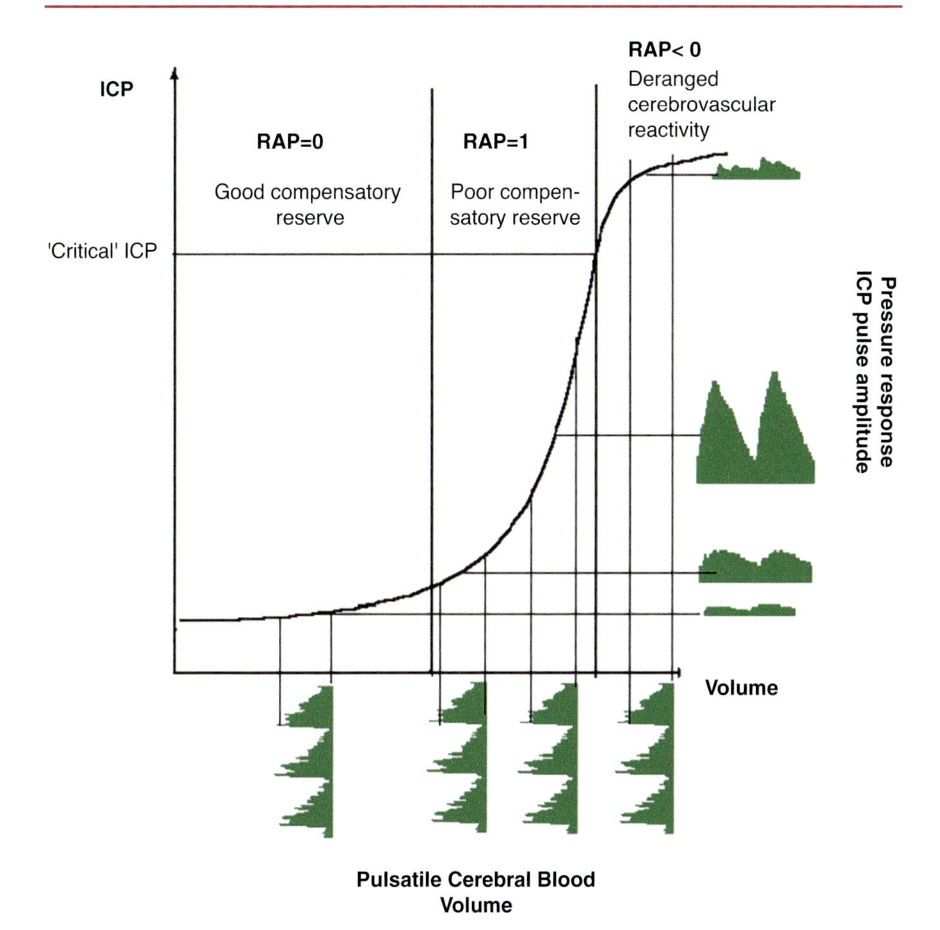

Fig. 7.9 RAP index is a correlation coefficient between mean intracranial pressure (ICP) and pulse amplitude of ICP. RAP equal to 0 at low ICP values shows good compensatory reserve. RAP close to +1 indicates that the current 'monitoring point' is on exponential part of the curve, thus associated with poor compensatory reserve. When ICP value reaches the level above the critical ICP threshold, when cerebral arterioles start to hypotgetically collapse, RAP decreases to negative values

References

1. Chesnut RM, Marshall LF, Klauber MR, Blunt BA, Baldwin N, Eisenberg HM, Jane JA, Marmarou A, Foulkes MA. The role of secondary brain injury in determining outcome from severe head injury. J Trauma. 1993;34(2):216–22.
2. Albeck MJ, Børgesen SE, Gjerris F, Schmidt JF, Sørensen PS. Intracranial pressure and cerebrospinal fluid outflow conductance in healthy subjects. J Neurosurg. 1991;74(4):597–600.
3. Welch K. The intracranial pressure in infants. J Neurosurg. 1980;52(5):693–9.
4. Mazzola CA, Adelson PD. Critical care management of head trauma in children. Crit Care Med. 2002;30(11):393–401.

5. Chapman PH, Cosman ER, Arnold MA. The relationship between ventricular fluid pressure and body position in normal subjects and subjects with shunts: a telemetric study. Neurosurgery. 1990;26(2):181–9.
6. Carney N, Totten AM, O'Reilly C, Ullman JS, Hawryluk GW, Bell MJ, Bratton SL, Chesnut R, Harris OA, Kissoon N, Rubiano AM, Shutter L, Tasker RC, Vavilala MS, Wilberger J, Wright DW, Ghajar J. Guidelines for the management of severe traumatic brain injury, fourth edition. Neurosurgery. 2017;80(1):6–15.
7. Sorrentino E, Diedler J, Kasprowicz M, Budohoski KP, Haubrich C, Smielewski P, Outtrim JG, Manktelow A, Hutchinson PJ, Pickard JD, Menon DK, Czosnyka M. Critical thresholds for cerebrovascular reactivity after traumatic brain injury. Neurocrit Care. 2012;16(2):258–66.
8. Monro A. Observations on the structure and function of the nervous system. Edinburgh: Creech & Johnson; 1783.
9. Mokri B. The Monro-Kellie hypothesis: applications in CSF volume depletion. Neurology. 2001;56(12):1746–8.
10. Klatzo I. Neuropathological aspects of brain edema. J Neuropathol Exp Neurol. 1967;26(1):1–14.
11. Hawthorne C, Piper I. Monitoring of intracranial pressure in patients with traumatic brain injury. Front Neurol. 2014;5:121.
12. Ocamoto GN, Russo TL, Mendes Zambetta R, Frigieri G, Hayashi CY, Brasil S, Rabelo NN, Spavieri Júnior DL. Intracranial compliance concepts and assessment: a scoping review. Front Neurol. 2021;12:756112.
13. Avezaat CJ, van Eijndhoven JH, Wyper DJ. Cerebrospinal fluid pulse pressure and intracranial volume-pressure relationships. J Neurol Neurosurg Psychiatry. 1979;42(8):687–700.
14. Rowed DW, Leech PJ, Reilly PL, Miller JD. Hypocapnia and intracranial volume-pressure relationship. A clinical and experimental study. Arch Neurol. 1975;32(6):369–73.
15. Marmarou A, Shulman K, Rosende RM. A nonlinear analysis of the cerebrospinal fluid system and intracranial pressure dynamics. J Neurosurg. 1978;48(3):332–44.
16. Harary M, Dolmans RGF, Gormley WB. Intracranial pressure monitoring—review and avenues for development. Sensors. 2018;18(2):465.
17. Lundberg N. Continuous recording and control of ventricular fluid pressure in neurosurgical practice. Acta Psychiatr Scand Suppl. 1960;36(149):1–193.
18. Czosnyka M, Pickard JD. Monitoring and interpretation of intracranial pressure. J Neurol Neurosurg Psychiatry. 2004;75(6):813–21.
19. Zakrzewska AP, Placek MM, Czosnyka M, Kasprowicz M, Lang EW. Intracranial pulse pressure waveform analysis using the higher harmonics centroid. Acta Neurochir. 2021;163(12):3249–58.
20. Dias C, Maia I, Cerejo A, Varsos G, Smielewski P, Paiva JA, Czosnyka M. Pressures, flow, and brain oxygenation during plateau waves of intracranial pressure. Neurocrit Care. 2014;21(1):124–32.
21. Martinez-Tejada I, Arum A, Wilhjelm JE, Juhler M, Andresen M. B waves: a systematic review of terminology, characteristics, and analysis methods. Fluids Barriers CNS. 2019;16(1):33.
22. Skippen P, Seear M, Poskitt K, Kestle J, Cochrane D, Annich G, Handel J. Effect of hyperventilation on regional cerebral blood flow in head-injured children. Crit Care Med. 1997;25(8):1402–9.
23. Cardoso ER, Rowan JO, Galbraith S. Analysis of the cerebrospinal fluid pulse wave in intracranial pressure. J Neurosurg. 1983;59(5):817–21.
24. Hu X, Glenn T, Scalzo F, Bergsneider M, Sarkiss C, Martin N, Vespa P. Intracranial pressure pulse morphological features improved detection of decreased cerebral blood flow. Physiol Meas. 2010;31(5):679–95.
25. Robertson CS, Narayan RK, Contant CF, Grossman RG, Gokaslan ZL, Pahwa R, Caram P Jr, Bray RS Jr, Sherwood AM. Clinical experience with a continuous monitor of intracranial compliance. J Neurosurg. 1989;71(5):673–80.

26. Kety SS, Schmidt CF. The nitrous oxide method for the quantitative determination of cerebral blood flow in man: theory, procedure and normal values. J Clin Invest. 1948;27(4):476–83.
27. Gibbs E, Lennox W, Nims L, Gibbs F. Arterial and cerebral venous blood: arterial-venous differences in man. J Biol Chem. 1942;144:325–32.
28. Winn HR. Youmans neurological surgery. 5th ed. Philadelphia: Elsevier; 2004.
29. Rowe GG, Maxwell GM, Castillo CA, Freeman DJ, Crumpton CW. A study in man of cerebral blood flow and cerebral glucose, lactate and pyruvate metabolism before and after eating. J Clin Invest. 1959;38(12):2154–8.
30. Robertson CS, Narayan RK, Gokaslan ZL, Pahwa R, Grossman RG, Caram P Jr, Allen E. Cerebral arteriovenous oxygen difference as an estimate of cerebral blood flow in comatose patients. J Neurosurg. 1989;70(2):222–30.
31. Bouma GJ, Muizelaar JP, Choi SC, Newlon PG, Young HF. Cerebral circulation and metabolism after severe traumatic brain injury: the elusive role of ischemia. J Neurosurg. 1991;75(5):685–93.
32. Lassen NA. Cerebral blood flow and oxygen consumption in man. Physiol Rev. 1959;39(2):183–238.
33. Rosner MJ, Coley IB. Cerebral perfusion pressure, intracranial pressure, and head elevation. J Neurosurg. 1986;65(5):636–41.
34. Donnelly J, Czosnyka M, Adams H, Cardim D, Kolias AG, Zeiler FA, Lavinio A, Aries M, Robba C, Smielewski P, Hutchinson PJA, Menon DK, Pickard JD, Budohoski KP. Twenty-five years of intracranial pressure monitoring after severe traumatic brain injury: a retrospective, single-center analysis. Neurosurgery. 2019;85(1):E75–82.
35. Kontos HA, Wei EP, Navari RM, Levasseur JE, Rosenblum WI, Patterson JL Jr. Responses of cerebral arteries and arterioles to acute hypotension and hypertension. Am J Physiol. 1978;234(4):H371–83.
36. Heistad D, Kontos H. Handbook of physiology. Bethesda: American Physiological Society; 1983.
37. Lang EW, Chesnut RM. Intracranial pressure. Monitoring and management. Neurosurg Clin N Am. 1994;5(4):573–605.
38. Sheinberg M, Kanter MJ, Robertson CS, Contant CF, Narayan RK, Grossman RG. Continuous monitoring of jugular venous oxygen saturation in head-injured patients. J Neurosurg. 1992;76(2):212–7.
39. Gopinath SP, Robertson CS, Contant CF, Hayes C, Feldman Z, Narayan RK, Grossman RG. Jugular venous desaturation and outcome after head injury. J Neurol Neurosurg Psychiatry. 1994;57(6):717–23.
40. Oertel M, Kelly DF, Lee JH, McArthur DL, Glenn TC, Vespa P, Boscardin WJ, Hovda DA, Martin NA. Efficacy of hyperventilation, blood pressure elevation, and metabolic suppression therapy in controlling intracranial pressure after head injury. J Neurosurg. 2002;97(5):1045–53.
41. Enevoldsen EM, Jensen FT. Autoregulation and CO2 responses of cerebral blood flow in patients with acute severe head injury. J Neurosurg. 1978;48(5):689–703.
42. Obrist WD, Langfitt TW, Jaggi JL, Cruz J, Gennarelli TA. Cerebral blood flow and metabolism in comatose patients with acute head injury. Relationship to intracranial hypertension. J Neurosurg. 1984;61(2):241–53.
43. Czosnyka M, Smielewski P, Kirkpatrick P, Laing RJ, Menon D, Pickard JD. Continuous assessment of the cerebral vasomotor reactivity in head injury. Neurosurgery. 1997;41(1):11–7.
44. Balestreri M, Czosnyka M, Steiner LA, Hiler M, Schmidt EA, Matta B, Menon D, Hutchinson P, Pickard JD. Association between outcome, cerebral pressure reactivity and slow ICP waves following head injury. Acta Neurochir Suppl. 2005;95:25–8.
45. Steiner LA, Czosnyka M, Piechnik SK, Smielewski P, Chatfield D, Menon DK, Pickard JD. Continuous monitoring of cerebrovascular pressure reactivity allows determination of optimal cerebral perfusion pressure in patients with traumatic brain injury. Crit Care Med. 2002;30(4):733–8.

46. Aries MJ, Czosnyka M, Budohoski KP, Steiner LA, Lavinio A, Kolias AG, Hutchinson PJ, Brady KM, Menon DK, Pickard JD, Smielewski P. Continuous determination of optimal cerebral perfusion pressure in traumatic brain injury. Crit Care Med. 2012;40(8):2456–63.
47. Czosnyka M, Smielewski P, Timofeev I, Lavinio A, Guazzo E, Hutchinson P, Pickard JD. Intracranial pressure: more than a number. Neurosurg Focus. 2007;22(5):E10.
48. Czosnyka M, Guazzo E, Whitehouse M, Smielewski P, Czosnyka Z, Kirkpatrick P, Piechnik S, Pickard JD. Significance of intracranial pressure waveform analysis after head injury. Acta Neurochir. 1996;138(5):531–41; discussion 541-2.

Non-invasive Neuromonitoring: Near Infrared Spectroscopy and Pupillometry

8

Etrusca Brogi

Abbreviations

%CH	Percent change in pupil size in %
AHA	American Heart Association
CA	Cerebral autoregulation
CBF	Cerebral blood flow
CI	Confidence interval
$CMRO_2$	Metabolic requirement
Cox	Cerebral oximetry index
CPR	Cardiopulmonary resuscitation
$CrSO_2$	Cerebral regional oxygen saturation
CT	Computed tomography
CV	Mean constriction velocity
CW-NIRS	Continuous wave NIRS
DCS	Diffuse correlation spectroscopy
DV	Velocity of dilatation
ECC	Emergency cardiovascular care
ED	Emergency department
END-PANIC	Establishing Normative Data for Pupillometer Assessments in Neuroscience Intensive Care
fNIRS	Functional NIRS
Hb	Deoxyhemoglobin
HbO_2	Oxyhemoglobin
ICH	Intracerebral hemorrhage
ICP	Intracranial pressure
ICU	Intensive care unit

E. Brogi (✉)
Department of Anesthesia and Intensive Care, Pisa University Hospital, Pisa, Italy

E. Brogi et al. (eds.), *Traumatic Brain Injury*, Hot Topics in Acute Care Surgery and Trauma, https://doi.org/10.1007/978-3-031-50117-3_8

ID	Identification number
LAT	Latency
MAX	The maximum diameter
MCV	Maximum constriction velocity
MD	Microdialysis
MIN	The minimum diameter of the pupils
MRI	Magnetic resonance imaging
NIRS	Near-infrared spectroscopy
NPi	Neurological pupilar index
OD	Optical density
OEF	Oxygen extraction fraction
ORANGE	Outcome pRognostication of Acute Brain Injury using the NeuroloGical Pupil IndEx study
$PbtO_2$	Brain oxygen tension
PD	Pupil diameter
PMS	Phase modulated spectroscopy
PRx	Pressure reactivity index
rCBFi	Cerebral blood flow index
rSO_2	Regional cerebral oxygen saturation
rSO_2	Regional oxygen saturation
rTHb	Relative total tissue hemoglobin concentration
SAH	Subarachnoid hemorrhage
$SjvO_2$	Jugular oxygen saturation
SRS	Partially resolved spectroscopy
TBI	Traumatic brain injury
TCD	Transcranial Doppler
THI	Tissue hemoglobin index
THx	Total hemoglobin reactivity index
TOI	Tissue oxygenation index
TOx	Tissue oxygen reactivity index
TRS-NIRS	Time-resolved spectroscopy
V_{max}	Maximum contraction velocity of the pupil

8.1 Introduction

Traumatic brain injury (TBI) remains a main cause of mortality and disability worldwide with important socioeconomic burdens, both in direct and indirect costs [1, 2]. The annual incidence rate of TBI varies between countries and it was estimated that the incidence increased up to 3.6% in the last decades [1]. For those patients who survive the primary insult, the major object of TBI management is represented by the prevention of secondary injuries that may arise after the initial traumatic event and exacerbate the brain injury [3]. Several factors may act as secondary insults to the brain (e.g., hypoxemia, hypercapnia, hypovolemia, and intracranial hypertension), with impairments in cerebral oxygenation and autoregulation. Consequently, it is extremely important to sustain adequate cerebral perfusion from the pre-hospital management through all the phases of hospital care. It has already been proved that early detection and management of the possible causes of secondary insult, already in the prehospital phases, could impact neurological outcomes and mortality [4].

Consequently, Neuromonitoring, with a multimodality approach, plays a crucial role for the rapid detection of altered cerebral perfusion, pressure parameters, oxygenation, metabolism, and brain electrophysiology [5, 6]. The aim of neuromonitoring is to provide a deep insight in the physio pathological mechanisms of traumatic brain injury for a tailored treatment. In the current clinical practice, the dynamic of the secondary insult is generally evaluated using invasive methods requiring probes or catheters. Examples of these kind of methods includes, but are not limited to, intracranial pressure (ICP), brain oxygen tension ($PbtO_2$), microdialysis (MD), and jugular oxygen saturation ($SjvO_2$). Some of these methods required neurosurgical intervention, may require imaging probe location control and may also carry the risk of infection and/or bleeding [7]. On the other hand, beside the unquestionable role of the neuroimaging (e.g., computerized tomography, magnetic resonance imaging, CT perfusion and angiography), these techniques are not available at bedside and they cannot provide continuous monitoring [8].

Noninvasive monitoring is rapidly emerging as applicable, and reliable tool for the bedside evaluation of patients with TBI and could represent a valuable option for the assessment of the trajectories of the secondary insults. Non-invasive methods include transcranial ultrasound, evoked potentials, electroencephalography, near-infrared spectroscopy (NIRS), Bispectral index and pupillometry. In this chapter, we aimed to provide an overview of the technological feature and of the clinical application both of NIRS and pupillometry in TBI patients.

8.2 NIRS: The Technology

Spectroscopy studies the compositions and structure of matter, at the atomic and molecular scale, based on the evaluation of its interaction with electromagnetic radiation. This kind of methodology is generally classified by the type of radiant energy used, the wavelength, the type of material evaluated, and by the nature of interaction between the energy and the material.

Near-infrared spectroscopy (NIRS) is a rising noninvasive monitoring modality with the capability of continuously monitoring perfusion of the brain at the bedside, providing information about oxygen saturation of hemoglobin within the microcirculation [9]. NIRS represents an analytic tool that can be classified as an absorption spectroscopic method that measures the chromophore absorption at a particular wavelength; the near-infrared region of the electromagnetic spectrum [10, 11]. The wavelengths utilized range between 700 nm and 1000 nm, where the absorption of chromophores (e.g., oxyhemoglobin, and deoxyhemoglobin) is maximized whereas the absorption of other molecules is diminished (e.g., water, lipid, melanin).

The near-infrared light is transmitted from NIRS sensors, applied on the forehead of the patients, and it can penetrate brain bone through cerebral tissue allowing the evaluation of tissue oxygenation 2–3 cm below NIRS sensors [9]. The light travels through the biological tissue not following a straight path from the sensor to the detector, but it rather depends on the scattering events; in the end, the light can be absorbed or reflected. Indeed, through the biological tissue, NIR photon propagation depends on reflection, absorption, and scattering following a wavelength-dependent process. Light absorption by tissue (i.e., light attenuation) can be quantified with the Beer-Lambert equation and it is directly proportional to the concentration of chromophores (i.e., oxyhemoglobin, deoxyhemoglobin, and cytochrome-c-oxidase) [12]. Even more, light attenuation depends on the light intensity, the distance traveled by the light and the extinction coefficient of the compounds [13]. The different absorption properties of these chromophores also influences light attenuation. The total light absorption can be obtained by the sum of the contribution of different compounds, when the tissue contains different kinds of chromophores [14]. Parallelly, scattering process consists of photon deviation from a straight trajectory, and depends on the size of the particles and the wavelength of the light. In biological tissue, scattering represents the dominating process (e.g., 80%), consequently, the modified Beer-Lambert equation, considering the effects of scattering, is applied in order to a more accurate quantification [15].

By the evaluation of the intensity of the light traveling through the tissue and the consequent information on light attenuation, healthcare personnel can obtain important information regarding cerebral concentrations of oxyhemoglobin (HbO_2) and deoxyhemoglobin (Hb) and, consequently, on regional oxygen saturation (rSO_2), cerebral regional oxygen saturation ($CrSO_2$) and the balance between oxygen delivery and consumption.

The regional oxygen saturation is calculated by the following formula:

$$rSO_2 = \frac{[HbO_2]}{[HbO_2]+[HbO_2]} \times 100\%$$

rSO_2 represents a mixed tissue saturation, because NIRS is not able to distinguish between arterial and venous blood.

It is important to highlight that nowadays several devices are available for clinical practice with different detection methods, strengths, and limitations. Consequently, they cannot be used interchangeably. Type of Spectroscopy techniques currently in use:

- Continuous wave NIRS (CW-NIRS): using a light of constant intensity. The attenuated light signal is measured at a fixed distance. This method assumes that light scattering over time is constant, and that changes in absorption are only due to HbO_2 and Hb;
- Spatially resolved spectroscopy (SRS): light attenuation is measurements using multiple light detectors placed at a certain distance from an incident light;

- Time-resolved spectroscopy (TRS-NIRS): light's intensity is detected as the temporal point spread function over time;
- Phase modulated spectroscopy (PMS): the frequency and the intensity of the light is modulated and light path length are measured at each wavelength [16].
- Diffuse correlation spectroscopy (DCS): use the intensity fluctuation of Near infrared light.

Some limitations of the measurement methods can be represented by the thickness of skull bones, myelin sheaths, skin pigmentation, wounds, medication on the scalp, and hematoma.

8.3 NIRS: Clinical Application

NIRS can be used in all the different phases of patient management: from prehospital care to the rehabilitation settings. The spatial and temporal analysis of tissue oxygenation performed by NIRS let to analyze the various dynamic pathophysiological states in TBI patients with important impact on patient management. NIRS can detect absorption characteristics in different brain regions at the bedside, providing information about microvascular and tissue oxygen metabolic status.

NIRS can be used in the detection of brain hematoma and it can also be used to identify delayed hematoma following TBI, thus representing a valuable triaging tool in TBI patients requiring urgent intervention [17]. The sensitivity of NIRS post-traumatic hematoma detection ranges from 68 to 95.5% between the published studies [18–21]. In intracranial hematoma, hemoglobin concentration is higher than in normal brain tissue, consequently, NIRS analyses are characterized by a greater light absorption at 760 nm on the side of the hematoma and asymmetry in the optical density (OD) between hemispheres [22, 23]. The OD differences between the two hemispheres increase with the size of the hematoma, however, the accuracy and reliability of the measurement are reduced in case of deep hematoma. OD differences seem to be more marked for epidural and subdural hematomas in comparison to ICH [24, 25]. It is also important to remember that scalp hematoma can obscure the readings [25]. NIRS evaluation cannot be used as an alternative method to other conventional techniques (i.e., TC, MRI) with higher sensitivity, however, it represents a valuable easy-to-use device characterized by a noninvasive nature for earlier detection of impending intracranial emergency [26]. This information can be really important in prehospital setting and ED department for a quick identification of patients that may need neurosurgical intervention and consequent centralization.

NIRS can be used for the early identification of impaired cerebral oxygenation. The evaluation of the concentration of HbO_2 and Hb allows the calculation of regional cerebral tissue oxygen saturation (rSO_2), consequently, it is possible to have an estimation of the cerebral oxygen extraction fraction (OEF) and of the balance between oxygen delivery and consumption. In case of increased oxygen demand, tissue brain extracts a bigger quantity of oxygen, thus venous oxygen saturation is reduced. rSO_2 represents mixed tissue saturation due to the fact that NIRS analyses are not able to differentiate between arterial, capillaries and venous blood. rSO_2 is approximately 70%, supposing a 75% of venous contribution and 25% of arterial contribution of NIRS measurement [27]. The evaluation of the absolute value of rSO_2 and its trend are currently used in cardiac surgery and carotid artery surgery to prevent episodes of decreased tissue hemoglobin oxygenation and rSO_2 from baseline thus preventing cerebral ischemia [28].

In TBI patients, the coupling between metabolic requirement ($CMRO_2$) and cerebral blood flow (CBF) is altered. A rising in ICP with reduced CBF lead to hypoperfusion episodes, with no consensual reduction in CMRO2; protracted periods of low level of rSO_2 (<60%) are associated with and impaired cerebral perfusion and higher mortality [29]. In TBI patients, rSO_2 has been shown to correlate with the measurement obtained with invasive methods of cerebral oxygenation such as $SjvO_2$, whereas conflicting results are obtained on the correlation between rSO_2 and $PbtO_2$ [30, 31]. In 2010, Leal-Noval et al. evaluated the correlation between invasive brain tissue oxygen pressure ($PbrO_2$) and rSO_2 in 22 TBI patients. They found a direct correlation between rSO_2 and $PbrO_2$ [beta coefficient and 95% CI = 0.36 (0.35–0.37)] [32]. However, they also found a low accuracy for detecting moderate brain hypoxia ($PbtO_2 < 15$ mmHg) and found a moderate accuracy for severe hypoxia ($PbtO_2 < 12$ mmHg) [32]. The correlation between rSO_2 and $PbtO_2$ was evaluated also by Esnault et al. in 2015 [33]. No correlation was found between rSO_2 and $PbtO_2$ ($r = 0.016$ [−0.103–0.134]) [33]. Even more, rSO_2 allowed the identification of fewer ischemic episodes in comparison with $PbtO_2$ (<15%). The authors concluded that rSO_2 cannot represent a substitute for $PbtO_2$. Contrarily, Brawanski et al. found a good correlation between the two methods in more than 90% of the cases [34]. These results were also confirmed in a group of severe TBI patients [35]. Interestingly, Budohoski et al. found that NIRS signal changed earlier than $PbtO_2$ following pressure changes [PtO_2: 39.6s (IQR 16.4–66.0) vs. NIRS:10.9s (IQR −5.9–39.6), $p < 0.001$] and ICP changes [PtO_2: 22.9s (IQR 11.0–53.0) vs. NIRS: 7.1s (IQR −8.8–195), $p < 0.001$] [36]. The heterogeneity of the findings can be explained by the fact that NIRS, SjO_2 and $PbtO_2$ represent different techniques and measure different parameters. In fact, NIRS measurements represent the average value of arterial, capillary, and venous blood, SjO_2 measures deoxygenated blood returning to the heart through the internal jugular veins and $PbtO_2$ evaluates a small area of tissue in the immediate vicinity of the probe. However, the integration of the data obtained from these modalities can provide a global detailed picture of oxygen metabolism.

Several attempts have been made to evaluate the role of NIRS as an alternative to conventional neuromonitoring methods to determine the degree of cerebral autoregulation (CA) and for the CBF evaluation [22, 37]. The assumption of a possible correlation between NIRS values and CBF lies on the assumption that changes in Hb concentration correlate with changes in CBF. However, the correlation between these parameters is not linear and is influenced by several confounding factors, leading to published conflicting results on this topic. Xenon CT studies failed to significantly find a correlation between CBF and NIRS measurements [38, 39]. Furthermore, Indocyanine green studies obtained contradictory results [37, 40, 41].

Consequently, the role of NIRS in the evaluation of CBF warrants further evaluation. Nevertheless, the assumption of a possible correlation between NIRS value and cerebral autoregulation lies on the fact that brain oximetry is related to arterial oxygen concentration, CBF and cerebral metabolism. As already stated, several NIRS devices are available and recent advantages in NIRS technologies can allow the measurements of various indexes useful for the continuous CA assessment.

Examples of proposed NIRS-indices of cerebrovascular reactivity:

- cerebral blood flow index (rCBFi), measured with diffuse correlation spectroscopy,
- tissue oxygenation index (TOI) = ratio of concentration of HbO_2 ad total hemoglobin (HbT);
- relative total tissue hemoglobin concentration (rTHb);
- tissue hemoglobin index (THI), measurement of hemoglobin signal strength;
- cerebral oximetry index (COx), correlation between $rScO_2$ and mean arterial pressure;
- tissue oxygen reactivity index (TOx);
- Total Hemoglobin reactivity index (THx), derived from total Hb, arterial blood pressure and tissue oxygen reactivity index (TOx).

Changes in the NIRS signal over time have been studied in order to assess the efficacy of CA evaluation. In 2010, Smielewski et al. analyzed data from different bedside monitors among 150 patients using a mathematical model [42]. They found a significant correlation between NIRS-derived reactivity indices (i.e., COx, TOx, THx) with Pressure reactivity index (PRx) and TCD-based indices. Furthermore, Computing correlation between blood flow velocity, NIRS parameters (i.e., TOI) and arterial blood pressure, performed in septic patients, showed abnormal CA in the vasodilatation state [43]. Highton et al. found a statistically significant correlation between PRx and THx ($rs = 0.63$, $P < 0.001$), PRx and Tox ($rs = 0.40$, $P = 0.04$) in a cohort of brain-injured patients [44]. Similarly, Zweifel et al. found a good correlation between THx and PRx in TBI patients [45]. The evidence, so far, seems to encourage the use of NIRS-derived parameters for CA evaluation. Further trials are needed for a deeper understanding of the effective role of NIRS in this setting.

NIRS has also been advocated as a noninvasive tool for ICP evaluation. However, the published articles lead to conflicting results. Zuluaga et al. evaluated the association between $CrSO_2$ and ICP in 30 children [46]. The authors found that the relation between these two parameters was influenced by the diagnosis. rSO_2 decreased in patients with brain tumor ($P = 0.05$) and hydrocephalus ($P < 0.001$) and increased ICP, whereas in patients with intracranial hemorrhage rSO_2 increased ($p < 0.001$). Muellner et al. did not find any statistical difference between healthy volunteers and patients with increased ICP. The authors concluded that the use of NIRS as a monitoring tool for increased ICP has to be discouraged [47]. Contrarily, Budohoski et al. found that NIRS derived parameters were able to fast detect ICP fluctuation [36]. It is important to note that NIRS has the potential to detect hypoxic events related to an increase in ICP, not to directly diagnose an increase in ICP. Even more, no validated threshold of rSO_2 is currently available to detect episodes of increased ICP.

Finally, NIRS can also have a promising and interesting role during the rehabilitation phases of TBI. NIRS not only can evaluate the recovery of cerebral oxygenation and autoregulation, but also can record the improvements in motor and cognitive function. Functional NIRS (fNIRS) is a high-density NIRS array that utilizes 47 NIRS channels allowing to map brain function. This multi-channel device analyzes changes in HbO in frontal and temporal lobes. Several studies have shown that NIRS can be used to evaluate different brain activation areas during motor and cognitive tasks and to track the evolution of the changes in neuronal activation during rehabilitation [48–50].

8.4 Pupillometry: The Technology

Examination of the pupil is an essential part of the neurological evaluation providing vital information regarding new or impeding intracranial pathology.

Pupillometer is a clinical method that can objectively analyze both static and dynamic pupillary data using a reflected light with the same size of the pupil, through measurement of the pupillary light reflex [51]. From the technological point of view, pupillometer can be classified as manual and automated. The manual method consists of a subjective evaluation of the pupil size and reaction of the pupil to the light performed by healthcare personnel generally using a penlight [52]. Otherwise, another kind of manual pupillometer is represented by a chart method for pupil size measurement. One of the most famous examples of manual pupillometry is represented by The Haab's pupillometer. In this method, the operator compares the pupil size with graduated filled circles on a slide rule, the "Haab' scale" [53]. Unfortunately, manual pupil measurements do not represent a quantitative method and therefore it is susceptible to intra and inter-observers variability.

An automated Pupillometer is a potable medical infrared technology with an optical scanner that objectively quantifies pupil diameter and reactivity, providing a numerical evaluation of the pupil characteristics, thus providing an objective and quantitative neurological pupil measurement [54, 55]. Besides providing an accurate measurement of pupil size, symmetry, and reactivity, automated Pupillometer can provide a measurement of the trend of pupil size and reactivity in order to have important feedback on neurological status [56]. An example of pupillometer evaluation and of pupillometry-related parameters in a healthy volunteer is shown in Fig. 8.1.

On the market, some instruments are offered. Even more, mobile smartphone digital pupillometry is increasingly available [57]. However, one of the most common types of pupillometer consists of a handheld infrared optics machine with a lithium battery (NeurOptics® NPi®-300 Pupillometer). This device can be recharged through a dedicated charging station base. After sending an infrared light, the reflected image is analyzed on an infrared sensor [58]. Then, the corresponding measurements are displayed on the touchscreen monitor. Even more, automated

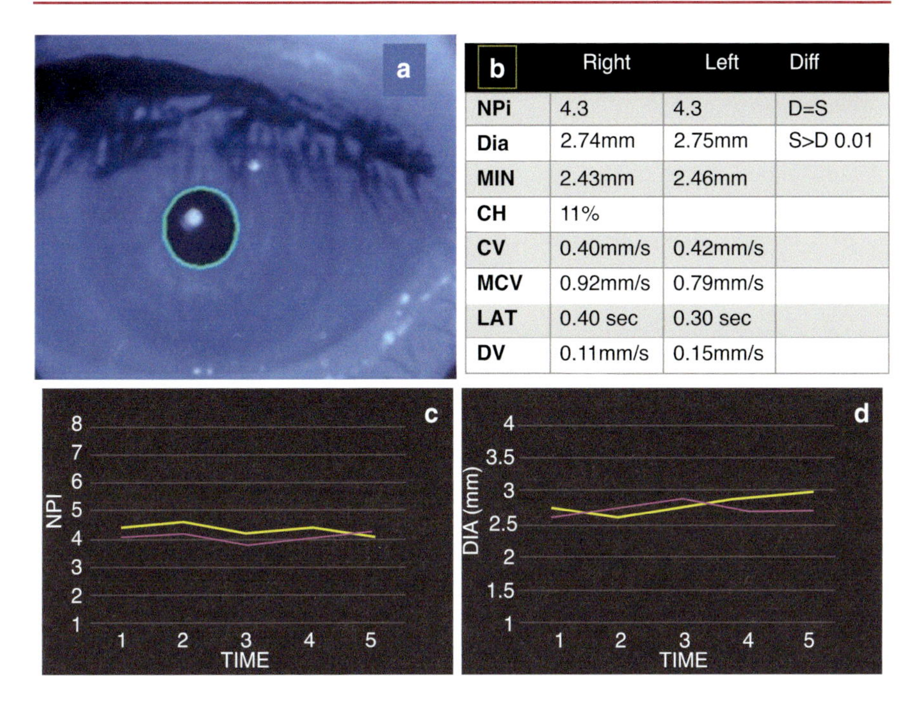

b	Right	Left	Diff
NPi	4.3	4.3	D=S
Dia	2.74mm	2.75mm	S>D 0.01
MIN	2.43mm	2.46mm	
CH	11%		
CV	0.40mm/s	0.42mm/s	
MCV	0.92mm/s	0.79mm/s	
LAT	0.40 sec	0.30 sec	
DV	0.11mm/s	0.15mm/s	

Fig. 8.1 Pupillometer evaluation of the left pupil (**a**). Pupillometer records in a healthy volunteer (**b**). Graphical representation of NPi and pupil size (Dia) trend for the left (yellow line) and right (pink line) pupil at different time point (vertical axis) in a healthy volunteer (**c**, **d** respectively)

Pupillometer is equipped with hardware that stores and processes the data and provides a graphical trend of the pupil measurements in order to evaluate pupil progress over time. The Pupillometer is also furnished with a disposable plastic device with a memory chip mounted on the lens of the Pupillometer with a corresponding reader. This device is intended for single-patient use, and it records all the measurements of a specific patient, linked with and identification number (i.e., ID) [56]. The single-user feature prevents the infection risk. The ID is entered on the memory chip of the disposable device during the first measurement. This plastic device allows also to deliver a constant light stimulus due to the fact that it keeps the device at a definite distance and also allows to stabilize the device on the patient during the measurement. This disposable plastic device can be connected to a corresponding reader in order to download the data stored. Pupillometer is not affected by ambient light.

From pre-hospital setting and during all the phases of hospital care, the pupillometer allows the registration of [59]:

- *MAX*: the maximum diameter, in mm, before light stimulus;
- *MIN*: the minimum diameter of the pupils, in mm;
- *%CH*: Percent change in pupil size in %, a value of <10% is considered an abnormal findings;

- *CV*: Mean constriction velocity, in mm/s, a value of C<0.8 mm/s is considered abnormal [60, 61];
- *MCV*: maximum constriction velocity, in mm/s;
- *LAT*: elapsed time between retinal stimulation and the onset of real pupillary constriction, in seconds;
- *DV*: velocity of dilatation, in mm/s;
- *NPi*: Neurological pupilar index, a dimensionless index obtained from an algorithm that takes into consideration all the aforementioned variables.

The average pupil diameter in healthy subjects ranges from 2.5 mm to 4 mm in bright light and from 4 to 8 mm in the darkness [59]. NPI score can range from 0 (absent reactivity) to 5 (a vivacious response) [62]. An asymmetry in NPi value between the right and left pupil equal and/or major of 0.7 can be considered an abnormal pupil finding. NPI can be classified in:

- Normal/"active response": NPi 3–5
- Abnormal/"slow response": NPi below 3
- Unresponsive/atypical response/not Measurable: NPi equal to 0.

Some contraindications on the usage of pupillometer warrant special considerations. Pupillometry cannot be used in patients with injured orbital and periorbital structure (i.e., edema, fractures, open wound). Possible limitations of pupillometer interpretation are represented by ophthalmological disease and ocular refractory abnormality in the patient's clinical history.

8.5 Pupillometry: Clinical Application

Neurological evaluation of the pupil has always been play a central role in clinical practice with vital prognostic implications [63]. The pupillary light reflex is an autonomic reflex in reaction to light and consists of adjustments of pupil size in order to control the amount of light that reaches the retina [64]. The parasympathetic system controls pupillary constriction (through the iris sphincter muscle). The afferent pupillary fibers are in thigh connection with the photoreceptors at the level of the retina and travel through the optic nerve, the optic chiasma and the optic tract [59]. At the midbrain level, the afferent pathways send fibers bilaterally to the Edinger-Westphal nucleus [61]. The efferent pupillary fibers consist of parasympathetic preganglionic fibers that exit the midbrain and travel through the oculomotor nerve (third cranial nerve) until the ciliary ganglion. From this ganglion, parasympathetic postganglionic axons reach and innervate the iris sphincter muscle leading to bilateral pupillary constriction after a light stimulus. An asymmetric response to light implies a lesion anywhere in the pupillary pathway. In case of focal or diffuse mass effect with midbrain compression and impending transtentorial herniation, alteration in pupils' size and reactivity may occur highlighting the importance of pupilar evaluation [62].

Pupillary light reflex can be used to detect second cranial (optic nerve) nerve injury, third cranial nerve injury and brain stem lesions. Even more, pupillary light reflex can be altered after several drugs administration (e.g., fentanyl, barbituric, morphine, midazolam) [59]. Consequently, automated pupillometry can be used to evaluate several diseases affecting the pupillary light reflex arch. Recently, automated pupillometry has been used in the evaluation of several medical conditions, such as brain tumors, Parkinson, autism, Alzheimer, autonomic dysfunction, diabetes mellitus, alcohol, toxins and recreational drugs [59, 65]. Even more, in 2020, the American Heart Association (AHA) Guidelines for Cardiopulmonary Resuscitation (CPR) and Emergency Cardiovascular Care (ECC) has introduced automated pupillometry as an objective evaluation of brain injury prognosis in patients following cardiac arrest [66]. After automated pupillometry assessment, pupillary light reflex values were higher in survivors and in patients with a good neurological outcome compared with non survivors [67]. In a 2019 systematic review assessing the use of pupillometry in NeuroICU, automated pupillometry showed to increase reproducibility in comparison to the standard pupillary evaluation, with the ability to detect earlier pupillary changes [68]. The authors also highlighted the importance of pupillometry to detect the impending rise of intracranial pressure and its role as a prognostic indicator in Neuro ICU [55, 69]. Several studies found that automated pupillometry is capable of detecting light reflex of pupils that were classified as non-reactive on manual evaluation by healthcare professional in up to 66.7% of the cases. The median absolute error in measuring pupil size using manual pupillometry in comparison to automated pupillometry varies between the studies, reaching 39% of cases [52, 54].

The clinical implication of pupillary changes on outcome has already been proved in TBI patients. Abnormal pupillary light response and pupillary asymmetry were correlated with outcome [70, 71]. NPi value of the automated pupillometer differs between patients with poor neurological outcomes in comparison to favorable outcomes in patients with acute brain injury [72]. Even more, in TBI patients, unilateral pupillary dilatation presents different outcomes in comparison to bilateral pupillary abnormalities [73]. Significant anisocoria (>0.5 mm) has been associated with intracranial hypertension and impending uncal herniation [74]. Even more, altered pupillary constriction velocity (e.g., <0.6 mm/s) and asymmetry in patients with severe head injury may represent a suggestive sign of increased ICP or intracranial hypertension [55, 74]. Further insight into the relation between Pupillometer value and 6-month mortality will be obtained after the publication of the data on the ongoing ORANGE study; a prospective, observational, and study that including patients with TBI, aSAH, and ICH [75].

Furthermore, quantitative pupillometry represents a potential monitoring method for following TBI patients from hospital admission to recovery across its spectrum of severity. Following concussive events in asymptomatic TBI patients, authors have found modifications in the pupillary light reflex with increased pupillary constriction and a decrease in dilation velocity and NPi. This represents a useful information for the diagnosis and rapid identification of subacute asymptomatic TBI patients in case of clinically asymptomatic high-acceleration head impacts cases

[76, 77]. In severe TBI, pupillometry has shown to play an important role in detecting increased intracranial pressure events and it can speed up the detection of neurological decompensation [78]. In 2011, Chen et al. observed that the finding of an abnormal NPi (<3) using an automated pupillometer may be suggestive of increased ICH in patients with different mechanisms of brain injury (i.e., TBI, SAH, ICH) [62]. The authors found an inverse correlation between ICP and NPi. Interestingly, the authors also observed that the first evidence of abnormal pupil occurs several hours earlier that the actual increase of ICP. In 2019, Al-Obaidi et al. analyzed 16,221 pupillary data from the END-PANIC registry in patients in Neurocritical care unit [79, 80]. The authors found that mean pupillometer values were lower in patients with increased ICP. Taylor et al. also found that a value CV below 0.6 mm/s might be suggestive of increased ICP. The authors observed that the CV value would further drop in case of ICP >30 mmHg [81]. Pupillometry and pupil reactivity can be also used to guide hypertonic therapy, acting as a noninvasive monitor of osmotic therapy's response [82]. Ong et al. observed an improvement in NPi value after the administration or both mannitol of hypertonic saline (e.g., 2 h) [82]. Furthermore, pupillometry may be useful in detecting intracranial midline shift with significant correlation between midline shift and the NPi, CV and pupillary asymmetry [83]. Consequently, Automated Pupillometer can be used as a triage tool in TBI patients requiring urgent intervention [84, 85].

Finally, pupillometry and pupillary reflex can serve as noninvasive monitoring for detecting level of analgesia, depth of sedation and response to analgesic drugs. During a noxious stimulus, pupillary size variation of 20% correlates with the presence of pain due to the evoked sympathetic system [86]. Emerging data showed that variation in the mean CH of the pupil diameter correlate with the depth of sedation, and maximum pupillary constriction velocity and diameter correlate with pain scores [87, 88]. Even more, the maximum contraction velocity of the pupil (V_{max}) and variation in pupil diameter (PD) correlated with the level of sedation [89]. Not surprisingly, the size values vary in relation to the administration of opioids.

8.6 Conclusions

Neuromonitoring can play a crucial role for the rapid detection of secondary insults and for continuous evaluation of patients with TBI at the bedside. NIRS and pupillometry can be used in all the different phases of patient management: from prehospital care to the rehabilitation settings. Both methods can represent a useful triaging tool for the rapid detection of impending neurological complications. Even more, these noninvasive methods can be implemented for the evaluation of cerebral hemodynamics, cerebral oxygen metabolism and cerebral functional state. Further studies are needed to deeper delineate the role of these methods in the current clinical practice.

References

1. BD 2016 Traumatic Brain Injury and Spinal Cord Injury Collaborators. Global, regional, and national burden of traumatic brain injury and spinal cord injury, 1990-2016: a systematic analysis for the Global Burden of Disease Study 2016. Lancet Neurol. 2019;18(1):56–87.
2. Dewan MC, Rattani A, Gupta S, Baticulon RE, Hung YC, Punchak M, et al. Estimating the global incidence of traumatic brain injury. J Neurosurg. 2018;130(4):1080–97.
3. Dearden NM. Mechanisms and prevention of secondary brain damage during intensive care. Clin Neuropathol. 1998;17(4):221–8.
4. Volpi PC, Robba C, Rota M, Vargiolu A, Citerio G. Trajectories of early secondary insults correlate to outcomes of traumatic brain injury: results from a large, single centre, observational study. BMC Emerg Med. 2018;18(1):52.
5. Feyen BF, Sener S, Jorens PG, Menovsky T, Maas AI. Neuromonitoring in traumatic brain injury. Minerva Anestesiol. 2012;78(8):949–58.
6. Karagianni MD, Brotis AG, Gatos C, Kalamatianos T, Vrettou C, Stranjalis G, et al. Neuromonitoring in severe traumatic brain injury: a bibliometric analysis. Neurocrit Care. 2022;36(3):1044–52.
7. Le Roux P, Menon DK, Citerio G, Vespa P, Bader MK, Brophy GM, et al. Consensus summary statement of the International Multidisciplinary Consensus Conference on Multimodality Monitoring in Neurocritical Care: a statement for healthcare professionals from the Neurocritical Care Society and the European Society of Intensive Care Medicine. Intensive Care Med. 2014;40(9):1189–209.
8. Douglas DB, Ro T, Toffoli T, Krawchuk B, Muldermans J, Gullo J, et al. Neuroimaging of traumatic brain injury. Med Sci. 2019;7(1):2.
9. Marin T, Moore J. Understanding near-infrared spectroscopy. Adv Neonatal Care. 2011;11(6):382–8.
10. Nilapwar SM, Nardelli M, Westerhoff HV, Verma M. Absorption spectroscopy. Methods Enzymol. 2011;500:59–75.
11. Beć KB, Huck CW. Breakthrough potential in near-infrared spectroscopy: spectra simulation. A review of recent developments. Front Chem. 2019;7:48.
12. Pellicer A, Bravo MC. Near-infrared spectroscopy: a methodology-focused review. Semin Fetal Neonatal Med. 2011;16(1):42–9.
13. Mayerhöfer TG, Popp J. Beer's law - why absorbance depends (almost) linearly on concentration. ChemPhysChem. 2019;20(4):511–5.
14. Murkin JM, Arango M. Near-infrared spectroscopy as an index of brain and tissue oxygenation. Br J Anaesth. 2009;103(Suppl 1):i3–13.
15. Rolfe P. In vivo near-infrared spectroscopy. Annu Rev Biomed Eng. 2000;2:715–54.
16. Levy WJ. The influence of demographic factors on phase-modulated spectroscopy in adults. Philos Trans R Soc Lond Ser B Biol Sci. 1997;352(1354):751–3.
17. Sen AN, Gopinath SP, Robertson CS. Clinical application of near-infrared spectroscopy in patients with traumatic brain injury: a review of the progress of the field. Neurophotonics. 2016;3(3):031409.
18. Kessel B, Jeroukhimov I, Ashkenazi I, Khashan T, Oren M, Haspel J, et al. Early detection of life-threatening intracranial haemorrhage using a portable near-infrared spectroscopy device. Injury. 2007;38(9):1065–8.
19. Robertson CS, Zager EL, Narayan RK, Handly N, Sharma A, Hanley DF, et al. Clinical evaluation of a portable near-infrared device for detection of traumatic intracranial hematomas. J Neurotrauma. 2010;27(9):1597–604.
20. Leon-Carrion J, Dominguez-Roldan JM, Leon-Dominguez U, Murillo-Cabezas F. The Infrascanner, a handheld device for screening in situ for the presence of brain haematomas. Brain Inj. 2010;24(10):1193–201.

21. Ghalenoui H, Saidi H, Azar M, Yahyavi ST, Borghei Razavi H, Khalatbari M. Near-infrared laser spectroscopy as a screening tool for detecting hematoma in patients with head trauma. Prehosp Disaster Med. 2008;23(6):558–61.
22. Gomez A, Sainbhi AS, Froese L, Batson C, Alizadeh A, Mendelson AA, et al. Near infrared spectroscopy for high-temporal resolution cerebral physiome characterization in TBI: a narrative review of techniques, applications, and future directions. Front Pharmacol. 2021;12:719501.
23. Zhang Q, Ma H, Nioka S, Chance B. Study of near infrared technology for intracranial hematoma detection. J Biomed Opt. 2000;5(2):206–13.
24. Gopinath SP, Robertson CS, Grossman RG, Chance B. Near-infrared spectroscopic localization of intracranial hematomas. J Neurosurg. 1993;79(1):43–7.
25. Robertson CS, Gopinath S, Chance B. Use of near infrared spectroscopy to identify traumatic intracranial hemotomas. J Biomed Opt. 1997;2(1):31–41.
26. Weigl W, Milej D, Janusek D, Wojtkiewicz S, Sawosz P, Kacprzak M, et al. Application of optical methods in the monitoring of traumatic brain injury: a review. J Cereb Blood Flow Metab. 2016;36(11):1825–43.
27. Sørensen H, Secher NH, Rasmussen P. A note on arterial to venous oxygen saturation as reference for NIRS-determined frontal lobe oxygen saturation in healthy humans. Front Physiol. 2013;4:403.
28. Nenna A, Barbato R, Greco SM, Pugliese G, Lusini M, Covino E, et al. Near-infrared spectroscopy in adult cardiac surgery: between conflicting results and unexpected uses. J Geriatr Cardiol. 2017;14(11):659–61.
29. Roldán M, Kyriacou PA. Near-infrared spectroscopy (NIRS) in traumatic brain injury (TBI). Sensors. 2021;21(5):1586.
30. Kirkpatrick PJ, Smielewski P, Czosnyka M, Menon DK, Pickard JD. Near-infrared spectroscopy use in patients with head injury. J Neurosurg. 1995;83(6):963–70.
31. Tateishi A, Maekawa T, Soejima Y, Sadamitsu D, Yamamoto M, Matsushita M, et al. Qualitative comparison of carbon dioxide-induced change in cerebral near-infrared spectroscopy versus jugular venous oxygen saturation in adults with acute brain disease. Crit Care Med. 1995;23(10):1734–8.
32. Leal-Noval SR, Cayuela A, Arellano-Orden V, Marín-Caballos A, Padilla V, Ferrándiz-Millón C, et al. Invasive and noninvasive assessment of cerebral oxygenation in patients with severe traumatic brain injury. Intensive Care Med. 2010;36(8):1309–17.
33. Esnault P, Boret H, Montcriol A, Carre E, Prunet B, Bordes J, et al. Assessment of cerebral oxygenation in neurocritical care patients: comparison of a new four wavelengths forehead regional saturation in oxygen sensor (EQUANOX®) with brain tissue oxygenation. A prospective observational study. Minerva Anestesiol. 2015;81(8):876–84.
34. Brawanski A, Faltermeier R, Rothoerl RD, Woertgen C. Comparison of near-infrared spectroscopy and tissue p(O2) time series in patients after severe head injury and aneurysmal subarachnoid hemorrhage. J Cereb Blood Flow Metab. 2002;22(5):605–11.
35. Holzschuh M, Woertgen C, Metz C, Brawanski A. Dynamic changes of cerebral oxygenation measured by brain tissue oxygen pressure and near infrared spectroscopy. Neurol Res. 1997;19(3):246–8.
36. Budohoski KP, Zweifel C, Kasprowicz M, Sorrentino E, Diedler J, Brady KM, et al. What comes first? The dynamics of cerebral oxygenation and blood flow in response to changes in arterial pressure and intracranial pressure after head injury. Br J Anaesth. 2012;108(1):89–99.
37. Weigl W, Milej D, Gerega A, Toczylowska B, Kacprzak M, Sawosz P, et al. Assessment of cerebral perfusion in post-traumatic brain injury patients with the use of ICG-bolus tracking method. NeuroImage. 2014;85(Pt 1):555–65.
38. Shafer R, Brown A, Taylor C. Correlation between cerebral blood flow and oxygen saturation in patients with subarachnoid hemorrhage and traumatic brain injury. J Neurointerv Surg. 2011;3(4):395–8.

39. Kim MN, Durduran T, Frangos S, Edlow BL, Buckley EM, Moss HE, et al. Noninvasive measurement of cerebral blood flow and blood oxygenation using near-infrared and diffuse correlation spectroscopies in critically brain-injured adults. Neurocrit Care. 2010;12(2):173–80.
40. Yoo KY, Baek HY, Jeong S, Hallacoglu B, Lee J. Intravenously administered indocyanine green may cause falsely high near-infrared cerebral oximetry readings. J Neurosurg Anesthesiol. 2015;27(1):57–60.
41. Hopton P, Walsh TS, Lee A. Measurement of cerebral blood volume using near-infrared spectroscopy and indocyanine green elimination. J Appl Physiol. 1999;87(5):1981–7.
42. Smielewski P, Czosnyka M, Zweifel C, Brady K, Hogue C, Steiner L, et al. Multicentre experience of using ICM+ for investigations of cerebrovascular dynamics with near-infrared spectroscopy. Crit Care. 2010;14(Suppl 1):P348.
43. Steiner LA, Pfister D, Strebel SP, Radolovich D, Smielewski P, Czosnyka M. Near-infrared spectroscopy can monitor dynamic cerebral autoregulation in adults. Neurocrit Care. 2009;10(1):122–8.
44. Highton D, Ghosh A, Tachtsidis I, Panovska-Griffiths J, Elwell CE, Smith M. Monitoring cerebral autoregulation after brain injury: multimodal assessment of cerebral slow-wave oscillations using near-infrared spectroscopy. Anesth Analg. 2015;121(1):198–205.
45. Zweifel C, Castellani G, Czosnyka M, Helmy A, Manktelow A, Carrera E, et al. Noninvasive monitoring of cerebrovascular reactivity with near infrared spectroscopy in head-injured patients. J Neurotrauma. 2010;27(11):1951–8.
46. Zuluaga MT, Esch ME, Cvijanovich NZ, Gupta N, McQuillen PS. Diagnosis influences response of cerebral near infrared spectroscopy to intracranial hypertension in children. Pediatr Crit Care Med. 2010;11(4):514–22.
47. Muellner T, Schramm W, Kwasny O, Vécsei V. Patients with increased intracranial pressure cannot be monitored using near infrared spectroscopy. Br J Neurosurg. 1998;12(2):136–9.
48. Kontos AP, Huppert TJ, Beluk NH, Elbin RJ, Henry LC, French J, et al. Brain activation during neurocognitive testing using functional near-infrared spectroscopy in patients following concussion compared to healthy controls. Brain Imaging Behav. 2014;8(4):621–34.
49. Hibino S, Mase M, Shirataki T, Nagano Y, Fukagawa K, Abe A, et al. Oxyhemoglobin changes during cognitive rehabilitation after traumatic brain injury using near infrared spectroscopy. Neurol Med Chir. 2013;53(5):299–303.
50. Rodriguez Merzagora AC, Izzetoglu M, Onaral B, Schultheis MT. Verbal working memory impairments following traumatic brain injury: an fNIRS investigation. Brain Imaging Behav. 2014;8(3):446–59.
51. Sirois S, Brisson J. Pupillometry. Wiley Interdiscip Rev Cogn Sci. 2014;5(6):679–92.
52. Meeker M, Du R, Bacchetti P, Privitera CM, Larson MD, Holland MC, et al. Pupil examination: validity and clinical utility of an automated pupillometer. J Neurosci Nurs. 2005;37(1):34–40.
53. Witting MD, Goyal D. Interrater reliability in pupillary measurement. Ann Emerg Med. 2003;41(6):832–7.
54. Couret D, Boumaza D, Grisotto C, Triglia T, Pellegrini L, Ocquidant P, et al. Reliability of standard pupillometry practice in neurocritical care: an observational, double-blinded study. Crit Care. 2016;20:99.
55. Taylor WR, Chen JW, Meltzer H, Gennarelli TA, Kelbch C, Knowlton S, et al. Quantitative pupillometry, a new technology: normative data and preliminary observations in patients with acute head injury. Technical note. J Neurosurg. 2003;98(1):205–13.
56. Nyholm B, Obling L, Hassager C, Grand J, Møller J, Othman M, et al. Superior reproducibility and repeatability in automated quantitative pupillometry compared to standard manual assessment, and quantitative pupillary response parameters present high reliability in critically ill cardiac patients. PLoS One. 2022;17(7):e0272303.
57. McGrath LB, Eaton J, Abecassis IJ, Maxin A, Kelly C, Chesnut RM, et al. Mobile smartphone-based digital pupillometry curves in the diagnosis of traumatic brain injury. Front Neurosci. 2022;16:893711.

58. Larson MD, Behrends M. Portable infrared pupillometry: a review. Anesth Analg. 2015;120(6):1242–53.
59. Hall CA, Chilcott RP. Eyeing up the future of the pupillary light reflex in neurodiagnostics. Diagnostics. 2018;8(1):19.
60. Ellis CJ. The pupillary light reflex in normal subjects. Br J Ophthalmol. 1981;65(11):754–9.
61. Shoyombo I, Aiyagari V, Stutzman SE, Atem F, Hill M, Figueroa SA, et al. Understanding the relationship between the neurologic pupil index and constriction velocity values. Sci Rep. 2018;8(1):6992.
62. Chen JW, Gombart ZJ, Rogers S, Gardiner SK, Cecil S, Bullock RM. Pupillary reactivity as an early indicator of increased intracranial pressure: The introduction of the Neurological Pupil index. Surg Neurol Int. 2011;2:82.
63. McCrary JA 3rd. Pupil in clinical diagnosis. Light reflex anatomy and the afferent pupil defect. Trans Sect Ophthalmol Am Acad Ophthalmol Otolaryngol. 1977;83(5):820–6.
64. Belliveau AP, Somani AN, Dossani RH. Pupillary light reflex. In: StatPearls. Treasure Island: StatPearls Publishing; 2023.
65. Bista Karki S, Coppell KJ, Mitchell LV, Ogbuehi KC. Dynamic pupillometry in type 2 diabetes: pupillary autonomic dysfunction and the severity of diabetic retinopathy. Clin Ophthalmol. 2020;14:3923–30.
66. Panchal AR, Bartos JA, Cabañas JG, Donnino MW, Drennan IR, Hirsch KG, et al. Part 3: adult basic and advanced life support: 2020 American Heart Association Guidelines for Cardiopulmonary Resuscitation and Emergency Cardiovascular Care. Circulation. 2020;142(16):S366–468.
67. Tamura T, Namiki J, Sugawara Y, Sekine K, Yo K, Kanaya T, et al. Quantitative assessment of pupillary light reflex for early prediction of outcomes after out-of-hospital cardiac arrest: a multicentre prospective observational study. Resuscitation. 2018;131:108–13.
68. Phillips SS, Mueller CM, Nogueira RG, Khalifa YM. A systematic review assessing the current state of automated pupillometry in the NeuroICU. Neurocrit Care. 2019;31(1):142–61.
69. Giede-Jeppe A, Sprügel MI, Huttner HB, Borutta M, Kuramatsu JB, Hoelter P, et al. Automated pupillometry identifies absence of intracranial pressure elevation in intracerebral hemorrhage patients. Neurocrit Care. 2021;35(1):210–20.
70. Morris GF, Juul N, Marshall SB, Benedict B, Marshall LF. Neurological deterioration as a potential alternative endpoint in human clinical trials of experimental pharmacological agents for treatment of severe traumatic brain injuries. Executive Committee of the International Selfotel Trial. Neurosurgery. 1998;43(6):1369–72; discussion 72-4.
71. Choi SC, Narayan RK, Anderson RL, Ward JD. Enhanced specificity of prognosis in severe head injury. J Neurosurg. 1988;69(3):381–5.
72. Park JG, Moon CT, Park DS, Song SW. Clinical utility of an automated pupillometer in patients with acute brain lesion. J Korean Neurosurg Soc. 2015;58(4):363–7.
73. Chesnut RM, Gautille T, Blunt BA, Klauber MR, Marshall LE. The localizing value of asymmetry in pupillary size in severe head injury: relation to lesion type and location. Neurosurgery. 1994;34(5):840–5; discussion 5-6.
74. Manley GT, Larson MD. Infrared pupillometry during uncal herniation. J Neurosurg Anesthesiol. 2002;14(3):223–8.
75. Oddo M, Taccone F, Galimberti S, Rebora P, Citerio G. Outcome prognostication of acute brain injury using the neurological pupil index (ORANGE) study: protocol for a prospective, observational, multicentre, international cohort study. BMJ Open. 2021;11(5):e046948.
76. Joseph JR, Swallow JS, Willsey K, Almeida AA, Lorincz MT, Fraumann RK, et al. Pupillary changes after clinically asymptomatic high-acceleration head impacts in high school football athletes. J Neurosurg. 2019;133(6):1886–91.
77. Master CL, Podolak OE, Ciuffreda KJ, Metzger KB, Joshi NR, McDonald CC, et al. Utility of pupillary light reflex metrics as a physiologic biomarker for adolescent sport-related concussion. JAMA Ophthalmol. 2020;138(11):1135–41.

78. Fischer VE, Boulter JH, Bell RS, Ikeda DS. Paradoxical contralateral herniation detected by pupillometry in acute syndrome of the trephined. Mil Med. 2020;185(3-4):532–6.
79. Al-Obaidi SZ, Atem FD, Stutzman SE, Olson DM. Impact of increased intracranial pressure on pupillometry: a replication study. Crit Care Explor. 2019;1(10):e0054.
80. Olson DM, Stutzman SE, Atem F, Kincaide JD, Ho TT, Carlisle BA, et al. Establishing normative data for pupillometer assessment in neuroscience intensive care: The "END-PANIC" registry. J Neurosci Nurs. 2017;49(4):251–4.
81. Taylor LA, Kreutzer JS, Demm SR, Meade MA. Traumatic brain injury and substance abuse: a review and analysis of the literature. Neuropsychol Rehabil. 2003;13(1-2):165–88.
82. Ong C, Hutch M, Barra M, Kim A, Zafar S, Smirnakis S. Effects of osmotic therapy on pupil reactivity: quantification using pupillometry in critically ill neurologic patients. Neurocrit Care. 2019;30(2):307–15.
83. Osman M, Stutzman SE, Atem F, Olson D, Hicks AD, Ortega-Perez S, et al. Correlation of objective pupillometry to midline shift in acute stroke patients. J Stroke Cerebrovasc Dis. 2019;28(7):1902–10.
84. El Ahmadieh TY, Bedros N, Stutzman SE, Nyancho D, Venkatachalam AM, MacAllister M, et al. Automated pupillometry as a triage and assessment tool in patients with traumatic brain injury. World Neurosurg. 2021;145:163–9.
85. Singer KE, Wallen TE, Jalbert T, Wakefield D, Spuzzillo A, Sharma S, et al. Efficacy of noninvasive technologies in triaging traumatic brain injury and correlating with intracranial pressure: a prospective study. J Surg Res. 2021;262:27–37.
86. Lukaszewicz AC, Dereu D, Gayat E, Payen D. The relevance of pupillometry for evaluation of analgesia before noxious procedures in the intensive care unit. Anesth Analg. 2015;120(6):1297–300.
87. Connelly MA, Brown JT, Kearns GL, Anderson RA, St Peter SD, Neville KA. Pupillometry: a non-invasive technique for pain assessment in paediatric patients. Arch Dis Child. 2014;99(12):1125–31.
88. Paulus J, Roquilly A, Beloeil H, Théraud J, Asehnoune K, Lejus C. Pupillary reflex measurement predicts insufficient analgesia before endotracheal suctioning in critically ill patients. Crit Care. 2013;17(4):R161.
89. Rouche O, Wolak-Thierry A, Destoop Q, Milloncourt L, Floch T, Raclot P, et al. Evaluation of the depth of sedation in an intensive care unit based on the photo motor reflex variations measured by video pupillometry. Ann Intensive Care. 2013;3(1):5.

9 Brain Ultrasonography

Gritti Paolo, Briolini Andrea, Chiara Robba, Rita Bertuetti, and Nicola Zugni

9.1 Introduction

Ultrasonography (US) has revolutionized monitoring in both acute and chronic clinical settings mostly because of its bedside applicability non-invasiveness, repeatability, low cost, no radiation risk and well tolerated by patients [1]. Even if it does not replace advanced static imaging exams, it adds dynamic information without displace patient from Intensive Care Unit (ICU), representing a bridge between clinical examination and other expensive and/or invasive methods [2, 3].

In the beginning of echographic era, brain US (BUS), was not considered feasible because intact skull was seen as a seemingly impenetrable obstacle; the first historical BUS was performed in 1942 by Karl Theodor Dussik, in Austria [2]. However, in 1952, Guttner et al. showed that Dussik method was of no value because of great absorption and reflection of US waves by the bone structure. In the following years, BUS was partially abandoned until the end of 1970s, when two-dimensional B-mode imaging was applied in young children to visualize the cerebral parenchyma through fontanels [1, 4, 5].

Actually, for BUS there are two main techniques: "blind" Transcranial Doppler (TCD) and Transcranial Color-Coded duplex Doppler Sonography (TCCD), both over 4 main acoustic windows (Fig. 9.1):

G. Paolo (✉) · B. Andrea
Neurointensive Care Unit, Department of Anaesthesia and Critical Care Medicine, Papa Giovanni XXIII Hospital, Bergamo, Italy

C. Robba
IRCCS, Policlinico San Martino, Genova, Italy

Department of Surgical Sciences and Diagnostic Integrated, University of Genoa, Genoa, Italy

R. Bertuetti · N. Zugni
Department of Aneasthesia, Intensive Care and Emergency Medicine, ASST Spedali Civili di Brescia University Hospital, Brescia, Italy

E. Brogi et al. (eds.), *Traumatic Brain Injury*, Hot Topics in Acute Care Surgery and Trauma, https://doi.org/10.1007/978-3-031-50117-3_9

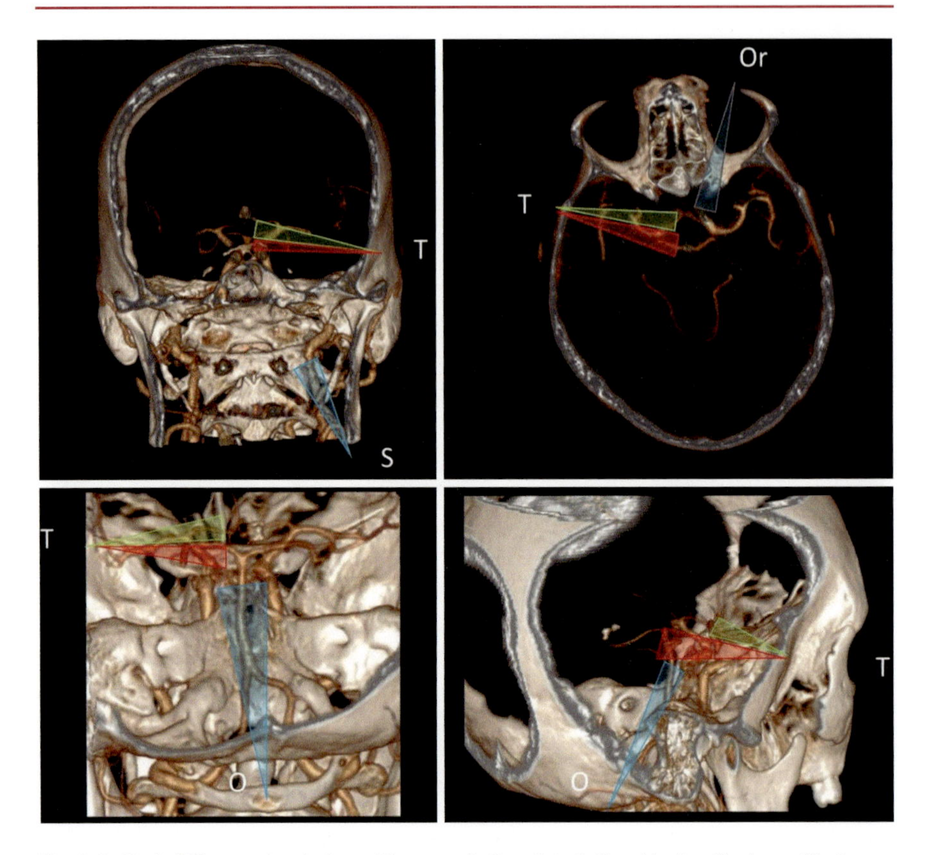

Fig. 9.1 Brain US acoustic windows. *T* temporal, *O* occipital, *Or* orbicular, *S* submandibular

- Transorbital;
- Transtemporal; the most important, correlates with pterion (the thinnest part of skull); junction of greater wing of sphenoid bone, squamous portion of temporal bone, frontal and parietal bone. It is clinically found cephalad to zygomatic arch and anterior to ear;
- Occipital-foramen magnum;
- Submandibular.

Patients who have had decompressive craniectomy or children with open fontanelle have additional bone-free acoustic windows [1, 4].

Although BUS is relatively easy technique, it is characterized by some important limitations such as necessity of patent transcranial acoustic windows and operator skillness acquired through knowledge of the various landmarks, parameters and especially through hands-on training and practice. In approximately 20% of patients, worst in aged woman, it is not possible to find transtemporal window. Recently an expert consensus agreement on how to define general skill recommendations and competency levels for BUS examination within the neurocritical care setting has been produced [3].

9.1.1 Transcranial Doppler (TCD)

TCD was codified in 1982 by Rune Aaslid at University of Berne, (Switzerland) and introduced into clinical practice in 1986, enabling the recording of blood velocities from intracranial arteries through insonation of low-frequency Pulsed Doppler (PD) waves of 2 MHz, Echoes reflected with different frequency—the Doppler shift, directly proportional to velocity of the object- are received by transducer probe and processed to produce a spectral waveform based on insonation depth, angle, and direction of blood flow, permitting artery identification and Cerebral Blood Flow (CBF) velocities analysis [1].

Conventionally, flows that move toward or away from transducer have respectively positive and negative directions of spectrograms. Newer US machines have colour M-Mode capabilities for easier detection of flow: red if moves toward transducer, blue if moves away [6].

The main TCD basic parameters are:

- Flow velocities:
  - Peak systolic velocity (SV)
  - Diastolic velocity (DV)
  - Mean velocity (MV)

CBF is equal to product of MV and Cross-Sectional Area (CSA); if CSA is normal and constant, CBF will be mainly dependent on MV, thus it can be considered a CBF surrogate. However, when CSA is reduced as in atherosclerotic stenosis or cerebral vasospasm, increase in MV is necessary to maintain CBF although is neither interchangeable nor surrogate of CBF, because cerebral perfusion down the stenosis can be critically compromised. Factors affecting MV are age, Cerebral Perfusion Pressure (CPP), haematocrit, core body temperature, arousal, pain and inflammation (e.g., meningitis) and it is paramount to perform TCD with mean arterial pressure (MAP) at least 60 mmHg, normal arterial blood gases (e.g. $PaCO_2$), core temperature normal, and appropriate sedation level [6]. Some other TCD derived indices frequently used to assess the resistance in the cerebrovascular system are the Gosling's pulsatility index:

$$P.I. = \frac{SV - DV}{MV} \tag{9.1}$$

SV peak systolic velocity, *DV* diastolic velocity, *MV* mean velocity.

The resistive index:

$$R.I. = \frac{SV - DV}{SV} \tag{9.2}$$

SV peak systolic velocity, *DV* diastolic velocity, *MV* mean velocity.

Velocities are dependent on insonation angle while Doppler indices are not, thus latest are preferable when velocities are not accurate (e.g., large insonation angles, like more than 30°) [5].

Factors that can modify Doppler velocities, mean velocities and indices are reported in Table 9.1.

Table 9.1 TCD/TCCD features and factors affecting TCD velocities and Doppler indices [4, 5]

TCD/TCCD features					Factors affecting TCD	
	TCD					
Windows	Settings	Vessels and depth (mm)	Flow direction and MV (cm/s)	TCCD main structures	Velocities	Doppler indices
Transtemporal	Depth 50–56 mm range 30–75 mm	MCA, 30–60 ACA, 60–80 MCA/ACA, 60–65 PCA p1, 60–70 PCA p2, 60–70 TICA, 55–65	Towards, 55 ± 12 Away, 50 ± 11 Bidirectional, 39 ± 10 Towards, 40 ± 10 Away, 39 ± 10 towards	Mesencephalic and diencephalic structures + circle of Willis – Mesencephalic plane: identification of controlateral skull and midbrain ("butterfly shape") – Diencephalic plane: from mesencephalic, beam cranial tilt approximately 10° allows third ventricle identification (two pulsating parallel lines slightly more cranial and anterior to midbrain) – Ventricular plane: further cranial tilting allows thalami and lateral ventricles frontal horns visualization	*Increase* – Reduced vessel area (e.g. vasospasm, atherosclerotic stenosis) – Hypoxemia – Hypercapnia – Hyperemia – Arterial hypertension – Hypertermia	*Increase* – Intracranial hypertension – Hypocapnia – Chronic arterial hypertension

TCD/TCCD features					Factors affecting TCD	
	TCD					
Windows	Settings	Vessels and depth (mm)	Flow direction and MV (cm/s)	TCCD main structures	Velocities	Doppler indices
Transorbital	Decrease power to minimum depth 50–52 mm range 40–80 mm	OA, 40–60 CS, 60–80	Towards, 21 ± 5 Bidirectional, 45 ± 15	Ophthalmic artery, CS and optic nerve sheath	*Decrease* – Advanced age – Low cardiac output – Arterial hypotension – Hypotermia – Sedative medications (not volatile anesthetics)	*Decrease* – Distal vasodilatation down to stenosis – Hypercapnia – Hyperemia
Suboccipital	Full power depth 75 mm	VA, 60–90 BA, 80–120	Away, 38 ± 10 Away, 41 ± 10	Foramen magnum, vertebral arteries and BA distal segments		
Submandibular	Depth 50 mm range 30–50 mm	ICA, 40–50	Away, 37 ± 8	ICA extracranial portion for Lindegaard Index calculation (mean flow velocity ratio between MCA and ICA)		

ACA anterior cerebral artery, *BA* basilar artery, *CS* carotid siphon, *ICA* internal carotid artery, *MCA* middle cerebral artery, *MV* mean velocities, *PCA* posterior cerebral artery (p1: first segment; p2: second segment), *TICA* terminal internal carotid artery, *VA* vertebral artery

9.1.2 How to Perform Transcranial Doppler (TCD)

Although the main technique involved to perform a complete TCD exams is not the current aim of this chapter, a simple example of blind exploration with a 2 MHz probe can start from the Transtemporal window where Middle Cerebral Artery (MCA) could be found at 50 mm depth, searching a toward flow to probe corresponding to main segment (M1) of MCA. Internal Carotid Artery (ICA) bifurcation and Anterior Cerebral Artery (ACA) where find set up 65 mm depth as a bidirectional flow (positive/negative) corresponding to ICA bifurcation into MCA and ACA. Moving the transducer slightly cephalad and anterior consent to insonate the first segment (A1) of ACA, which flow directed away from probe.

Carotid Siphon (CS) and Posterior Cerebral Artery (PCA) where funded returning to ICA bifurcation without changing depth and with slightly caudal angulation for register CS flow moving toward the transducer. From ICA bifurcation, orientating the probe slightly posterior and caudal at 70 mm depth, should be revealed first segment (P1) of PCA flow toward the probe. At 80 mm depth P2 flow is normally registered, moving away from transducer.

Through the Transorbital window, CS is found at 80 mm depth with flow toward or toward/away from probe. Ophthalmic artery (OA) is normally located at 40 mm depth with flow toward transducer and has high-resistance velocity profile, differently from intracranial arteries. Place the probe through the Transforaminal window and aim at the bridge of the noise is possible to detect at 75 mm depth the terminal of both vertebral artery (VA) and the begin of the basilar artery (BA).

For Submandibular approach the position of the probe is laterally under the jaw, anterior and medial to sternocleidomastoid, with transducer aims upwards and slightly medially; dept is set at 50 mm and range at 30–50 mm; ICA will be found at 40–50 mm depth [5].

9.1.3 Transcranial Color-Coded Duplex Doppler Sonography (TCCD)

TCCD combines Doppler pulse wave technology with B-mode, which is 2-dimensional imaging of parenchymal structures. The main advantages over blind TCD are an easier identification of intracranial vessels, in relation to pivotal anatomic landmarks and the visualization of brain anatomy and potential pathological states, like mass-occupying lesions, brain midline shift (BMLS), hydrocephalus and others (Fig. 9.2) [1, 5].

TCCD uses the same transducers and equipment of focused echocardiography (cardiac 3–5 MHz probe), however in paediatric patients or small adults population optimal imaging may be possible using higher frequency probes [7]. The TCCD use is very practical in various settings and situations as in acute ischemic stroke, non-invasive estimation of ICP and BMLS evaluation in Intracranial Haemorrhage (ICH) or other intracranial lesions such as tumor, abscess, and advanced brain edema, ICP and CBF monitoring in Traumatic Brain Injury (TBI) and Subarachnoid

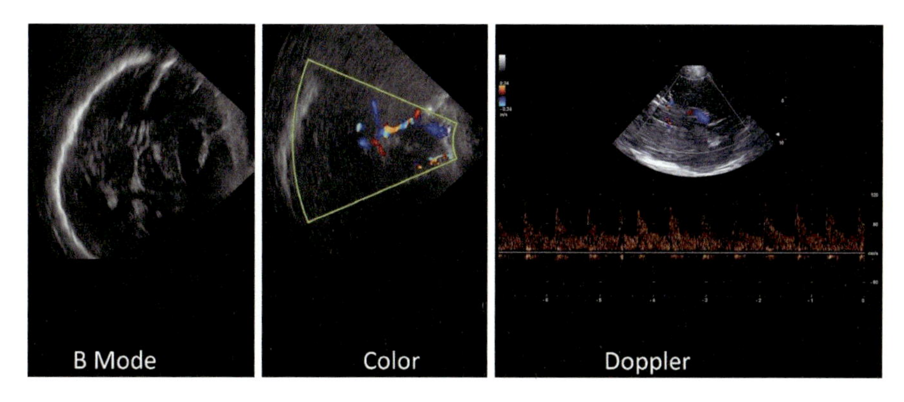

Fig. 9.2 TCCD, color and B-mode. TCCD combines B-mode with Doppler pulse wave technology. The B-mode imaging displays 2-dimensional image of skull, brain and blood vessels as seen by ultrasound probe. Once the desired blood vessel is found with the color function

Haemorrhage (SAH). Finally, the use of TCCD could be performed in the setting of clinical diagnosis of Brain Death (BD) [1, 5].

More advanced techniques such as contrast-enhanced and three-dimensional TCCD are available but have not been used widely in clinical settings as yet.

9.1.4 TCCD Basic Parameters and Practical Use

In addition at the traditional TCD basic parameters, TCCD consent to correct electronically the insonation angle, thus obtaining more accurate and higher velocities. Moreover, the use of MicroVascularization (MicroV) technology, based on signal amplitude width algorithm for achieve higher morphological resolution, consent to improve representation of vessel morphology in comparison to conventional CD allowing a furthered examination of Circle of Willis (like for anastomotic vessels through anterior or posterior communicating arteries) and improved assessments of intracranial stenosis (Fig. 9.3) [8].

The TCCD exams start, as for the TCD, from the traditional windows.

9.1.4.1 Transtemporal Window

From the transtemporal window maintaining index mark pointed towards patient's anterior/front, starts the brain exploration through three plans: mesencephalic and diencephalic (commonly used for vascular diagnosis, because located the Circle of Willis) and ventricular (Fig. 9.3).

The procedure must be performed for each hemisphere.

Mesencephalic Plane:

- Start identifying ipsilateral/contralateral temporal bones and third ventricle (midline structure).

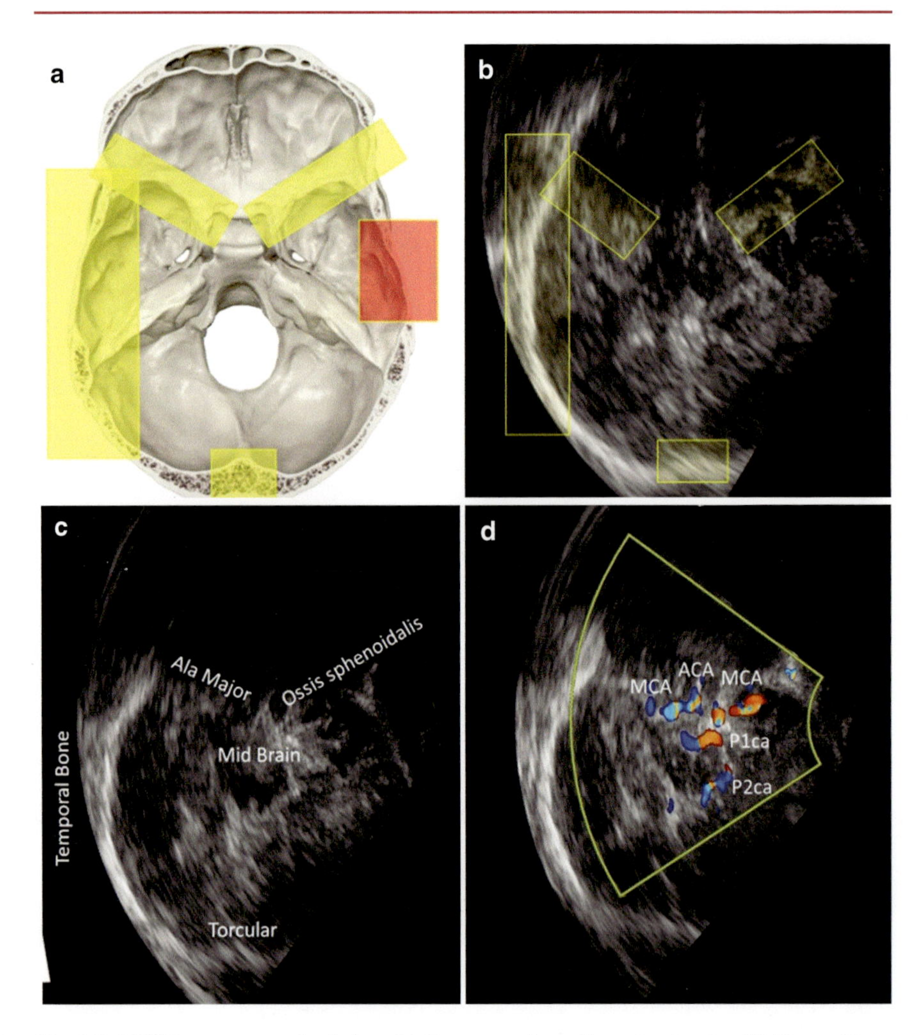

Fig. 9.3 TCCD transtemporal window. (**a**) Representation of bone landmarks. (**b**) View of bone landmarks in brain US. (**c**) Relationship between bone landmarks, midbrain and confluence of sinuses. (**d**) Circle of Willis insonation. *MCA* medium cerebral artery, *ACA* anterior

- Decrease depth to third ventricle in far-field and recognized mesencephalic plane by butterfly-shaped hypoechoic cerebral peduncles surrounded by hyperechoic star-shaped basal cisterns, forming an overall heart-shape form.
- MCA analysis: place Color Doppler box over top-half screen (near field) just lateral to cerebral peduncles. Identify MCA by red coded zone, then obtain waveform through Pulse Wave Doppler with assistance of insonation angle correction. M1 segment obtained at 50 mm depth and M2 at 40 mm depth. Most distal sampleable point is proximal ICA bifurcation (red coded) into MCA and ACA, useful in focal vasospasm screen.

- ACA analysis: anterior angulation of probe with 6–7 cm depth; A1-precommunicating segment is normally blue coded. Accurate view of Anterior Communicating Artery is not feasible because of its short length.
- PCA analysis: posterior angulation of probe with 55–75 mm depth; P1-precommunicating segment is normally red coded and P2-postcommunicating segment blue coded. Posterior Communicating Artery is infrequently seen because of its perpendicular course to insonation angle and frequently hypoplastic (50% of cases).

Diencephalic Plane:
- Angulating the transducer 10° cephalad and recognized it by two centrals hyperechoic lines corresponding to third ventricle, with hypoechoic thalami on each side and hyperechoic pineal gland on the right

Ventricular Plane:
- With further cephalad angulation, the plane is demarcated by frontal horns of lateral ventricles [9].

9.1.4.2 Transorbitary Window

Using high-frequency linear probe it is shows anechoic ocular globe and echogenic retrobulbar area, with possibility for Optic Nerve Sheath Diameter (ONSD) measurement as non-invasive ICP assessment.

Moreover, a vascular evaluation consents the identification of Carotid Siphon (CS) at 80 mm depth, Ophthalmic Artery (OA) at 40 mm depth and red-coded, a terminal ICA branch that passes over Optic Nerve (ON) and supplies ocular globe circulation with important anastomoses from ipsilateral ECA, relevant in cases of ipsilateral ICA obstruction. This approach also permits Central Retinal Artery (CRA, an OA branch within ON) evaluation, important when its occlusion is suspected (with presentation of acute painless monocular blindness).

Images must be obtained at reduced power output with mechanical index not exceeding 0.23 for increased theoretical safety (risks of capillary bleeding for values exceeding this threshold) [10].

9.1.4.3 Transforaminal Window

Allows Posterior Cerebral Circulation (PCC) assessment: transducer is positioned over upper neck at base of skull, angled cephalad toward the nose, with probe indicator to right. Anatomical reference landmark is foramen magnum, a central hypoechoic structure; Color Doppler shows an inside "v-shaped" coded blue, corresponding to intracranial segment of Vertebral Arteries (VAs) extend cephalad to constitute Basilar Artery (BA).

9.1.4.4 Submandibular Window

Assessment of distal extracranial ICA, with lowest Nyquist level selected (~20 cm/s) and probe indicator directed anteriorly: ICA is commonly posterolateral to

ECA (both blude-coded) and, differently from this latter, lacks of cervical branches and has low-resistance velocity profile [1, 4, 10].

9.1.5 Altered Anatomy: Intracranial Haemorrhage, Hydrocephalus and Midline Shift

9.1.5.1 Intracranial Haemorrhage

TCCD allows identification of both supratentorial and infratentorial Intracerebral Haemorrhage (ICH) and indirect assessment of intracranial hypertension and mass effect (Fig. 9.4).

It could be part of multimodal diagnosis and monitoring process of ICH: after initial CT scan, a baseline TCCD could be performed analyzing the hematoma volume (independently associated with early neurological deterioration and mortality) and Cerebral Blood Flow (CBF) doppler, then repeated regularly to evaluate early hematoma expansion, a strong determinant of mortality and poor outcome [9, 11]. CT angiography spot sign may predict hematoma expansion, but CT information's are static and frequent studies are not practical in these patients, mostly in ICU admitted [12].

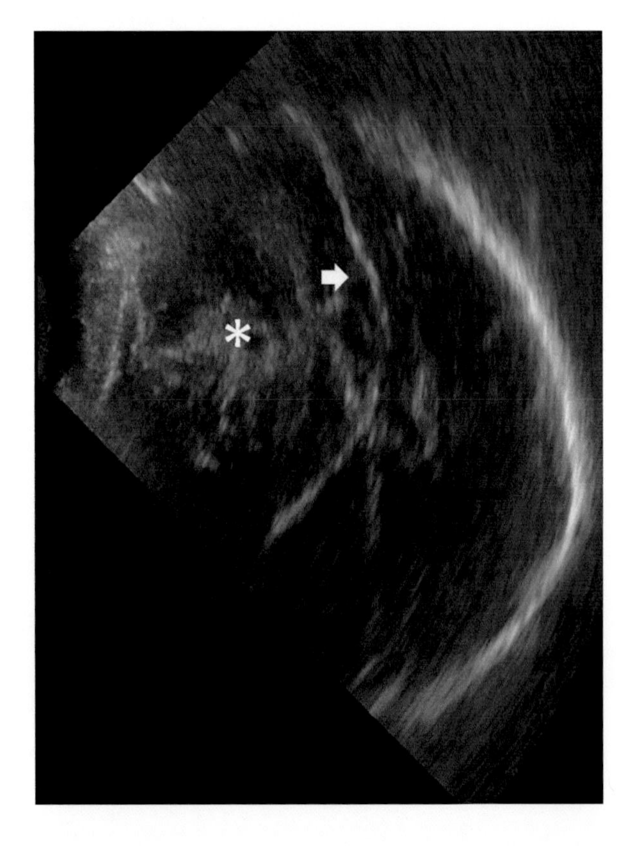

Fig. 9.4 Large spontaneous ICH of right hemisphere (*). To note right to left brain shift (white arrow)

TCCD ICH detection sensitivity and specificity are respectively 94% and 95%, with positive predictive value of 91% and negative of 95%; detection of extra-axial hematomas was 88% in one study [1]; early monitoring in first 7 days from ICH showing good correlation between TCCD and CT measurements [11]. A recent study showed that in decompressive craniectomy TCCD was as effective as CT assessing hyperdense focal lesions, other than Midline Shift (MLS), ventricular system dimensions and position of ventricular monitoring catheters [13]. Both intra/extra-axial hematomas are initially seen as hyperechoic masses demarcated from brain parenchyma; after about 5 days they become hypoechoic, surrounded by hyperechoic halo [11]. Volume hematoma and its expansion can be evaluated using the same CT equation for ICH volume estimation:

$$\frac{A \cdot B \cdot C}{2} \tag{9.3}$$

where A is the greatest haemorrhage diameter by CT, B the largest diameter 90° to A on the same slice, C the approximate number of 10-mm slices on which ICH was seen [14].

TCCD limitations for ICH analysis are a lack of specificity for hyperechoic Ultrasound (US) lesions, that may also be caused by arteriovenous malformations or tumours, so initial CT scan is required to confirm ICH diagnosis; moreover hematomas could not be visible within transtemporal window, the most common approach, leading to the risk of misdiagnosis.

TCCD can evaluate hematoma per se, but also give functional information about ICH repercussions on cerebral hemodynamic. Pulsatility Index (PI) strongly reflects the increased flow resistance downstream and elevated values can be used as surrogate marker of cerebral hemodynamic compromise due to intracranial hypertension, allowing non-invasive Intracranial Pressure (ICP) estimation; as ICP increase, Cerebral Perfusion Pressure (CPP) decrease causing diastolic and mean CBF decreasing and PI increasing [2, 15]; furthermore hematoma expansion could be predicted monitoring PI ratios of unaffected hemisphere. Impaired Cerebral Autoregulation (CA) is associated with larger hematoma volumes, signs of elevated ICP and worse outcomes; when detected with TCCD, patients require stricter Blood Pressure (BP) control. Finally, Optical Nerve Sheath Diameter (ONSD) measurement can identify increased ICP hematoma-related, generally expected for hematomas larger than 25 ml [2].

9.1.5.2 Hydrocephalus

Hydrocephalus is a common complication of subarachnoid hemorrhage (SAH), occurring up to 30% of patient, but can also presents in ICH or mass lesions of posterior fossa, in acute meningeal diseases and as NCH complication [2, 16].

Non-invasive bedside monitoring of ventricular system could be useful in disturbances of cerebrospinal fluid (CSF) circulation, first when clinical examination is not feasible (patient comatose or sedated) and CSF spaces appear anechoic, surrounded by hyperechoic borders of cerebral ventricles. However, in adults only partial evaluation of ventricular system can be realized, due to cranial sutures, [13] and the correlation between TCCD and CT measurements is higher for third ventricle rather than for lateral ones because ventricle diameters depend on probe orientation angle [2]. Otherwise in fetus and newborn the entire ventricular system is analysable through fontanelles, so TCCD is mostly used in paediatric population, additionally taking advantage of X-ray sparing method, for ventricular size measurement, indirect ICP monitoring, decrease of intracranial compliance analysis and follow up of shunts in patients with hydrocephalus [17].

In patient underwent decompressive craniectomy the entire ventricular system is analysable with different probe and quality (Fig. 9.5).

Moreover, TCCD can be used in hypertensive hydrocephalus to evaluate flow velocity alterations of intracranial cerebral arteries, resistivity index (RI) or PI and could help to predict the need for External Ventricular Drain (EVD) insertion and for safe EVD removal after a clamping trial with high sensitivity and negative predictive value (both 100%) and 83% specificity [2, 16, 18]: an increase in lateral ventricular width lower than cut-of value (5.5 mm) after 24 h from clamping is a good indication for safe removal. An acoustic window can also be used as a guide for insertion or repositioning of ventricular catheter during ventriculostomy, shown to help reduce multiple attempts and confirm correct placement, especially in patients with distorted anatomy [19].

Hydrocephalus assessment in adults is done at diencephalic plane, viewing third ventricle, and measuring the largest transverse diameter from inner-to-inner borders; normal size may vary with age (<60 years: 1.2–5.1 mm; >60 years: 3.3–9.2 mm) but in absence of hydrocephalus third ventricle is often fairly small visible as two parallel hyperechoic ventricular walls.

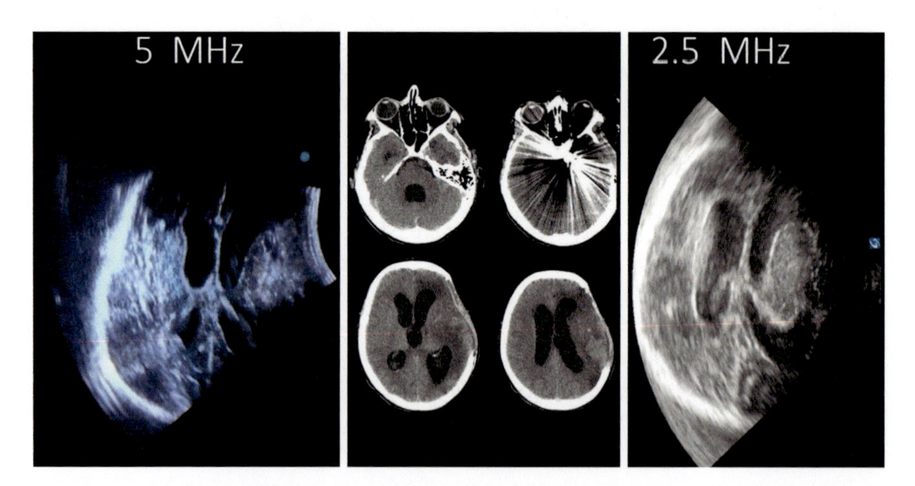

Fig. 9.5 Transtemporal window in decompressive craniectomy patients and hydrocephalus. Visualization of all ventricular system with better resolution using higher frequency probe (5 MHz convex vs 2.5 MHz cardiac probe); CT brain scan in the center of the figure

9.1.5.3 Midline Shift

Any amount of Midline Shift (MLS) is abnormal, but poor neurological outcome is associated with "clinically significant" MLS, defined as size >0.5 cm on CT imaging (gold standard technique); it can be caused by severe Traumatic Brain Injury (TBI), stroke and haemorrhage (extradural, subdural or intracerebral).

Early MLS detection is thus very important because allows implementation of appropriate treatment plan and for MLS > 0.5 cm surgical evacuation is recommended; if CT scan is not immediately available in a patient with deteriorating neurological status, TCCD could be a feasible bedside item for monitoring MLS and mass effect, showing positive and satisfying correlation with CT-MLS albeit US-MLS measurement relies heavily on finding a proper transtemporal window [18, 20, 21], and has the tendency to slightly underestimate the measure, including patients submitted to decompressive craniectomy: US-MLS > 0.35 cm predicts CT-MLS > 0.5 cm with good sensitivity, specificity and positive likelihood ratio of more than 5 [20, 21].

There are not data correlating angle of insonation and accuracy of US-MLS measurements, but 2012 AIUM guidelines state that upward angle should be no greater than 10–15°, even that may not always be possible [18]. Presence of third ventricle hydrocephalus does not condition MLS measurement, because done to the centre of ventricle, not to its outer walls [17].

US-MLS measurements begin on diencephalic plane through temporal window, with identification of ipsilateral and contralateral bone table and third ventricle (double hyperechogenic line over midbrain). There are two methods to quantify MLS [18, 22]:

- Measure distance from external bone table to the center of third ventricle; distance A from ipsilateral side, B from contralateral side; equation used to calculate MLS deviation is:

$$\text{MLS} = \frac{\text{distance A} - \text{distance B}}{2} \tag{9.4}$$

Distance A: from ipsilateral side. Distance B: from controlateral side.

This technique has good correlation with CT values and is the least vulnerable to operator error; however, accuracy is limited with decompressive craniectomy.

- For expedited investigation, measure from ipsilateral side to third ventricle (distance A) and the full distance of ipsilateral-contralateral temporal bone (distance D), using the formula: distance A – (distance D/2)

$$\text{MLS} = \text{distance A} - \frac{\text{distance D}}{2} \tag{9.5}$$

Distance D: full distance of ipsilateral-contralateral temporal bone. Distance A: from the center of third ventricle to ipsilateral side.

With either method, if result number is positive the MLS is away from ipsilateral side, if negative the MLS is toward.

9.2 Vasospasm

Different pathological conditions, like aneurismatic subarachnoid hemorrhage (aSAH), are complicated by severe narrowing of main cerebral arteries; however, also head injury patients with traumatic SAH may develop cerebral vasospasm (it occurs in up to 30–40% of the patients after severe traumatic brain injury) [23].

Worldwide, 500,000 subarachnoid hemorrhages occur annually secondary to ruptured aneurysms. Incidence of SAH has been showing a deflecting curve during past recent years, however it remains high with 8 cases of spontaneous SAH per 100,000 person-year as reported in a meta-analysis including 75 studies from 32 countries [24, 25]. Fifty percent of survivors make incomplete recovery and 35% (20–50%) die [26]. Thirty percent of deaths generally occurs within 48 h of admission (26% do not arrive at the hospital or die in the emergency room [25]), 56% of deaths happens by day 7 from bleeding, and 76% by SAH day 14. The most common adjudicated primary cause of death is direct effect of the primary hemorrhage (i.e. severe cerebral hypoperfusion and elevated intracranial pressure). Vasospasm and delayed cerebral ischemia (DCI) continue to have an important impact on neurological outcome (being responsible for 5% of mortality) [26]. Angiographic vasospasm is associated with DCI, but other factors are hypothesized to contribute to DCI pathophysiology, including microcirculatory constriction, microthrombosis, cortical spreading ischemia, and delayed cell apoptosis [27].

Vasospasm is defined as narrowing of cerebral vessels resulting in reduced cerebral blood flow (CBF). Vasospasm occurs most frequently 7–10 days after aneurysm rupture and resolves spontaneously after 21 days. Only 50% of vasospasm is also clinically relevant, displaying neurological symptoms. Probably, many factors contribute to the development of ischemia and infarction including: distal microcirculatory failure, poor collateral anatomy and genetic or physiological variation in cellular ischemic tolerance [28]. Digital subtraction angiography (DSA) is the gold standard examination for diagnosis of cerebral vasospasm, nevertheless, transcranial Color Doppler (TCCD) ultrasonography finds its role in the bed side monitoring of these patients [29, 30]. Guidelines for the management of aneurysmal subarachnoid hemorrhage recommend with class IIa monitoring of vasospasm by transcranial doppler (TCD) [28].

On a TCCD examination vessel narrowing reveals itself by showing an increase in focal cerebral blood flow velocity (CBFV): according to the Bernoulli principle [31]. the pressure drop at the end of the stenotic tract is translated in an increase in the flow velocity. A flow velocity increase >25–40 cm/s and/or a 50% increase in velocity compared to baseline conditions over 24 h is considered a ringing bell for the development of vasospasm. Vasospasm in middle cerebral artery (MCA) can be classified into mild, moderate and severe based on the flow velocity increases of 80–120 cm/s, 120–200 cm/s, >200 cm/s, respectively. While a blood flow velocity >85 cm/s is considered for the diagnosis of vasospasm of the basilar artery [1, 32].

Increased flow velocities in cerebral vessels occur not only in cases of vasospasm, but also in the presence of other causes: hyperemia, increased $PaCO_2$ values, loss of autoregulation, arteriovenous malformations. Therefore, it is important to integrate the ultrasound examination with the assessment of the Lindegaard ratio: defined as the ratio of the mean FV of the MCA to mean FV of the extracranial portion of the ipsilateral Intra Cerebral Artery (ICA). A value greater than 3 indicates vasospasm, conversely, values less than 3 suggest hyperemia. For the evaluation of vasospasm in the basilar artery, a modified Lindegaard ratio (Sviri ratio) has been proposed, calculated as the ratio between the mean FV in basilar and vertebral artery [33]. A mean velocity above 85 cm/s and a Sviri ratio >3 are suggestive of vasospasm (50% occlusion) with a sensitivity of 92% and specificity of 97% [34] (Table 9.2).

Washington et al. study compared reliability of TCD with angiographic studies for diagnosis of vasospasm in different cerebral vessels and found that TCD performs best on MCA (sensitivity 38–91% and specificity 94–100%) [32, 35]. Furthermore, a 2018 meta-analysis confirmed the data obtained in the mentioned previous study and underlines that the use of TCCD rather than blind TCD improves diagnostic performance, in fact authors calculated a sensitivity and specificity averaging 81.5% (95% confidence interval [CI] 66.0–90.0) and 96.6% (95% confidence interval [CI] 93.0–98.0), respectively when using TCCD for assessment of vasospasm in MCA.

This meta-analysis also concluded that TCCD may be used to identify and follow up patients with vasospasm (high positive predictive value (PPV): 98.2% (95% confidence interval [CI] 96.4–99.1), but it should not be used to rule-out patients without vasospasm (low negative predictive value (NPV) 69.1% (95% confidence interval [CI] 56.1–80.9) [36].

As shown in the meta-analysis by Kumar et al. vasospasm diagnosed with TCCD is predictive of DCI diagnosis. Pooled estimates for TCCD diagnosis of vasospasm (for DCI) were sensitivity 90% (95% confidence interval [CI] 77–96%), specificity 71% (95% CI 51–84%), positive predictive value 57% (95% CI 38–71%), and negative predictive value 92% (95% CI 83–96%) [37] (Table 9.3).

Table 9.2 Lindegaard ratio and Sviri ratio

Vasospasm	Mean flow velocity (cm/s)	Lindegaard index or Sviri ratio
Middle cerebral artery		
Mild	80–120	3–4
Moderate	120–200	4-5
Severe	>120	>5
Basilar artery velocity		
Mild	70–80	>2
Moderate	>85	2.5–3
Severe	>85	>3

Table 9.3 Sensitivity, specificity, positive predictive value (PPV), and negative predictive value (NPP) of TCD in the detection of vasospasm in circle of Willis arteries

Vessels	Sensitivity (%)	Specificity (%)	PPV (%)	NPV (%)
Anterior cerebral artery	13–82	65–100	41–100	37–80
Middle cerebral artery	38–91	94–100	83–100	29–98
Posterior cerebral artery	48	69	37	78
Basilar artery velocity	73–76.9	79	63	88

9.3 Intracranial Pressure Estimation

Many acute brain injuries can be complicated by intracranial hypertension, if not promptly recognized and treated, this condition can lead to secondary damage and ominous consequences. Elevated intracranial pressure (ICP) causes the development of diffuse swelling, subfalcine herniation, transforaminal herniation or transtentorial herniation according to the type of primary injury, those in turn determine hypoperfusion, vessels compressions and structure stretching ending up then in extension of neurological deficits, formation of new ischemic areas, worse outcome and increased mortality rate [38].

Monitoring and optimization of both cerebral perfusion pressure (CPP) and intracranial pressure (ICP) play a central role in severe traumatic brain injury, hemorrhagic stroke (aSAH, intraparenchimal bleeding), ischemic stroke, hydrocephalus, hepatic encephalopathy, and alterations in venous outflow. A variety of techniques can be used to monitor intracranial pressure: clinical examination, radiological examinations, measurement of intracranial pressure by invasive and non-invasive methods. At present, the gold standard for continuous ICP monitoring is invasive measurement through insertion of a catheter directly into the brain ventricles (external ventricular drain—EVD) that is connected to an external pressure transducer. However, EVD placement is not without complications: cerebral hemorrhages (2–10%, although clinically evident hemorrhages is between 0.5% and 1%), infection (5–20%) and catheter obstruction are described [39, 40]. Brain intraparenchymal catheters, despite being safer, still require an invasive procedure and cannot be recalibrated once inserted, rendering the measurements prone to imprecision throughout time owing to zero drift (Table 9.4).

Available non-invasive methods are not able to replace invasive methods (intraparenchymal and intraventricular) but can find a place in clinical practice in patients with contraindications to invasive methods or in situations where invasive methods are not available. In recent decades, there has been an increase in the use of brain ultrasound in intensive care units and in emergency rooms. The possibility of using ultrasound based non-invasive methods is an attractive prospect for the following reasons:

- rapid screening and identification of patients requiring invasive ICP monitoring;
- no risk of complications related to invasive procedures;
- ultrasound can be repeated at the patient's bedside, evaluating the evolution and effectiveness of the response to the administered therapy.

Table 9.4 Complications of invasive monitoring

	Intraparenchymal catheters (%)	EVD (%)
Cerebral hemorrhages	2.5	2–10
Clinically evident hemorrhages	0.15–0.47	0.5–1
Infection	0–1	5–20
Technical complications	2.37	
Transducer disconnection	0.15	
Optical fibre rupture	0.31	
Malfunctions and obstructions	0.31	
Mispositioning	1.4–3.1	

Ultrasound assessment of ICP includes:

- Analysis of cerebral blood flow velocity waveform assessed by TCD or TCCD;
- Optic nerve sheath diameter (ONSD) measurement;
- Brain Midline Shift (MLS) measurement.

9.3.1 Analysis of Cerebral Blood Flow Velocity Waveform Assessed by TCD or TCCD

Cerebral vessels are surrounded by brain parenchyma which is enclosed within the skull. This system is an excellent example of a Starling resistor, therefore increases in ICP or reduction in CPP determine an increase in the arterial transmural pressure and an increase in the resistivity for the flow. When assessing CBFV with TCD, all this translates into a drop in the diastolic FV (FVd) and increase in the Pulsatily Index (PI). Patients with TBI (Traumatic Brain Injury) show a significantly reduced diastolic flow velocity (FVd) and increased PI in 70% of cases [41].

TCD-derived methods for calculating non-invasive ICP (nICP) can be classified into the following three categories:

- Methods based on the TCD-derived PI,
- Methods based on calculation of noninvasive cerebral perfusion pressure (nCPP),
- Methods based on mathematical models associating cerebral blood flow velocity and arterial blood pressure.

9.3.1.1 Pulsatily Index

The Gosling PI is a ratio derived from the difference between the systolic and diastolic FV over mean FV (Eq. (9.1)).

T The effect of the increase in ICP results in a reduction in FVd (earlier than changes in systolic flow velocity (FVs)), with a consequent increase in PI. However, the use of this parameter is controversial, as the value depends not only on the change in resistance (increase in ICP), but also on CPP, systemic blood pressure and changes in $PaCO_2$. A formula (Eq. (9.6)) was proposed to transform the PI value into a ICP value (sensitivity 89% and specificity 92%) [18]:

$$ICP = (10.93 \times PI) - 1.28 \tag{9.6}$$

Formula for estimating ICP.

According to this formula, a value of PI of 2.13 should be the cut off for intracranial hypertension as it yields an ICP value of 22 mmHg or more; nevertheless, PI <1.2 are usually considered normal, such value corresponds to an ICP value of 12 mmHg with the formula. In view of this wide range of values compared to ICP values, the use of PI must be interpreted with caution. The main advantage of PI is that it is not dependent on the angle of insonation. Under physiological conditions, PI appears to have good ability to estimate ICP, but these are lost under pathological conditions in which the parameters modulating flow and radius of the MCA are altered. A loss of the autoregulatory mechanism, inadequate mean artery pressure (MAP), the presence of vasospasm, CO_2 concentration and advanced diabetes mellitus, the presence of stiff arteries can alter the linearity of the relationship between PI (vascular resistance index) and ICP, changing PI values independently of ICP values. Since in patients with acute brain damage the autoregulatory mechanism is often impaired, this means that PI cannot be considered a reliable parameter in estimating ICP.

Literature suggests that accuracy of PI based nICP estimation greatly varies from ±5 to ±43.8 mmHg. Bellner et al. described most favorable results, with a 95% confidence interval for prediction of ±4.2 mmHg and strong correlation coefficient with ICP, $R = 0.94$ ($p < 0.05$). However, such results were never replicated by other authors [42, 43]. A recent 2019 meta-analysis, again, highlighted the poor accuracy of PI in detecting increased intracranial pressure, AUROC curves ranged from 0.550 and 0.718 [44]. Recently, Chang et al. demonstrated that PI assessment together with measurement of optic nerve sheath diameter improves accuracy (AUC 0.943) [45].

Finally, some studies have shown a correlation between PI and neurological outcome. In traumatic brain injury patients, a PI > 1.25 correlates with secondary neurological deterioration within 1 week after trauma [46]. A study of 46 patients with spontaneous intracerebral hemorrhage, increased PI proved a positive correlation with poor outcome measured with the modified Ranking Scale (mRS) at 6 months after the acute event ($R = 0846$, $p = 0.002$) [15]. In ischemic stroke patients PI (Odds ratio (OR) 0.057, 95% CI 0.007–0.494) is independently associated with unfavorable outcomes [47].

9.3.1.2 Methods Based on the Calculation of Non Invasive CPP (nCPP)

Many authors have proposed mathematical formulas to estimate CPP (nCPP). Knowing the CPP, it is possible to estimate ICP according to the following relationship (Eq. (9.7)):

$$\mathrm{ICP} = \mathrm{MAP} - \mathrm{nCPP} \tag{9.7}$$

ICP intracranial pressure, *MAP* mean artery pressure, *nCPP* noninvasive cerebral perfusion pressure.

Aaslid et al. were the first to propose this approach by presenting a formula for the estimation of CPP based on the spectral PI and the first harmonic component of the ABP (Eq. (9.8)), which demonstrated to be quite sensitive to the variation of CPP but limited in accuracy [33].

$$\text{nCPP} = \text{FVm} \times \frac{A}{f} \tag{9.8}$$

FV mean, *f* pulsatile amplitude, *A* first harmonic of ABP.

Czosnyka et al. used the following formula (Eq. (9.9)):

$$\text{nCPP} = \text{MAP} \times \left(\frac{\text{FVd}}{\text{FVm}} \right) + 14 \tag{9.9}$$

MAP mean artery pressure, *FVd* diastolic flow velocity, *FVm* mean flow velocity.

In their studies, they observed a difference between actual CPP and nCPP <10 mmHg in 89% of measurements and <13 mmHg in 93% of measurements [48]. In 2022, the results of the international multicenter IMPRESSIT-2 study were published, this trial aimed at the diagnostic accuracy of nICP in assessing or ruling out intracranial hypertension. This study showed that the formula proposed by the Cambridge group (Eq. (9.5)) had a high negative predictive value (91.3%) indicating high discriminant accuracy of nICP in excluding intracranial hypertension [49].

The value of arterial blood pressure (ABP) below which he collapses and cessation of blood flow occurs is referred to as critical closing pressure (CrCP). CrCP is equal to the sum of ICP with vascular wall tension (WT). In view of this association, the following formula for estimating nCPP has been proposed [50]:

$$\text{nCPP} = \text{ABP} \times 0.734 - \frac{0.266}{\sqrt{1 + \left(\frac{\text{CPP}}{\text{FV}} \times \frac{\text{CaBV1}}{a1} \times \text{HR} \times 2\pi \right)^2}} - 7.26 \tag{9.10}$$

HR heart rate given in beat/s, a1 represents the pulse amplitude of the first harmonic of the FV waveform, *CaBV1* pulse amplitude of the first harmonic of the cerebral arterial blood volume waveform (CaBV).

The formula proposed by Varsos et al. (Eq. (9.10)) correlated well with invasive CPP ($R = 0.851$) with a bias of 4.02, 6.01, and in 83.3% of the cases with an estimation error below 10 mmHg. nCPP accurately predicted low CPP (<70 mmHg) with an area under the curve of 0.913 (95% CI 0.883–0.944) [50].

Edouard et al. estimated the CPP (nCPP) using formula combining the phasic values of flow velocities and arterial pressure (Eq. (9.11)):

$$nCPP = \left(\frac{FVm}{FVm - FVd} \right) \times \left(ABPm - ABPd \right) \text{mmHg} \tag{9.11}$$

ABPm mean arterial blood pressure, *ABPd* diastolic arterial blood pressure.

In this study, patients were divided into two groups: in group A the comparison was performed repeatedly under stable conditions and in group B the comparison was performed during a CO_2 reactivity test. In stable condition (group A) the nCPP and invasive CPP are correlated (slope 0.76; intercept, +10.9; 95% CI −3.5 to 25.4).

The relationship persisted during ICP increase (group B) (slope, 0.55; intercept, +32.6; 95% CI, +16.3 to +48.9) but discrepancy between the two variables increased as reflected by the increase in bias variability [51].

9.3.1.3 Methods Based on Mathematical Models Associating Cerebral Blood Flow Velocity and Arterial Blood Pressure

Methods based on mathematical models are very elegant and sophisticated, however they require monitoring and processing signals (cerebral blood velocity and artery blood pressure (ABP)) by means of dedicated and experimental systems making thus such techniques not suitable yet for clinical application but for research only.

9.3.1.4 Black-Box Model for Estimation of ICP (nICP_BB)

According to this model, the intracranial compartment is thought as a black-box (BB) system, where ICP is a system response to the incoming signal ABP [52]. The system response is described in terms of a transfer function between ABP and ICP [53]. The rules of the function-relationship between CBV waveform and ABP-ICP in this system is linear and was validated using multiple regression models on datasets of reference patients. The output data provide continuous full waveform of nICP (in mmHg).

9.3.1.5 Cerebrovascular Dynamics Model for Estimation of ICP (nICP_Heldt) [43, 50]

This model infers nICP from continuous monitoring of ABP and FV in MCA and then plotting this input variables into a specific algorithm which takes into account the relationship between the tree major intracranial compartments—brain tissue, vasculature, and cerebrospinal fluid. This physiological model of cerebrovascular dynamics [54] is represented by a circuit analog and provides mathematical limits that relate the measured waveforms to ICP.

9.3.1.6 Modified Black-Box Model

The previously described black-box model for nICP estimation [52] adopts a linear relationship among ABP, ICP, and FV. Xu et al. [55] assuming that the relationships among these three signals are more complex than linear models, investigated the adoption of several nonlinear regression approaches. The ICP estimation showed that the mean ICP error by the nonlinear approaches can be reduced compared to the original approach. Statistical tests also demonstrated that the ICP estimation error by the proposed nonlinear kernel approaches is statistically smaller than that obtained with nICP_BB.

9.3.2 Optic Nerve Sheath Diameter

Increased ICP, no matter what the cause, is transmitted to the subarachnoid compartment of the nerve, causing enlargement of the optic nerve sheath and thereby enlargement of the ONSD (Fig. 9.6).

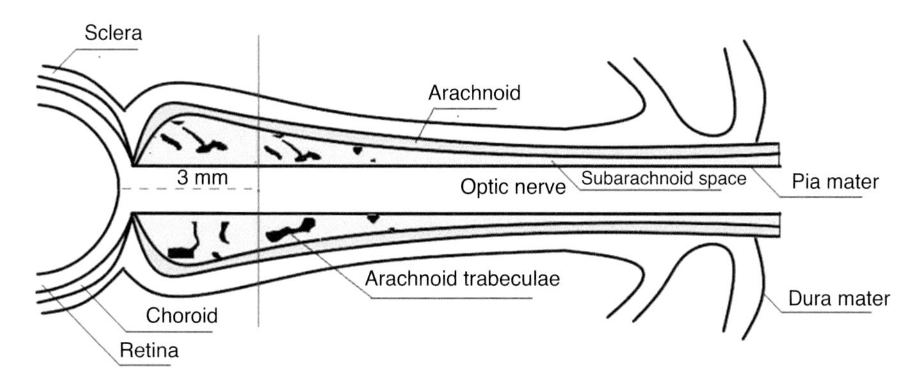

Fig. 9.6 Anatomy of the optic nerve. CSF, cerebrospinal fluid [56]

The possibility of using the optic nerve sheath diameter (ONSD), for the measurement of ICP, had already been considered using other radiological methods: CT, MRI [57]. However, the use of such investigations was very costly and involved moving the patient from the intensive care unit. The use of ultrasonography overcomes these disadvantages by performing the examination at the patient's bedside, at low cost, without radiation or side effects.

The learning curve of the technique is rapid; 17–25 examinations are required. Attention must be paid to false images that could lead to false measurements [58]. The most frequent errors are:

- Sampling of the retinal artery running close to the nerve (hypoechogenic image), which is difficult to distinguish from the optic nerve guineas themselves. To remove this doubt, it is advisable to use the colour mode of the ultrasound scanner, discriminating false images.
- The retina itself can sometimes project a conical shadow behind the eyeball, which mimics the optic nerve sheath.

Validation of this method has been achieved by comparison with invasive ICP measurements. In adult patients with signs of intracranial hypertension on CT, the ONSD value ranged between 4.84 and 6.4 mm; in contrast, in patients without radiological signs of intracranial hypertension, measurements ranged between 3.49 and 4.94 mm, with good sensitivity and specificity [1]. In a recent meta-analysis by Robba et al., measurements by ONSD showed good accuracy (range 0.811–0.954) for the diagnosis of intracranial hypertension, with a ROC curve of 0.938 [59]. A new meta-analysis published in 2022 that included 619 patients found sensitivity was 90% (95% CI: 85–94%], specificity was 85% (95% CI: 80–89%) [60].

The measurement of the ONSD was also studied in the pediatric population, showing a different cutoff; the upper limit of normality under 1 year of age is 4.99 mm (sensibility 50%, specificity 58.8%, positive predicted value 22.2%, negative predicted value 83.3%), while at older ages it is 5.75 mm (sensibility 91.7%, specificity 66.7%, positive predicted value 45.8%, negative predicted value 96.3%) [56]. In support of the validity of this measurement as an indirect ICP parameter, the administration of hypertonic solution in patients with intracranial hypertension correlates with a reduction in ONSD at the end of the infusion itself, with concomitant reduction in invasively measured ICP and increase in CPP [57]. However, the ONSD value cannot be used as a dynamic ICP monitoring. The study by Wu et al. found little correlation between changes in ICP and ONSD ($R = 0.358$) [61]. Other potential application include the evaluation of intracranial hypertension in hypoxic ischemic brain injury after cardiac arrest. In a study of Cardim et al. ONSD showed a linear relationship between ICP ($R = 0.53$), with a strong ability to predict intracranial hypertension (ICP $\geq$ 20 mmHg) in this population (AUC = 0.96 (95 CI%: 0.90–1.00) [62].

Despite the results of these studies, the diagnostic cutoff for intracranial hypertension is still much debated, with many studies reporting an optimal cutoff ranging from 5 to 6 mm.

9.3.3 Brain Midline Shift

As early as 1977, Becker et al. noted that patients with midline shift (MLS) greater than 1 cm had a higher mortality rate than without it and represents a factor correlated with increased ICP (53 vs. 25%) [63, 64]. As described in the previous subchapter, measurement of the MLS by CT is the gold standard; however, measurements by TCCD showed good correlation, with a tendency to underestimate measurements. The cutoff of 2.5 mm MLS by TCCD showed a sensitivity of 78% and specificity of 89%, with positive predictive value of 86% and negative predictive value of 83% in patients with cerebral hemorrhage [1]. Furthermore, in a 2014 study Motuel et al. confirmed that the MLS measured with TCCD underestimates when compared with CT (3.2 vs. 4.2 mm); this result can be explained in the different location of the measurements in the two methods (CT at the level of the septum pellucidum, while with TCCD at the level of the III ventricle). Despite this underestimation, the ability to detect an MLS > 0.5 cm and increases ICP has a sensitivity and specificity of 85%, when using a cutoff of 3.5 mm [20]. The good correlation between the two methods also remains in patients with head trauma, as demonstrated in the 2004 study by Pou et al. These authors found a correlation between the two methods of 0.88 with an error of 1.2 mm [22]. Therefore, midline shift assessment should be integrated also in the estimation of non invasive ICP at the patient bedside.

9.4 Brain Death

The criteria for the diagnosis of brain death vary in different states of the world. The demonstration of the absence of cerebral blood flow is always mandatory in France and Italy under 1 year of age. It is also essential when a thorough clinical neurological examination is not possible. Brain stem reflexes cannot be fully reliable in the presence of: eye injuries, metabolic disorders, skull fractures, sedatives, hypothermia. In these cases, the assessment of cerebral blood flow (CBF) is of paramount

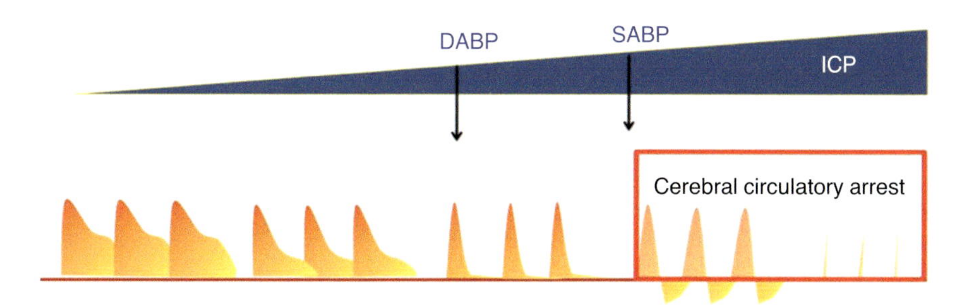

Fig. 9.7 Doppler signal during cerebral circulatory arrest

importance. Digital Subtraction Angiography (DSA) represents the gold standard for the diagnosis of cerebral blood flow arrest. DSA is an invasive examination that requires transferring the patient to radiology as well as Brain CT angio. TCD/TCCD is able to assess CBF non invasively at the bedside, in order to standardize and optimize the performance of the technique, the patient must be kept normocapnic, heart rate should be below 120/min bpm and systolic blood pressure should be >90 mmHg. Both supratentorial and infratentorial blood flow is to be evaluated by insonating both the MCA through the trans-temporal window and the vertebro-basilar axis through the trans-foraminal window. Growing intracranial hypertension is associated with progressive reduction in diastolic flow velocity. When ICP equals systemic diastolic pressure, the disappearance of the diastolic flow velocity is observed. A further increase in ICP leads to the appearance of reverberant flow (negative diastolic flow velocity), until the appearance of systolic spikes (systolic flow velocity peaks of low amplitude and present only in the proto-systolic phase) followed by the complete disappearance of the Doppler signal (Fig. 9.7) [1, 65].

A recent meta-analysis exploring the accuracy of TCD for diagnosing brain death (BD) found pooled sensitivity and specificity estimates of 90% (95% CI, 87–0.92%) and 98% (95% CI, 96–99%), respectively. These results suggest that TCD is a highly accurate ancillary test in the context of suspected BD [66].

There are situation when typical TCD waveforms indicative of cerebral circulatory arrest are not identified: decompressive craniectomies, skull fractures and intraventricular drains, newborn with open fontanelle or patients with brainstem injuries [67]. False positive TCD findings may also be seen in rupture of cerebral aneurysm and momentary sudden intracranial hypertension, return of cerebral blood flow after cardiac arrest, ICA distal occlusion and aortic insufficiency [68].

9.5 Cerebral Autoregulation

Cerebral autoregulation (CA) is the capability of the brain to maintain blood flow constant despite changes in cerebral perfusion pressure (within a range of 50–150 mmHg in healthy subjects).

CA can be impaired in many cerebral and systemic syndromes such as TBI, stroke (either ischemic and hemorrhagic), carotid disease and sepsis. When CA is compromised brain tissue is susceptible to pressure changes and thus at risk of developing ischemia or edema.

CA can be codified into: (a) pressure type regulation, which means that changes in CBF are kept to a minimum even when CPP varies, as long as the variations are within 50 and 150 mmHg, and (b) vasomotor reactivity, which is the response of the cerebral circle to changes in $aPCO_2$ and aPO_2. Pressure regulation can be further subdivided into dynamic regulation, involving brisk response of the vasomotor tone, on behalf of CBF, to fluctuations in arterial pressure or its pulsatile nature, and static autoregulation, involving a rapid response to slow changes in average arterial pressure, mean arterial pressure (MAP), in order to maintain CBF constant [69, 70].

TCD allows both testing and monitoring several components of CA by application of different techniques.

Changes in flow velocity (FV) in MCA in response to fluctuations in blood pressure and arterial carbon dioxide tension have been used as markers of cerebrovascular regulation. Thus autoregulation of the cerebral circulation can be assessed by examining the changes in FV in response to changes in $PaCO_2$ and MAP. Assessment of autoregulation in response to changes in $PaCO_2$ is termed CO_2 reactivity. In the range of $PaCO_2$ between 20 and 60 mmHg, CBF changes by approx. 3%/mmHg change in $PaCO_2$ [71, 72].

The static component of CA is measured by observing changes in flow velocity caused by pharmacologically/mechanically induced episodes of hypertension and hypotension: MCA FV is initially measured under normal conditions and then remeasured once a steady state has been achieved following a 20–30 mmHg induced increase in mean arterial blood pressure. In order to quantify and test autoregulatory response, the static rate of autoregulation (SRoR) is calculated as the percent change in estimated cerebrovascular resistance (eCVR calculated as MAP/FV) over the percent change in CPP or MAP. When autoregulation is maintained, FV change should be negligible and the value of the index should be 100%. A value of autoregulatory index less than 40% suggests impaired autoregulation [69].

The dynamic component of autoregulation can be tested or monitored.

"Test" techniques comprise:

- *Aaslid 'cuff test' method*, according to this, arterial hypotension is induced by placing thigh cuffs on each thigh and then tightening them up to 50mmHg above the PAS for 3 min and then quickly releasing them, all this while measuring MCA flow velocity by using TCD [73].This transition allows calculation of both the dynamic rate of regulation, dRoR, whose normal value is 20%/s (percentage per second), that indicates how quickly the velocity of cerebral flow returns to its starting level after the hypotensive stimulus, and of the index of dynamic autoregulation (dARI). Dynamic ARI is a dimensionless index ranging from 0 to 9 that describes the response of CBF to a steep decrease in ABP; the threshold value for a preserved autoregulation is around 5. However, inducing rapid changes in systemic arterial pressure in patients who are already seriously compromised could be harmful, so this limits the application of the cuff test.

- *Transient hyperaemic response test (THRT)* [74, 75] is based on the compensatory vasodilatation of the cerebral distal arterioles occurring after a brief compression of the common carotid artery. The test involves measuring systolic speed of flow in the MCA at basal conditions first, then the ipsilateral common carotid is compressed for 5–8 s causing a reduction in CPP. If autoregulation is intact, the cerebral arterioles respond to the reduction in CPP through vasodilatation able to reduce resistance and keep the CBF constant, so once the compression is released, we there is a temporary increase in blood flow as CPP acts on a dilated vascular bed. The increase in flow translates as an increase in velocity of MCA flow. Autoregulation integrity can be assessed by calculating the THRR, which is defined as the ratio between the velocity of systolic flow during the hyperaemic phase (two cycles after the compression release excluding the very first cycle) and the velocity of basic systolic flow (five cycles before compression). The normal THRR range is between 1.105 and 1.29 (average (95% CI) 1.2 (1.17–1.24)), a threshold of 1.10 has been approved as the lower limit for a normal response. The strength and duration of the carotid compression are the two variables that make THRR unreliable as a quantitative indicator. Current literature disagree about how long the compression phase needs to be in order to get the maximum hyperaemic response. Some authors consider 5 s whereas others consider 10 s. As far as the strength of the compression is concerned, it needs to be sufficient to cause a reduction in cerebral flow of at least 40% [76, 77].

Continuous monitoring of cerebral autoregulatory function, entails the availability of a dedicated TCD machine for monitoring sessions and a dedicated software for FV wave and CPP or ABP signals collection and analysis. The "mean flow velocity index" (Mx index) expresses the correlation (coefficient) between CPP and TCD detected mean flow velocity in the MCA: a positive correlation means that blood flow is pressure-dependent and absent autoregulation, a negative correlation is found when autoregulatory function is preserved. Mxa is the correlation coefficient between ABP and FV. Analogously to Mx, Mxa close to +1 denotes impaired autoregulation. In patients with TBI, negative values or values <0.3 indicate intact autoregulation, whereas values >0.3 failure of cerebral autoregulation [69, 78–80].

9.6 Conclusion

Brain Ultrasonography is becoming an important tool for the bedside assessment of cerebrovascular physiology at patients bedside. It is safe, non invasive, repeatable, and can be performed using any ultrasound machine currently available in the intensive care unit. At present, brain ultrasonography application is limited mainly to the neurocritical care settings, but it is starting to expand in other clinical settings such as perioperative period and general intensive care unit population.

References

1. Rasulo FA, Bertuetti R. Transcranial doppler and optic nerve sonography. J Cardiothorac Vasc Anesth. 2019;33(1):38–52. Available from: http://www.ncbi.nlm.nih.gov/pubmed/31279352.
2. Bittencourt Rynkowski C, Caldas J. Ten good reasons to practice neuroultrasound in critical care setting. Front Neurol. 2022;12:799421. Available from: https://pubmed-ncbi-nlm-nih-gov.proxy.unibs.it/35095741/.
3. Robba C, Poole D, Citerio G, Taccone FS, Rasulo FA. Consensus on brain ultrasonography in critical care group. Brain ultrasonography consensus on skill recommendations and competence levels within the critical care setting. Neurocrit Care. 2019. Available from http://www.ncbi.nlm.nih.gov/pubmed/31264072.
4. Dinsmore M, Venkatraghavan L. Clinical applications of point-of-care ultrasound in brain injury: a narrative review. Anaesthesia. 2022;77(Suppl 1):69–77. Available from: https://pubmed-ncbi-nlm-nih-gov.proxy.unibs.it/35001377/.
5. Bertuetti R, Gritti P, Pelosi P, Robba C. How to use cerebral ultrasound in the ICU. Minerva Anestesiol. 2020;86(3):327–40.
6. Blanco P, Abdo-Cuza A. Transcranial Doppler ultrasound in neurocritical care. J Ultrasound. 2018;21(1):1–16. Available from: https://pubmed-ncbi-nlm-nih-gov.proxy.unibs.it/29429015/.
7. Blanco P, Blaivas M. Applications of transcranial color-coded sonography in the emergency department. J Ultrasound Med. 2017;36(6):1251–66. Available from: https://pubmed-ncbi-nlm-nih-gov.proxy.unibs.it/28240783/.
8. Malferrari G, Pulito G, Pizzini AM, Carraro N, Meneghetti G, Sanzaro E, et al. MicroV technology to improve transcranial color coded Doppler examinations. J Neuroimaging. 2018;28(4):350–8. Available from: https://pubmed-ncbi-nlm-nih-gov.proxy.unibs.it/29727515/.
9. Camps-Renom P, Méndez J, Granell E, Casoni F, Prats-Sánchez L, Martínez-Domeño A, et al. Transcranial duplex sonography predicts outcome following an intracerebral hemorrhage. AJNR Am J Neuroradiol. 2017;38(8):1543–9. Available from: https://pubmed-ncbi-nlm-nih-gov.proxy.unibs.it/28619839/.
10. Blanco P. Transcranial color-coded duplex sonography: another option besides the blind method. J Ultrasound Med. 2016;35(3):669–71. Available from: https://pubmed-ncbi-nlm-nih-gov.proxy.unibs.it/26892825/.
11. Pérez ES, Delgado-Mederos R, Rubiera M, Delgado P, Ribó M, Maisterra O, et al. Transcranial duplex sonography for monitoring hyperacute intracerebral hemorrhage. Stroke. 2009;40(3):987–90. Available from: http://stroke.ahajournals.org.
12. Wada R, Aviv RI, Fox AJ, Sahlas DJ, Gladstone DJ, Tomlinson G, et al. CT angiography "spot sign" predicts hematoma expansion in acute intracerebral hemorrhage. Stroke. 2007;38(4):1257–62. Available from: https://pubmed-ncbi-nlm-nih-gov.proxy.unibs.it/17322083/.
13. Caricato A, Mignani V, Bocci MG, Pennisi MA, Sandroni C, Tersali A, et al. Usefulness of transcranial echography in patients with decompressive craniectomy: a comparison with computed tomography scan. Crit Care Med. 2012;40(6):1745–52. Available from: https://pubmed-ncbi-nlm-nih-gov.proxy.unibs.it/22610180/.
14. Webb AJS, Ullman NL, Morgan TC, Muschelli J, Kornbluth J, Awad IA, et al. Accuracy of the ABC/2 score for intracerebral hemorrhage: systematic review and analysis of MISTIE, CLEAR-IVH, and CLEAR III. Stroke. 2015;46(9):2470–6. Available from: https://pubmed-ncbi-nlm-nih-gov.proxy.unibs.it/26243227/.
15. Park J, Hwang S-K. Transcranial Doppler study in acute spontaneous intracerebral hemorrhage: the role of pulsatility index. J Cerebrovasc Endovasc Neurosurg. 2021;23(4):334–42. Available from: https://pubmed.ncbi.nlm.nih.gov/34579508/.
16. Kiphuth IC, Huttner HB, Struffert T, Schwab S, Köhrmann M. Sonographic monitoring of ventricle enlargement in posthemorrhagic hydrocephalus. Neurology. 2011;76(10):858–62. Available from: https://pubmed-ncbi-nlm-nih-gov.proxy.unibs.it/21288979/.

17. de Oliveira RS, Machado HR. Transcranial color-coded Doppler ultrasonography for evaluation of children with hydrocephalus. Neurosurg Focus. 2003;15(4):3. Available from: https://pubmed-ncbi-nlm-nih-gov.proxy.unibs.it/15344902/.
18. Lau VI, Arntfield RT. Point-of-care transcranial Doppler by intensivists. Crit Ultrasound J. 2017;9(1):21. Available from: https://pubmed-ncbi-nlm-nih-gov.proxy.unibs.it/29030715/.
19. Strowitzki M, Komenda Y, Eymann R, Steudel WI. Accuracy of ultrasound-guided puncture of the ventricular system. Childs Nerv Syst. 2008;24(1):65–9. Available from: https://pubmed-ncbi-nlm-nih-gov.proxy.unibs.it/17609966/.
20. Motuel J, Biette I, Srairi M, Mrozek S, Kurrek MM, Chaynes P, et al. Assessment of brain midline shift using sonography in neurosurgical ICU patients. Crit Care. 2014;18(1):676.
21. Hakim Sameh M, Abdellatif AA, Ali MI, Ammar MA. Reliability of transcranial sonography for assessment of brain midline shift in adult neurocritical patients: a systematic review and meta-analysis. Minerva Anestesiol. 2021;87(4):467–75. Available from: https://pubmed-ncbi-nlm-nih-gov.proxy.unibs.it/33054015/.
22. Llompart Pou J, Abadal Centellas J, Palmer Sans M, Prez Brcena J, Casares Vivas M, Homar Ramrez J, et al. Monitoring midline shift by transcranial color-coded sonography in traumatic brain injury. A comparison with cranial computerized tomography. Intensive Care Med. 2004;30(8):1672–5. Available from: https://pubmed-ncbi-nlm-nih-gov.proxy.unibs.it/15197433/.
23. Perrein A, Petry L, Reis A, Baumann A, Mertes PM, Audibert G. Cerebral vasospasm after traumatic brain injury: an update. Minerva Anestesiol. 2015;81(11):1219–28. Available from: https://pubmed.ncbi.nlm.nih.gov/26372114/.
24. Macdonald RL, Schweizer TA. Spontaneous subarachnoid haemorrhage. Lancet. 2017;389(10069):655–66. Available from: https://pubmed-ncbi-nlm-nih-gov.proxy.unibs.it/27637674/.
25. Korja M, Lehto H, Juvela S, Kaprio J. Incidence of subarachnoid hemorrhage is decreasing together with decreasing smoking rates. Neurology. 2016;87(11):1118–23. Available from: https://pubmed-ncbi-nlm-nih-gov.proxy.unibs.it/27521438/.
26. Lantigua H, Ortega-Gutierrez S, Schmidt JM, Lee K, Badjatia N, Agarwal S, et al. Subarachnoid hemorrhage: who dies, and why? Crit Care. 2015;19(1):309. Available from: https://pubmed-ncbi-nlm-nih-gov.proxy.unibs.it/26330064/.
27. Macdonald RL. Delayed neurological deterioration after subarachnoid haemorrhage. Nat Rev Neurol. 2014;10(1):44–58. Available from: https://pubmed-ncbi-nlm-nih-gov.proxy.unibs.it/24323051/.
28. Connolly ES, Rabinstein AA, Carhuapoma JR, Derdeyn CP, Dion J, Higashida RT, et al. Guidelines for the management of aneurysmal subarachnoid hemorrhage: a guideline for healthcare professionals from the American Heart Association/american Stroke Association. Stroke. 2012;43(6):1711–37. Available from: https://pubmed-ncbi-nlm-nih-gov.proxy.unibs.it/22556195/.
29. Rasulo FA, De Peri E, Lavinio A. Transcranial Doppler ultrasonography in intensive care. Eur J Anaesthesiol Suppl. 2008;42(42):167–73. Available from: https://pubmed-ncbi-nlm-nih-gov.proxy.unibs.it/18289437/.
30. Li K, Barras CD, Chandra RV, Kok HK, Maingard JT, Carter NS, et al. A review of the management of cerebral vasospasm after aneurysmal subarachnoid hemorrhage. World Neurosurg. 2019;126:513–27.
31. Aaslid R. Transcranial Doppler assessment of cerebral vasospasm. Eur J Ultrasound. 2002;16(1–2):3–10. Available from: https://pubmed.ncbi.nlm.nih.gov/12470845/.
32. Washington CW, Zipfel GJ. Detection and monitoring of vasospasm and delayed cerebral ischemia: a review and assessment of the literature. Neurocrit Care. 2011;15(2):312–7. Available from: https://pubmed-ncbi-nlm-nih-gov.proxy.unibs.it/21748499/.
33. Aaslid R, Lundar T, Lindegaard KF, Nornes H. Estimation of cerebral perfusion pressure from arterial blood pressure and transcranial Doppler recordings. In: Intracranial press VI. Cham: Springer; 1986. p. 226–9. Available from: https://link.springer.com/chapter/10.1007/978-3-642-70971-5_43.

34. Sviri GE, Ghodke B, Britz GW, Douville CM, Haynor DR, Mesiwala AH, et al. Transcranial Doppler grading criteria for basilar artery vasospasm. Neurosurgery. 2006;59(2):360–5. Available from: https://pubmed.ncbi.nlm.nih.gov/16883176/.
35. Kalanuria A, Nyquist PA, Armonda RA, Razumovsky A. Use of transcranial Doppler (TCD) ultrasound in the neurocritical care unit. Neurosurg Clin N Am. 2013;24(3):441–56. https://doi.org/10.1016/j.nec.2013.02.005.
36. Mastantuono JM, Combescure C, Elia N, Tramèr MR, Lysakowski C. Transcranial Doppler in the diagnosis of cerebral vasospasm: an updated meta-analysis. Crit Care Med. 2018;46(10):1665–72. Available from: https://pubmed-ncbi-nlm-nih-gov.proxy.unibs.it/30080684/.
37. Kumar G, Shahripour RB, Harrigan MR. Vasospasm on transcranial Doppler is predictive of delayed cerebral ischemia in aneurysmal subarachnoid hemorrhage: a systematic review and meta-analysis. J Neurosurg. 2016;124(5):1257–64. Available from: https://pubmed.ncbi.nlm.nih.gov/26495942/.
38. Dostovic Z, Dostovic E, Smajlovic D, Ibrahimagic OC, Avdic L. Brain edema after ischaemic stroke. Mediev Archaeol. 2016;70(5):339–41. Available from: http://www.ncbi.nlm.nih.gov/pubmed/27994292.
39. Bauer DF, McGwin G, Melton SM, George RL, Markert JM. The relationship between INR and development of hemorrhage with placement of ventriculostomy. J Trauma. 2011;70(5):1112–7. Available from: http://www.ncbi.nlm.nih.gov/pubmed/20805772.
40. Martínez-Mañas RM, Santamarta D, de Campos JM, Ferrer E. Camino intracranial pressure monitor: prospective study of accuracy and complications. J Neurol Neurosurg Psychiatry. 2000;69(1):82–6. Available from: http://www.ncbi.nlm.nih.gov/pubmed/10864608.
41. Czosnyka M, Richards HK, Whitehouse HE, Pickard JD. Relationship between transcranial Doppler-determined pulsatility index and cerebrovascular resistance: an experimental study. J Neurosurg. 1996;84(1):79–84.
42. Bellner J, Romner B, Reinstrup P, Kristiansson KA, Ryding E, Brandt L. Transcranial Doppler sonography pulsatility index (PI) reflects intracranial pressure (ICP). Surg Neurol. 2004;62(1):45–51. Available from: https://pubmed-ncbi-nlm-nih-gov.proxy.unibs.it/15226070/.
43. Cardim D, Robba C, Bohdanowicz M, Donnelly J, Cabella B, Liu X, et al. Non-invasive monitoring of intracranial pressure using transcranial Doppler ultrasonography: is it possible? Neurocrit Care. 2016;25(3):473–91. Available from: http://www.ncbi.nlm.nih.gov/pubmed/26940914.
44. Fernando SM, Tran A, Cheng W, Rochwerg B, Taljaard M, Kyeremanteng K, et al. Diagnosis of elevated intracranial pressure in critically ill adults: systematic review and meta-analysis. BMJ. 2019;366:4225. Available from: https://pubmed.ncbi.nlm.nih.gov/31340932/.
45. Chang T, Yan X, Zhao C, Zhang Y, Wang B, Gao L. Noninvasive evaluation of intracranial pressure in patients with traumatic brain injury by transcranial Doppler ultrasound. Brain Behav. 2021;11(12):e2396. Available from: https://pubmed.ncbi.nlm.nih.gov/34725957/.
46. Bouzat P, Almeras L, Manhes P, Sanders L, Levrat A, David JS, et al. Transcranial Doppler to predict neurologic outcome after mild to moderate traumatic brain injury. Anesthesiology. 2016;125(2):346–54. Available from: https://pubmed-ncbi-nlm-nih-gov.proxy.unibs.it/27224640/.
47. Sato T, Niijima A, Arai A, Maku T, Motegi H, Takahashi M, et al. Middle cerebral artery pulsatility index correlates with prognosis and diastolic dysfunctions in acute ischemic stroke. J Stroke Cerebrovasc Dis. 2022;31(3):106296. Available from: https://pubmed.ncbi.nlm.nih.gov/35033988/.
48. Schmidt EA, Czosnyka M, Gooskens I, Piechnik SK, Matta BF, Whitfield PC, et al. Preliminary experience of the estimation of cerebral perfusion pressure using transcranial doppler ultrasonography. J Neurol Neurosurg Psychiatry. 2001;70(2):198–204.
49. Rasulo FA, Calza S, Robba C, Taccone FS, Biasucci DG, Badenes R, et al. Transcranial Doppler as a screening test to exclude intracranial hypertension in brain-injured patients:

the IMPRESSIT-2 prospective multicenter international study. Crit Care. 2022;26(1):110. Available from: https://pubmed-ncbi-nlm-nih-gov.proxy.unibs.it/35428353/.
50. Varsos GV, Kolias AG, Smielewski P, Brady KM, Varsos VG, Hutchinson PJ, et al. A noninvasive estimation of cerebral perfusion pressure using critical closing pressure. J Neurosurg. 2015;123(3):638–48. Available from: https://pubmed.ncbi.nlm.nih.gov/25574566/.
51. Edouard AR, Vanhille E, Le Moigno S, Benhamou D, Mazoit JX. Non-invasive assessment of cerebral perfusion pressure in brain injured patients with moderate intracranial hypertension. Br J Anaesth. 2005;94(2):216–21. Available from: https://pubmed.ncbi.nlm.nih.gov/15591334/.
52. Schmidt B, Klingelhöfer J, Schwarze JJ, Sander D, Wittich I. Noninvasive prediction of intracranial pressure curves using transcranial Doppler ultrasonography and blood pressure curves. Stroke. 1997;28(12):2465–72. Available from: https://pubmed-ncbi-nlm-nih-gov.proxy.unibs.it/9412634/.
53. Kasuga Y, Nagai H, Hasegawa Y, Nitta M. Transmission characteristics of pulse waves in the intracranial cavity of dogs. J Neurosurg. 1987;66(6):907–14. Available from: https://pubmed-ncbi-nlm-nih-gov.proxy.unibs.it/3572519/.
54. Ursino M, Lodi CA. A simple mathematical model of the interaction between intracranial pressure and cerebral hemodynamics. J Appl Physiol. 1997;82(4):1256–69. Available from: https://pubmed-ncbi-nlm-nih-gov.proxy.unibs.it/9104864/.
55. Xu P, Kasprowicz M, Bergsneider M, Hu X. Improved noninvasive intracranial pressure assessment with nonlinear kernel regression. IEEE Trans Inf Technol Biomed. 2010;14(4):971–8. Available from: https://pubmed-ncbi-nlm-nih-gov.proxy.unibs.it/19643711/.
56. Cannata G, Pezzato S, Esposito S, Moscatelli A. Optic nerve sheath diameter ultrasound: a noninvasive approach to evaluate increased intracranial pressure in critically ill pediatric patients. Diagnostics. 2022;12(3):767. Available from: https://pubmed.ncbi.nlm.nih.gov/35328319/.
57. Launey Y, Nesseler N, Le Maguet P, Mallédant Y, Seguin P. Effect of osmotherapy on optic nerve sheath diameter in patients with increased intracranial pressure. J Neurotrauma. 2014;31(10):984–8.
58. Ballantyne SA, O'Neill G, Hamilton R, Hollman AS. Observer variation in the sonographic measurement of optic nerve sheath diameter in normal adults. Eur J Ultrasound. 2002;15(3):145–9. Available from: https://pubmed.ncbi.nlm.nih.gov/12423741/.
59. Robba C, Santori G, Czosnyka M, Corradi F, Bragazzi N, Padayachy L, et al. Optic nerve sheath diameter measured sonographically as non-invasive estimator of intracranial pressure: a systematic review and meta-analysis. Intensive Care Med. 2018;44:1284–94.
60. Aletreby W, Alharthy A, Brindley PG, Kutsogiannis DJ, Faqihi F, Alzayer W, et al. Optic nerve sheath diameter ultrasound for raised intracranial pressure: a literature review and meta-analysis of its diagnostic accuracy. J Ultrasound Med. 2022;41(3):585–95. Available from: https://pubmed.ncbi.nlm.nih.gov/33893746/.
61. Wu GB, Tian J, Liu XB, Wang ZY, Guo JY. Can optic nerve sheath diameter assessment be used as a non-invasive tool to dynamically monitor intracranial pressure? J Integr Neurosci. 2022;21(2):54. Available from: https://pubmed.ncbi.nlm.nih.gov/35364642/.
62. Cardim D, Griesdale DE, Ainslie PN, Robba C, Calviello L, Czosnyka M, et al. A comparison of non-invasive versus invasive measures of intracranial pressure in hypoxic ischaemic brain injury after cardiac arrest. Resuscitation. 2019;137:221–8. Available from: https://pubmed.ncbi.nlm.nih.gov/30629992/.
63. Becker DP, Miller JD, Ward JD, Greenberg RP, Young HF, Sakalas R. The outcome from severe head injury with early diagnosis and intensive management. J Neurosurg. 1977;47(4):491–502. Available from: http://www.ncbi.nlm.nih.gov/pubmed/903803.
64. Gerriets T, Stolz E, Modrau B, Fiss I, Seidel G, Kaps M. Sonographic monitoring of midline shift in hemispheric infarctions. Neurology. 1999;52(1):45–9. Available from: http://www.ncbi.nlm.nih.gov/pubmed/9921847.
65. Robba C, Goffi A, Geeraerts T, Cardim D, Via G, Czosnyka M, et al. Brain ultrasonography: methodology, basic and advanced principles and clinical applications. A narrative review. Intensive Care Med. 2019;45:913–27.

66. Chang JJ, Tsivgoulis G, Katsanos AH, Malkoff MD, Alexandrov AV. Diagnostic accuracy of transcranial doppler for brain death confirmation: systematic review and meta-analysis. AJNR Am J Neuroradiol. 2016;37(3):408–14. Available from: https://pubmed.ncbi.nlm.nih.gov/26514611/.
67. Cabrer C, Domínguez-Roldan JM, Manyalich M, Trias E, Paredes D, Navarro A, et al. Persistence of intracranial diastolic flow in transcranial Doppler sonography exploration of patients in brain death. Transplant Proc. 2003;35(5):1642–3. Available from: https://pubmed.ncbi.nlm.nih.gov/12962741/.
68. Dominguez-Roldan JM, Jimenez-Gonzalez PI, Garcia-Alfaro C, Rivera-Fernandez V, Hernandez-Hazañas F. Diagnosis of brain death by transcranial Doppler sonography: solutions for cases of difficult sonic windows. Transplant Proc. 2004;36(10):2896–7. Available from: https://pubmed.ncbi.nlm.nih.gov/15686655/.
69. Panerai RB. Assessment of cerebral pressure autoregulation in humans–a review of measurement methods. Physiol Meas. 1998;19(3):305–38. Available from: https://pubmed-ncbi-nlm-nih-gov.proxy.unibs.it/9735883/.
70. Paulson OB, Strandgaard S, Edvinsson L. Cerebral autoregulation. Cerebrovasc Brain Metab Rev. 1990;2(2):161–92.
71. Stocchetti N, Maas AIR, Chieregato A, Van Der Plas AA. Hyperventilation in head injury: a review. Chest. 2005;127(5):1812–27. Available from: https://pubmed-ncbi-nlm-nih-gov.proxy.unibs.it/15888864/.
72. Maeda H, Matsumoto M, Handa N, Hougaku H, Ogawa S, Itoh T, et al. Reactivit of cerebral blood flow to carbon dioxide in various types of ischemic cerebrovascular disease: evaluation by the transcranial doppler method. Stroke. 1993;24(5):670–5.
73. Giller CA. A bedside test for cerebral autoregulation using transcranial Doppler ultrasound. Acta Neurochir. 1991;108(1–2):7–14. Available from: https://pubmed-ncbi-nlm-nih-gov.proxy.unibs.it/2058430/.
74. Czosnyka M, Kirkpatrick PJ, Pickard JD. Multimodal monitoring and assessment of cerebral haemodynamic reserve after severe head injury. Cerebrovasc Brain Metab Rev. 1996;8(4):273–95.
75. Smielewski P, Czosnyka M, Kirkpatrick P, Pickard JD. Evaluation of the transient hyperemic response test in head-injured patients. J Neurosurg. 1997;86(5):773–8. Available from: https://pubmed-ncbi-nlm-nih-gov.proxy.unibs.it/9126891/.
76. Cavill G, Simpson EJ, Mahajan RP. Factors affecting assessment of cerebral autoregulation using the transient hyperaemic response test. Br J Anaesth. 1998;81(3):317–21. Available from: https://pubmed-ncbi-nlm-nih-gov.proxy.unibs.it/9861111/.
77. Ursino M, Giulioni M, Lodi CA. Relationships among cerebral perfusion pressure, autoregulation, and transcranial Doppler waveform: a modeling study. J Neurosurg. 1998;89(2):255–66. Available from: https://pubmed-ncbi-nlm-nih-gov.proxy.unibs.it/9688121/.
78. Czosnyka M, Smielewski P, Lavinio A, Pickard JD, Panerai R. An assessment of dynamic autoregulation from spontaneous fluctuations of cerebral blood flow velocity: a comparison of two models, index of autoregulation and mean flow index. Anesth Analg. 2008;106(1):234–9. Available from: https://pubmed-ncbi-nlm-nih-gov.proxy.unibs.it/18165583/.
79. Budohoski KP, Czosnyka M, De Riva N, Smielewski P, Pickard JD, Menon DK, et al. The relationship between cerebral blood flow autoregulation and cerebrovascular pressure reactivity after traumatic brain injury. Neurosurgery. 2012;71(3):652–60. Available from: https://pubmed-ncbi-nlm-nih-gov.proxy.unibs.it/22653390/.
80. Czosnyka M, Brady K, Reinhard M, Smielewski P, Steiner LA. Monitoring of cerebrovascular autoregulation: facts, myths, and missing links. Neurocrit Care. 2009;10(3):373–86. Available from: https://pubmed-ncbi-nlm-nih-gov.proxy.unibs.it/19127448/.

Neurophysiology in Traumatic Brain Injury

10

F. Fossi, F. Zumbo, S. M. Carenini, and A. Chieregato

10.1 Introduction

Electrophysiological monitoring can be considered an offshoot of neurological examination and neuroimaging in the intensive care unit [1]. Electroencephalogram (EEG) and evoked potentials (EP) are cheap and non-invasive. EEG helps the clinical evaluation of comatose patients and helps in predicting outcome [2].

Electroencephalogram records the activity of cortical neurons, specifically of pyramidal neurons (which ride orthogonally to the surface), tracking both excitatory and inhibitory postsynaptic potentials. EEGs are obtained by recording spontaneous electrical activity with metal electrodes on the scalp usually employing 8–24 channels, with the electrodes interconnected in two directions.

EEG rhythms are classified by frequency bands: ranging from a higher frequency to a lower one: δ 1–4 Hz, θ 4–7 Hz, α 8–13 Hz and β <13 Hz. The amplitude is usually between 20 and 200 mV. In normal EEGs the activity is symmetrical with α rhythm. As subjects become drowsy, θ and δ activity increases; α rhythm is absent in sleeping subjects.

Evoked potentials, instead, are the potentials recorded after electrical stimulation of peripheral nerves, generated in the cerebral cortex, subcortical nuclei, brainstem or spinal cord. Brainstem auditory evoked potentials (BAEP) are produced by the brainstem after auditory stimulus.

Somatosensory evoked potentials (SEP) are the electrical activity recorded in the brain after electrical stimulation of a peripheral sensory nerve.

EP waveforms are first marked "P" if positive or "N" if negative, then by the milliseconds of latency between the sensory stimulus and their appearance.

F. Fossi (✉) · F. Zumbo · S. M. Carenini · A. Chieregato
Grande Ospedale Metropolitano Niguarda, Milan, Italy
e-mail: francesca.fossi@ospedaleniguarda.it

E. Brogi et al. (eds.), *Traumatic Brain Injury*, Hot Topics in Acute Care Surgery and Trauma, https://doi.org/10.1007/978-3-031-50117-3_10

SEP are produced by stimulation of peripheral nerves and generated by sequential activation of the ascending volley. The N20/P22 complexes are generated by the somatosensory cortex (N20 and N38/P38) and motor and premotor cortex (P22).

BAEPs are produced by applying a simple auditory stimulus, like clapping, and feature five waves.

Immediately after traumatic brain injury, electrophysiological tests are usually more complex to be interpreted than in other acute brain injuries (e.g., hypoxic coma or stroke), because sedation interferes with EEG interpretation [3]. During a traumatic coma, the EEG pattern is usually composed by delta waves; and less frequently in "alpha-like coma", an alpha rhythm unreactive to sensory stimulation (i.e., different from the normal alpha rhythm). Burst suppression or brief bursts of activity may be seen. A higher proportion of delta waves correlates with poorer prognosis; focal abnormalities are more typical of mild and moderate TBI.

To evaluate EEG without the confounding effect of sedation, it is useful to look back at 1970s studies submitted by Bricolo et al. The two hemispheres are usually asymmetric, with the more severely damage one lower and monotonous [2]. Unilateral slowing which is later associated with flattening, indicates extradural or subdural hematoma or severe brain ischemia [2]. In general, asymmetries are correlated to worse outcomes.

Taking this into account, it is also possible to study the effect of medical acts; for example, intravenous benzodiazepines increase the amount of alpha and beta frequencies: prognosis is good if they induce an increase of spindle activity, in a "sleep-like" pattern [2]. When benzodiazepines do not induce any changes of frequency, prognosis is unfavorable [2]. Hyperventilation can flatten and slow the electrical activity in the healthy hemisphere and, to a lesser degree, in the ischemic hemisphere [1].

TBI patients can present a change in the frequency or amplitude of the background electroencephalographic activity, detected within a few seconds from stimulus, which is strongly related to recovery of consciousness [4]. Bilateral absence of SEP is associated to a 90–95% chance of non-awakening, unilateral or bilateral absence is associated to 100% severe disability [5].

After TBI electroclinical seizures are not rare, as they are present in 5–12% patients [6]; the incidence is higher when the TBI is severe [7].

Post-traumatic seizures are usually classified as immediate, early, or late when they occur respectively within 24 h, 7 days, or more than 7 days after injury.

Seizures can be associated with high intracranial pressure (HICP) and a high mean lactate/pyruvate ratio according to microdialysis data [8]. Different types and lengths of seizures were compared, finding no differences; patients were however shown to have higher mean ICP during and after seizures (even 10 h later). Mean ictal ICP was higher than the mean interictal ICP (in the 12 h preceding the seizure) [8].

Claassen found a 18% of seizuring patients during continuous EEG (cEEG) monitoring, including NCSE and NCS. Every patient did not have any sign nor symptom and 8% had nonconvulsive status epilepticus.

Risk of seizures is higher [9] in:

- Neurosurgery for hematoma either subdural or epidural
- Neurosurgery for an intracerebral hematoma
- GCS lower than 8
- Depressed skull fracture
- Dural penetration
- One unreactive pupil
- Cortical contusion and parietal lesions

It is also true that the incidence of electroencephalographic seizure is very low or absent when a patient is subjected to sedation for the control of intracranial hypertension [10].

In many studies seizures are associated with worse outcomes, therefore early diagnosis and treatment could be important [11, 12].

Periodic and rhythmic patterns like Lateralized Periodic Discharge Amplitude (LPDS or PLEDs) can be found in TBI. They are described as large, sharp and repetitive potentials, typical of brains with acute damage; they signify an unstable brain [13]; the risks and benefits of treatment are still not known.

Early seizures increase the risk of late seizures [11, 12].

A qualitative approach useful for the clinician can be based on EEG patterns classified by Synek [14]. These patterns link prognostic capability with outcome quality:

- Optimal: dominant alpha activity with theta, reactive
- Benign: dominant theta activity with alpha, reactive; delta activity with sleep spindles; high amplitude rhythmic frontal delta in theta-delta background
- Uncertain significance: dominant theta activity with delta, not reactive; diffuse delta reactive or not reactive; slow theta reactive with delta and epileptiform discharges; alpha pattern coma, reactive
- Malignant: dominant slow delta, not reactive, with burst-suppression <1 s; dominant theta or delta, not reactive, with burst-suppression >1 s, with or without epileptiform discharges; alpha or theta pattern coma, not reactive
- Fatal: diffuse low amplitude delta, not reactive; isoelectric activity

The predictive ability of EEG is superior to that of clinical scales, especially regarding certain groups of disabilities.

Disorders of consciousness (DoC) after TBI can include unresponsive wakefulness syndrome (UWS) or minimally conscious state (MCS). It is easy to imagine how important is to diagnose and predict these two outcomes both from clinical and social/ethical perspectives. Clinical neurological scales (GCS, pupils' reactivity to light) can predict binary outcomes with an accuracy of about 90%. However, both high-density EEG and functional MRI are promising techniques to further improve prognostic accuracy. Patients with reactive EEG signal to external stimuli, larger

EEG amplitudes, and stronger activity in the higher-frequency bands (alpha and beta) are more likely to have a positive outcome after 6 months [15, 16]; they used CRS-R score (Coma Recovery Scale—Revised) from 0 (comatose patients) to 23. Disorders of consciousness patients often show severe functional and structural thalamocortical lesions and disconnections with a drop in the EEG coherence in the damaged hemisphere. Coherence (Coh) is the mathematical measure of degree of similarity of the EEG recorded at two sensors, it ranges ranges from 0 to 1. If variations of the two signals are more similar over time, then it suggests functional connectivity, meaning that two areas of the brain are working together.

The aim of this chapter is to describe the usefulness of quantitative EEG and its clinical applications and to fully explain EP as a fundamental tool in neuromonitoring.

10.2 Quantitative EEG

Direct visual analysis of raw EEG data remains the gold standard for electrophysiology in the ICU, not only for traumatic brain injury (TBI). Unfortunately, standard raw EEG interpretation has numerous disadvantages for a diffused, worldwide adoption as a standard for TBI neuromonitoring, such as difficult and highly subjective interpretation, time-consuming data analysis and the need for cumbersome equipment.

Quantitative EEG [17], defined by Nuwer in 1997 as "the mathematical processing of digitally recorded EEG in order to highlight specific waveform components, transform the EEG into a format or domain that elucidates relevant information, or associate numerical results with the EEG data for subsequent review or comparison". The qEEG may help to overcome the EEG disadvantages, allowing rapid screening of patient neurological status.

Quantitative EEG is based on the mathematical analysis of the frequency, amplitude, and time domain of raw EEG, and offers to clinicians different graphs such as suppression ratio (BSR), compressed and density spectral array (CSA and CDSA), fast Fourier transformation (FFT), asymmetry, alpha/delta ratio, and amplitude EEG as showed in Table 10.1 [18].

In addition, the Bispectral Index™ (BIS™ Monitoring System, Medtronic Minneapolis, MN), developed to assist the anesthesiologists in the operating room in monitoring deep of anesthesia and based on quantitative EEG processing, has been used in ICU [19, 20], despite its limitations on long term use. Some of known limits of Bispectral Index™ are those related to the confounding effects of some drugs like Ketamine (which produces a state of dissociative anesthesia without reduction in BIS values), electromyography interference with EEG signal acquisition, interpreted as high-frequency, low-amplitude waves and falsely elevating the BIS, insufficient data on BIS application in patients with neurologic disease [21].

One of the first qEEG techniques was amplitude EEG, developed by Prior and Maynard [22] in the 1960s for use in adult intensive care patients. It consists of a system in which the EEG signal from a single pair of electrodes is amplified and

Table 10.1 Summary of main qEEG techniques and characteristics

Compressed spectral array (CSA)	Compressed spectral array (CSA) it's a frequency analysis technique that compresses the raw EEG to provide a 3D graphical display of frequency and power against time
Color density spectral array (CDSA)	CDSA applies a fast Fourier transformation (FFT) to convert raw EEG signals into a time-compressed and color-coded display, also known as color spectrogram. Graphical representation of the CDSA is constituted by EEG power (amplitude^2/Hz, by color) and frequency (y-axis) over time (x-axis)
Asymmetry	Difference between right and left cerebral hemisphere EEG frequency and/or power
Alpha/delta ratio (ADR)	Moving average of the ratio of 8–13 Hz band power divided by 1–4 Hz band power
Burst suppression ratio (BSR)	Measure of the percentage of time within an interval spent in the suppressed state
Amplitude EEG	Processed EEG signal and displayed on a semilogarithmic amplitude and time-compressed scale
Bispectral Index™	Derived from EEG signal processing techniques including bispectral analysis, power spectral analysis, and time domain analysis, combined via a complex proprietary algorithm to optimize the correlation between the EEG and the clinical effects of anesthesia
Total power (TP)	Express the power in the measured frequency band
Spectral edge frequency (SEF)	Is the frequency below a certain perceptual (generally 95% or 90%) of the total EEG power is located

passed through a special wide-band filter, subjected to logarithmic amplitude compression and then passed into a peak-sensitive rectifier. This has a short time constant so that it follows short-term fluctuations in the amplitude of the activity. This result corresponded to the amplitude distribution of the signals.

Compressed Spectral Array [23] (CSA) and Color density spectral array [24] (CDSA) are two of the most used qEEG techniques. CDSA applies a fast Fourier transformation (FFT) to convert raw EEG signals into a time-compressed and color-coded display, also known as color spectrogram. Graphical representation of the CDSA is constituted by EEG power (amplitude^2/Hz, by color) and frequency (y-axis) over time (x-axis). For example, most EEG seizures are characterized by increases in frequency and amplitude compared to the baseline EEG, which are displayed in CDSA as changes in color (power increase) compared to the baseline or shifts of power into higher frequency ranges (upward arches of color). As with every qEEG method, CDSA is prone to false negatives (not all seizures display frequency and power increases and may be under-recognized) and false positives (generally due to artifacts that produce frequency and power increases) [25].

The burst suppression ratio (BSR) is a measure of the percentage of time within an interval spent in the suppressed state and is widely used as an indicator of the depth of suppression of cortical electrical activity. BSR is helpful for the management of patients requiring deep sedation, such as those with status epilepticus or barbiturate coma. Historically, BSR have been manually calculated, but technical improvements have led to the possibility of automatic segmentation and calculation [26].

Currently, several qEEG techniques are experimentally applied on some aspects of TBI management: seizure and status epilepticus detection [8, 27–29], monitoring of depth of sedation [19, 20, 30] until barbiturate coma [31, 32] and outcome prediction [33–35].

10.2.1 Seizure and Status Epilepticus Detection

In a cohort of 94 patients with moderate and severe TBI, Vespa and colleagues [27] found that approximately 20% of the patients experienced clinically and electroencephalographically detected seizures during acute intensive care periods. The total power trend increase (subsequently confirmed by an independent electroencephalographer on continuous EEG recording) was one of the methods used to identify possible seizures, also by inexperienced clinicians. However, different patient management protocols may have led to different results. Olivecrona et al. [10], on a population of 47 TBI patients deeply sedated (intravenous Midazolam, Propofol, Thiopental or a combination thereof), reports no EEG seizures on prolonged cEEG and Amplitude-integrated EEG data monitoring.

Williamson et al. [28] tested the ability of CDSA to detect seizures in a mixed ICU population of 118 adult patients (in addition to TBI). The CDSA reviewers were two neurology residents, blinded to primary cEEG data, after receiving a 2-h tutorial on the basic theory of spectral EEG analysis and an example review of CDSA displays of seizures. Combined, the two reviewers correctly identified 98.7% of patients with seizures and a median of 94.2% of seizures per patient, with a mean CDSA review time of 10.3 min, indicating that CDSA could be used as a screening tool for seizures despite a high rate of false positives.

10.2.2 Monitoring the Depth of Sedation

Another field in which qEEG has been explored is monitoring depth of sedation. The Bispectral Index™ uses a complex proprietary algorithm to analyze electric signals recorded from four electrodes placed on the forehead, displaying a number ranging from 0 (isoelectric EEG) to 100 (awake patient). Values between 60 and 80 indicate light sedation, whereas values between 40 and 60 generally reflect a deeper level of unconsciousness suitable for surgery. Lower values of the BIS index correlate with a greater effect of anesthetic on EEG, until the degree of EEG suppression becomes the primary determinant of the BIS value [36].

The Bispectral Index™ has been used to monitor sedation levels in TBI patients. Yan et al. [30] evaluated the therapeutic effectiveness of different BIS values in patients with severe TBI in a prospective observational study. Patients were randomly assigned to one of three groups: two groups consisted of patients in whom sedative depth was maintained within a BIS range of 40–50 and 50–60 respectively, while in the third group (control group) sedation was set to maintain a Richmond Agitation-Sedation Score [37] (RASS) score within −2 and −3. Patients in the two

BIS groups showed a more stable sedation status and ICP values, but no differences in outcome or length of stay in the neurocritical care unit were observed.

10.2.3 Barbiturate Coma

As for monitoring depth of sedation, Bispectral Index™ has been used to assess the effectiveness of barbiturate coma in terms of depression of electrical activity. Cottenceau et al. [32] compared the number of bursts and the suppression ratio derived from EEG recording (suppression ratio from EEG [SR_{EEG}]: percentage of the last 60 s in cortical silence) to concomitant data from the BIS-XP™ (BIS and suppression ratio [SR_{BIS}]) in eleven patients with TBI. The optimal level of barbiturate coma was defined as 2–5 bursts/min in the EEG, with a strong statistical agreement between SR_{BIS} and SR_{EEG} (intraclass correlation coefficient of 0.94, 95% CI, 0.90–0.96) and optimal BIS values between 6 and 15.

10.2.4 Outcome Prediction

Outcome prediction is another field in which qEEG may help to identify patients with poor outcomes. Haveman [34] and Tewarie [35] both used a combination of qEEG features and variables derived from the International Mission for Prognosis and Clinical Trial Design [38] (IMPACT) predictor for neurologic outcome prediction in patients with moderate to severe TBI. Both researchers reported a higher sensitivity and specificity in outcome prediction with respect to IMPACT score alone, with mean amplitude of EEG, Spectral Edge Frequency [39] (SEF, the highest frequency at which a significant amount of power is present in the EEG) and BSI [40] (Brain Symmetry Index, estimate the symmetry of power between pairs of electrodes from left and right hemispheres) being the most relevant features of the models among the others.

Despite is a promising and evolving technology, it should be noted that qEEG and its application in TBI has been surrounded by some skepticism. The main concerns are the high percentage of false-positive findings principally due to artifact contamination (eye movements, muscle activity), normal variation of EEG between patients or misinterpretation of qEEG graphs by personnel poorly trained in EEG readings, as pointed out by Nuwer [17] in 1997 and Haneef [41] in 2013.

10.3 Evoked Potentials monitoring in Traumatic Brain Injury

Evoked potentials (EPs) are progressively become a fundamental tool in intensive care multimodal neuromonitoring [42]. Nowadays, they are of mainstem importance in integrating clinical and neuroradiological data obtain from patients suffering TBI. Their impact in prognostication after such an event have been largely investigated [43–45].

The term evoked potential refers to an electroencephalographic event, related to different applied stimuli, able to reveal the integrity of a neurological pathway. The electrical potential is obtained by filter random scalp EEG activity and extracting lesser amplitude signals, applied with constant intensity and frequency. The most common modalities of evoked potentials are referred as

- Somatosensory Evoked Potentials (SSEP), obtained by electrical stimuli applied to median, ulnar or tibial nerve [46, 47]
- Brainstem evoked potentials (BAEPs), auditory stimuli applied by special ear/headphone [46, 47]
- Visual Evoked Potential (VEP), obtain with special masks that can reproduce light stimulation of known intensity and frequency [47]

10.3.1 SSEPs

To measure SSEPs different electrodes are applied in crucial points. Erb's point (at the conjunction between the sternocleidomastoid muscle and the clavicula), C2, C7; C3 and C4 (located in parietal sensitive areas), according to the 10–20 International System.

A square-wave pulse of known intensity, duration and amplitude, is applied to the wrist with the cathode placed cranially, until a twitch is observed at the thumb, or a potential is recorded at the neck. Related to different levels, many EPs can be observed: N10, N12 and N14, when recorded from the neck, and P15, N20, P20, N25, P25, P30, N35 and P45 when recorded from the scalp. Some authors refer to central conduction times (CCT), that is the differences in peak latency between N14 and N20, and the amplitude ratios (AR) between the peak of N14 and the subsequent positivity and the peak of N20 [46]. Some of the most clinically important SSEPs are reported in the Table 10.2:

10.3.2 BAEPs

They consist in acoustic stimuli applied alternatively to both ears by special headphones or earphones, and the other one masked with white noise. Usual recording is

Table 10.2 Summary of the most clinically important SSEPs

SSEP wave	Generator source	Level
N9	Brachial plexus	Erb's Point
N12	Dorsal Horn C6	Lower cervical plexus
N13/P14	Medial lemniscus	Cervicomedullary junction
N18	Thalamus	
N20	Sensory cortex	posterior edge of the central fissure
P2	Primary motor cortex	Motor cortex
P30/P30	Medial lemniscus	Cervicomedullary junction
P45	Postcentral somatosensory cortex	Postcentral cortex

Table 10.3 Sources and levels of BAEP waves

BAEP wave	Generator source	Level
I	Auditory nerve	Cochlea-pontemedullary entry
II	Auditory nerve/cochlear nucleus	Pontomedullary
III	Olivary complex	Caudal pontine
IV	Lateral lemniscus	Rostral pontine midbrain
V	Inferior colliculus	Midbrain
VI	Medial geniculate body	Thalamic
VII	Thalamocortical radiation	Thalamic/thalamocortical

caught from Fz (10–20 International System). Five waves can be detected and named with Roman types from I to V, with I wave corresponding to acoustic nerve, III to bulb-pontine junction and the V to the midbrain (see Table 10.3). Various interpeak latencies can be measured to evaluate and localized possible focuses of brain injury.

10.3.3 VEPs

Few authors report VEPs as routine monitoring in brain injury, thus their impact in term of outcome determinant is yet to establish. Nonetheless, VEPs can be evaluated for possible visual deficit after mild or severe traumatic brain injury.

10.3.4 Technical Considerations and Clinical Issues

EPs describe specific anatomical pathways, potentially affected by specific brain injury, therefore a thorough anatomical knowledge is crucial in interpreting and integrating the data obtain from this monitoring and applying this information to complex central nervous system events [43].

SSEPs e BAEPs have been shown to be correlated with prognosis, better than the isolated values of pupil abnormalities, GCS or motor GCS, EEG or CT scan. Obviously, this aspect should encourage the highest grade in integration of data deriving from different diagnostic test, and not rely on just one, as international recommendations suggest [42]. The great advantage of EPs is that they are not altered by deep sedation or curarization, thus they allow clinicians to obtain information about outcome, working as an important neuromonitoring as well. Furthermore, they are not altered by progressive hypothermia [45, 46, 48, 49].

In general terms, the presence of early SSEPs after TBI well correlates with favourable outcomes, whereas bilateral absence correlates with unfavourable outcome.

These findings could correspond either to brainstem damage and/or diffuse cortical damage.

Conversely, the absence of a cortical responses should be correlated with focal EEG and CT scan abnormalities in association with focal cerebral contusion or damage in white matter underlying the cortical mantle or deep thalamic lesions. The analisys of SSEPs wave in combination with CT for deep contusion of midbrain, or local traumatic intracerebral hematomas, can allow the physicians to contextualize the meaning of absent cortical signal [50, 51]. Some authors report that with monolateral lack of response and without focal contusions, presence of SSEPs on the left, and not on the right, hemisphere correlates with good outcome [46, 51–53].

Regarding BAEPs, altered responses, especially with an increase of interpeak latency between III and V wave can suggest midbrain lesions, which correlate with poor prognosis [46, 54].

The early absence of a response does not necessarily correlate with unfavourable outcome. Many authors noted that EPs may return after few days after TBI, possibly as expression of the reversibility of the neuronal injury in penumbral areas. For example, the appearing or the disappearing of the cortical responses correlates respectively are associated with favourable or unfavourable prognosis [55]. Therefore, it should be preferable to administer EPs more times during the clinical evolution of the patient although, but up to date, in the knowledge of the authors, no standardization exists to uniform the timing in EPs recording.

Of mention, patients who underwent a recent decompressive craniectomy (within 48 h), or in other circumstances, as in case of subdural or extradural effusion and deep skin wounds, may present dynamical changes in SSEP due the changes of local impedance. In the former case, patients may present a transient lack of SSEPs, or augmented amplitude with normal amplitude ratio may be observed from the decompressed side. In the latter, persistent absence of cortical responses may represent a false negative result [56, 57].

SSEPs and BAEPs analysis may also reveal variable correlations with different parameters, like interpeak latencies, or amplitude ratios between different waves, as well as for central conduction time. Unfortunately, literature does not always restitute clear and univocal data.

One of the most frequent problems in comparing different studies is due to extreme heterogeneity in the pattern of TBI, with different anatomical impairment to SSEPs and BAEPs. Furthermore, the adopted parameters in composing EPs often differ in term of technical setting [58].

Data about sensibility and specificity, with an obvious impact in term of predictive power, may be influenced by study design itself, as the clinical decision to prosecute or not the care of the patient is a complex process that consider many other factors.

In the aim to overtake problems of technical nature, different authors have proposed scores to improve sensibility and specificity of these tests. Rumpl et al. [46] proposed scales that take into account the presence/absence of cortical response and possible variations in conduction time/latency, creating a scale for intermediate grading of outcome [58].

EPs represent a fundamental tool in neuromonitoring and prognostication in patients suffering from traumatic brain injury. Nonetheless, an integrated approach, considering clinical, neurophysiological and neuroimaging data, is advisable to better depict a realistic outcome of the patient. In the future, it should be advisable that international scientific societies provide adequate recommendations to standardize timing and modalities in EPs recording.

10.4 Conclusions

Electrophysiological monitoring is a key feature of a routine neurological examination. It is important for both EEG and EP testing to be repeated; EEG duration especially should be prolonged. qEEG might be a useful instrument, but it is necessary to be aware the possibility of false positives.

Clinical, neurophysiological and neuroimaging exams should be integrated in a multimodal approach to complex patients such as those suffering TBI.

References

1. Duff J. The usefulness of quantitative EEG (QEEG) and neurotherapy in the assessment and treatment of post-concussion syndrome. Clin EEG Neurosci. 2004;35(4):198–209.
2. Bricolo A, Turazzi S, Faccioli F, Odorizzi F, Sciaretta G, Erculiani P. Clinical application of compressed spectral array in long-term EEG monitoring of comatose patients. Electroencephalogr Clin Neurophysiol. 1978;45(2):211–25.
3. Amantini A, Carrai R, Lori S, Peris A, Amadori A, Pinto F, et al. Neurophysiological monitoring in adult and pediatric intensive care. Minerva Anestesiol. 2012;78(9):1067–75.
4. Logi F, Pasqualetti P, Tomaiuolo F. Predict recovery of consciousness in post-acute severe brain injury: the role of EEG reactivity. Brain Inj. 2011;25(10):972–9.
5. Amantini A, Grippo A, Fossi S, Cesaretti C, Piccioli A, Peris A, et al. Prediction of 'awakening' and outcome in prolonged acute coma from severe traumatic brain injury: evidence for validity of short latency SEPs. Clin Neurophysiol. 2005;116(1):229–35.
6. Annegers JF, Hauser WA, Coan SP, Rocca WA. A population-based study of seizures after traumatic brain injuries. N Engl J Med. 1998;338(1):20–4.
7. Englander J, Bushnik T, Duong TT, Cifu DX, Zafonte R, Wright J, et al. Analyzing risk factors for late posttraumatic seizures: a prospective, multicenter investigation. Arch Phys Med Rehabil. 2003;84(3):365–73.
8. Vespa PM, Miller C, McArthur D, Eliseo M, Etchepare M, Hirt D, et al. Nonconvulsive electrographic seizures after traumatic brain injury result in a delayed, prolonged increase in intracranial pressure and metabolic crisis. Crit Care Med. 2007;35(12):2830–6.
9. Claassen J, Mayer SA, Kowalski RG, Emerson RG, Hirsch LJ. Detection of electrographic seizures with continuous EEG monitoring in critically ill patients. Neurology. 2004;62(10):1743–8.
10. Olivecrona M, Zetterlund B, Rodling-Wahlstrom M, Naredi S, Koskinen LO. Absence of electroencephalographic seizure activity in patients treated for head injury with an intracranial pressure-targeted therapy. J Neurosurg. 2009;110(2):300–5.
11. Wang HC, Chang WN, Chang HW, Ho JT, Yang TM, Lin WC, et al. Factors predictive of outcome in posttraumatic seizures. J Trauma. 2008;64(4):883–8.
12. Chiaretti A, Piastra M, Pulitano S, Pietrini D, De Rosa G, Barbaro R, et al. Prognostic factors and outcome of children with severe head injury: an 8-year experience. Childs Nerv Syst. 2002;18(3-4):129–36.
13. Kalamangalam GP, Slater JD. Periodic lateralized epileptiform discharges and afterdischarges: common dynamic mechanisms. J Clin Neurophysiol. 2015;32(4):331–40.

14. Synek VM. EEG abnormality grades and subdivisions of prognostic importance in traumatic and anoxic coma in adults. Clin Electroencephalogr. 1988;19(3):160–6.
15. Bagnato S, Boccagni C, Sant'Angelo A, Prestandrea C, Mazzilli R, Galardi G. EEG predictors of outcome in patients with disorders of consciousness admitted for intensive rehabilitation. Clin Neurophysiol. 2015;126(5):959–66.
16. Estraneo A, Fiorenza S, Magliacano A, Formisano R, Mattia D, Grippo A, et al. Multicenter prospective study on predictors of short-term outcome in disorders of consciousness. Neurology. 2020;95(11):e1488–e99.
17. Nuwer M. Assessment of digital EEG, quantitative EEG, and EEG brain mapping: report of the American Academy of Neurology and the American Clinical Neurophysiology Society. Neurology. 1997;49(1):277–92.
18. Alkhachroum A, Appavu B, Egawa S, Foreman B, Gaspard N, Gilmore EJ, et al. Electroencephalogram in the intensive care unit: a focused look at acute brain injury. Intensive Care Med. 2022;48(10):1443–62.
19. De Deyne C, Struys M, Decruyenaere J, Creupelandt J, Hoste E, Colardyn F. Use of continuous bispectral EEG monitoring to assess depth of sedation in ICU patients. Intensive Care Med. 1998;24(12):1294–8.
20. Simmons LE, Riker RR, Prato BS, Fraser GL. Assessing sedation during intensive care unit mechanical ventilation with the Bispectral Index and the Sedation-Agitation Scale. Crit Care Med. 1999;27(8):1499–504.
21. Johansen JW, Sebel PS. Development and clinical application of electroencephalographic bispectrum monitoring. Anesthesiology. 2000;93(5):1336–44.
22. Maynard D, Prior PF, Scott DF. Device for continuous monitoring of cerebral activity in resuscitated patients. Br Med J. 1969;4(5682):545–6.
23. Bickford R, Billinger T, Fleming NI, Stewart L. The compressed spectral array (CSA): a pictorial EEG. Proc San Diego Biomed Symp; 1972.
24. Salinsky M, Sutula T, Roscoe D. Representation of sleep stages by color density spectral array. Electroencephalogr Clin Neurophysiol. 1987;66(6):579–82.
25. Topjian AA, Fry M, Jawad AF, Herman ST, Nadkarni VM, Ichord R, et al. Detection of electrographic seizures by critical care providers using color density spectral array after cardiac arrest is feasible. Pediatr Crit Care Med. 2015;16(5):461–7.
26. Brandon Westover M, Shafi MM, Ching S, Chemali JJ, Purdon PL, Cash SS, et al. Real-time segmentation of burst suppression patterns in critical care EEG monitoring. J Neurosci Methods. 2013;219(1):131–41.
27. Vespa PM, Nuwer MR, Nenov V, Ronne-Engstrom E, Hovda DA, Bergsneider M, et al. Increased incidence and impact of nonconvulsive and convulsive seizures after traumatic brain injury as detected by continuous electroencephalographic monitoring. J Neurosurg. 1999;91(5):750–60.
28. Williamson CA, Wahlster S, Shafi MM, Westover MB. Sensitivity of compressed spectral arrays for detecting seizures in acutely ill adults. Neurocrit Care. 2014;20(1):32–9.
29. Swisher CB, White CR, Mace BE, Dombrowski KE, Husain AM, Kolls BJ, et al. Diagnostic accuracy of electrographic seizure detection by neurophysiologists and non-neurophysiologists in the adult ICU using a panel of quantitative EEG trends. J Clin Neurophysiol. 2015;32(4):324–30.
30. Yan K, Pang L, Gao H, Zhang H, Zhen Y, Ruan S, et al. The influence of sedation level guided by bispectral index on therapeutic effects for patients with severe traumatic brain injury. World Neurosurg. 2018;110:671–83.
31. Prins SA, de Hoog M, Blok JH, Tibboel D, Visser GH. Continuous noninvasive monitoring of barbiturate coma in critically ill children using the Bispectral index monitor. Crit Care. 2007;11(5):R108.
32. Cottenceau V, Petit L, Masson F, Guehl D, Asselineau J, Cochard JF, et al. The use of bispectral index to monitor barbiturate coma in severely brain-injured patients with refractory intracranial hypertension. Anesth Analg. 2008;107(5):1676–82.

33. Vespa PM, Boscardin WJ, Hovda DA, McArthur DL, Nuwer MR, Martin NA, et al. Early and persistent impaired percent alpha variability on continuous electroencephalography monitoring as predictive of poor outcome after traumatic brain injury. J Neurosurg. 2002;97(1):84–92.
34. Haveman ME, Van Putten M, Hom HW, Eertman-Meyer CJ, Beishuizen A, Tjepkema-Cloostermans MC. Predicting outcome in patients with moderate to severe traumatic brain injury using electroencephalography. Crit Care. 2019;23(1):401.
35. Tewarie PKB, Beernink TMJ, Eertman-Meyer CJ, Cornet AD, Beishuizen A, van Putten M, et al. Early EEG monitoring predicts clinical outcome in patients with moderate to severe traumatic brain injury. Neuroimage Clin. 2023;37:103350.
36. Kelley S. Monitoring consciousness. Using the Bispectral Index™ during anesthesia. 2007.
37. Ely EW, Truman B, Shintani A, Thomason JW, Wheeler AP, Gordon S, et al. Monitoring sedation status over time in ICU patients: reliability and validity of the Richmond Agitation-Sedation Scale (RASS). JAMA. 2003;289(22):2983–91.
38. Murray GD, Butcher I, McHugh GS, Lu J, Mushkudiani NA, Maas AI, et al. Multivariable prognostic analysis in traumatic brain injury: results from the IMPACT study. J Neurotrauma. 2007;24(2):329–37.
39. Rampil I, Sasse F, Smith NT, Hoff B, Flemming D, editors. Spectral edge frequency—a new correlate of anesthetic depth. Washington: The American Society of Anesthesiologists; 1980.
40. Sheorajpanday RV, Nagels G, Weeren AJ, van Putten MJ, Deyn D. Reproducibility and clinical relevance of quantitative EEG parameters in cerebral ischemia: a basic approach. Clin Neurophysiol. 2009;120(5):845–55.
41. Haneef Z, Levin HS, Frost JD Jr, Mizrahi EM. Electroencephalography and quantitative electroencephalography in mild traumatic brain injury. J Neurotrauma. 2013;30(8):653–6.
42. Le Roux P, Menon DK, Citerio G, Vespa P, Bader MK, Brophy GM, et al. Consensus summary statement of the International Multidisciplinary Consensus Conference on Multimodality Monitoring in Neurocritical Care: a statement for healthcare professionals from the Neurocritical Care Society and the European Society of Intensive Care Medicine. Intensive Care Med. 2014;40(9):1189–209.
43. Fossi S, Amantini A, Grippo A, Innocenti P, Amadori A, Bucciardini L, et al. Continuous EEG-SEP monitoring of severely brain injured patients in NICU: methods and feasibility. Neurophysiol Clin. 2006;36(4):195–205.
44. Attia J, Cook DJ. Prognosis in anoxic and traumatic coma. Crit Care Clin. 1998;14(3):497–511.
45. Carter BG, Butt W. Are somatosensory evoked potentials the best predictor of outcome after severe brain injury? A systematic review. Intensive Care Med. 2005;31(6):765–75.
46. Rumpl E, Prugger M, Gerstenbrand F, Hackl JM, Pallua A. Central somatosensory conduction time and short latency somatosensory evoked potentials in post-traumatic coma. Electroencephalogr Clin Neurophysiol. 1983;56(6):583–96.
47. Amantini A, Amadori A, Fossi S. Evoked potentials in the ICU. Eur J Anaesthesiol Suppl. 2008;42:196–202.
48. Azabou E, Rohaut B, Heming N, Magalhaes E, Morizot-Koutlidis R, Kandelman S, et al. Early impairment of intracranial conduction time predicts mortality in deeply sedated critically ill patients: a prospective observational pilot study. Ann Intensive Care. 2017;7(1):63.
49. Markand ON, Warren C, Mallik GS, King RD, Brown JW, Mahomed Y. Effects of hypothermia on short latency somatosensory evoked potentials in humans. Electroencephalogr Clin Neurophysiol. 1990;77(6):416–24.
50. Xu W, Jiang G, Chen Y, Wang X, Jiang X. Prediction of minimally conscious state with somatosensory evoked potentials in long-term unconscious patients after traumatic brain injury. J Trauma Acute Care Surg. 2012;72(4):1024–9.
51. Morgalla MH, Tatagiba M. Long-term outcome prediction after a traumatic brain injury using early somatosensory and acoustic evoked potentials: analysis of the predictive value of the different single components of the potentials. Neurodiagn J. 2014;54(4):338–52.
52. Guerit JM. Evoked potentials in severe brain injury. Prog Brain Res. 2005;150:415–26.
53. Robinson LR, Micklesen PJ, Tirschwell DL, Lew HL. Predictive value of somatosensory evoked potentials for awakening from coma. Crit Care Med. 2003;31(3):960–7.

54. Wedekind C, Hesselmann V, Lippert-Gruner M, Ebel M. Trauma to the pontomesencephalic brainstem-a major clue to the prognosis of severe traumatic brain injury. Br J Neurosurg. 2002;16(3):256–60.
55. Schorl M, Valerius-Kukula SJ, Kemmer TP. Median-evoked somatosensory potentials in severe brain injury: does initial loss of cortical potentials exclude recovery? Clin Neurol Neurosurg. 2014;123:25–33.
56. Bethune A, Scantlebury N, Potapova E, Dinn N, Yang V, Mainprize T, et al. Somatosensory evoked potentials after decompressive craniectomy for traumatic brain injury. J Clin Monit Comput. 2018;32(5):881–7.
57. Carter BG, Butt W. Review of the use of somatosensory evoked potentials in the prediction of outcome after severe brain injury. Crit Care Med. 2001;29(1):178–86.
58. Kaplan PW. Electrophysiological prognostication and brain injury from cardiac arrest. Semin Neurol. 2006;26(4):403–12.

11 Integration of Brain Oxygen Measurement and Cerebral Metabolism: Brain Tissue Oxygenation, Jugular Bulb Oximetry, Intracerebral Microdialysis and Brain Neuromarkers

Arturo Chieregato and Lorenzo Querci

Abbreviation

AVDL	Arteriovenous difference in lactate
$AVDO_2$	Arteriovenous oxygen difference
$AVDpCO_2$	Arteriovenous pCO_2 difference
BBB	Brain-blood barrier
CaO_2	Arterial oxygen content
CBF	Cerebral blood flow
CBV	Cerebral blood volume
CMD	Cerebral microdialysis
$CMRO_2$	Cerebral metabolic rate oxygen
CO_2D	Cerebral oxygen delivery
CPP	Cerebral perfusion pressure
CT	Computed tomography
CTp	CT perfusion
GCS	Glasgow Coma Scale
ICP	Intracranial pressure
MRI	Magnetic resonance imaging
OEF	Oxygen extraction fraction
PET	Positron-emission tomography
PRx	Pressure reactivity index
rCBF	Regional cerebral blood flow
rCBV	Regional cerebral blood volume
SjO_2	Oxygen saturation at the jugular bulb
Xe-CT	Xenon-CT

A. Chieregato (✉) · L. Querci
Terapia intensiva ad indirizzo neurologico/neurochirurgico, ASST Grande Ospedale Metropolitano Niguarda, Milano, Italy
e-mail: arturo.chieregato@ospedaleniguarda.it

E. Brogi et al. (eds.), *Traumatic Brain Injury*, Hot Topics in Acute Care Surgery and Trauma, https://doi.org/10.1007/978-3-031-50117-3_11

11.1 Aims of Monitoring in the Patient with Traumatic Brain Injury

Intensive care physicians must recognise that TBI is not a homogeneous syndrome but a heterogeneous one [1, 2]. Don't recognise the variances, improperly using monitoring, letting therapy be guided by monitoring rather than anatomical-pathological-age-related patterns, and patient's problems can be associated with iatrogenic complication [3]. A further fundamental aspect in neuromonitoring selection is the availability of economic and human resources suitable for implementing the monitoring and, subsequently, for its constant interpretation. Once dealing with neuromonitoring, we must consider the ability to identify pathological aspects and that therapies could improve the physiopathologically altered target. Our knowledge of pathophysiology is the way that, together with empirical observation, leads us to improve medicine. However, the capability to reconstruct the physiological reality depends on the instruments we have and our abilities to interpret them. Physicians should always consider that every medical intervention can be associated with iatrogenic complications or that an increased treatment intensity is more associated with a higher incidence of complications. An aspect that can modulate these aspects and sustain the benefit of the control—monitoring—is the attempt at its integrated analysis rather than the gestures following interpretation. Most of the findings described in this chapter are probably in full use in a few centres worldwide. One of the purposes of this chapter is to describe these neuromonitoring to help translate the insights into actual practice when these data monitors are unavailable. The three physiological dimensions the clinician applies his interpretative efforts are brain volume, cerebral blood flow (CBF), and cerebral (oxygen) metabolism.

11.2 The Brain Volume(s)

An increase in brain volume for any reason produces an increase in intracranial pressure (ICP) related to intracranial compliance. Since the measurement of the ICP is an essential monitoring in TBI and is widespread, the brain volume is the physiological object of most significant interest to the clinician. A progressive acute increase of ICP, in minutes or hours, is undoubtedly a phenomenon that could produce brain damage due to microvascular hypoperfusion after low cerebral perfusion pressure (CPP) or due to macrovascular hypoperfusion by direct compression of arterial vessels after coning due to high ICP. Elevated ICP values can be obtained with different temporal kinetics. The slow increase (hours, days), notwithstanding appropriate therapies, of ICP, is usually due to an increase of brain volume due to evolving mass lesions or the worsening of focal oedema or diffuse swelling. An intermittent short-term increase (minutes) of ICP (hyperemia waves) [4], often self-limited, can have a very different meaning and must be faced either by tolerating it and waiting for its self-resolution or by acting through the prevention of the avoidable secondary causes of ICP increase. The slow pattern of progressive increase in hours or days must be interpreted as an indicator of TBI severity and a potential carrier of new additional severity. Whatever the context, slow or intermittent ICP elevation, the first interpretative approach to brain volume is the evaluation of computed tomography (CT). Symmetric reduction of basal cisterns indicates increased overall volume (swelling). Compression of the third ventricle can express an increase in the volume of the basofrontal portion of frontal lobes and precede the effacement of the basal cisterns. Focal oedema, representing non- normal water accumulation, may be associated with an increase in the volume of the whole brain. A midline shift expresses an asymmetrical supratentorial volume increase at the expense of a less affected brain. Repetition of CT is the first monitoring in TBI, observing the trend of these parameters (focal edema, basal cisterns, III ventricle and shift) over time. Age is obviously not a monitoring tool but has to be considered to interpretate every monitoring results. In older people, neuronal loss is associated with greater intracranial compliance [5] (Fig. 11.1) and therefore, the extent of brain volume increase can be in part dissociated from any eventual increase in ICP. Global brain volume can be distinguished by added extra-vessels blood volume (intraparenchymal blood), cell volume, interstitial space volume, cerebral blood volume (CBV), and cerebral cerebrospinal fluid volume. The presence of intraparenchymal blood is the expression of a traumatic-lacerative phenomenon [6] in which the blood leaves from multiple precapillary and capillary lesions and which can evolve into coalescence or, sometimes, into traumatic intraparenchymal hematomas. In this lesion, the trauma produces a rupture of arterioles and the blood floods into the parenchyma. Of these lesions, CT monitoring at the onset can provide an

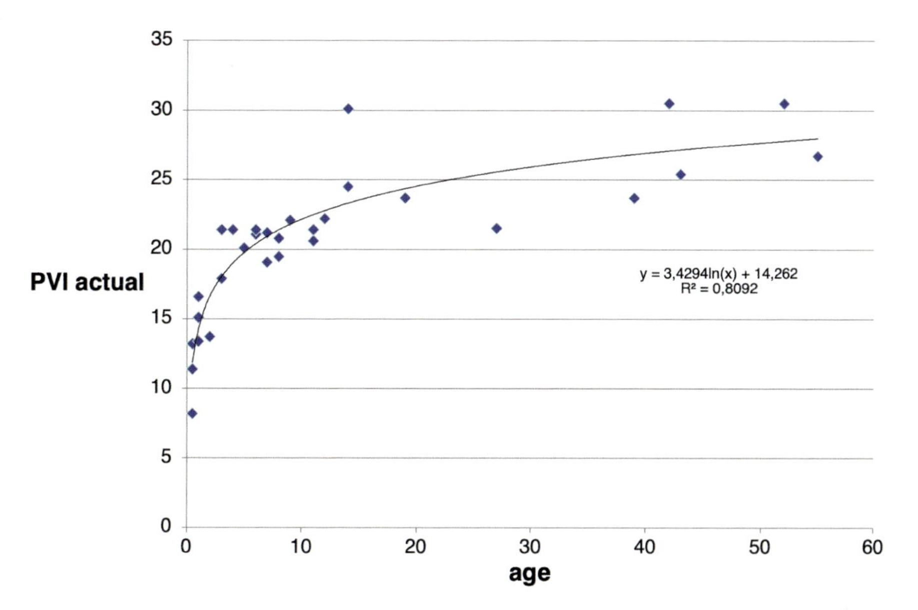

Fig. 11.1 Normal values of pressure volume index according to the age rewritten from Shapiro [5]. Low compliance is found in the younger subjects, while a slow increase is found in the adult epochs

identification of an immediate surgical indication or a waiting-and-see situation to be re-evaluated after the worsening of ICP values or the need for a higher therapeutic level or after a neuroworsening [7]. Smaller contusions or scissural subarachnoid haemorrhages may occur early in CT [6, 8–10] and both can be predictors of evolution-evolving lesions. Evolution may consist in the growth of the hematoma and, therefore, subsequently of the oedema. The expansion of the hematoma can be anticipated by measuring abnormalities on focal CBV, currently measurable with another diagnostic-imaging monitoring method, the CT-perfusion (CTp) [11, 12]. The presence of areas of reduced CBV in regions typically associated with the onset of contusions, such as frontal-basal and temporal lobes, even once not initially associated with hypoattenuation in non-contrast CT can indicate and predict the presence of evolving lesions [13]. The CTp also allows the study of the state of the blood-brain barrier. Therefore, CBV, the amount of blood in the brain volume unit, was pioneristically introduced with Xe-CT [14, 15] and now entered in clinical routine during CTp results evaluation. While focal or regional CBV (rCBV) reduction is usually due to a derangement of microcirculation, a reduction of global CBV can be functional. In fact, a global CBV reduction may be attributable to decreased $CMRO_2$, spontaneous or more often induced by sedative drugs or hypothermia. A rCBV reduction can be secondary to uncompensated or not-compensable ischemia (for example, from an artery compression due to high ICP) or to a mortification of the tissue due to direct or countercoup traumatic energy, eg, traumatic laceration [13]. In addition to be informative in the single study, the CTp can monitor the progress of the CBV over time. From a therapeutic standpoint of view, in the context of decreased regional cerebral blood flow (rCBF), the need for therapies to increase regional perfusion may emerge. Less frequently CBV may be increased. With increased global CBV and ICP, we must look for a status epilepticus, a post-anoxic syndrome, and other secondary causes such as hyperthermia, hypercapnia, or anaemia. More focal forms of increased rCBF and rCBV usually fade over time and belong to a normal postischemic reaction to repair damaged tissue [16]. In such conditions, the increase of rCBV might be coupled with amd increase of regional cerebral metabolism for glucose (cCMRGG) due to restorative phenomena. With CT and CTp, we can only suppose whether water accumulation tends to be intracellular, extracellular in the interstitium, or free in a chaotic manner in the damaged parenchyma. For example, when oedema progressively grows over the days around a traumatic intraparenchymal hematoma, we can suppose that water is usually in the interstitial space (vasogenic oedema). Inflammatory factors released by the hematoma produce an inflammatory phenomenon that increases permeability to water. Initially, the water collects centripetally only around the hematoma but over the time also follows the myelinated pathways as a way of least resistance. When this oedema is near the cortex follows the fibres of the white matter and enters between the convolutions without involving the cortical layers. Unlike a traumatic parenchymal hematoma, the oedema of a true laceration usually increases just in the first days as an expression of direct traumatic oedema [17]. About the latter, it is probably an osmotic oedema due to the osmotic power of cellular fragments (released from the laceration) that attract water [18]. These assessments of applied traumatic neuropathology can only be confirmed using magnetic resonance imaging (MRI). Increasing its availability, MRI can distinguish between cytotoxic oedema and vasogenic oedema. This knowledge can guide therapy and prognosis prediction. In the presence of an intraparenchymal lesion with mass effect and an increase in ICP that appears malignant the question is if surgery could be the more appropriate therapy. Considering that vasogenic oedema is potentially reversible, a MRI can guide the clinician on a conservative medical attitude (for example when edema in predominantly vasogenic) or toward a more aggressive surgical approach (for example once edema in predominantly cytotoxic).

In fact, the demonstration of blood in the core and cytotoxic oedema can suggest removing the hemorrhagic core utilising an image-guided precision surgery resectioning brain parenchyma no longer functionally useful. Therefore, by means of CTp, we can measure CBV, and with MRI, we can establish where extravascular water is displaced. Brain volume is determined even by cells volume. The monitoring of serum sodium plays a role so elementary as it is of enormous physiological importance. As a consequence of the selective control of the water entry into the interstitium, thanks to the integrity of the endothelial and cellular tight junctions, the aquaporins and the role of the sodium-potassium pump, sodium is by far the leading generator of the transmembrane gradient that determines the cell volume. Not only a sodium reduction in hyponatremia but also an uncontrolled reduction, albeit in the range of normal sodium, can generate cellular swelling. In daily clinical practice, many conditions can alter natremia: the reversal of therapy with hypertonic saline, a diabetes insipidus, improper management of total parenteral nutrition, the use of hypotonic crystalloids, the overcorrection of a diabetes insipidus, the cerebral wasting syndrome, the syndrome of inappropriate ADH secretion and a natriuresis from arterial hypertension with aldosterone escape (Fig. 11.2). The knowledge of these dynamics and their prevention anticipates most of the unwanted cellular effects of sodium. Conversely, osmolarity variations may have a therapeutic effect by stitching up brain volume. In recent years, advanced monitoring (as MRI) has been beneficial for personalising hyperosmolar therapy with sodium or with mannitol

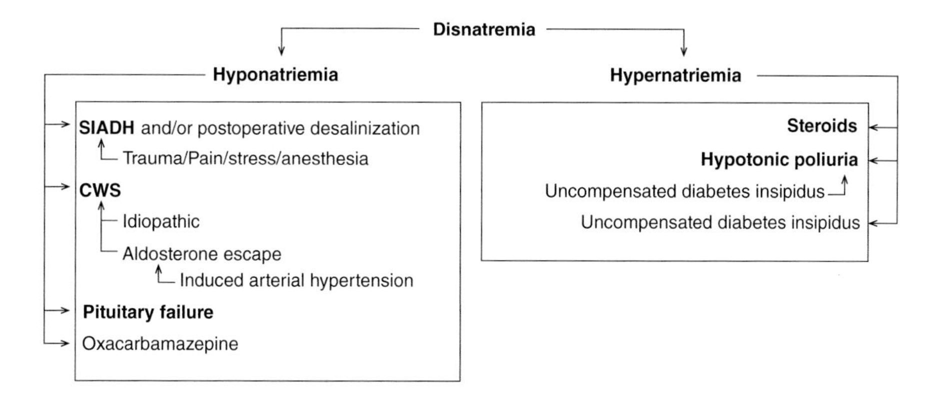

Fig. 11.2 The most frequent syndromic causes of hyponatremia and hypernatremia

showing that the osmotic agents reduce the water content more in the brain territories with an intact blood-brain barrier (BBB) [19]. This contrasts with the common belief that mannitol and hypertonic saline are aimed at reducing oedema in lesioned areas, but this is not the case. Excluding the vascular constricting bolus effect [20] of mannitol, the use of osmotics reduces the volume of regions with preserved BBB and therefore reduces ICP allowing better toleration of the pathological areas' mass effect. Conversely, in the diseased areas, the presence of opened tight junctions, which is at the basis of vasogenic oedema allowing the entry of reparative cells, and the diffusion of osmotic molecules can increase the focal oedema [21]. It is the balance between the size and extent of the alteration of the barrier and the extent of the lesions with respect to healthy areas that determines the net effect of the mannitol administration. An extended clinical application of CTp in the study of BBB could potentially be helpful in monitoring to target osmotic therapy. Besides the CBV and oedema, ICP, together with the monitoring of the Glasgow Coma Scale (GCS) and pupillary status, are the other cornerstones along with CT monitoring. GCS is a measure of the level of integration and connectivity of the consciousness. GCS grade is susceptible to diffuse and traumatic-hypoxic damage TBI, while it is less sensitive in focal low-energy impact lesions, for example, due to a fall of an elderly patient. Initially, these types of patients can present with focal symptoms, but with the evolution of the lesion, their neurological performance can decline and, therefore, could be more detectable by GCS. A specific case study is bifrontal contusions which tend to present with hyperactive delirium and only subsequently with motor alterations and neuroworsening. The meaning of GCS in a subchapter dealing with brain volume concerns the relation of neurological evaluation with neuronal activity, that one with $CMRO_2$, and a consequence with CBF and finally with CBV. This is the matter of the following subchapter. Cerebral blow volume and cerebral oedema have been discussed here as causes of increases in ICP. These changes and, therefore, changes in CPP could increase or reduce either CBV or cell volume and viability by acting on oxygen delivery. Therefore, the second aim of monitoring is CBF and $CMRO_2$.

11.2.1 Cerebral Blood Flow and Cerebral Metabolic Rate of Oxygen

Intuitively, if we focus on cellular vitality, this depends on the supply of nutrients and metabolic capacity. Therefore, we are interested in cerebral oxygen delivery (CO_2D)—availability of nutrients—and $CMRO_2$. Monitoring of CO_2D has always been more concerned with CBF than with the role of arterial oxygen content (CaO_2), which results from the product between haemoglobin concentration and oxygen saturation. Before going into the topic, we need to explore which clinical information and which more simplified monitoring could have some relationship with these dimensions. In a 1984 study by Obrist (with intravenous Xenon-133), a graph clearly expresses the direct relationship between $CMRO_2$ and GCS [22]. These results are reported in Fig. 11.3a, based on our unpublished data similar to that reported by

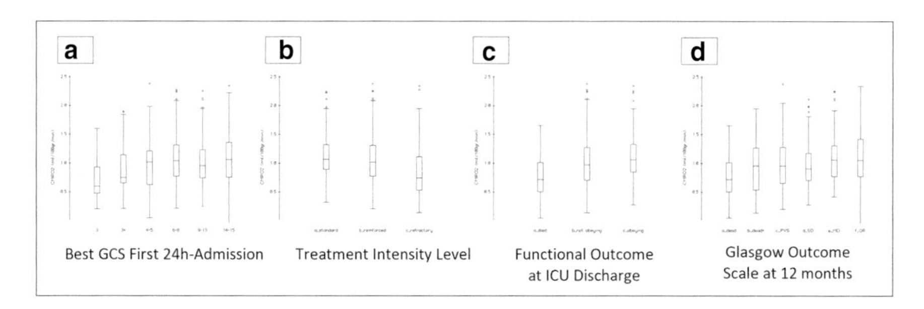

Fig. 11.3 Cerebral metabolic rate of oxygen ($CMRO_2$) and (**a**) Glasgow Coma Scale (GCS) on day 1 (GCS 3*: GCS 3 in association with pupils alteration). Higher GCS values are non-statistically associated with an improvement of $CMRO_2$. Original data from A. Chieregato, not published. (**b**) Treatment Intensity Level (TIL) on the day of the XeCT study. A not significant decline in $CMRO_2$ is associated with a higher level of treatment of intracranial hypertension. Remains to be established if due to the severity of the injury or as a consequence of the metabolic suppression due to the therapies. (**c**) Outcome at ICU discharge: a not significantly higher value of $CMRO_2$ is found in patients who obey simple orders at discharge. (**d**) Glasgow Outcome Scale (GOS) outcome at one year: "a_dead": died in ICU; "b_dead*" died after ICU discharge. *GOS PSV* persistent vegetative state, *GOS SD* severe disability, *GOS MD* moderate disability, *GOS GR* good recovery. Original data from A. Chieregato, not published

Robertson [23]. $CMRO_2$ seems to be GCS-dependent: in other words, the more neuronal function is damaged or underactive, the less oxygen is consumed. According to these data, $CMRO_2$ is more an effect than a cause of secondary injuries. It is a severity indicator. In parts, it is related to the age of the patients, with a decline of $CMRO_2$ during the ageing (Fig. 11.4). In the years that followed the '80, perhaps with the spread of sedation in the pre-hospital practice for TBI or perhaps with the restriction of studies to the most severe cases, this relationship was partially reduced. On the other hand, the existence of a metabolic rate linking to the electrical activity, allows sedation to produce a coupled reduction of CBF. This intervention is the base of sedative treatments, especially the treatment of refractory intracranial hypertension with barbiturate [24], and hypothermia. The relationships between $CMRO_2$ and the therapeutic level, barbiturate therapy or hypothermia are reported in the studies by Cormio [24], Robertson [25], and Chieregato [26]. In severely ill patients undergoing therapies for refractory intracranial hypertension, the strongest relationship with $CMRO_2$ may no longer be with GCS but instead with the therapeutic level (TIL) (Fig. 11.3b) itself [27]. In a review Robertson and Cormio reported that average $CMRO_2$ was 1.74 mmol/l/min and that $CMRO_2$ values lower than 1.5 ml/100 g/min were frequently associated with unfavourable outcomes [28, 29]. It is interesting to note how we found a mean value of $CMRO_2$ of 1.0 ml/100 g/min (SD 0.4) in severe TBI cases collected in the 2000s (Fig. 11.3a). In our patients, 94.3% of patients who died in ICU had at least one $CMRO_2$ value below 1.5 mnl/100gr/min compared to only 77.6% of those who survived with a good recovery at one year. Therefore it seems that in most recent years, $CMRO_2$ was depressed as an effect of sedation used to control intracranial hypertension [30]. Therefore, the predictive threshold 1.5 ml/100gr/min can be less informative than in the past. Our data show that, even

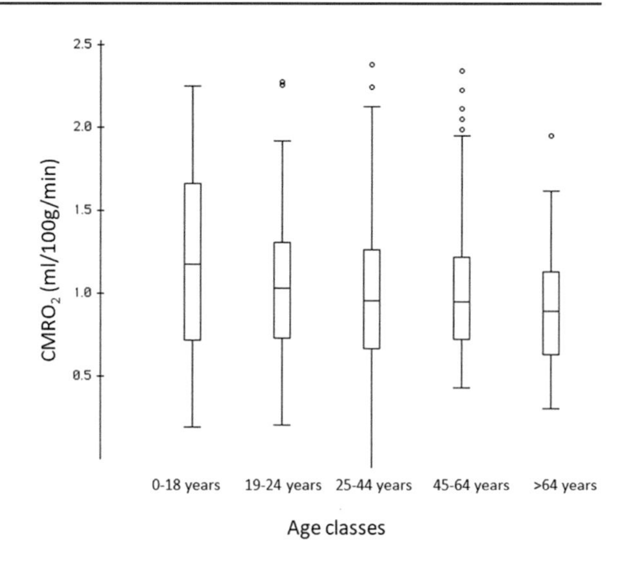

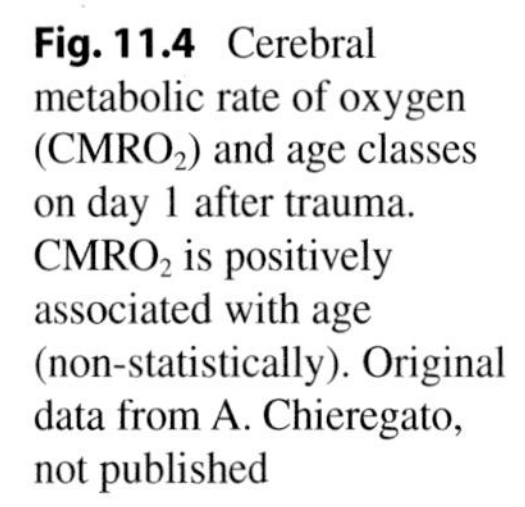

Fig. 11.4 Cerebral metabolic rate of oxygen ($CMRO_2$) and age classes on day 1 after trauma. $CMRO_2$ is positively associated with age (non-statistically). Original data from A. Chieregato, not published

with $CMRO_2$ values in ranges below those previously reported by literature, a relationship between $CMRO_2$ short-term outcome at patient discharge from ICU (Fig. 11.3c) and the one-year Glasgow Outcome Scale (Fig. 11.3d) can be appreciated. The meaning of reduced $CMRO_2$ was investigated in the following decades using the application of positron emission tomography (PET), which, differently from older global $CMRO_2$ evaluation, has led to the quantification of the ischemic voxels and a detailed regional assessment of the study of perilesional oedema. In this field, the Cambridge group studies are the reference. They propose a setting in which the PET scanner is located at the same flat as the neuro-ICU, favouring clinical research and translation in patient management. Besides GCS, age, and TIL, another proxy of $CMRO_2$ is electrophysiology and its synthetic quantifications, while sensory-evoked potentials explore the viability of neuronal networks. Whether the measured $CMRO_2$ is a cause, or an effect of patient severity is still unresolved, but anyway, the cell to consume O_2 needs a carrier of O_2 that is CBF. Cerebral blood flow, although it has long been considered one of the first targets of monitoring and treatment, has always had difficulties in clinical translation. After Xenon-133, radioactive and with CBF derivation from multiple regional measurements, the study of global CBF was obtained with nitrous oxide — Kety and Schmidt technique [31] — and after that with Xe-CT [26, 32–34]. The measurement of CBF, in association with the measurement of the arteriovenous oxygen difference ($AVDO_2$), have brought $CMRO_2$ measurement closer to clinical practice. Among the exciting data that emerged from the study of CBF with Xe-CT, we can remember the detection of low CBF values in the very early stages of the trauma [35–38], which coincides with that very early secondary damage, seen, for example from the low values of SjO_2. Xe-CT also made it possible to bring a much more affordable method than PET to bring the functional correlates of CT lesions to the clinic with regional CBF observation. For example, in focal lesions in SDH [39], in evacuated SDH [16], in traumatic hematomas [6], in differentiating the rCBF between contusions/lacerations and traumatic hematomas [6], or inverse steal phenomena [40], correlating the pericontusional microvascular ischemia with the topographic values of rCBF [41], or observing the effects of hypocapnia on CBF [42] and up to the correlates of acute rCBF with long-term atrophy [43]. It was also possible to apply Xe-CT to the pediatric population [44]. In the acute phase, Xe-CT allowed the knowledge of early ischemia in patients (and not in the laboratory like for Xe-133) [37, 41]. One limitation of Xe-CT is the static nature of the examination that can only be overcome with the not- easy double test manoeuvres in the same session, for example, testing high levels of CPP [45] or hypocapnia [46]. During the acute elevation of CPP through norepinephrine, just a minor improvement has been observed for rCBF in the edematous perilesional area. These results have been confirmed even by PET studies by the Cambridge group [47]. Conversely, a more pronounced reduction of rCBF was found when the baseline rCBF is relatively high [45] highlighting the benefit of measuring the CPP effect on rCBF instead of theorising it. A similar result, the paradox reduction or more elevated rCBF values after CPP elevation, was reported even using Xe-CT by Darby [48] in patients with subarachnoid haemorrhage post aneurysm rupture. Hypocapnia could demonstrate the lability of the rCBF in the traumatic penumbra [46]. Nowadays, no methodology measures bedside either the $CMRO_2$ or the CBF. Being semi-quantitative [49], the CTp suffers from an important imprecision in the measurement of CBF and, therefore cannot be used reliably to define $CMRO_2$. A few years ago, an exciting device was introduced for measuring local blood flow with the thermodilution method (Hemedex-Bowman) [50], but its diffusion remains limited. In clinical practice, the measurement of CPP guides the presumed management of CBF. Using Xe-CT, we [27] found that after the first few days of the management of the TBI patients allowing a CPP between 50 and 90 mmHg, the global CBF is, on average not affected by the lowest or the highest CPP values. This means that in the overall TBI-ICP population, modern neurocritical care is not associated with overt low global flow state during the instantaneous picture of the Xe-CT study, probably thanks to an autoregulation which is on average preserved. Indirect signs of pressure autoregulation are the relationship between mean arterial pressure (MAP) and ICP indicating whether ICP acts passively or actively: passively once an ICP increase follows the increase in blood pressure, showing a self-regulation deficit; or actively once an ICP decrease is observed with the increase in blood pressure indicating that myogenic vasoconstriction reduces CBV to keep CBF stable and to protect the blood-brain barrier. The possibility of observing changes in ICP due to changes in CBV is linked to the extent of cerebral compliance. Once cerebral compliance is low, the ICP changes reflect that of MAP and CPP. The Cambridge group [51] systematized this approach by observing a relationship between the pressure reactivity (PRx) index (a mobile correlation between ICP and MAP) and patient outcome.

11.2.2 The Dynamic Modifications of the Cerebral Metabolic Rate of Oxygen

As it was introduced above, studies of autoregulation and studies of CBF with Xe-CT have suggested that after the first day global CBF does not look to be an overt problem, and therefore probably, $CMRO_2$ is not dependent on CBF. There were intrinsic limits in $CMRO_2$ estimation as for the Kety and Schmidt method which was calculated by multiplying CBF by $AVDO_2$. Therefore, each relationship with calculated $CMRO_2$ was affected by the phenomenon of the mathematical coupling with CBF. Therefore the question regarding if $CMRO_2$ could be focally CBF dependent remained unsolved until the advent of PET. Almost all studies in this field have been conducted in Cambridge: a summary of their clinical results is described in the Menon review [52]. PET focuses on the value of the oxygen extraction fraction (OEF), the noble sister of SjO_2 (or $AVDO_2$) [53], but differently from SjO_2 or $AVDO_2$, it is measured regionally. Wide OEF values (a proxy for the ischemia) were unexpectedly frequent, even in apparently normal tissue, and frequently associated with normal SjO_2 values [54].

Therefore, the authors argued that ischemia, explained by a local increase in OEF, is much more frequent than expected once only global measures are considered. In an even more complex study, identifying the apparently normal areas on late MRI and, in the same way, the pathological areas and comparing them with the values measured in the acute phase, the Cambridge authors [55] highlight that contused brain regions are characterised by markedly reduced CBF, $CMRO_2$, and OEF. However, their data clearly show that there are also marked derangements in the physiology of those regions that ultimately appear structurally normal, suggesting once again that normal CT or MRI, or normal high SjO_2 do not exclude a more widespread focal mismatch. It is extremely important to observe that the control subjects displayed a close flow-metabolism coupling with OEF varying relatively little in respect to the variability of either CBF or $CMRO_2$. In control subjects, it is the $rCMRO_2$ that induces an increase in rCBF as a function of the required metabolism, and in this context, the rOEF remain stable. In contrast, in TBI patients, there was a significantly wider distribution of OEF values due to the heterogenous disruption of the CBF-$CMRO_2$ relationship both in lesion and in non-lesion regions. The progressive scientific process of the Cambridge group identifies how the dose and the diffusion of these alterations are associated with the patients outcome. More recently, the authors [52] hypothese that these diffused micro-ischemia areas are one of the bases of impaired connectivity due to the selective neuronal loss or the disruption of white matter neuronal tracts. Similarly, PET allowed them to cross-validate the significance of brain tissue oxygen ($PbtO_2$) [56]. A complex inductive analysis led Rosenthal [57] to propose the best possible explanation of what means values collected using $PbtO_2$. The $PbtO_2$ catheter is a sensor so small that it measures the O_2 that crosses many different compartments (arterial phase capillaries, venous phase capillaries, interstitial space, cellular space, mitochondria) but is relatively too large to be positioned in each of these compartments. The complexity of the physiological nature of $PbtO_2$ has led to unexpected results once physiological variables were therapeutically manipulated [58]: for example, an increase of $PbtO_2$ was observed after an increase of haemoglobin after blood transfusion however without any lactate-to-pyruvate ratio (will be better illustrated in the section of the cerebral microdialysis) improvement. Therefore, the transfusion of packed red blood cells acutely results in improved $PbtO_2$ but without any appreciable effects on cerebral metabolism. On the contrary, the same group shows an increase in regional $CMRO_2$ with normobaric hyperoxia [59] while a marked reduction in regional $CMRO_2$ with hypocapnia [60]. On induced arterial hypertension tests, [61], Coles shows a reduction of ischemic voxels in those with widely altered initial values, but a reduction of $CMRO_2$ and OEF. Chieregato in TBI [45] and Darby [48] in aneurysmal subarachnoid haemorrhage saw a reduction of CBF in areas with less reduced rCBF values and minor improvement in areas with overt pathological low rCBF values. The work of Coles [54] is beginning to reduce the asymptote that improving the microcirculation beyond supra-normal levels would improve CBF and, therefore $CMRO_2$. The same response of a modest increase in rCBF was obtained by Steiner when the measurement is centred on the perilesional tissue [47]. Finally, with Cunningham [62], the Cambridge group introduced the probabilistic threshold of irreversible ischemia concept by cross-referencing CBF, OEF, and $CMRO_2$ data with gliosis outcome measured at a distance from the acute phase by MRI. Although the probabilistic approach disappoints the physicians' natural desire for highly discriminative thresholds, it reflects much more the clinical uncertainty due to the biological complexity and the inevitable characteristic of functional imaging of being, inevitably, a single shot examination. While the Cambridge group initially guided their analysis supposing the classic concepts of interplay in pathological conditions between CBF (independent variable) and $CMRO_2$ (dependent variable), mediated by the ability to adapt thanks to the increase in OEF (dependent variable), they introduced the concept of O_2 diffusion limitation [63] once they compared PET data with $PbtO_2$ physiology. In such direction, Vespa [64] proposed a slightly different conception of ischemia. After the first 36 h, in which ischemia is more possible, TBI is associated with a reduction in oxidative metabolism and metabolic crisis (defined as elevated lactate/pyruvate ratio (LPR) above 40) that, however, is long-lasting [65]. In this study, Vespa used PET combined with cerebral microdialysis to study the regional and temporal course of this disturbance. The principal findings of this study were that the incidence of post-traumatic regional ischemia was low, accounting for just a minority of the metabolic disturbance. Subsequently, in 2016 Veenith of the Cambridge group completed the picture by introducing a marker that traces the hypoxic cells and demonstrating that the ischemic zones, those with tissue oxygen below 15 mmHg estimated at PET, can also be irreversibly hypoxic, even if the tissue could be apparently normal [66]. The Cambridge group, therefore, perfected the idea, already hypothesised in 2004, [63] that there is a difficulty in extracting O_2, due to a deranged microcirculation and/or to a limitation of oxygen diffusion to the cells [66]. Using the words of Lazaridis, "ischemia" was defined as a state of reduced CBF, decreased $CMRO_2$, and increased OEF while "non-ischemic (yet hypoxic)" areas had similar reductions in the same direction in $CMRO_2$ and CBF. However, "non-ischemic (yet hypoxic)" areas distinctly had not yet achieved an increase in OEF, a feature of O_2 shunt physiology [67]. Paul Vespa, in the associated editorial [68] therefore suggested that "hypoxia" and "ischemia" both appear in the post-TBI brain, but regions of the brain can be hypoxic but not ischemic, and vice versa [64]. This suggests that hypoxia could be unrelated to CBF deficit, but related to other mechanisms, such as a limitation to oxygen diffusion into edematous tissue despite adequate CBF. In this way, they reopened the debate about whether the brain is deprived of oxygen or whether the reduction in the $CMRO_2$ is due to a non-ischemic metabolic crisis. In 2021 the

Cambridge group [69] showed that in TBI patients, CBF and glucose metabolism tend to be reduced in apparently healthy brain regions. However, in some areas in apparently healthy tissue, particularly nearest brain lesions at risk of evolution, an increase in glucose utilisation was associated with non-ischemic reductions in CBF (without increased OEF) consistent with microvascular ischemia, oxygen diffusion limitation and mitochondrial dysfunction. This study highlights the possibility that "hypoxia" is associated with increased regional glucose utilization. In 2020, the Cambridge group completed its research cycle by associating outcome data with pathophysiological results [70]. In this context, the group highlights a prognostic association between the extent of ischemia within 24 h and a worse outcome (measured by mean of the Glasgow Outcome Scale, GOS). This association is not confirmed when the same physiological data are collected after the first 24 h. The lack of correlation between delayed (after the first 24 h) "ischemia" and GOS worst values probably raises the possibility that diffusion hypoxia and mitochondrial dysfunction (namely "hypoxia") contribute more after the early hours and days to the outcome than pure "ischemia". The study also confirms, as in previous papers, the high heterogeneity among different patients and within the same patients in different areas and lesions of rCBV, rCBF, $rCMRO_2$, and rOEF but focuses on the association of high CBV, disproportionate to CBF, to intracranial hypertension. Finally, they suggest that both global (SjO_2) and focal ($PbtO_2$) monitoring underestimate ischemia and have limited chances to depict the physiological heterogeneity of the traumatised brain and therefore dictate that these should be interpreted with caution. We must recognise that almost all the field research on the relationship among $CMRO_2$, CBF and OEF, thanks to PET come, over two decades, from a single centre, limiting the transition to clinical practice and the external validity of the results.

11.3 From Basic Knowledge to Bedside Monitoring

In the previous initial paragraphs, we have described how basic monitoring (ICP and CPP), together with neurological evaluation and interpretation of images from CT, MRI and CTp, help us to interpret brain volume and their relationship with brain compliance. With the study of global CBF and $CMRO_2$, we have seen that global brain data, after the first days of the trauma, when CPP is maintained in the range of 50–90 mmHg, are not usually suggestive of particularly pathological values. However, PET studies have made us discover, on the one hand, the existence of islands of mismatch (ischemia) not evident with global measurements. Other cerebral tissue, apparently norma tissue, could not be affected by mismatch (ischema) but could be any way affected by cellular suffering (hypoxia), suggesting a diffusion deficit or a deficit in oxygen utilisation. The presence of a defective O_2 request and/or its defective use can also be seen from the relationships already highlighted, years ago, by the calculation of the global $CMRO_2$ by means of the global CBF calculation and $AVDO_2$. Despite these enormous steps, the translation to daily clinical practice remains precarious as the related technologies still need to be widespread. It is now necessary to analyse in the next paragraphs step by step the monitors available at beside and how to apply and interpret them by incorporating the acquired knowledge.

11.4 Jugular Venous Oxygen Saturation Monitoring

The first step to translate bedside CBF (and $CMRO_2$) knowledge was in the 1980s the measurement of the oxygen saturation at the jugular bulb (SjO_2) and the associated value of arteriovenous oxygen difference ($AVDO_2$). This important innovation is due to Julio Cruz [71, 72], co-author of Obrist's work, who systematised the use of this technique in clinical practice. As it will similarly happen one decade later for $PbtO_2$, SjO_2 was not a measurement of one *pure*, *isolated*, or *specific* physiological entity because it interferes with two variables simultaneously, $CMRO_2$ and CBF, without being able to distinguish them except unless thanks to clinical and therapy information. SjO_2 is the oxygen saturation in venous blood sampled at the jugular bulb and reflects the balance between $CMRO_2$ and CBF and, indirectly, measuring the oxygen venous pO_2 value, the oxygen partial pressure in the tissue. Usually, the preferred side where the catheter is placed is the right sided jugular vein due to its dimensional dominance, but side-to-side differences are inevitable [73, 74]. Wrong positioning can occur [75], and it is necessary to check the position, which can be performed with anteroposterior and lateral cervical X-ray [76] or with a CT scan of the skull base. In Fig. 11.5, the correct positioning on lateral X-ray and in Fig. 11.6 on basal skull CT. Contrast injection into the catheter may help to distinguish the proper placement (Fig. 11.7). Misplacement in the low jugular vein or the inferior petrosal sinus (Fig. 11.8) can be associated with extracerebral contamination with

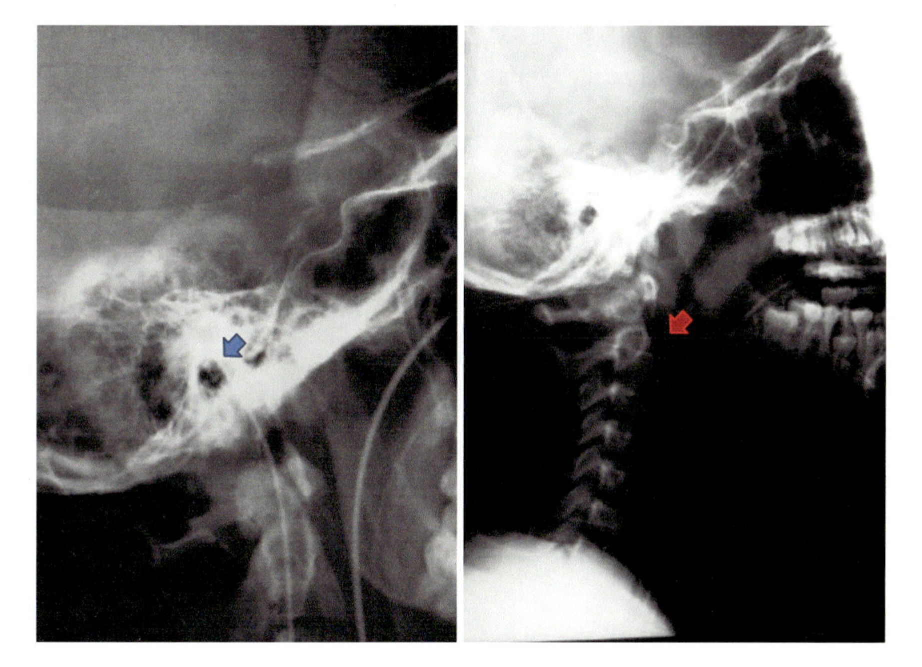

Fig. 11.5 Plain X-ray to evaluate the placement of the tip of the retrograde jugular catheter in the jugular bulb: the left panel highlights the correct positioning in the jugular bulb (blue arrow). In the right panel the catheter tip is high in the jugular vein (red arrow) but not in the jugular bulb and therefore the sample is contaminated by extracranial blood

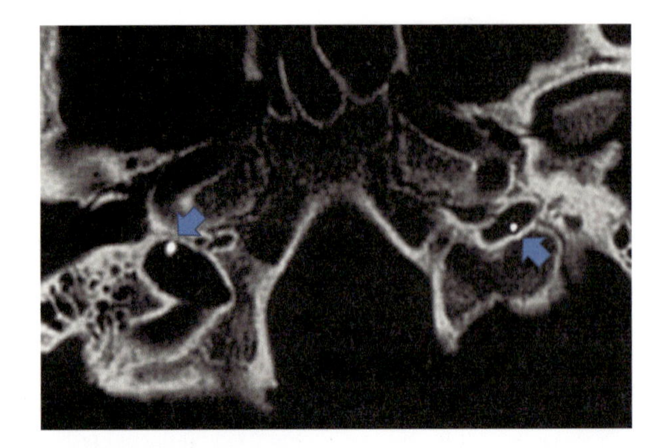

Fig. 11.6 CT scan of the skull base to evaluate the placement of the tips (blue arrows) in the jugular bulb. The size of the jugular bulbs is variable, with the right side being significantly larger than the left in two-thirds of people

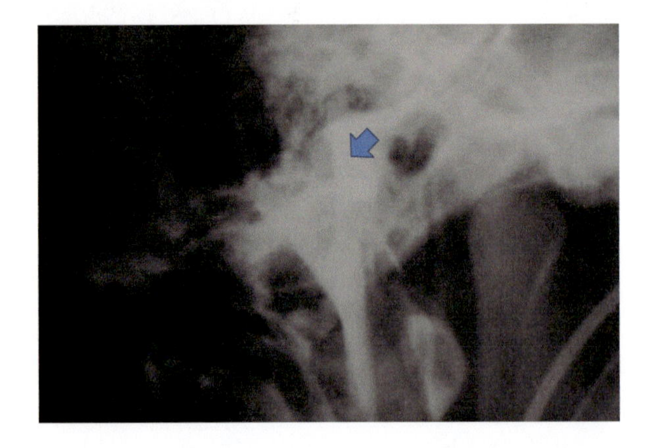

Fig. 11.7 Plain X-ray after medium contrast injection with the visualisation of the jugular bulb (blue arrow)

fictitiously high SjO_2 values. The most serious complications are venous thrombosis (Fig. 11.9) and misplacement in spinal space (Fig. 11.10). A further difficulty was defining normal values in the population. In fact, in the work of Gibbs in 1942 [77] and Dastur in 1963 [78], the sampling was obtained with the direct transcutaneous puncture of the jugular bulb, without radiological confirmation of the needle's tip, as initially described by Myerson [79]. The placement of the catheter in the jugular bulb is considered a more reliable technique, and normal values were obtained during the venography of endocrinological patients undergoing angiographic studies [80]. In this study, the SjO_2 values in normal subjects were lower, 57.1% (CI 52.3–61.6%). However, another level of normality occurs in TBI, which is characterised by higher levels of SjO_2 [81], and this value changes according to the time elapsed from trauma. The values for normal subjects and TBI patients are described in Table 11.1 [82–86]. Table 11.1 also describes the values with normal distribution expected in pathology compared to those expected in subjects without TBI. The jugular bulb is physiologically contaminated by 2.7% of extracerebral blood [87], and a slow aspiration rate is important to minimise the risk of further extracerebral blood aspiration [88]. In clinical use, the limits related to the impossibility of seeing

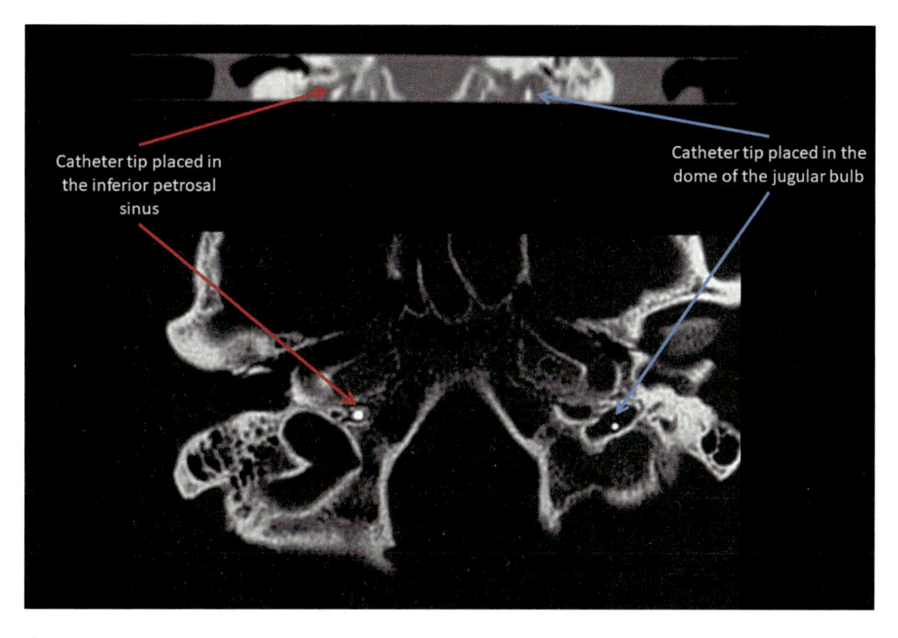

Fig. 11.8 Incorrect placement of a jugular bulb catheter in the right inferior petrosal sinus in comparison with the correct placement in the left jugular bulb

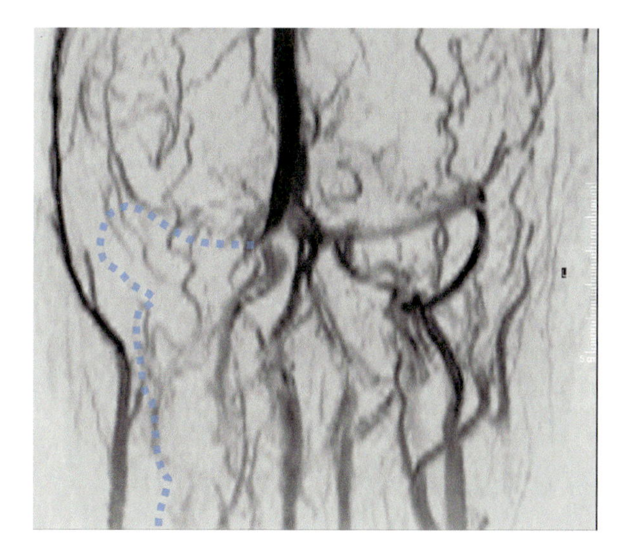

Fig. 11.9 AngioMRI showing the retrograde thrombosis of the right jugular vein and the intracranial venous system until the torcular (all dashed in blue)

focal phenomena have always been evident [89, 90]. The $AVDO_2$ and the SjO_2 do not only express the coupling between $CMRO_2$ and CBF, but in the lower values, they are in relation with the PjO_2 (the partial pressure of oxygen in the venous blood) and, therefore, with the tissue pressure of O_2 in turn in connection with the mitochondrial oxygen pressure. The relationships between low SjO_2 values and

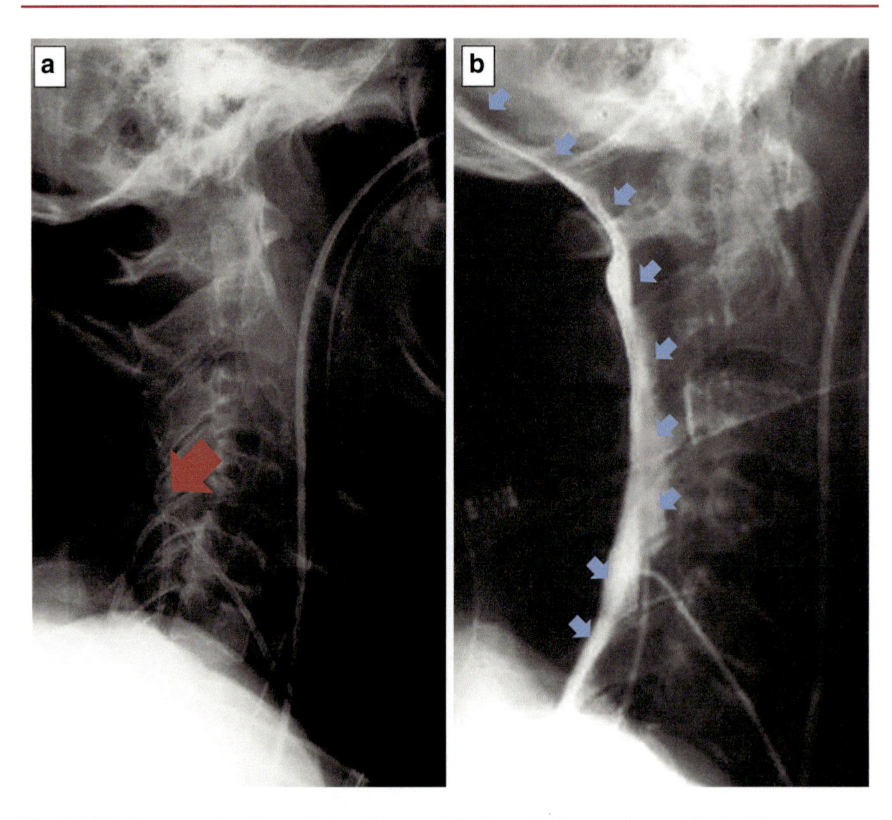

Fig. 11.10 Incorrect jugular catheter placement in the spinal space in a patient with an aneurysmatic subarachnoid haemorrhage. The aspiration of a bloody spinal blood apparently indicated correct venous positioning. Low haemoglobin values and radiological images with (**b**) and without (**a**) contrast injection. The red arrow indicate the tip of the catheter in the spinal space. The spinal space opacization is indicated by the multiple smaller blue arrows

Table 11.1 Oxygen saturation values in the jugular bulb (SjO_2)

		SjO_2 (%)		
	n	Mean (95% C.I.)	Upper limit (95% C.I.)	Lower limit (95% C.I.)
Normal subjects				
Gibbs 1942 [77]	50	62.0 (61.0–63.1)	69.4 (67.6–71.2)	54.6 (52.8–56.5)
Datsur 1963 [78]	26	64.3 (62.4–66.2)	73.7 (70.4–76.9)	55.0 (51.7–58.2)
Chieregato 2003 [81]	9	57.1 (52.3–61.6)	69.5 (61.2–77.7)	44.7 (36.5–53.0)
Severe head injury (Chieregato 1994–1997 unpublished data)				
All ICU data [80]	71	62.9 (60.6–65.2)	82.5 (78.5–86.6)	43.2 (39.2–47.3)
First 24 h post injury	71	59.2 (56.7–61.7)	80.2 (75.9–84.6)	38.1 (33.8–42.4)
24–48 h post injury	57	65.9 (64.3–67.5)	78.1 (75.3–80.8)	53.7 (51–56.5)
Post 48 h post injury	54	65.5 (64.1–66.9)	75.8 (73.4–78.3)	55.1 (52.6–57.5)
Brain death patients (Chieregato 1994–1997 unpublished data)	26	90 (87.9–92.0)	100 (96.5–103.5)	79.9 (76.4–83.4)

Gibbs [77] and Datsur [78] measurements were done using the blind percutaneous puncture of the jugular bulb according to Myerson [79]. Chieregato [81] sampled the blood into the jugular bulb under angiographic controlled catheterisation

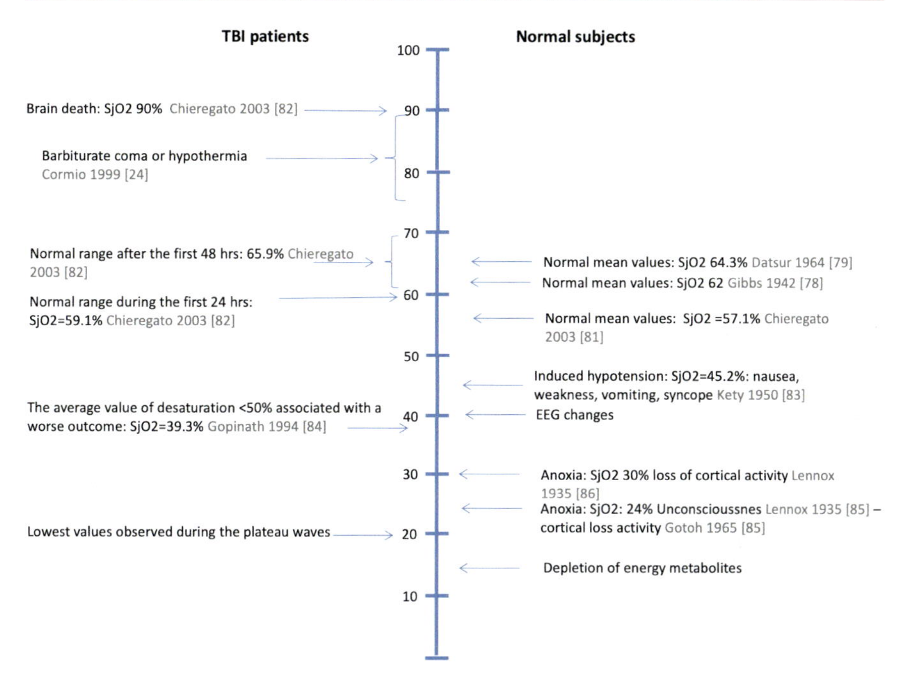

Fig. 11.11 The diagram represents in a schematic and semi-quantitative way the relationship between SjO_2 values and neurological deficits in normal subjects. The opposite side shows the SjO_2 levels in trauma patients

neurological symptoms and signs are shown in Fig. 11.11. As we said, the main expectation from $AVDO_2$, especially in centres without any chance to measure CBF, is to estimate CBF and $CMRO_2$. Therefore, from data on 546 Xe-CT studies on 260 patients with data obtained after the first 24 h, $AVDO_2$ and CBF seem to be strictly coupled (Fig. 11.12). These findings confirm that in stabilised patients, the coupling between CBF and $AVDO_2$ is preserved, and therefore $AVDO_2$ could give insights into CBF values. Conversely, the scatterplots show that in the usual CPP range, intended to be one of the cornerstones in ICP management, neither CBF, $AVDO_2$, nor $CMRO_2$ shows a dependency on CPP. That could be interpreted as an achieved new homeostasis in the acute plateau phase of trauma. Considering now the meaning of $AVDO_2$ and SjO_2 as a proxy of $CMRO_2$, for example, a very high value of SjO_2 can be observed in hypothermia or barbiturate coma, which is explained by a reduction in $CMRO_2$ [25]. However, high values of SjO_2 could be due also due to a spontaneous post-traumatic depression of $CMRO_2$ rather than an increase in CBF and that explains the prognostic association was observed between lower $AVDO_2$ values and the worst outcome (Fig. 11.13) [91, 92]. These observations of a few years ago are well connected with the most recent hypotheses based on the combined study of OEF, $PbtO_2$ and L/P ratio on the hypoxic state in the presence of sufficient O_2 availability. Conversely, after the first few days, larger $AVDO_2$ values can result from a more efficient oxygen extraction and a higher $CMRO_2$ which

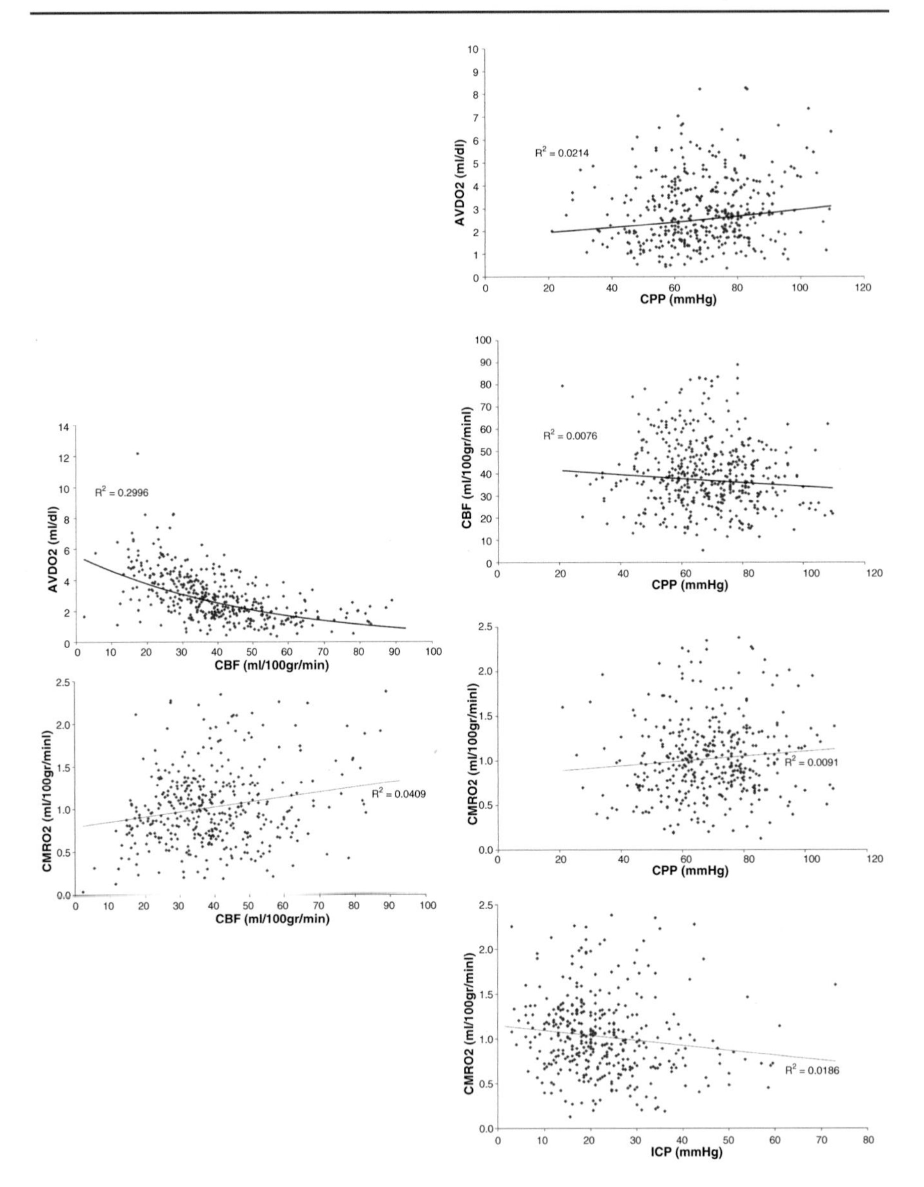

Fig. 11.12 Scatterplot between CBF (independent variable) and $AVDO_2$ (dependent variable). The scatterplot between CBF and $CMRO_2$ shows the independency of $CMRO_2$ from CBF albeit a potential mathematical coupling. No correlation is shown among ICP or CPP and $AVDO_2$ or CBF, or $CMRO_2$. Original data from A. Chieregato, not published

correlated with better outcome because the brain that extracts more works better. The spontaneous and induced sedation reduction of $CMRO_2$-is well described in Fig. 11.14 from unpublished data of 260 patients with Xe-CT and $AVDO_2$ studies. Once again, it can be appreciated as the first 8–16 h are the most critical because low

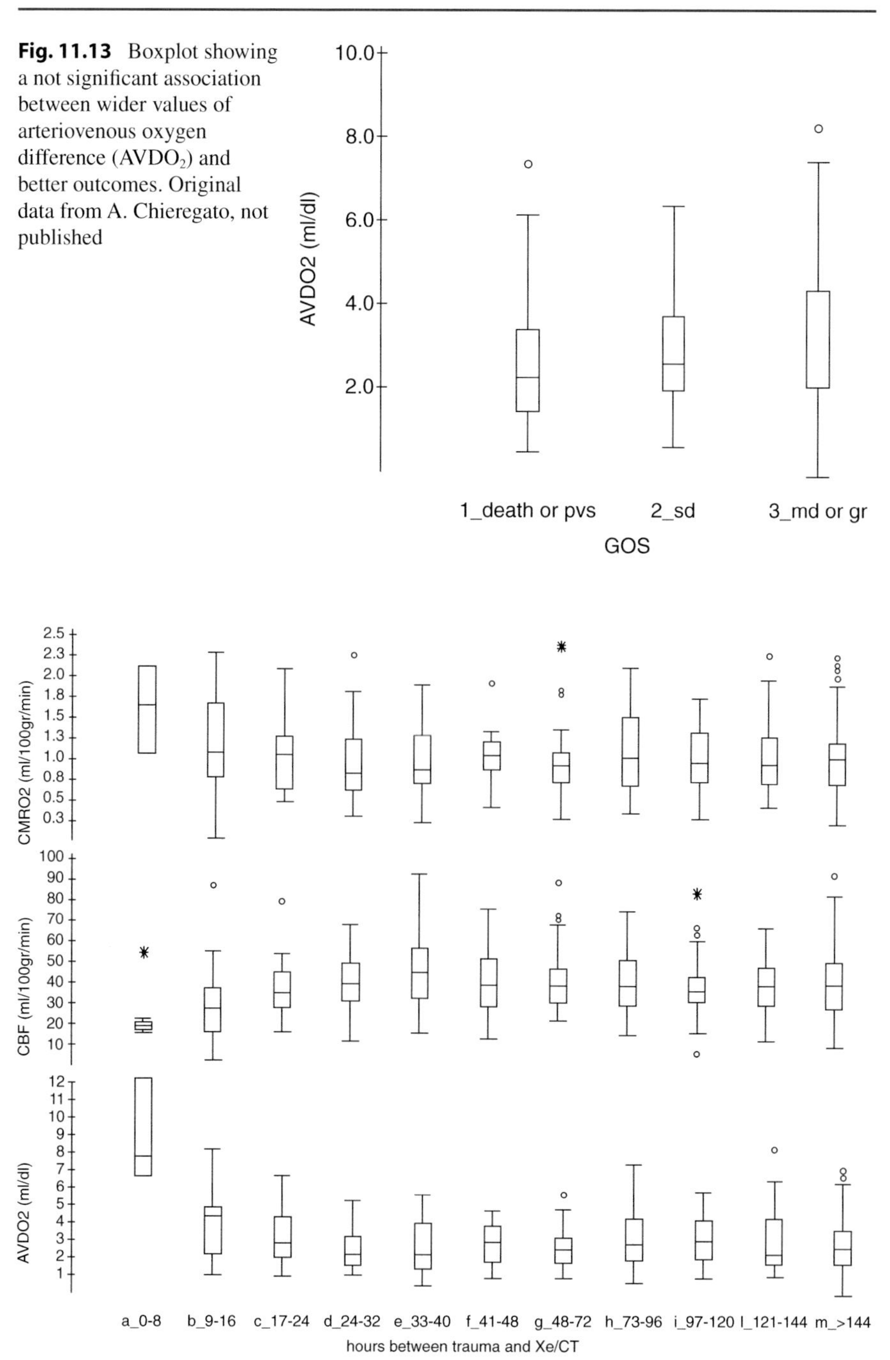

Fig. 11.13 Boxplot showing a not significant association between wider values of arteriovenous oxygen difference ($AVDO_2$) and better outcomes. Original data from A. Chieregato, not published

Fig. 11.14 Cerebral metabolic rate of oxygen ($CMRO_2$), cerebral blood flow (CBF) and arteriovenous oxygen difference ($AVDO_2$) trends in the first six days after TBI. Original data from A. Chieregato, not published

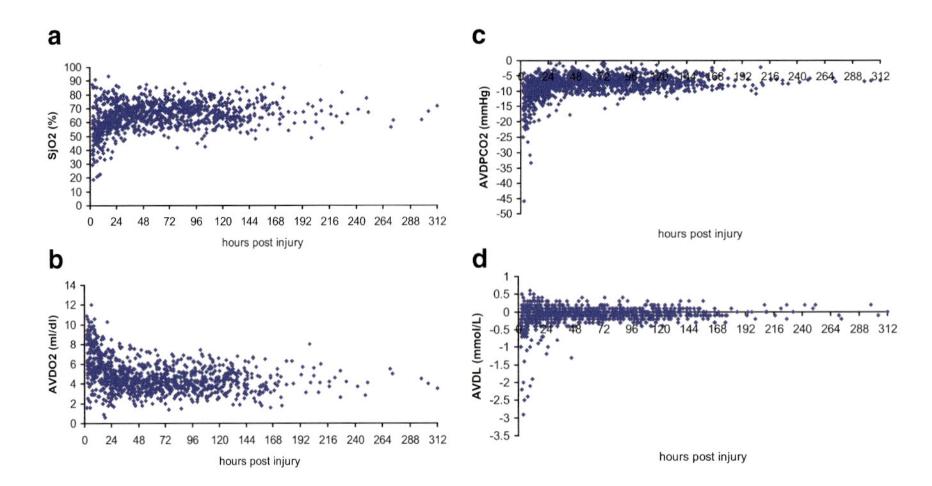

Fig. 11.15 Trend shows physiological variables during the first-thirteen days after TBI. A wide data dispersion is observed during the first 24 h. Original data from A. Chieregato, not published. (**a**) Jugular venous oxygen saturation (SjO_2), (**b**) arteriovenous PaO_2 difference ($AVDO_2$), (**c**) arteriovenous $PaCO_2$ difference ($AVDPCO_2$) and (**d**) arteriovenous lactate difference (AVDL) trend

CBF is associated with higher $CMRO_2$ and lower CBF values. The reduction of $CMRO_2$ and its independency from CPP values corroborates the hypothesis of a spontaneous decline in $CMRO_2$ to the changing of oxygen extraction shown by PET studies. The observation of the relationships between $CMRO_2$, $AVDO_2$ and outcome, together with independence from the CPP, shows that during the state phase, after the first 24 h, the $AVDO_2$ seems more informative for the definition of the prognosis than for the treatment of the patient. Nevertheless, these limitations leave open the use of $AVDO_2$ and SjO_2 as monitoring in the very complex hyperacute phase in which CO_2D is limited by trauma-associated hypotension, hypoxia, hypercapnia, anaemia and ICP is under active management and on the other side, the $CMRO_2$ shutdown has not yet occurred. Figure 11.15 from 79 patients obtained during the first 48 h shows the complex dynamics of this phase. Large $AVDO_2$ values in the first 24 h associated with low CPP values and widening of AVDL and $AVDCO_2$ suggest compensated or uncompensated hypoperfusion and are associated with a poorer outcome. In the early 1980 and until ten years ago, SjO_2 was the first, inexpensive window on brain metabolism available to any neurointensivist and neurosurgeon. The persistently high SjO_2 after the first days and the rarity of the interventions following its measurement have led to a gradual abandonment of the technique [93]. In the same way, the ultra-early use of SjO_2 is cumbersome from an operative point of view. Even if highly informative, in the first 24 h the use of SjO_2 in the emergency room has been abandoned. The relevance of early SjO_2 measurement relay on the observation that initially the $CMRO_2$ is higher, which goes hand in hand with the trend of SjO_2 which in the first 24 h is often below the normal values. The causes of this phenomenon can be multiple, for example, the effect of sedatives, a down-regulation associated with the severity of the coma (remember the

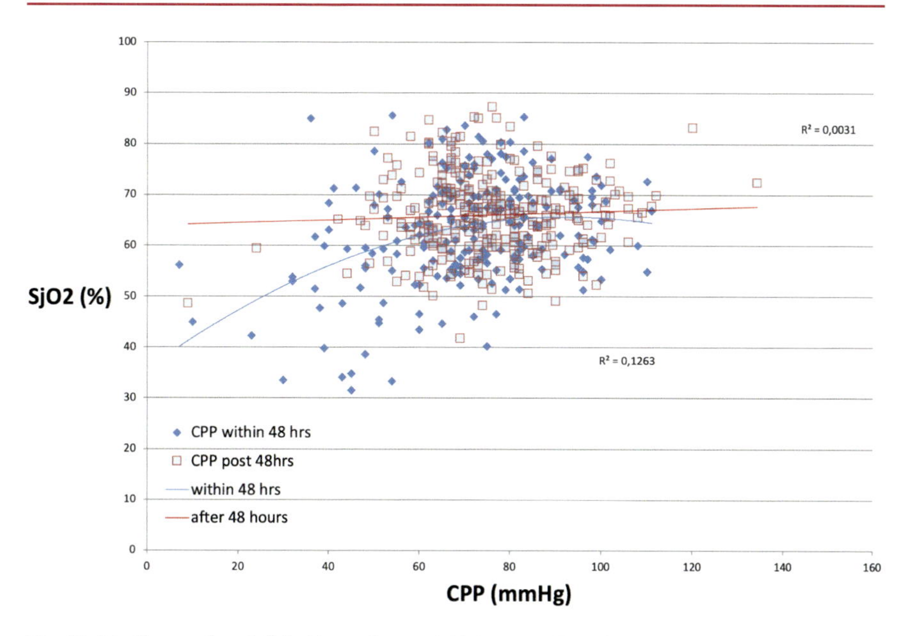

Fig. 11.16 Scatterplot of SjO_2 (dependent variable) versus CPP (independent variable). A dependency could be observed during the first 48 h but not in the following days

$CMRO_2$/GCS scatterplot by Obrist), or an actual alteration of O_2 metabolism [63, 65, 92] perhaps present in the most severe cases. The significance of SjO_2 in the first 24 h, a phase in which $CMRO_2$ is not depressed, has been underestimated [94]. In this time window, CBF could be critical and occult ICP not yet measured, hypotension and/or anaemia could be present. Figure 11.16 describes the different SjO_2 dependencies from CPP in the first 48 h with respect to phase post the first 48 h when SjO_2 is substantially independent of CPP values. Unpractical aspects in early patient management may have reduced its diffusion in the emergency room. Still, its measurement and information are not very dissimilar to those gathered by Verweij and Muizelaar [95] when they placed an ICP catheter before the evacuation of an acute subdural hematoma or when Schroder and Muizelaar [38] performed a Xe-CT with the hematoma still to be evacuated, and showed very elevated ICP values and highly depressed CBF and rCBF values. This physiological knowledge is the basis of the empirical therapy that is performed in patients with pupillary dilation with high-dose mannitol and hyperventilation, with or without barbiturate, which, at least in patients with mass, can reduce ICP levels reducing biological damage before the evacuation of the hematoma [96]. This therapy acts by reducing the CBV in the brain contralateral the hematoma through coupled vasoconstriction (barbiturate), hypocapnic direct vasoconstriction (hyperventilation) and autoregulatory vasoconstriction (bolus effect of mannitol). One of the intrinsic limits of SjO_2 is that its measure alone does not explain if its values are associated with a derangement of cellular metabolism. When the mismatch has already produced its damage (extensive cerebral infarction or post-traumatic alteration of O_2 metabolism, for example), the supervened extraction difficulty allows that high SjO_2 values can be associated with cellular anaerobiosis. In those years, Claudia Robertson [97] introduced the measurement of the arteriovenous difference in lactate (AVDL) and its relationship with $AVDO_2$ to compensate for these limitations. With this approach, she could distinguish early ischemia with low SjO_2 and normal AVDL, suggesting a CO_2D reduction but a preserved $CMRO_2$ [98], from definitive ischemia, with higher SjO_2 and high pathological AVDL. Robertson introduced a new index: the Lactate Oxygen Index (LOI), the ratio between AVDL and $AVDO_2$. Some reports showed informative findings from $AVDO_2$, SjO_2 and AVDL, especially in the first 24–48 h post-injury [83, 94, 99, 100]. The main results are the association between wide AVDL measured during the first 48 h post-injury with poorer outcomes, specifically in patients who developed refractory intracranial hypertension and cerebral dead in the first 48 h. Lactate is so well managed by the astrocyte-neuron unit that its spread beyond the blood-brain barrier denotes severe damage, manifesting as a late sign [94]. Conversely, positive AVDL values seem more frequent in TBI patients with a good recovery or a moderate disability at 1 year (Fig. 11.17). That can be explained by the role of lactate as an energy substrate for the brain [101], especially during peritraumatic arterial hyperlacticaemia [102]. In the early 90', the limited availability at bedside of the lactic acid analyser and the fact that delays in the execution of the test could be associated with the accumulation of lactate produced by the same erythrocytes reduced the use of AVDL in the acute phase. To compensate for these lactate limits, the arteriovenous CO_2 difference ($AVDpCO_2$) was explored [99, 103, 104], aware that an increase in the CO_2-delta could again potentially recognise two

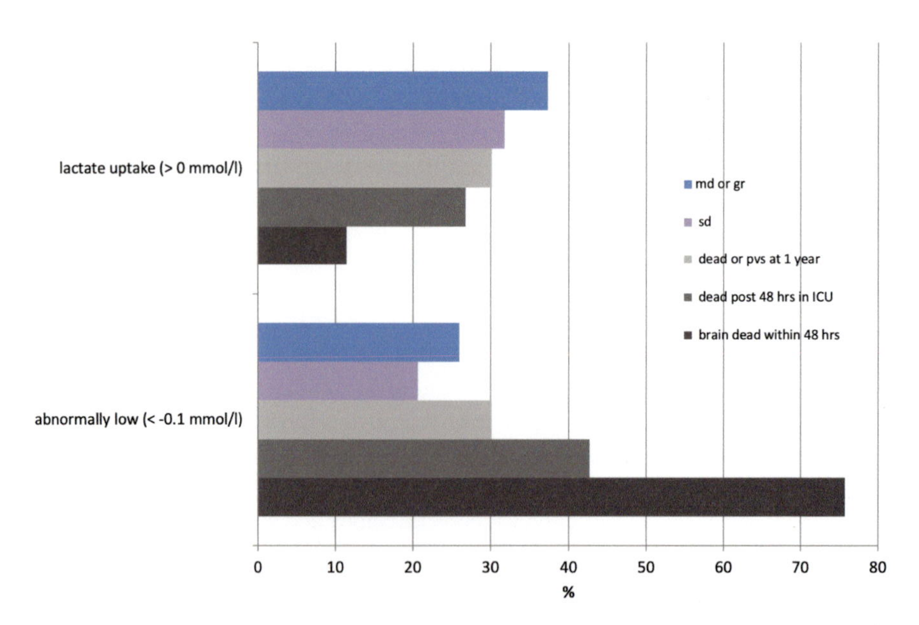

Fig. 11.17 Bar chart showing the association of AVDL categories and outcome. An association can be observed between the uptake of lactate and improved outcomes

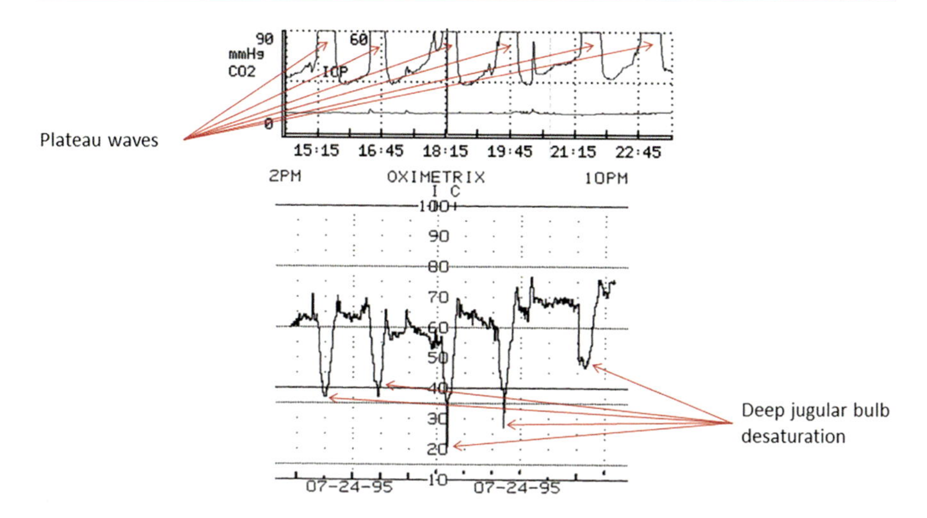

Fig. 11.18 The deep jugular bulb desaturation during plateau waves as evaluated by a fiberoptic catheter

causes: according to Fick's law, a reduction in CBF or a net production of CO_2 as the result of the buffering of the hydrogen ions produced by lactate. This limit was approached by relativising $AVDpCO_2$ and $AVDO_2$ with a simplified respiratory quotient (eQR) [99]. Although prognostic relationships have been described, use in clinical practice has not spread. In the 1990s, at a time when there were highly supported guidelines in favour of high levels of CPP based on the studies of Rosner [105], regardless of patient age and previous history of arterial hypertension, Claudia Robertson conducted a randomised controlled trial on two different therapeutic aims, guided or not by the achievement of target values of SjO_2. Infact, the study was supported by the observation that jugular bulb desaturations were associated with an unfavourable outcome [83]. This study did not obtain outcome benefits for the patient in whom the target SjO_2 values were obtained[106] but fivefold more medical complications [107]. The use of optical fibre catheters could have been of considerable support for continuously monitoring the relationship between interventions and ICP. However, the instability of the position of the catheter with respect to the vessel lumen often led to unreliable signals [108]. After the first post-trauma days, the persistently high characteristic of SjO_2 levels sampled episodically as well as the rarity of the interventions following its measurement [93], the relative reliability of continuous sampling with optical fibres and the appearance of the new sensors for measuring PtO_2 have led to a gradual abandonment of the technique notwithstanding its high potentiality. Figure 11.18 reported the extremely low values of SjO_2 measured employing a fiberoptic catheter during an ICP plateau wave. For an attending physician, observing a signal of this type at the bedside strengthens attention by identifying the metabolic crisis during the plateau wave. In less dramatic conditions, the SjO_2 fiberoptics catheter highlights the sensitivity of SjO_2 to $EtCO_2$ changes (Fig. 11.19). For those who have used SjO_2 in clinical practice, the

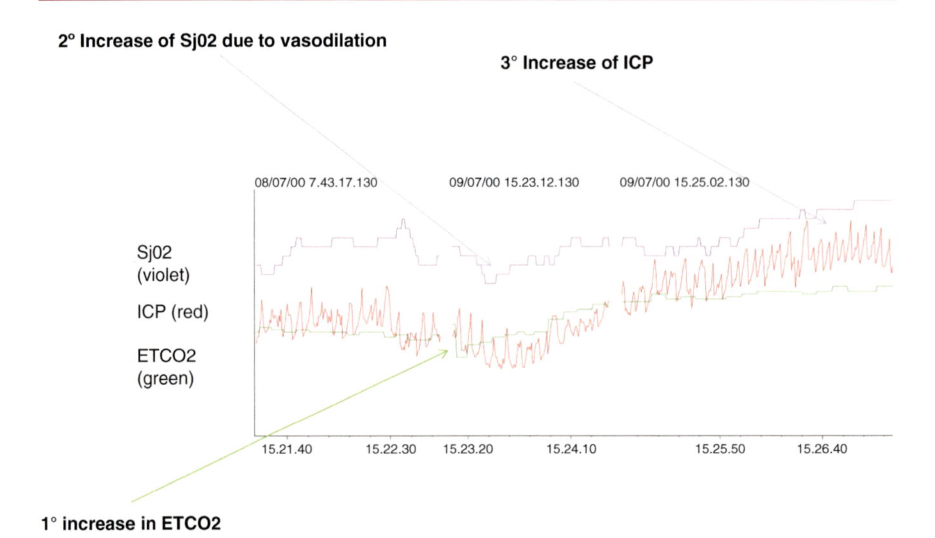

Fig. 11.19 The sensitivity of SjO_2 continuous measurement to changes in $EtCO_2$

perfusion and metabolic dimension has opened up and still resides in their cultural heritage [93]. It is the writer's opinion that the positioning in the first hours after the trauma of a SjO_2, as of an ICP, can identify underestimated damage in a phase of greater brain vulnerability. In intensive care, SjO_2 can still be useful for the non-blind use of hyperventilation among the second-level therapies of ICP. SjO_2 might also be useful for applying the minimum dose of barbiturate therapy to control refractory ICP along with ICP and EEG monitoring [24].

11.4.1 Brain Tissue Oxygen Monitoring

The $PbtO_2$ was born in the early 90s with the Clark-type polarographic partial pressure of oxygen probe (LICOX. GMS mbH, Kiel, Germany). The value measured must not be considered an intracellular PO_2 but more an interstitial PO_2. According to the Krogh theory, the values of interstitial PO_2 are heterogeneous as a function of the distance from the arteriolar bed and from the capillary itself (Fig. 11.20). LICOX is a tiny sensor (diameter 0.8 mm) that measures the voltage of dissolved oxygen at the tip, with the possibility of correcting the value according to the cerebral temperature. Initially, a second type of catheter (PARATREND) measured $PbtO_2$ with further intriguing measures such as PCO_2 and pH. Procedural complications are truly anecdotal, but the costs of the device are not marginal. The sampling area around the LICOX catheter is 13 mm^2. Therefore, in choosing the positioning, the clinician must decide which is the focus of greatest interest: the apparently healthy brain or the perilesional normal appearing area or the perilesional area surrounding the hemorrhagic core. A centrifugal evolution of rCBF

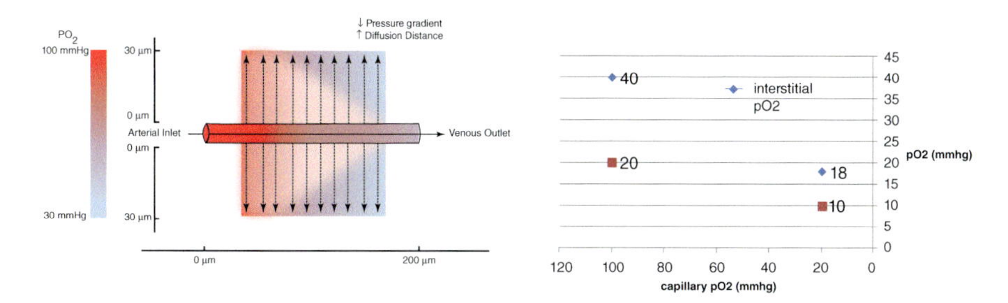

Fig. 11.20 The value measured by $PbtO_2$ is not intracellular PO_2 but more interstitial PO_2. According to the Krogh theory, the values of interstitial PO_2 are in continuous variation as a function of the distance from the arteriolar bed and from the capillary itself

anomalies is observed in focal pathologies such as traumatic hematoma [9]. In patients with diffuse injury, the $PbtO_2$ sensor is positioned in the subcortical white matter (a structure with a CBF about 33% lower than the cortex). For example, in a patient with diffuse injury (Fig. 11.21), the rCBF in the region of interest around the $PbtO_2$ is equivalent to that of the hemisphere. The positioning in the perilesional hypodense area or outside this area is obviously less simple. For example, this attempt can be burdened by inaccuracy as the probe may be placed erroneously inside the hemorrhagic core, instead of the edematous area. Figure 11.22 shows the placement of a $PbtO_2$ catheter in a lesion affected by vasogenic oedema. $PbtO_2$ arrives as a technological advance following SjO_2, and therefore SjO_2 was surpassed. The different behaviours concerning SjO_2 were rapidly clarified by studies demonstrating a good correlation in the apparently healthy tissue [109] and a poor correlation in the pathological tissue at CT scan [89]. Thresholds for ischemia were estimated using converging data from infarct determination after permanent middle cerebral artery occlusion in a feline model [110], from double measurement with Xe-CT and comparing to the ischemic threshold for CBF, comparing with known thresholds of SjO_2 or CPP [111] with outcome analysis in severely TBI patients [110, 112]. In apparently healthy tissue, after a secondary insult, SjO_2 for values of 40–50% correspond to $PbtO_2$ values among 5–8 mmHg [109, 113]. Some studies have established a relationship between the rCBF and the $PbtO_2$. In the work of Menzel [114] on TBI patients, by interpolating the $PbtO_2$ value of 20 mmHg in the curve, the value of rCBF measured with Xe- CT seems to be below 15 ml/100gr/min. Conversely, in the Valadka study [115], higher values of rCBF (less than 30 ml/100gr/min) can be interpolated for values of $PbtO_2$ of 20 mmHg. We must also consider that the rCBF changes over time, and the duration of the low rCBF is a cofactor in the result of ischemia [116]. The study by Cunningham and Menon [62] introduces the concept of a probabilistic threshold for irreversible damage associated with CBF levels below 15 ml/100 g/min. Furthermore, we need to consider that $PbtO_2$ is usually located in the white matter where the rCBF is physiologically lower as well as the threshold for ischemia that according to an old study, appears to be

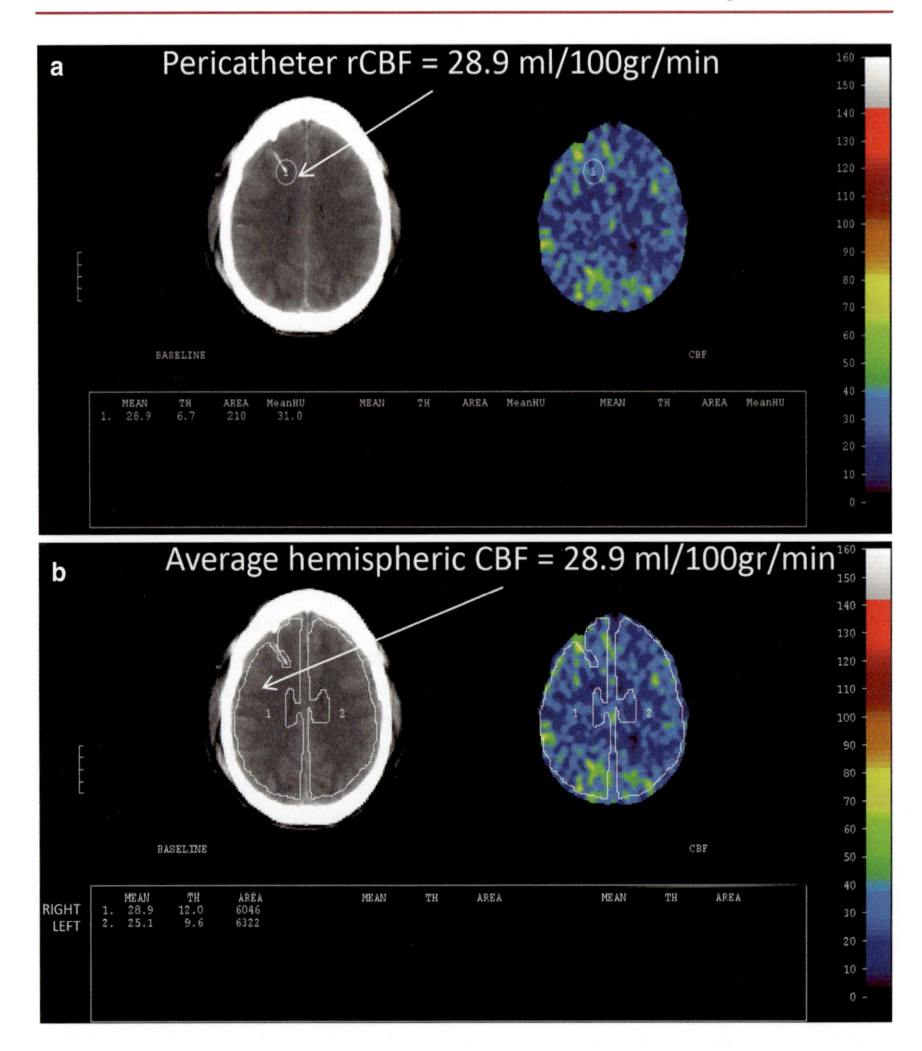

Fig. 11.21 Regional cerebral blood flow (rCBF) for (**a**) peri-catheter $PbtO_2$ tip and (**b**) hemispheric cerebral blood flow (1: right and 2: left) measured by XeCT. In a patient with diffuse injury, the $PbtO_2$ catheter placed in a normal-appearing healthy-brain area is a proxy for hemispheric evaluation

below 7.4 ml/100g/min [117]. According to the review by Stocchetti and colleagues [1] higher values of $PbtO_2$, between 15 and 20 mmHg, are associated with worse long-term outcome [63, 113]. Having defined what the critical values could be, the researchers have long wondered what could be the dominant role of determining the value of $PbtO_2$: the arteriolar side, the haemoglobin dissociation curve, the amount of haemoglobin, the regional blood flow, the irregularity of the capillaries, the compression by the swelling of the capillaries, the oxygen consumption, the mitochondrial oxygen extraction, the resistance to diffusion of oxygen from the capillary to the mitochondria? These aspects await more advanced research, and, in this

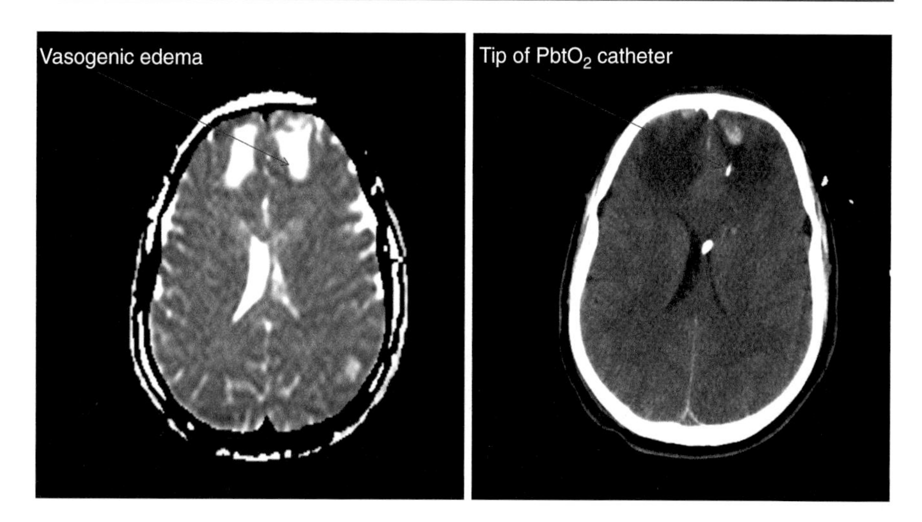

Fig. 11.22 A catheter correctly placed inside a vasogenic edematous area to observe penumbra

direction, we suggest reading the papers of Rosenthal [57] and Menon [63]. Rosenthal's combined the measurement of rCBF by thermodilution (Hemedex) with $PbtO_2$ measured by LICOX in the frontal white matter, apparently normal to the CT scan. He measured the effect of increased CPP obtained with catecholamines, of an increased PaO_2 (obtained by means of hyperoxia) and the induction of hypocapnia. The authors well recognised that manipulating PaO_2 can dramatically affect the value of $PbtO_2$. Using multivariate statistics, Rosenthal found that the coupled changes in rCBF and $AVDO_2$ offer the best association with $PbtO_2$ variations. The authors postulate that $PbtO_2$ may indicate oxygen accumulated in the tissue and that $PbtO_2$ it is not strictly the result of a balance between delivery and consumption. "the only statistically significant relationship was that between $PbtO_2$ and the product of CBF and cerebral arteriovenous oxygen tension difference ($AVTO_2$) suggesting a strong association between brain oxygen tension and diffusion of dissolved oxygen across the blood-brain barrier". And again "Local brain tissue oxygen tension is closely related to the product of local CBF and arteriovenous oxygen tension difference, suggesting that $PbtO_2$ may better reflect diffusion of dissolved plasma oxygen rather than total oxygen delivery or cerebral oxygen metabolism". They highlight a functional interplay between rCBF and PaO_2: hyperoxia produces vasoconstriction, and therefore the hypothesis that hyperoxia increased $PbtO_2$ is not sustainable during normobaric hyperoxia. On the contrary, when both rCBF and PaO_2 are reduced, certainly $PbtO_2$ is, in that setting, an indicator of reduced delivery. $PbtO_2$ must therefore be considered a *warning* indicator sensitive to the drop of PaO_2 (and SpO_2), of $PaCO_2$ (and $EtCO_2$), of CPP, of hemoglobinemia and to the increase in temperature but not specific to interpret one or the other physiological component. The association between $PbtO_2$ values ranging from 15 to 20 mmHg and negative outcome led, as happened for SjO_2, to perform studies to maintain $PbtO_2$ values above certain thresholds [118]. It is quite different to

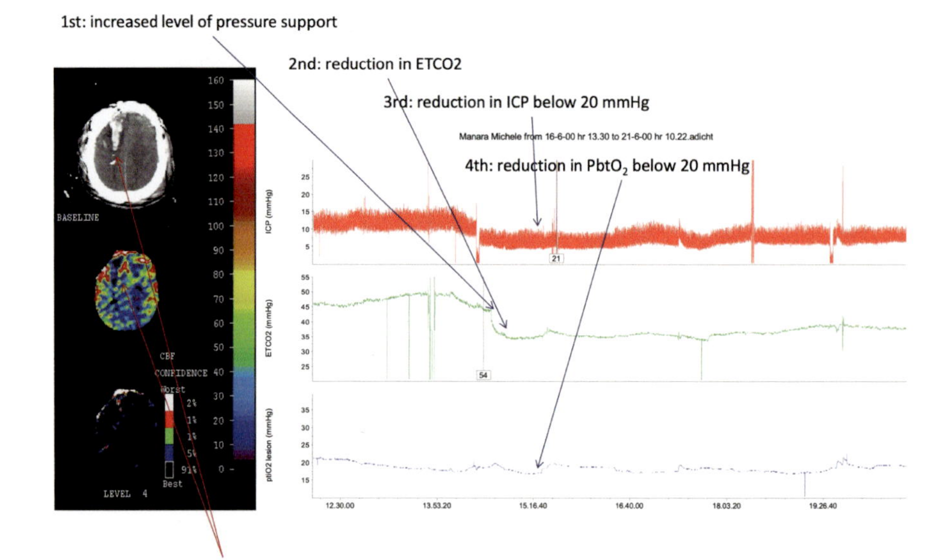

Fig. 11.23 The combined effect of hyperventilation on ICP and PbO_2

understand whether these strategies have any relevance in influencing the outcome of patients. Meixensberger, for example, by piloting the CPP, obtained success on the $PbtO_2$ values but without the possibility of verifying correspondents in terms of outcome [118]. More recently, Spiotta [119] showed, in a pre-post comparison, an association with an improvement in the long-term outcome when patients were not only cared according to an ICP-CPP-oriented protocol but also directed to achieve $PbtO_2$ values above 20 mmHg. The review of Nangunoori [120] well represents the state of the art on the subject and suggests a benefit from management which includes $PbtO_2$ monitoring. All the studies included were observational, and the evaluation of outcomes was not standardised for initial severity. Hays performed a systematic review and a meta-analysis which identified only three randomised controlled trials comparing strategies based on the control of $PbtO_2$ [121]. Randomised controlled trials [122–124] did not found an association between the addition of PbO_2-guided management and improved neurological outcome but found an association with increased survival. This is not new in traumatology or critical care medicine. Improving technology and monitoring can save a life but cannot improve, for example, an expected severe disability to a good recovery. Currently, the use of $PbtO_2$ helps to evaluate the impact of secondary insults at the bedside in a rather regional way, but technologically more reliable than SjO_2. Some of the changes in $PbtO_2$ can be explained (Fig. 11.23), others not (Fig. 11.24). It should be considered that among the variables conditioning $PbtO_2$, there is PaO_2 which can fluctuate based on ventilation/lung recruitment.

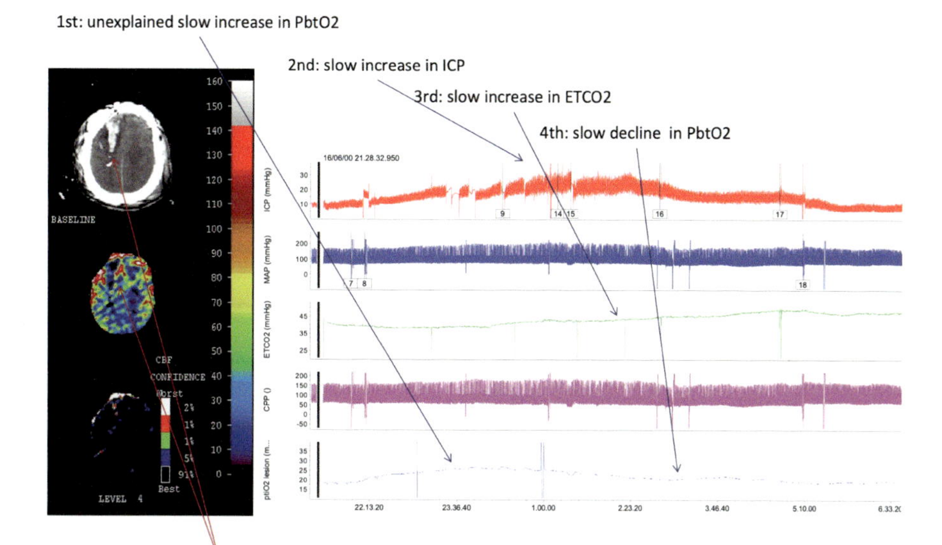

Fig. 11.24 Changes of $PbtO_2$ which the other variables cannot explain

11.5 Cerebral Microdialysis

The picture of cerebral monitors (Table 11.2) ends with the microdialysis. Cerebral microdialysis (CMD) is a micro-invasive technology that monitors semi-continuous extracellular interstitial fluid. It was introduced in advanced centres approximately 30 years ago [125], usually in combination with $PbtO_2$. A thin CMD catheter (diameter 0.6 mm) with a dialysis membrane at its tip is introduced into brain tissue. The CMD catheter may be tunnelled under the scalp and introduced into the brain tissue through a burr hole drilled in the cranium or directly through a bolt fixed to the skull in the usual manner. A CMD pump perfuses the interior of the catheter with an artificial cerebrospinal fluid, which equilibrates with the interstitial tissue surrounding the catheter. The equilibration takes place by diffusion of chemicals over the dialysis membrane without the need to remove any fluid from the organ. Using a 10-mm dialysis membrane and a perfusion flow of 0.3 l/min, glucose, lactate, pyruvate, and glutamate concentration in the dialysate becomes approximately 70% of the concentration in the interstitial fluid. The samples are continuously collected and analysed by a CMD analyser at the bedside, usually every hour or as needed. The analysis results are displayed as trend curves on the analyser. The authors suggest reading the report of the 2004 [126] and 2014 [127] consensus conference to observe the evolution of the knowledge. While $PbtO_2$, although non-specific, increases the insight into tissue oxygen storage and oxygen delivery, CMD adds information on substrate delivery and metabolism at the cellular level. It thus provides the most

Table 11.2 Neuromonitoring modalities for traumatic brain injury

	ICP	PRx	TCCD	$PbtO_2$	SjO_2	Cerebral microdialysis	EEG/SSEP/BAER
Variable observed and derived	Intracranial pressure → intracranial volume, intracranial compliance and cerebral perfusion pressure	High density ICP and MAP → autoregulation	Cerebral blood velocity → critical closing pressure and cerebral arterial impedance	Brain tissue partial tension of oxygen → oxygen diffusion and balance between CO_2D and $CMRO_2$	Oxygen saturation of venous jugular haemoglobin → balance between CO_2D and $CMRO_2$	Brain metabolite → aerobic or anaerobic metabolism, brain injury severity and inflammation	Cortical electrical activity → seizure activity, cellular disfunction
Type of measure	Global	Global	Global	Focal/global	Global	Focal	Global
Time resolution	Continuous	Continuous	Intermittent	Continuous	Intermittent/continuous	Intermittent	Continuous/ intermittent
PROs	Availability Price Waves analysis, more than pressure	Objective evaluation of cerebral reactivity Tailored CPP approach	Non-invasive monitoring High-ICP estimation Evaluation of cerebral reactivity	Surrogate for brain ischemia Peri-lesion monitoring or global monitoring	Availability Price (not for continuous monitoring)	Brain metabolism analysis Cellular dimension monitoring "mitochondrial approach"	Proxy for cellular integrity Availability (less for qEEG monitoring or intermittent SSEP/ BAER) NCSE detection Low-price
CONs	Risk of brain damage	Availability	Operator-dependent Transtemporal insonation not feasible PI depend also on several systemic and cerebral variables	Two variables analysed together Price Availability Risk of brain damage Difficult to focal position	Two variables analysed together Drug-pathophysiologic reduction of $CMRO_2$ → Low sensitivity to detect brain ischemia Price (for continuous monitoring)	Time-consuming Availability High price Risk of brain damage	Advanced skills for interpretation Bias of sedation for EEG

ICP intracranial cerebral pressure, *PRx* pressure reactivity index, *TCCD* transcranial color-coupled doppler, *EEG* electroencephalogram, *SSEP* somatosensory evoked potential, *BAER* brain stem auditory evoked response, *qEEG* quantitative-EEG, *CPP* cerebral perfusion pressure, *PI* pulsatility index direct means to monitor the fundamental process of energy failure. Not differently from $PbtO_2$, the technique of CMD is safe for the patient. As with all monitoring devices, including ICP electronic catheter, the risk related to the monitoring could be therapies directed by an inappropriate monitoring interpretation and not by the placement of the monitoring itself. Unlike $PbtO_2$, in TBI patients with diffuse injury, one catheter may be placed in the right frontal region. One catheter should be placed in the penumbra, the pericontusional tissue in patients with focal mass lesions. A second catheter could be placed in normal tissue in such patients. However, only in isolated publications [128] were two microdialysis catheters positioned in the edematous and apparently healthy areas, showing a higher metabolic vulnerability due to CPP reductions. No catheter should be placed in contusional-necrotic core tissue as for the $PbtO_2$ catheter. An editorial by Menon [3] highlights the heterogeneity of the TBI patients and different brain areas, and in particular the sensitivity of the traumatic penumbra. Biochemical changes that accompany brain tissue ischemia are well-known in animal studies. The worsening in redox state evident from an increase in the lactate/pyruvate ratio is particularly important. Furthermore, the lactate/pyruvate ratio was a more reliable marker than lactate alone. In TBI patients, a high lactate/pyruvate ratio is correlated with the severity of clinical symptoms and fatal outcome after severe trauma. The pattern of biochemical changes is detected at the bedside before that causes secondary injuries. Ischemia eventually leads to cell damage and decomposition of cell membranes. This is evident from an increase in whole-tissue levels of glycerol originating from the breakdown of glycerol-phospholipids, a constituent of cell membranes. An increase in glycerol has also been found in CMD samples of TBI patients, indicating that tissue ischemia has progressed to cell damage. Glutamate, another well-known marker of cell damage, has been studied extensively in animal models; for example, an increase during an epileptic crisis is well known. CMD is used clinically to estimate extracellular interstitial concentrations of small molecules but can also recover much larger molecules, such as inflammatory mediators, from the interstitial fluid. Instead of the standard 20-kDa molecular weight cut-off membrane, which recovers glucose, pyruvate, lactate, glycerol, glutamate, and other small hydrophilic molecules, a 100-kDa molecular weight cut-off membrane is used also to sample larger molecules, including cytokines. The experts recognise that most experience of CMD in neurocritical care has been obtained with hourly measurements, although more frequent sampling is possible. Hourly sampling appears insufficient to observe dynamic changes in brain chemistry, for example, due to spreading depolarization. While more frequent CMD analysis might help to predict adverse events, the costs due to increasing staff dedicated to the monitoring will increase, limiting the diffusion of the technique to research centres only. Zeiler [129] published a complete revision of this subject. We report his data in an extremely synthetic way. Low CMD glucose (range 0.46–1.39 mmol/L), high glutamate value above 20 μmol/l, high value of glycerol (range 83.0–150.0 μmol/l), and lactate to pyruvate ratio (LPR) within the range of 25–40 are associated with the poorer outcome while potassium level below 1.8 mmol/L is associated with good outcomes. Once considering the association with ICP increases (and CPP declines) changes in both LPR, glutamate and glycerol have often been followed by an increase of ICP. Similar cross-association has been observed in several studies measuring $PbtO_2$ and CMD. Fewer studies have been conducted with SjO_2 observing a similar association with low SjO_2 values. There is an association between worse PRx and elevated LPR, glutamate, and glycerol. There is an association between low rCBF (measured employing CTp or Xe- CT) and low glucose levels, high LPR, and elevated glutamate. The CBF and oxygen extraction fraction measured by PET, the most integrated finding among delivery and metabolism, showed a positive correlation between LPR and oxygen extraction fraction [130] and a negative correlation between LPR and $CMRO_2$ [64]. One considering the association with CT, a relevant study associated the level of chronic frontal lobe atrophy and the extent and duration of abnormal LPR levels. The review's authors reported that a minority of the studies reported an association between CMD and outcome, neuro-physiological measures, or imaging. The collaborative aspect between centres, which use CMD, is necessary to standardise the case mix, the measure of outcomes and the diffusion of similar monitoring packages (for example, CMD and $PbtO_2$ are always associated), as well as the region of interest explored by CMD, pathological or not. It is also necessary to overcome the isolated interpretation of anomalies associated with a certain outcome. We must ask ourselves if CMD adds anything to the already known predictive models. In a less evidence-based vision, imaging in the post-acute phase could be useful for establishing more direct connections with CMD values.

11.6 Neuromarkers

Imaging, monitoring of GCS over time, prompt observation of pupillary status, ICP and CPP, $PbtO_2$ and microdialysis provide useful information to reduce the factors determining secondary damage. Still, these methods do not provide sufficient information concerning primary injury (irreversible neuron, astrocyte, and glia damage). These damages have no therapy today. It is possible that in some phenotypes of TBI, the efforts to control ICP and perfusion could avoid death and further disability, but the functional outcome depends on the primary damage, perhaps identifiable early with the use of neuromarkers. On the contrary, there may be cases potentially evidenced by favourable neuromarkers patterns in which the trend of elevated ICP values could be more of an epiphenomenon. In these cases, it could be that an unnecessary strict treatment of ICP while treating the abnormal values introduces iatrogenic phenomena. Biomarkers are objective, reproducible, and quantifiable. Biomarkers have multiple uses: diagnostic, prognostic, and predictive biomarkers. Biomarkers may support clinical risk analysis, and decision-making and can be used to stratify patients into pathobiological defined (endophenotype-guided) subpopulations. Monitor biomarkers can screen and identify patients who may expect an altered, delayed, or complicated recovery or might later develop progressive neurobehavioral symptoms and deficits. Biomarkers should be specific, sensitive, rapidly, easily accessed, minimally invasive, cost-effective, and bidirectionally translatable for clinical and research use. One limitation of current TBI

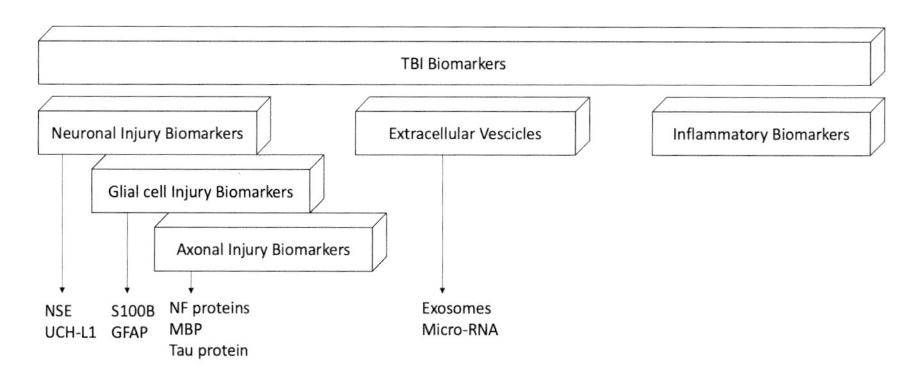

Fig. 11.25 Available neuromarkers in TBI. *NSE* neuron-specific enolase, *UCH-L1* ubiquitin C-terminal hydrolase L1, *S100B* S100 calcium-binding protein B, *GFAP* glial fibrillary acidic protein, NFs protein: Neurofilament proteins, *MBP* myelin basic protein

neuromarkers is that they exist in minimal concentrations and, therefore, require sensitive assay, which is not easily accessible. Furthermore, they might be undetectable in many cases owing to the limitations in their diffusion across the blood- brain and the cerebrospinal fluid flow limitations inflicted by the brain injury. TBI neuromarkers can characterise acute, sub-acute, and chronic post-injury stages capturing the initial damage, escalation, and progressive tissue loss. The complex and heterogeneous nature of TBI and the pathophysiological progression through primary and secondary injury cascades make it difficult to identify a single protein that can represent a signature of TBI complexity. Biological complexity in nature is so high that there is unlikely to be either a diagnostic or a prognostic marker, but associations of markers could sample complexity in the best way possible (Fig. 11.25 represents available TBI neuromarkers). Studies have demonstrated that Ubiquitin C-terminal Hydrolase L1 (UCHL1) levels increased significantly in patients with TBI injuries compared to controls after the first 24 h. A significant association was also found between UCH-L1 levels and measures used to assess the severity of TBI, including GCS, the evolution of lesions on CT scans and 6-week mortality of patients with TBI. This study also reported that UCH-L1 levels were significantly higher in patients with unfavourable outcomes four and eight days after TBI [131]. UCHL1 and GFAP have been reported to predict mortality six months after TBI [132]. UCH-L1 is detectable as early as 1 h after TBI, peaks at 8 h, and then declines slowly 48 h after injury. A high level of S100B during the initial TBI can predict a poor outcome, especially if it is accompanied by a second increase in levels of serum S100B that occurs during the subacute phase [132, 133]. This second peak can be due to ongoing damage to the astroglial cells exhibiting excitotoxicity and inflammation. In contrast, an initial lower level, and the lack of a second peak and other clinical measures suggest a moderate TBI and a good functional recovery. The levels may also increase due to a BBB dysfunction. Glial Fibrillary Acidic Protein (GFAP) is more brain-specific, and its concentration is less likely to increase during trauma to other body parts. It is not a good predictor for return to work and Glasgow outcome score [134, 135]. Neurofilament proteins (NFs) are specific neuronal and axonal proteins. NFs release lasts for days after the trauma, which may predict the occurrence of chronic morbidities and cognitive disability [136]. Studies reported that NF-L and NF-H increase in the first two weeks after severe TBI, indicating poor outcomes [137]. Inflammatory neuromarkers measurement after TBI could potentially help in disease progression monitoring, injury diagnosis, and prediction of long-term outcomes. The inflammatory blood neuromarkers could be elevated in response to any disease- causing cellular injury, so they are not highly specific for TBI. However, few studies have reported that these neuromarkers could possess a potential clinical utility for TBI patients [138]. The prolonged release of these cytokines contributes to neurodegenerative diseases [139]. Previously, adiponectin, a marker of inflammation, was reported to be elevated in the plasma of TBI patients and was found to be an independent predictor of unfavourable outcomes and mortality [140]. Also, high-mobility group box 1 (HMGB1), a marker of inflammation and a cytokine, was an important predictor for 1- year mortality in TBI patients [141, 142]. Taken together, these observations suggest that simultaneous assessment of neuromarkers reflecting different pathophysiological mechanisms and injury types would provide complementary information and increase diagnostic and prognostic accuracy, enabling clinicians to effectively stratify TBI patients. Consequently, one of the key questions is how best to determine and quantify the improvement in risk prediction offered by the combination of different markers. New statistical techniques must therefore be developed to identify general prognostic packages or focal damage prognostic packages or for example diffuse damage and connectivity or late ischemic damage, or neuronal loss. The recent study of Gradiseck [143] is a good example of this approach. Another approach combines monitoring types like neuroimaging and neuromarkers, as performed by Graham [144, 145] in a recent study to investigate the relationship between MRI diffusion tensor imaging and neuromarkers (NFs) in moderate and severe TBI. The use of neuromarkers in clinical practice nowadays is more in the rule-out of moderate TBI (FDA-approved package) than in the phenotyping of severe TBI. Still, with the advancement of technology, neuromarkers should become part of multimodal bedside monitoring.

11.7 Conclusion

We are faced with a declining trend of the medicine invasiveness (as for example the initial attempts to refine the evaluation of ICP by transcranial doppler or pupillometry) in association with a reduced confidence in the effectiveness of intensive treatment in a more general context in which the protocolled, tight treatments on intracranial pressure, seem to produce more complications rather than benefits. In this scenario, the interest in focal monitoring seems to decrease over time: the associated figure highlights these trends of reduction in scientific interest in SjO_2, $PbtO_2$ and CMD while an increase in interest in neuroimaging, primarily MRI, but also CTp and neuromarkers (Fig. 11.26). Simultaneously excluding the first temporal phases, which is highly dependent on the appropriateness and the timeliness of the first aid, trauma management and neurosurgical timing, the average TBI patient

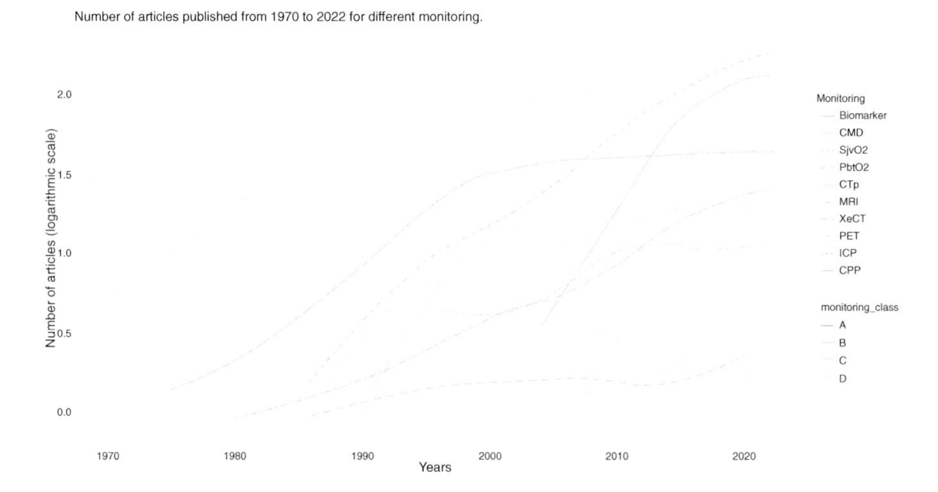

Fig. 11.26 Number of articles published from 1970 to 2022 for different monitoring.

seems to be more affected by a metabolic syndrome and axonal damage than by an ischemic pathophysiology. Or rather, in conditions of refractory ICP, global ischemic suffering can occur in the perilesional penumbra where the sensitivity to secondary insult is high, but in other areas, tolerant management of the ICP values might be adequate. Over the last 30 years in which the bedside tools SjO_2, $PbtO_2$ and CMD have spread, they have represented the willingness of high-income countries to explore and combat secondary damage. The teachings have been many, but the most important translation is to focus the clinical attention on those variables such as blood pressure, natremia, temperature control and management of $PaCO_2$ that can greatly afflict penumbra, much more than the apparently healthy brain. A paradigmatic example is the work of Nordström [128], in which CMD catheters are placed in both apparently healthy and diseased brains, and a wide dispersion of the L/P ratio in the pathological zone was observed, particularly in conditions of low CPP. These methods teach those who do not have these technologies that penumbra is more sensitive to insults. Let's consider, for example, that CMD requires an hourly sample and reasonably a nurse-to-patient ratio of 1:1, but we know that in many countries, even at a very high-level income, the ratio is 1:2 or 1:4. We are far from using these methods as daily bedside diagnostic tool. Another example of high scientific value, but of low applicability is the use of PET in the Cambridge centre [59]. Perhaps today, only PET with O_2 can try to establish any potential relationship between the increase in PaO_2, the increase in $PbtO_2$ and a reduction of OEF, demonstrating a delivery dependency. PET with 2-3-FDG is a widespread technique in large hospitals, while PET with O_2 requires a cyclotron in place due to the high instability of marked oxygen and a setting suitable for the reception of complex patients. These technologies today should be considered more for transitional medicine. In this sense, the researchers should force their observations into clinical patterns recognisable even by the standard centres so that the basic concepts can be translated even without advanced monitoring. The epidemiological evolution of traumatology with a reduction of high-impact trauma with the introduction of the helmet and car safety systems which mostly affected young people, and on the other hand, the increase in low trauma kinetic energy involving the elderly, often in association with the use of anticoagulants and antiplatelet agents, has perhaps reduced the scientific investment in head trauma, at least on several of the techniques described in this chapter. Symmetrically, the growing interest in neuroimaging and neuromarkers seems to be directed more towards a prognostic definition as early as possible, perhaps aimed at providing information to families on the prognosis and focus efforts on traditional therapies with more hope of recovering or resulting in an acceptable disability. In the present chapter, specific advanced monitoring has been described in association with standard ones. A visual integration of their relationship is shown in Fig. 11.27. Figure 11.28 shows a staircase approach to monitoring according to available resources and aims to evaluate more global physiology or focal lesion. The minimum monitoring setting that could be recommended today is ICP [1, 146, 147] and CPP in association with high-density monitoring [148]. The high-density monitoring teaches on a case-by-case basis the triggers of the ICP increase and allows a continuous review of the same case during treatment. Simple indicators like the PRx can help, despite phases of inaccuracy in ICP and CPP recording. SjO_2 monitoring is still of potential use, perhaps more to allow a window on metabolism. In a well-organized trauma team, the procedure may not be time-consuming. Isolated studies with SjO_2 [99] and studies with early CBF [35] and early PET [70] argue that in this phase, uncoupling is more frequent, and influences the outcome. The ultra-early positioning of an ICP sensor should be highly relevant,

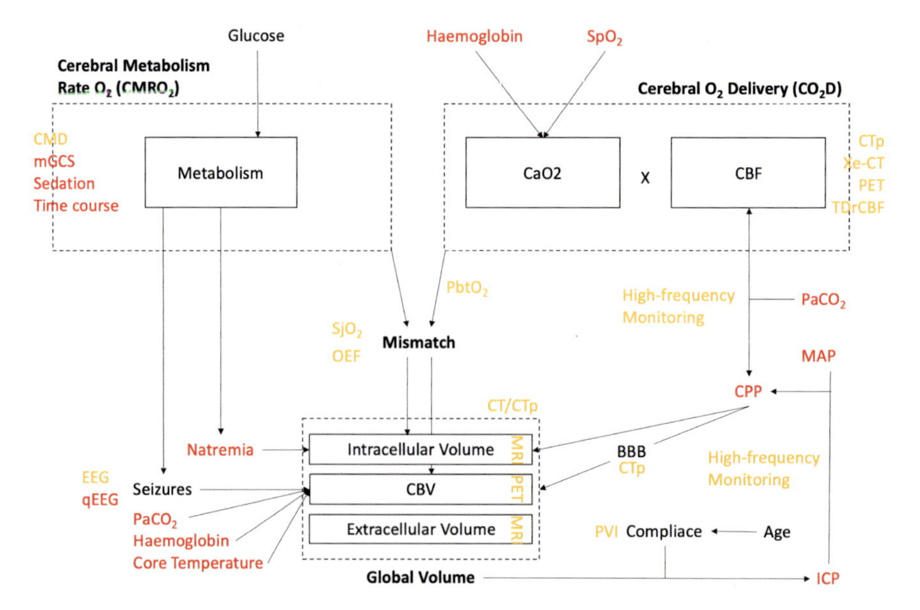

Fig. 11.27 Integration of neuromonitoring and relationship to physiological variables and determinants

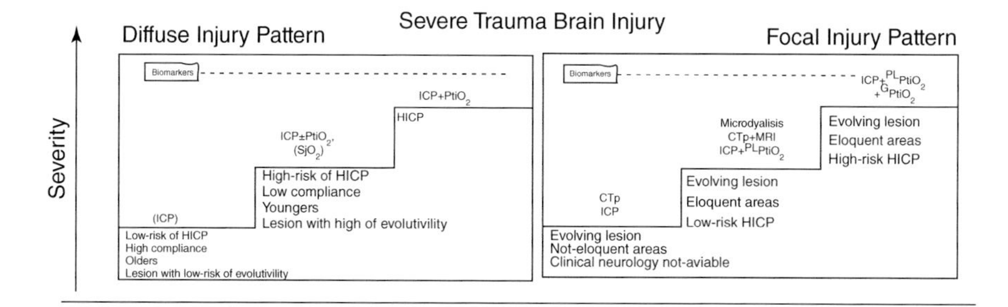

Fig. 11.28 Staircase approach to monitoring according to available resources and aims to evaluate diffuse injury pattern (left panel) or focal lesion (right panel). *HICP* high intracranial pressure; *G* global; *PL* peri-lesion

but could conflict with, for example, acquired coagulopathies [95]. A suggested second higher level of monitoring could be, in cases with refractory intracranial hypertension, the association, to ICP-CPP monitoring, of $PbtO_2$ placed in the apparently healthy brain at CT to identify critical CPP levels for oxygen perfusion/diffusion. At a third level of complexity, using $PbtO_2$ could be suggested in the hypodense areas of a contusion in eloquent areas for which a conservative, non-surgical treatment seems the best strategy. This monitoring, which must be positioned very accurately, can increase the information on the vulnerability of the injured areas [149]. If we decide to preserve the lesion at the cost of the high-intensity level of treatment to control high ICP levels, we have to be sure that any reduction of CPP did not impair the local $PbtO_2$. In a recent consensus, Chesnut [150] identifies with the co-authors a sequential approach in which the measurement of ICP and $PbtO_2$ are integrated into a reasonable approach. In cases where the control of ICP could be as important as the preservation of penumbral areas, $PbtO_2$ measurements should be guided on the base of functional imaging, for example, CTp [149].

References

1. Stocchetti N, Carbonara M, Citerio G, Ercole A, Skrifvars MB, Smielewski P, Zoerle T, Menon DK. Severe traumatic brain injury: targeted management in the intensive care unit. Lancet Neurol. 2017;16:452–64.
2. Saatman KE, Duhaime A-C, Bullock R, AIR M, Valadka A, Manley GT, Workshop Scientific Team and Advisory Panel Members. Classification of traumatic brain injury for targeted therapies. J Neurotrauma. 2008;25:719–38.
3. Menon DK. Procrustes, the traumatic penumbra, and perfusion pressure targets in closed head injury. Anesthesiology. 2003;98:805–7.
4. Czosnyka M, Smielewski P, Piechnik S, Schmidt EA, Al-Rawi PG, Kirkpatrick PJ, Pickard JD. Hemodynamic characterization of intracranial pressure plateau waves in head-injury patients. J Neurosurg. 1999;91:11–9.
5. Shapiro K, Marmarou A, Shulman K. Characterization of clinical CSF dynamics and neural axis compliance using the pressure-volume index: I. The normal pressure-volume index. Ann Neurol. 1980;7:508–14.

6. Chieregato A, Compagnone C, Tanfani A, Ravaldini M, Tagliaferri F, Pascarella R, Servadei F, Targa L, Fainardi E. Cerebral blood flow mapping in two different subtypes of intraparenchymal hemorrhagic traumatic lesions. Acta Neurochir Suppl. 2005;95:159–64.
7. Compagnone C, Murray GD, Teasdale GM, Maas AI, Esposito D, Princi P, D'Avella D, Servadei F, European Brain Injury Consortium. The management of patients with intradural post-traumatic mass lesions: a multicenter survey of current approaches to surgical management in 729 patients coordinated by the European Brain Injury Consortium. Neurosurgery. 2005;57:1183–92; discussion 1183-1192.
8. Chieregato A, Fainardi E, Morselli-Labate AM, Antonelli V, Compagnone C, Targa L, Kraus J, Servadei F. Factors associated with neurological outcome and lesion progression in traumatic subarachnoid hemorrhage patients. Neurosurgery. 2005;56:671–80; discussion 671-680.
9. Chieregato A, Fainardi E, Servadei F, Tanfani A, Pugliese G, Pascarella R, Targa L. Centrifugal distribution of regional cerebral blood flow and its time course in traumatic intracerebral hematomas. J Neurotrauma. 2004;21:655–66.
10. Kurland D, Hong C, Aarabi B, Gerzanich V, Simard JM. Hemorrhagic progression of a contusion after traumatic brain injury: a review. J Neurotrauma. 2012;29(1):19–31. https://doi.org/10.1089/neu.2011.2122. Epub 2011 Dec 5. PMID: 21988198; PMCID: PMC3253310.
11. Patchana T, Dorkoski R, Zampella B, Wiginton JG, Sweiss R, Menoni R, Miulli DE (2019) The use of computed tomography perfusion on admission to predict outcomes in surgical and nonsurgical traumatic brain injury patients. Cureus. https://doi.org/10.7759/cureus.5077.
12. Alcock S, Batoo D, Ande SR, et al. Early diagnosis of mortality using admission CT perfusion in severe traumatic brain injury patients (ACT-TBI): protocol for a prospective cohort study. BMJ Open. 2021;11:e047305.
13. Wintermark M, van Melle G, Schnyder P, Revelly J-P, Porchet F, Regli L, Meuli R, Maeder P, Chioléro R. Admission perfusion CT: prognostic value in patients with severe head trauma. Radiology. 2004;232:211–20.
14. Schroder ML, Muizelaar JP, Fatouros PP, Kuta AJ, Choi SC. Regional cerebral blood volume after severe head injury in patients with regional cerebral ischemia. Neurosurgery. 1998;42:1276–80.
15. Muizelaar JP, Fatouros PP, Schröder ML. A new method for quantitative regional cerebral blood volume measurements using computed tomography. Stroke. 1997;28:1998–2005.
16. Chieregato A, Noto A, Tanfani A, Bini G, Martino C, Fainardi E. Hyperemia beneath evacuated acute subdural hematoma is frequent and prolonged in patients with an unfavorable outcome: a xe-computed tomographic study. Neurosurgery. 2009;64:705–17; discussion 717-718.
17. Ribas GC, Jane JA. Traumatic contusions and intracerebral hematomas. J Neurotrauma. 1992;9(Suppl 1):265–78.
18. Kawamata T, Katayama Y, Aoyama N, Mori T. Heterogeneous mechanisms of early edema formation in cerebral contusion: diffusion MRI and ADC mapping study. Acta Neurochir Suppl. 2000;76:9–12.
19. Videen TO, Zazulia AR, Manno EM, Derdeyn CP, Adams RE, Diringer MN, Powers WJ. Mannitol bolus preferentially shrinks non-infarcted brain in patients with ischemic stroke. Neurology. 2001;57:2120–2.
20. Muizelaar JP, Wei EP, Kontos HA, Becker DP. Mannitol causes compensatory cerebral vasoconstriction and vasodilation in response to blood viscosity changes. J Neurosurg. 1983;59:822–8.
21. Zornow MH, Prough DS. Fluid management in patients with traumatic brain injury. New Horiz. 1995;3:488–98.
22. Obrist WD, Langfitt TW, Jaggi JL, Cruz J, Gennarelli TA. Cerebral blood flow and metabolism in comatose patients with acute head injury. Relationship to intracranial hypertension. J Neurosurg. 1984;61:241–53.
23. Robertson CS, Contant CF, Gokaslan ZL, Narayan RK, Grossman RG. Cerebral blood flow, arteriovenous oxygen difference, and outcome in head injured patients. J Neurol Neurosurg Psychiatry. 1992;55:594–603.

24. Cormio M, Gopinath SP, Valadka A, Robertson CS. Cerebral hemodynamic effects of pentobarbital coma in head-injured patients. J Neurotrauma. 1999;16:927–36.
25. Robertson CS, Cormio M. Cerebral metabolic management. New Horiz. 1995;3:410–22.
26. Chieregato A, Tanfani A, Fainardi E. A practical approach to interpretation of CBF measured by mean of xenon-CT in patients with traumatic brain injury. Open Neurosurg J. 2010;3:28–58.
27. Chieregato A, Tanfani A, Compagnone C, Turrini C, Sarpieri F, Ravaldini M, Targa L, Fainardi E. Global cerebral blood flow and CPP after severe head injury: a xenon-CT study. Intensive Care Med. 2007;33:856–62.
28. Shalit MN, Beller AJ, Feinsod M. Clinical equivalents of cerebral oxygen consumption in coma. Neurology. 1972;22:155–60.
29. Jaggi JL, Obrist WD, Gennarelli TA, Langfitt TW. Relationship of early cerebral blood flow and metabolism to outcome in acute head injury. J Neurosurg. 1990;72:176–82.
30. Cruz J. Low clinical ischemic threshold for cerebral blood flow in severe acute brain trauma. Case report. J Neurosurg. 1994;80:143–7.
31. Kety SS, Schmidt CF. The determination of cerebral blood flow in man by the use of nitrous oxide in low concentration. Am J Physiol. 1945;143:53–66.
32. Lassen NA. Cerebral blood flow tomography with xenon-133. Semin Nucl Med. 1985;15:347–56.
33. Yonas H, Pindzola RP, Johnson DW. Xenon/computed tomography cerebral blood flow and its use in clinical management. Neurosurg Clin N Am. 1996;7:605–16.
34. Yonas H, Darby JM, Marks EC, Durham SR, Maxwell C. CBF measured by Xe-CT: approach to analysis and normal values. J Cereb Blood Flow Metab. 1991;11:716–25.
35. Hlatky R, Contant CF, Diaz-Marchan P, Valadka AB, Robertson CS. Significance of a reduced cerebral blood flow during the first 12 hours after traumatic brain injury. Neurocrit Care. 2004;1:69–83.
36. Bouma GJ, Muizelaar JP, Choi SC, Newlon PG, Young HF. Cerebral circulation and metabolism after severe traumatic brain injury: the elusive role of ischemia. J Neurosurg. 1991;75:685–93.
37. Bouma GJ, Muizelaar JP, Stringer WA, Choi SC, Fatouros P, Young HF. Ultra-early evaluation of regional cerebral blood flow in severely head-injured patients using xenon-enhanced computerized tomography. J Neurosurg. 1992;77:360–8.
38. Schröder ML, Muizelaar JP, Kuta AJ. Documented reversal of global ischemia immediately after removal of an acute subdural hematoma. Report of two cases. Neurosurgery. 1994;80:324–7.
39. Salvant JB, Muizelaar JP. Changes in cerebral blood flow and metabolism related to the presence of subdural hematoma. Neurosurgery. 1993;33:387–93.
40. Darby JM, Yonas H, Marion DW, Latchaw RE. Local "inverse steal" induced by hyperventilation in head injury. Neurosurgery. 1988;23:84–8.
41. Schröder ML, Muizelaar JP, Bullock MR, Salvant JB, Povlishock JT. Focal ischemia due to traumatic contusions documented by stable xenon-CT and ultrastructural studies. J Neurosurg. 1995;82:966–71.
42. Marion DW, Bouma GJ. The use of stable xenon-enhanced computed tomographic studies of cerebral blood flow to define changes in cerebral carbon dioxide vasoresponsivity caused by a severe head injury. Neurosurgery. 1991;29(6):869–73.
43. Astrup J, Bergholt B, Gyldensted C, Bogesvang A, Holdgaard HO, Dahl B. Ischemic focal lesions in acute head injury: correlation to late focal atrophy. Scand Suppl Acta Neurol. 1996;1996:118–9.
44. Adelson D, Clyde B, Kochanek PM, Wisniewski SR, Marion DW, Yonas H. Cerebrovascular response in infants and young children following severe traumatic brain injury: a preliminary report. Pediatr Neurosurg. 1997;26:200–7.
45. Chieregato A, Tanfani A, Compagnone C, Pascarella R, Targa L, Fainardi E. Cerebral blood flow in traumatic contusions is predominantly reduced after an induced acute elevation of cerebral perfusion pressure. Neurosurgery. 2007;60:115–2; discussion 123.

46. McLaughlin MR, Marion DW. The use of xenon cerebral blood flow computed tomography to evaluate perfusion and vasoresponsivity of cerebral contusions. Acta Neurol Scand. 1996;93:117.
47. Steiner LA, Coles JP, Johnston AJ, et al. Responses of posttraumatic pericontusional cerebral blood flow and blood volume to an increase in cerebral perfusion pressure. J Cereb Blood Flow Metab. 2003;23:1371–7.
48. Darby JM, Yonas H, Marks EC, Durham S, Snyder RW, Nemoto EM. Acute cerebral blood flow response to dopamine-induced hypertension after subarachnoid hemorrhage. J Neurosurg. 1994;80:857–64.
49. Wintermark M, Thiran JP, Maeder P, Schnyder P, Meuli R. Simultaneous measurement of regional cerebral blood flow by perfusion CT and stable xenon CT: a validation study. AJNR Am J Neuroradiol. 2001;22:905–14.
50. Rosenthal G, Sanchez-Mejia RO, Phan N, Hemphill JC, Martin C, Manley GT. Incorporating a parenchymal thermal diffusion cerebral blood flow probe in bedside assessment of cerebral autoregulation and vasoreactivity in patients with severe traumatic brain injury: clinical article. J Neurosurg. 2011;114:62–70.
51. Steiner LA, Czosnyka M, Piechnik SK, Smielewski P, Chatfield D, Menon DK, Pickard JD. Continuous monitoring of cerebrovascular pressure reactivity allows determination of optimal cerebral perfusion pressure in patients with traumatic brain injury. Crit Care Med. 2002;30:733–8.
52. Menon DK. Brain ischaemia after traumatic brain injury: lessons from $15O_2$ positron emission tomography. Curr Opin Crit Care. 2006;12:85–9.
53. Coles JP, Fryer TD, Smielewski P, Rice K, Clark JC, Pickard JD, Menon DK. Defining ischemic burden after traumatic brain injury using 15O PET imaging of cerebral physiology. J Cereb Blood Flow Metab. 2004;24:191–201.
54. Coles JP, Fryer TD, Smielewski P, et al. Incidence and mechanisms of cerebral ischemia in early clinical head injury. J Cereb Blood Flow Metab. 2004;24:202–11.
55. Coles JP, Cunningham AS, Salvador R, Chatfield DA, Carpenter A, Pickard JD, Menon DK. Early metabolic characteristics of lesion and nonlesion tissue after head injury. J Cereb Blood Flow Metab. 2009;29:965–75.
56. Gupta AK, Hutchinson PJ, Fryer T, et al. Measurement of brain tissue oxygenation performed using positron emission tomography scanning to validate a novel monitoring method. J Neurosurg. 2002,96:263–8.
57. Rosenthal G, Hemphill JC, Sorani M, Martin C, Morabito D, Obrist WD, Manley GT. Brain tissue oxygen tension is more indicative of oxygen diffusion than oxygen delivery and metabolism in patients with traumatic brain injury. Crit Care Med. 2008;36:1917–24.
58. Zygun DA, Nortje J, Hutchinson PJ, Timofeev I, Menon DK, Gupta AK. The effect of red blood cell transfusion on cerebral oxygenation and metabolism after severe traumatic brain injury. Crit Care Med. 2009;37:1074–8.
59. Nortje J, Coles JP, Timofeev I, et al. Effect of hyperoxia on regional oxygenation and metabolism after severe traumatic brain injury: preliminary findings. Crit Care Med. 2008;36:273–81.
60. Coles JP, Fryer TD, Coleman MR, et al. Hyperventilation following head injury: effect on ischemic burden and cerebral oxidative metabolism. Crit Care Med. 2007;35:568–78.
61. Coles JP, Steiner LA, Johnston AJ, et al. Does induced hypertension reduce cerebral ischaemia within the traumatized human brain? Brain. 2004;127:2479–90.
62. Cunningham AS, Salvador R, Coles JP, et al. Physiological thresholds for irreversible tissue damage in contusional regions following traumatic brain injury. Brain J Neurol. 2005;128:1931–42.
63. Menon DK, Coles JP, Gupta AK, et al. Diffusion limited oxygen delivery following head injury. Crit Care Med. 2004;32:1384–90.
64. Vespa P, Bergsneider M, Hattori N, Wu H-M, Huang S-C, Martin NA, Glenn TC, McArthur DL, Hovda DA. Metabolic crisis without brain ischemia is common after traumatic brain injury: a combined microdialysis and positron emission tomography study. J Cereb Blood Flow Metab. 2005;25:763–74.

65. Verweij BH, Muizelaar JP, Vinas FC, Peterson PL, Xiong Y, Lee CP. Impaired cerebral mitochondrial function after traumatic brain injury in humans. J Neurosurg. 2000;93:815–20.
66. Veenith TV, Carter EL, Geeraerts T, et al. Pathophysiologic mechanisms of cerebral ischemia and diffusion hypoxia in traumatic brain injury. JAMA Neurol. 2016;73:542–50.
67. Lazaridis C. Diffusion hypoxia and/or primary mitochondrial failure? JAMA Neurol. 2016;73:1372–3.
68. Vespa PM. Brain hypoxia and ischemia after traumatic brain injury: is oxygen the right metabolic target? JAMA Neurol. 2016;73:504.
69. Hermanides J, Hong YT, Trivedi M, et al. Metabolic derangements are associated with impaired glucose delivery following traumatic brain injury. Brain J Neurol. 2021;144:3492–504.
70. Launey Y, Fryer TD, Hong YT, et al. Spatial and temporal pattern of ischemia and abnormal vascular function following traumatic brain injury. JAMA Neurol. 2020;77:339–49. https://doi.org/10.1001/jamaneurol.2019.3854. PMID: 31710336; PMCID: PMC6865302.
71. Cruz J, Allen SJ, Miner ME. Hypoxic insults in acute brain injury. Crit Care Med. 1985;13:284.
72. Cruz J. The first decade of continuous monitoring of jugular bulb oxyhemoglobinsaturation: management strategies and clinical outcome. Crit Care Med. 1998;26:344–51.
73. Scheinberg P. Simultaneous bilateral determinations of cerebral blood flow and arterial-cerebral venous oxygen and glucose differences. Proc Soc Exp Biol Med Soc Exp Biol Med. 1950;74:575–8.
74. Stocchetti N, Paparella A, Bridelli F, Bacchi M, Piazza P, Zuccoli P. Cerebral venous oxygen saturation studied with bilateral samples in the internal jugular veins. Neurosurgery. 1994;34:38–43; discussion 43-44.
75. Chieregato A, Veronesi V, Calzolari F, Marchi M, Targa L. Prematurely detected traumatic carotid-cavernous sinus fistula, by means of unintentional contralateral inferior petrosal sinus catheterization: bilateral jugular bulb oxygen saturation findings. J Neurosurg Anesthesiol. 1998;10:16–21.
76. Bankier AA, Fleischmann D, Windisch A, Germann P, Petritschek W, Wiesmayr MN, Hübsch P. Position of jugular oxygen saturation catheter in patients with head trauma: assessment by use of plain films. AJR Am J Roentgenol. 1995;164:437–41.
77. Gibbs EL, Lennox WG, Nims LF, Gibbs FA. Arterial and cerebral venous blood. J Biol Chem. 1942;144:325–32.
78. Dastur DK, Lane MH, Hansen DB, Kety SS, Butler RN, Perlin S, Sokoloff L. Effects of aging on cerebral circulation and metabolism in man. In: Birren JE, Butler RN, Greenhouse SW, Sokoloff L, Yarrow MR, editors. Hum. aging Biol. Behav. study. Bethesda: US Dept of Health, Education, & Welfare; 1963. p. 59–76.
79. Myerson A. Technic for obtaning blood from the internal jugular vein and internal carotid artery. Arch Neurol Psychiatr. 1927;17:807.
80. Chieregato A, Calzolari F, Trasforini G, Targa L, Latronico N. Normal jugular bulb oxygen saturation. J Neurol Neurosurg Psychiatry. 2003;74:784–6.
81. Chieregato A. How much normal are the normal SjO_2 values? Minerva A. 2003;2003:301–6.
82. Kety SS, King BD, Horvath SM, Jeffers WS, Hafkenschiel JH. The effects of an acute reduction in blood pressure by means of differential spinal sympathetic block on the cerebral circulation of hypertensive patients. J Clin Invest. 1950;29:402–7.
83. Gopinath SP, Robertson CS, Contant CF, Hayes C, Feldman Z, Narayan RK, Grossman RG. Jugular venous desaturation and outcome after head injury. J Neurol Neurosurg Psychiatry. 1994;57:717–23.
84. Gotoh F, Meyer JS, Takagi Y. Cerebral effect of hyperventilation in man. Arch Neurol. 1965;12:410–23.
85. Lennox WG. Relationship of unconsciusness to cerebral blood flow and to anoxemia. Arch Neurol Psychiatr. 1935;34:1001.
86. Lennox WG, Gibbs FA, Gibbs EI. The relationship in man of cerebral activity to blood flow and to blood constituents. J Neurol Psychiatry. 1938;1:211–25.
87. Shenkin HA, Harmel MH, Kety SS. Dynamic anatomy of the cerebral circulation. Arch Neurol Psychiatr. 1948;60:240–52.

88. Matta BF, Lam AM. The rate of blood withdrawal affects the accuracy of jugular venous bulb. Oxygen saturation measurements. Anesthesiology. 1997;86:806–8.
89. Gupta AK, Hutchinson PJ, Al-Rawi P, Gupta S, Swart M, Kirkpatrick PJ, Menon DK, Datta AK. Measuring brain tissue oxygenation compared with jugular venous oxygen saturation for monitoring cerebral oxygenation after traumatic brain injury. Anesth Analg. 1999;88:549–53.
90. Chieregato A, Targa L, Zatelli R. Limitations of jugular bulb oxyhemoglobin saturation without intracranial pressure monitoring in subarachnoid hemorrhage. J Neurosurg Anesthesiol. 1996;8:21–5.
91. Stocchetti N, Canavesi K, Magnoni S, Valeriani V, Conte V, Rossi S, Longhi L, Zanier ER, Colombo A. Arterio-jugular difference of oxygen content and outcome after head injury. Anesth Analg. 2004;99:230–4.
92. Cormio M, Valadka AB, Robertson CS. Elevated jugular venous oxygen saturation after severe head injury. J Neurosurg. 1999;90:9–15.
93. Latronico N, Beindorf AE, Rasulo FA, Febbrari P, Stefini R, Cornali C, Candiani A. Limits of intermittent jugular bulb oxygen saturation monitoring in the management of severe head trauma patients. Neurosurgery. 2000;46:1131–8; discussion 1138-1139.
94. Chieregato A, Marchi M, Zoppellari R, Fabbri E, Cianchi G, Forini E, Targa L. Detection of early ischemia in severe head injury by means of arteriovenous lactate differences and jugular bulb oxygen saturation. Relationship with CPP, severity indexes and outcome. Preliminary analysis. Acta Neurochir Suppl. 2002;81:289–93.
95. Verweij BH, Muizelaar JP, Vinas FC. Hyperacute measurement of intracranial pressure, cerebral perfusion pressure, jugular venous oxygen saturation, and laser Doppler flowmetry, before and during removal of traumatic acute subdural hematoma. J Neurosurg. 2001;95:569–72.
96. Chieregato A, Venditto A, Russo E, Martino C, Bini G. Aggressive medical management of acute traumatic subdural hematomas before emergency craniotomy in patients presenting with bilateral unreactive pupils. A cohort study. Acta Neurochir. 2017;159:1553–9.
97. Robertson CS, Narayan RK, Gokaslan ZL, Pahwa R, Grossman RG, Caram P, Allen E. Cerebral arteriovenous oxygen difference as an estimate of cerebral blood flow in comatose patients. J Neurosurg. 1989;70:222–30.
98. Cruz J. Relationship between early patterns of cerebral extraction of oxygen and outcome from severe acute traumatic brain swelling: cerebral ischemia or cerebral viability? Crit Care Med. 1996;24:953–6.
99. Chieregato A, Marchi M, Fainardi E, Targa L. Cerebral arterio-venous pCO_2 difference, estimated respiratory quotient, and early posttraumatic outcome: comparison with arterio-venous lactate and oxygen differences. J Neurosurg Anesthesiol. 2007;19:222–8.
100. Robertson CS, Grossman RG, Goodman JC, Narayan RK. The predictive value of cerebral anaerobic metabolism with cerebral infarction after head injury. J Neurosurg. 1987;67:361–8.
101. Magistretti PJ, Pellerin L. Cellular mechanisms of brain energy metabolism and their relevance to functional brain imaging. Philos Trans R Soc Lond Ser B Biol Sci. 1999;354:1155–63.
102. Nemoto EM, Hoff JT, Severinghaus JW. Lactate uptake and metabolism by brain during hyperlactatemia and hypoglycemia. Stroke. 1974;5:48–53.
103. Chieregato A, Zoppellari R, Targa L. Cerebral arteriovenous PCO_2 difference and early global cerebral ischemia in a patient with acute severe head injury. J Neurosurg Anesthesiol. 1997;9:256–62.
104. Stocchetti N, Zanier ER, Nicolini R, Faegersten E, Canavesi K, Conte V, Gattinoni L. Oxygen and carbon dioxide in the cerebral circulation during progression to brain death. Anesthesiology. 2005;103:957–61.
105. Rosner MJ, Rosner SD, Johnson AH. Cerebral perfusion pressure: management protocol and clinical results. J Neurosurg. 1995;83:949–62.
106. Robertson CS, Valadka AB, Hannay HJ, Contant CF, Gopinath SP, Cormio M, Uzura M, Grossman RG. Prevention of secondary ischemic insults after severe head injury. Crit Care Med. 1999;27:2086–95.

107. Contant CF, Valadka AB, Gopinath SP, Hannay HJ, Robertson CS. Adult respiratory distress syndrome: a complication of induced hypertension after severe head injury. J Neurosurg. 2001;95:560–8.
108. Sheinberg M, Kanter MJ, Robertson CS, Contant CF, Narayan RK, Grossman RG. Continuous monitoring of jugular venous oxygen saturation in head-injured patients. J Neurosurg. 1992;76:212–7.
109. Kiening KL, Unterberg AW, Bardt TF, Schneider GH, Lanksch WR. Monitoring of cerebral oxygenation in patients with severe head injuries: brain tissue PO_2 versus jugular vein oxygen saturation. J Neurosurg. 1996;85:751–7.
110. Doppenberg EM, Zauner A, Watson JC, Bullock R. Determination of the ischemic threshold for brain oxygen tension. Acta Neurochir Suppl. 1998;71:166–9.
111. Sarrafzadeh AS, Kiening KL, Bardt TF, Schneider GH, Unterberg AW, Lanksch WR. Cerebral oxygenation in contusioned vs. nonlesioned brain tissue: monitoring of $PtiO_2$ with Licox and Paratrend. Acta Neurochir Suppl. 1998;71:186–9.
112. Valadka AB, Goodman JC, Gopinath SP, Uzura M, Robertson CS. Comparison of brain tissue oxygen tension to microdialysis-based measures of cerebral ischemia in fatally head-injured humans. J Neurotrauma. 1998;15:509–19.
113. Gopinath SP, Valadka AB, Uzura M, Robertson CS. Comparison of jugular venous oxygen saturation and brain tissue PO_2 as monitors of cerebral ischemia after head injury. Crit Care Med. 1999;27:2337–45.
114. Menzel M, Doppenberg EM, Zauner A, Soukup J, Reinert MM, Clausen T, Brockenbrough PB, Bullock R. Cerebral oxygenation in patients after severe head injury: monitoring and effects of arterial hyperoxia on cerebral blood flow, metabolism and intracranial pressure. J Neurosurg Anesthesiol. 1999;11:240–51.
115. Valadka AB, Hlatky R, Furuya Y, Robertson CS. Brain tissue PO_2: correlation with cerebral blood flow. Acta Neurochir Suppl. 2002;81:299–301.
116. Jones TH, Morawetz RB, Crowell RM, Marcoux FW, FitzGibbon SJ, DeGirolami U, Ojemann RG. Thresholds of focal cerebral ischemia in awake monkeys. J Neurosurg. 1981;54:773–82.
117. Bell BA, Symon L, Branston NM. CBF and time thresholds for the formation of ischemic cerebral edema, and effect of reperfusion in baboons. J Neurosurg. 1985;62:31–41.
118. Meixensberger J, Jaeger M, Väth A, Dings J, Kunze E, Roosen K. Brain tissue oxygen guided treatment supplementing ICP/CPP therapy after traumatic brain injury. J Neurol Neurosurg Psychiatry. 2003;74:760–4.
119. Spiotta AM, Stiefel MF, Gracias VH, Garuffe AM, Kofke WA, Maloney-Wilensky E, Troxel AB, Levine JM, Le Roux PD. Brain tissue oxygen-directed management and outcome in patients with severe traumatic brain injury. J Neurosurg. 2010;113:571–80.
120. Nangunoori R, Maloney-Wilensky E, Stiefel M, Park S, Andrew Kofke W, Levine JM, Yang W, Le Roux PD. Brain tissue oxygen-based therapy and outcome after severe traumatic brain injury: a systematic literature review. Neurocrit Care. 2012;17:131–8.
121. Hays LMC, Udy A, Adamides AA, et al. Effects of brain tissue oxygen ($PbtO_2$) guided management on patient outcomes following severe traumatic brain injury: a systematic review and meta-analysis. J Clin Neurosci. 2022;99:349–58.
122. Lee H-C, Chuang H-C, Cho D-Y, Cheng K-F, Lin P-H, Chen C-C. Applying cerebral hypothermia and brain oxygen monitoring in treating severe traumatic brain injury. World Neurosurg. 2010;74:654–60.
123. Lin C-M, Lin M-C, Huang S-J, et al. A prospective randomized study of brain tissue oxygen pressure-guided management in moderate and severe traumatic brain injury patients. Biomed Res Int. 2015;2015:529580.
124. Okonkwo DO, Shutter LA, Moore C, et al. Brain oxygen optimization in severe traumatic brain injury phase-II: a phase II randomized trial. Crit Care Med. 2017;45:1907–14.
125. Ungerstedt U, Pycock C. Functional correlates of dopamine neurotransmission. Bull Schweiz Akad Med Wiss. 1974;30:44–55.
126. Bellander B-M, Cantais E, Enblad P, et al. Consensus meeting on microdialysis in neurointensive care. Intensive Care Med. 2004;30:2166–9.

127. Hutchinson PJ, Jalloh I, Helmy A, et al. Consensus statement from the 2014 International Microdialysis Forum. Intensive Care Med. 2015;41:1517–28.
128. Nordström C-H, Reinstrup P, Xu W, Gärdenfors A, Ungerstedt U. Assessment of the lower limit for cerebral perfusion pressure in severe head injuries by bedside monitoring of regional energy metabolism. Anesthesiology. 2003;98:809–14.
129. Zeiler FA, Thelin EP, Helmy A, Czosnyka M, Hutchinson PJA, Menon DK. A systematic review of cerebral microdialysis and outcomes in TBI: relationships to patient functional outcome, neurophysiologic measures, and tissue outcome. Acta Neurochir. 2017;159:2245–73.
130. Hutchinson PJ, Gupta AK, Fryer TF, et al. Correlation between cerebral blood flow, substrate delivery, and metabolism in head injury: a combined microdialysis and triple oxygen positron emission tomography study. J Cereb Blood Flow Metab. 2002;22:735–45.
131. Papa L, Akinyi L, Liu MC, et al. Ubiquitin C-terminal hydrolase is a novel biomarker in humans for severe traumatic brain injury. Crit Care Med. 2010;38:138–44.
132. Mondello S, Papa L, Buki A, Bullock MR, Czeiter E, Tortella FC, Wang KK, Hayes RL. Neuronal and glial markers are differently associated with computed tomography findings and outcome in patients with severe traumatic brain injury: a case control study. Crit Care. 2011;15:R156.
133. Thelin EP, Nelson DW, Bellander B-M. Secondary peaks of S100B in serum relate to subsequent radiological pathology in traumatic brain injury. Neurocrit Care. 2014;20:217–29.
134. Papa L, Lewis LM, Falk JL, et al. Elevated levels of serum glial fibrillary acidic protein breakdown products in mild and moderate traumatic brain injury are associated with intracranial lesions and neurosurgical intervention. Ann Emerg Med. 2012;59:471–83.
135. Metting Z, Wilczak N, Rodiger LA, Schaaf JM, van der Naalt J. GFAP and S100B in the acute phase of mild traumatic brain injury. Neurology. 2012;78:1428–33.
136. Wang KK, Yang Z, Zhu T, Shi Y, Rubenstein R, Tyndall JA, Manley GT. An update on diagnostic and prognostic biomarkers for traumatic brain injury. Expert Rev Mol Diagn. 2018;18:165–80.
137. Lambertsen KL, Soares CB, Gaist D, Nielsen HH. Neurofilaments: the C-reactive protein of neurology. Brain Sci. 2020;10:56.
138. Visser K, Koggel M, Blaauw J, van der Horn HJ, Jacobs B, van der Naalt J. Blood- based biomarkers of inflammation in mild traumatic brain injury: a systematic review. Neurosci Biobehav Rev. 2022;132:154–68.
139. Johnson VE, Stewart JE, Begbie FD, Trojanowski JQ, Smith DH, Stewart W. Inflammation and white matter degeneration persist for years after a single traumatic brain injury. Brain. 2013;136:28–42.
140. Luo D, Chen P, Yang Z, Fu Y, Huang Y, Li H, Chen J, Zhuang J, Zhang C. High plasma adiponectin is associated with increased pulmonary blood flow and reduced right ventricular function in patients with pulmonary hypertension. BMC Pulm Med. 2020;20:204.
141. Wang K-Y, Yu G-F, Zhang Z-Y, Huang Q, Dong X-Q. Plasma high-mobility group box 1 levels and prediction of outcome in patients with traumatic brain injury. Clin Chim Acta. 2012;413:1737–41.
142. Gao T-L, Yuan X-T, Yang D, Dai H-L, Wang W-J, Peng X, Shao H-J, Jin Z-F, Fu Z-J. Expression of HMGB1 and RAGE in rat and human brains after traumatic brain injury. J Trauma Acute Care Surg. 2012;72:643–9.
143. Gradisek P, Carrara G, Antiga L, et al. Prognostic value of a combination of circulating biomarkers in critically ill patients with traumatic brain injury: results from the European CREACTIVE Study. J Neurotrauma. 2021;38:2667–76.
144. Graham NSN, Zimmerman KA, Moro F, et al. Axonal marker neurofilament light predicts long-term outcomes and progressive neurodegeneration after traumatic brain injury. Sci Transl Med. 2021;13:eabg9922.
145. Graham NSN, Zimmerman KA, Bertolini G, et al. Multicentre longitudinal study of fluid and neuroimaging BIOmarkers of AXonal injury after traumatic brain injury: the BIO-AX-TBI study protocol. BMJ Open. 2020;10:e042093.

146. Stocchetti N, Zanaboni C, Colombo A, Citerio G, Beretta L, Ghisoni L, Zanier ER, Canavesi K. Refractory intracranial hypertension and "second-tier" therapies in traumatic brain injury. Intensive Care Med. 2008;34:461–7.
147. Stocchetti N, Maas AIR. Traumatic intracranial hypertension. N Engl J Med. 2014;370:2121–30.
148. Zanier ER, Ortolano F, Ghisoni L, Colombo A, Losappio S, Stocchetti N. Intracranial pressure monitoring in intensive care: clinical advantages of a computerized system over manual recording. Crit Care. 2007;11:R7.
149. Valadka AB, Robertson CS. Surgery of cerebral trauma and associated critical care. Neurosurgery. 2007;61:203–20; discussion 220-221.
150. Chesnut R, Aguilera S, Buki A, et al. A management algorithm for adult patients with both brain oxygen and intracranial pressure monitoring: the Seattle International Severe Traumatic Brain Injury Consensus Conference (SIBICC). Intensive Care Med. 2020;46:919–29.

Future Directions: Multimodality Monitoring and Machine Learning

12

Wellingson Silva Paiva, Raphael Bertani, Sávio Batista, and Guilherme Melo Silva

12.1 Introduction

Historically, severe traumatic brain injury (TBI) has been considered fatal and unrepairable. Documents from the American Civil War state that the leading cause of death from penetrating TBI at that time (1861–1865) was infections [1]. Although this scenario vastly improved with the advent of antiseptics [1], the idea that neurological patients required specific, specialized care only began to rise between the 1910s and 1930s, concomitantly with the development of Neurosurgery as a specialty, mainly by Drs. Harvey Cushing and Walter Dandy [2]. Actual intensive care units only began appearing around the 1950s, when the term "critical care" was coined, possibly by Dr. Max Harry Weil [2]. Finally, in the 1980s and 1990s, neurocritical care became organized as a medical specialty with formal training, guidelines, and best practices. This process was likely the result of the efforts of passionately engaged healthcare professionals related to neurology, neurosurgery, and critical care that dedicated their time and passion to furthering their understanding of neurophysiology and pathophysiology, dramatically improving the prognosis of neurocritical patients who have built a legacy that is continuously benefiting patients all over the world.

Currently, neurocritical care has evolved dramatically, becoming globally recognized as a medical specialty, with its own societies, journals, meetings, and community. With technological developments came improved neurosurgical approaches and better patient management guidelines, powered mostly by innovations such as advanced imaging and improved multimodality monitoring, which has been currently evolving to be ever less invasive. Another rising star in the armamentarium of the neurointensivist is machine learning, which has the potential to alleviate the burden caused by excessive information extracted from patients and our inability to

W. S. Paiva (✉) · R. Bertani · S. Batista · G. M. Silva
Division of Neurosurgery, University of Sao Paulo Medical School, São Paulo, Brazil

E. Brogi et al. (eds.), *Traumatic Brain Injury*, Hot Topics in Acute Care Surgery and Trauma, https://doi.org/10.1007/978-3-031-50117-3_12

interpret this information with precision and celerity [3]. These rising stars come with many new potential benefits and, of course, hurdles and challenges, which will be both discussed in this chapter.

12.2 Multimodal Monitoring

Intensive care is essential in managing moderate and severe traumatic brain injury patients (mTBI, sTBI). In recent years, it has become widely recognized by medical practitioners that physical examination alone relays insufficient and delayed information on the dynamic, ever-changing physiology of the nervous system. Based on this new understanding, multimodality monitoring in the neurological intensive care unit (neuroICU) has become a standard of care [4]. As the possibilities of acquiring information from the intricate functioning of the brain from different sources increased, thus multimodality rose.

By combining information from blood arterial pressure (BAP) and intracranial pressure (ICP), insight into cerebral perfusion pressure (CPP), and autoregulation (AR), can be gained. A doppler ultrasound can be added so that cerebral blood flow (CBF) can be measured. Through an ICP catheter, brain temperature and tissue oxygen pressure (PtO_2) (Fig. 12.2) can be obtained [5]. Microdialysis catheters (MD) can give further insight into cerebral metabolism by continuously sampling analytes (hormones, neurotransmitters, glycine, glutamate, metabolites, etc.) at the interstitial space [6].

Although a vast amount of information can be obtained, interpreting and analyzing such data is also challenging, with the end goal being allowing clinicians to take a tailored approach to each patient by making treatment decisions that are guided by dynamic physiological changes and not mere, predetermined thresholds [7]. Below, you will find how the aforementioned parameters are currently being used and examples of research being done for future uses:

12.2.1 Intracranial Pressure (ICP)

Invasive monitoring of intracranial pressure through intraparenchymal, subdural, or intraventricular catheter is, globally, a mainstay of most NeuroICU units. Increased ICP, mainly in acute brain injury patients, has been independently associated with increased mortality risk and poor outcomes [8], prompting its monitoring and attempts to aggressively treat its increase. Although ICP monitoring is currently recommended for treating intracranial hypertension (IH) in TBI patients [9], the benefits of the intervention are still questioned [10], which may be due to the significant variation in ICP monitoring and management in different centers and countries [8]. Nonetheless, the benefits of monitoring ICP lie in the possibility of early detection of IH to guide early and, possibly, aggressive treatment, as well as allowing the determination of parameters such as the CPP, found by subtracting the value for ICP from the value for mean arterial pressure (MAP). Despite the historical controversy, many recent studies have shown benefits in ICP monitoring, mainly for severe TBI but also spontaneous intracranial hemorrhage (ICH) patients [11–14] and others.

Yet, the required procedure to insert a catheter is still required and is not free of complications, mainly infection, and hemorrhage that may cause significant, irreversible damage [15]. These complication rates vary significantly in the literature [15], and these risks limit the use of ICP monitoring, which causes invasive monitorization to be more widely used in more severe cases.

This may change significantly with the advent and establishment of non-invasive methods of ICP monitoring. Several methods have been proposed and are currently being used that vary from electroencephalography (EEG), ultrasound (such as optic nerve sheath and transcranial doppler), optic coherence tomography, pupillometry, strain-gauge sensors to measure skull deformation, and others [16–18]. Although most of these methods do not provide numerical values for ICP, they provide estimations and associated parameters [18], and increasing attention has been given to waveform analysis. Yet, not providing absolute numerical values can be considered a significant disadvantage of those methods. Fortunately, studies that compare invasive and non-invasive methods are being carried out more frequently.

Recent studies have suggested that noninvasive ICP waveform analysis can act as a surrogate for values given by invasive ICP monitoring by comparing results from invasive and non-invasive analysis in neurocritical patients with subarachnoid hemorrhage (SAH), intracerebral hemorrhage (ICH), ischemic stroke and TBI [19]. Although the authors have acknowledged the limitations of such studies, this could pave the way for increased accessibility of non-invasive monitoring in different scenarios, such as low-middle income countries (LMIC), rural or isolated areas, and prehospital settings. The reduced or even absent surgical complications could improve not only patient management in all settings but also make multimodal monitoring economically viable and therefore improve results in areas where resources are scarce and reduce economic burden in general.

There is still significant work to be done on developing non-invasive ICP and ICP waveform monitoring methods and on comparing these methods with the gold standard. As these developments occur, a trend of the increasing presence of non-invasive monitoring devices may be seen in NeuroICUs throughout the globe (Fig. 12.1).

12.2.2 Autoregulation

Cerebral autoregulation (CAR) is the physiological mechanism through which brain tissue maintains adequate cerebral blood flow (CBF) despite variations in arterial blood pressure [19]. This is achieved by adjusting vascular resistance according to such variations [7]. It is worth noting brain injury will disrupt CAR [7] and that ICP elevations that happen in the setting of impaired autoregulation or low CCP are less tolerable by brain tissue, as well as the higher the ICP elevation, the less tolerable it is in general [19].

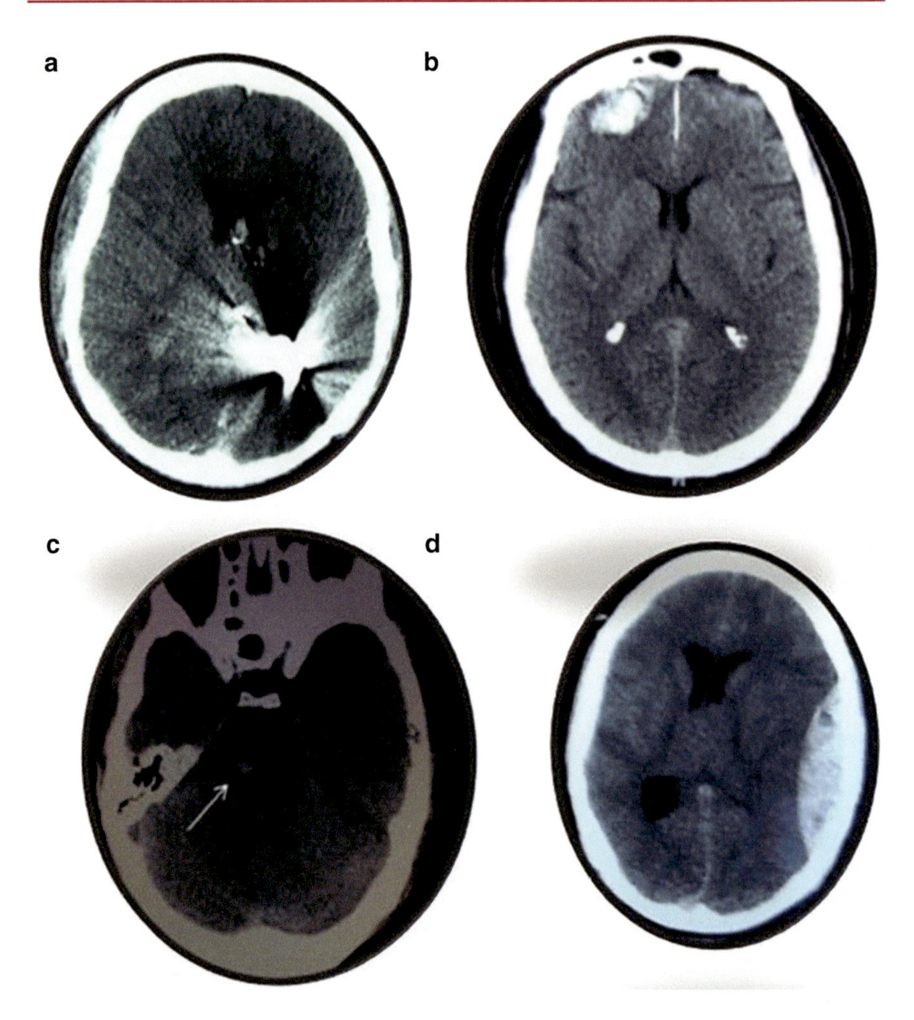

Fig. 12.1 Head CT from different patients with severe traumatic brain injury submitted to multi-monitoring management in NeuroICU setting. In (**a**) penetrating brain injury (gunshot wound to the head). In (**b**) frontal brain contusion. In (**c**) diffuse axonal injury. In (**d**) acute epidural hematoma

Optimal CCP can be achieved by observing changes caused to CAR when PPC changes, thus finding the CCP range in which the patient presents with the most preserved CAR. For such means, CAR is calculated by invasive methods, using the pressure reactivity index (PRx), the moving Pearson's correlation coefficient between 30 consecutive measurements of ICP, and mean arterial blood pressure (MAP). The PRx will be expressed in values ranging from − 1 (negative PRx, inverse correlation), which translates to a mostly preserved CAR, and +1 (positive PRx, nonreactive cerebral vascular responses despite changes in MAP and ICP) signaling disrupted CAR [19]. CAR can also be expressed with the Pulse Amplitude Index (PAx), which is the correlation between ICP pulse amplitude and MAP.

This allows CAR to be estimated by means of invasive (PAx) non-invasive methods (nPAx) that do not yield numerical values for ICP, but its waveform and, therefore, a relative pulse amplitude [20, 21]. Studies have shown that PAx and nPAx may be strongly correlated.

With the development and improvement of non-invasive devices, as mentioned before, not only the monitoring of ICP but also of cerebrovascular reactivity, estimated by monitoring CAR with PAx, will become even more feasible and accessible, allowing for more information to be obtained with reduced cost and for a wider range of patients.

12.2.3 Brain Tissue Oxygenation

Brain hypoxia is a well known issue following both traumatic and non-traumatic acute brain injury, as well as many other situations [22]. Continuous brain tissue oxygen monitoring offers the opportunity to gain better insight into complex brain physiology in order to optimize the management and potentially improve patient outcomes after the acute brain injury. In this context, Brain tissue oxygenation ($PbtO_2$) can be measured as a part of neurological multimodal neuromonitoring. Low $PbtO_2$ levels have been associated with poor neurologic outcomes in several neurocritical pathologies, such as SAH and TBI [7, 23, 24]. Interestingly, the difference in outcomes seem to be independent of CPP and ICP levels and several studies suggest benefits of combining ICP/CPP guided monitoring with brain tissue $PbtO_2$-directed therapy with a target $PbtO_2$ of more than 20 mmHg, having this been also suggested by guidelines [7, 25, 26].

Effort has also been made to implement non-invasive strategies to measure $PbtO_2$. Near-infrared spectroscopy is a possible non-invasive monitoring method that may be able to acquire information on $PbtO_2$, CBF, CAR and ICP [7, 27–29]. Despite some limitations of the method, such as confounding signals from extracranial tissues and the presence of intracranial hematomas or edema possibly invalidating readings [7], current and future improvements of the NIRS technology may allow it to be fully implemented in TBI care, as another non-invasive monitoring tool [27] (Fig. 12.2).

12.2.4 Cellular Metabolism: Cerebral Microdialysis

The study of brain metabolism allows us to assess the conditions of the different cerebral physiological pathways, analyze the changes that occur when these pathways shift towards energetically less efficient mechanisms, and detect waste products secondary to tissue damage [7, 30]. Cerebral Microdialysis (CMD) normally utilizes a catheter with a double-lumen probe coated at its tip by a dialyzing semipermeable membrane. The probe is implanted in the brain tissue, and an isotonic solution of known characteristics is then perfused through one of the two channels

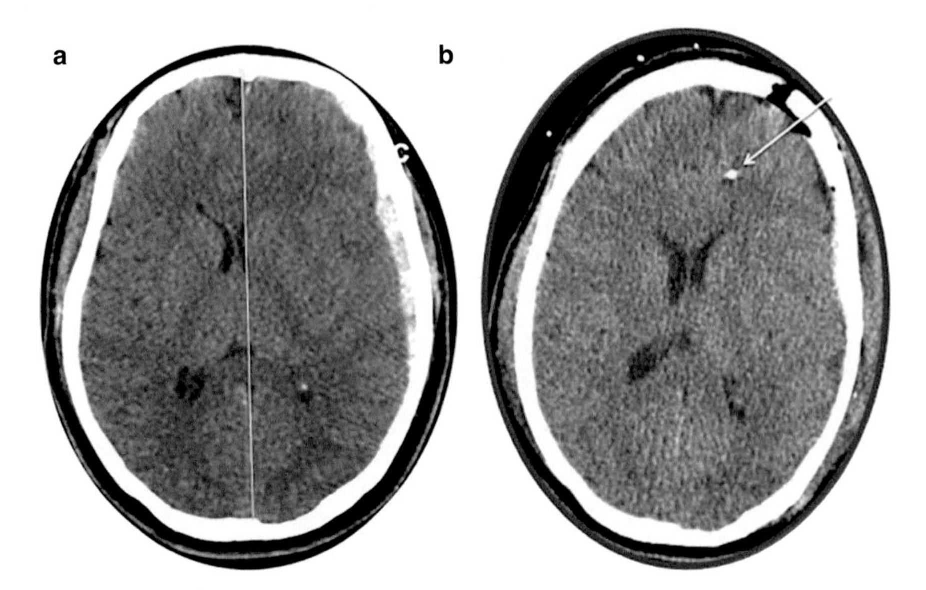

Fig. 12.2 Head CT of a severe traumatic brain injury patient. In (**a**) Preoperative CT showing acute subdural hematoma with midline shift. In (**b**) postoperative CT showing complete evacuation of subdural hematoma and the arrow marks a tissue oxygen pressure (PtO_2) catheter

at a programmable rate (0.1–5μl/min). It is worth noting that a single catheter may contain probes for microdialysis, ICP and $PtbO_2$ [31]. Once this solution comes into contact with the tissue interstice, substance exchange takes place through the semipermeable membrane, and the second catheter channel accumulates the microdialysate. Diffusion allows passage of molecules across the semipermeable membrane according to their concentration gradient from the brain extracellular fluid into the isotonic dialysis fluid [7, 32]. This allows monitoring of the concentration of glucose, pyruvate, glutamate, and glycerol, reflecting the brain's energetic metabolism [7].

Energetic dysfunction is known to be a major issue in TBI. Both ischemic and hemorrhagic pathologies can trigger metabolic crisis by causing an imbalance of supply and demands of glucose and microdialysis can identify both [33]. Studies in neurocritical patients variations in glucose, glutamate and glycine, as well as altered lactate/pyruvate (L/P) ratio through microdialysis, which have shown the following correlations [7, 33–35].

12.2.4.1 Glucose

Following TBI, serum glucose concentrations, overall glycemic control and its homeostasis with brain glucose may be lost, causing brain glucose to fail to supply metabolic demand even when serum glucose concentration is within a normal range [34]. This could be the cause of a metabolic collapse (not caused by ischemia) and is termed neuroglycopenia. This phenomenon is identified by CMD and has been correlated with poor outcomes in both interventional and observational studies, as well as increased glucose levels have been shown to have negative effects [35].

12.2.4.2 Lactate: Pyruvate Ratio

The lactate: pyruvate (L/P) ratio is an indicator of balance between oxidative and anaerobic metabolisms [35]. An increased L/P ratio with low pyruvate indicates diminished supply of energy substrate, suggestive of ischemia. An elevated LP ratio in the presence of normal or high pyruvate (higher levels of lactate in relation to pyruvate) suggests mitochondrial dysfunction [7, 36]. When combined with low glucose levels, increased L/P ratios suggest severe ischemia and correlate with poorer outcomes [37]. Changes in brain oxygenation, perfusion and glucose availability, therefore, seem to reflect changes in L/P ratios [35]. Sustained increased L/P ratios have been associated with poor outcomes in severe TBI in several studies [35, 38–41].

12.2.4.3 Glutamate and Glycerol

Glutamate is a marker of hypoxia/ischemia and excitotoxicity, and glycerol is a (nonspecific) marker of hypoxia/ischemia-related cell membrane breakdown [41, 42]. Although studies have shown these metabolites to be increased in groups of patients with worse outcomes, correlation seems to be weaker when compared to other parameters [35].

CMD may also be able to detect changes before they are observed in other monitoring methods, since the changes are measured at the cellular levels [43]. CMD may provide invaluable information for research, since it may help establish whether systemically administered agents cross the blood–brain barrier to their site of action and monitor the cascade effects of drug actions directly, as well as changes caused by other interventions [39, 44]. Unfortunately, CMD is still highly invasive as it requires implantation of a catheter directly into the brain tissue and still has very limited temporal resolution (results can mostly be measured hourly), which may miss several short-lived events and minute-changes [7, 31].

Further development of CMD may involve usage biosensors so that CMD via jugular or subcutaneous microdialysis would be made possible, thus not requiring the insertion of a catheter to the brain tissue, as well as development of biosensors to be used in conjunction with CMD to detect spreading depolarization waves (spreading depression) and detection of other substances, possibly even entering the realm of proteomics. Optical sensors could help diminish the need for reagents and also improve temporal resolution, allowing for better correlations and further understanding of the dynamics between cerebral metabolism changes and ICP, CPP and CAR [31, 39].

With further development of the above mentioned techniques, increasingly larger volumes of data will be generated. For this data to be processed, a data ecosystem is required. A data ecosystem is a platform that allows combination and processing of data from multiple sources [45]. For this end, machine-learning algorithms may be a promising solution.

12.3 Machine-Learning: Concepts and Definitions

Considered an advanced statistical technique [46], Machine learning (ML) is the use and development of computer systems to automate data analysis, creating analytical models with algorithms and statistics. Without specific instructions, these systems are expected to draw inferences from patterns found in the data, capable of "learning" from that data and identifying patterns with minimal to zero human intervention [47]. It is, therefore, an aspect of artificial intelligence (AI), a broader concept that concerns the ability of a machine to make decisions based on "reasoning" that resembles human thinking.

In the service sector, "robots" are replacing humans in customer service, as can be seen with the use of "chatbots" or virtual assistants [48]. Most of the time, "robots" or "bots" are just software: sets of codes built to handle a certain task automatically. It is worth noting that the goal is not merely to reduce hiring costs. AI and ML could benefit the market not only by reducing prices, but also by improving the quality, customization or speed of delivery of products and services, since ML can be much more effective than humans in some tasks, which is especially true for learning and identifying patterns from the large amounts of data being produced nowadays [49].

The end goal is to create software that, when exposed to new data, can adapt independently. This data, added to previous calculations and sometimes subjected to repetition, produces reliable decisions and results, born from the idea that machines could learn to perform specific tasks without being programmed to do so. Although some people see AI and machine learning as trends that bring robots closer to what is most human and subjective in us, the basis of everything is still the exact sciences. What allows a machine to have anything like intelligence are algorithms [50].

As novel as the concept sounds, the concept of ML is almost 70 years old. In the 1950s, when the first computer models were being developed, Alan Turing, considered the precursor of computing, began to carry out the first tests to analyze the reasoning power of machines [51]. At that time, this resulted in the mere repetition of simple sequences of commands, but it was the beginning of what we today know as ML.

Later, using Turing's discoveries as a reference, an American computer scientist named Arthur Lee Samuel went further and created the first software capable of learning [52]. The experiment consisted of a virtual checkers game, in which the system improved performance as the games passed. That is, the machine specialized, learning moves and creating strategies from its history, and it became increasingly difficult for someone to overcome it in a match.

Samuel was also responsible for using the term ML for the first time in 1959. Since then, technology has evolved a lot, and so has the amount and complexity of information. As a result, new concepts and tools are also introduced, such as AI, Big Data, and the Internet of Things, among others. Although benchmarking exactly what innovations these technologies will bring is difficult, they will most likely be increasingly integrated into our daily lives.

Currently, ML research is linked to the concept of Industry 4.0, also called the Fourth Industrial Revolution. The concept relates to the more widespread use of automation and information technology in the service sector and in the production of consumer goods. Automation, although not innovative, when implemented together with artificial intelligence, Big Data, the Internet of Things, and ML, allows for innovation [53]. This new reality of automation facilitates a leap in productivity worldwide.

Although humans can also process data and then complete tasks, information and data are produced increasingly faster, which can be explained by the crescent use of sensors or electronic devices connected through the web, allied with the less expensive prices of data storage [54]. Enter Big Data—there's so much information that it's humanly impossible to harness all that data, which is why we turn to machines. A great example is applications for driving: users are providing data on the speed of travel on the route they took, as well as time spent. Based on this information and the data collected from users traveling on the same road, the application will recommend whether or not other drivers should take the same route. A huge team of human beings could not possibly collect this data and make constant, real-time route suggestions. The application's algorithm, which works 24 h a day, can. Despite the creation of algorithms designed to take advantage of this immense amount of data, there is a significant amount of lost information, meaning there is significant room for improvement [55].

While multimodality monitoring provides a vast amount of patient information, it can become excessive. Magnetic Resonance Imaging (MRI) images, physiological waveforms, continuous electroencephalograms, laboratory tests, clinical findings, genetic information, and patient demographics are examples of data acquired. This vast amount of data becomes overwhelming to humans and barely usable since we cannot process all of it. This chaotic data pile becomes an issue instead of a solution. Thus, neurocritical care in neurotrauma can be seen as a "Big Data problem" [56]. With ML algorithms, automatic interpretation of the information collected is made possible in an effective approach for better resource management and patient care [3].

In a similar fashion to satellite navigation software provided by cellphone map applications used for driving, ML algorithms are able to trace "optimized routes" for healthcare professionals when dealing with both the diagnosis and prognosis of different illnesses. Even more so, some algorithms can predict complications of specific diseases or situations, allowing for early prophylactic treatment or time-efficient decisions in emergencies [3].

When assisted with phenotyping techniques, which are complex algorithms that allow the software to identify changes in a spectrum (such as mild versus moderate TBI), ML can also characterize the progression of diseases (even if subclinical), therefore enabling comprehensive risk assessment [57]. In the same manner, ML has been used to uncover different phenotypes, or clusters of patients that share similar characteristics. In a cohort of TBI patients followed for 3 and 6 months after the injury, certain patients were presenting phenotype-specific disparities related to their hematological profiles and 3 different clusters were found. One cluster presented with anemia with low hemoglobin and hematocrit; a second cluster had normal hematological values with a lower platelet count and elevated prothrombin time, and a third cluster had findings suggestive thrombocytopenia, anemia and coagulopathy.

These differences would otherwise go unnoticed, but were successfully determined by an ML model [58]. Further phenotyping and clustering of patients may need more effective and tailored approaches for each individual patient in the future. In fact, this type of algorithm may benefit patients by optimizing procedure parameters and, possibly, minimizing side effects and maximizing treatment efficiency [59].

There are several examples of successful use of ML for predictions in the neurocritical care setting. In a study, ICH was successfully detected by an ML algorithm built to identify them in computed tomography (CT) scans. The algorithm not only detected missed hemorrhages but also did so faster—the median time of diagnosis was 25 times faster [60]. In another study, several ML algorithms trained with an extensive TBI registry could properly prognosticate neurological function at discharge with reasonable accuracy, using patient information such as a history of present illness, age, gender, drugs in use, vital signs, and glucose levels at admission [61].

Another example is the prediction of in-hospital hypokalemia, a common complication. A study using five ML algorithms analyzed information included on the first hospitalization day, which was composed primarily of demographic data, weight, patient's medical history, vital signs, laboratory results, Glasgow Coma Scale (GCS), and treatment procedures. Increased risk of in-hospital mortality and a higher ratio of mechanical ventilation (MV) requirement on admission were also noticed in patients with hypokalemia [62]. Another study enrolled 785 TBI patients that were in MV in an attempt to predict in-hospital mortality. ML algorithms were given demographic characteristics, sustained injuries, and CT findings, and, with those predictors, outcomes were anticipated with an accuracy of over 80% [63]. Finally, an international study trained algorithms in a 686 cohort from 4 University Hospitals in one country and retrained the algorithms with 636 patients from 2 different countries for external validation, in an attempt to predict risk of 30-day all-cause mortality from admission. based on ICP and CPP values [64].

Regarding ICP, an ML-based method was modeled to predict increased ICP after TBI. By recording dynamic MAP and ICP monitoring changes, the algorithm predicted increases in ICP 30 min before they actually happened. It was also capable of predicting long-term neurological outcomes at 6 months by collecting data during the first 24 h of monitoring [65]. While increasing ICP represents a concerning risk, impending hypotension does not fall short, being one of the most worrisome secondary insults of TBI [46]. Since the duration of these events is an important prognostic factor, its prediction through an ML algorithm trained with data such as age, sex, systolic blood pressure, and heart rate can represent meaningful improvements in patient outcomes. Results from a study using data from 22 neurointensive care units in Europe show that ML algorithms might be able to predict episodes of hypotension 15 min ahead of onset [46]. Moreover, there are also algorithms for the prediction of intraoperative hypotension, featuring both intraoperative and preoperative predictors [66].

In offset, a study used ML to attempt to predict hemorrhagic contusion progression using data from a radiomics analysis of 107 TBI patients with ICH [67]. A radiomics analysis consists of using specific software to extract information of interest from medical imaging that is not visible to the human eye, using algorithms [68]. The study showed that using radiomics analysis of patient's admission CT scans and clinical information, predicting hemorrhagic progression and poor neurological outcome is more feasible and effective than using clinical information alone [67].

A major concern regarding research in ML is whether or not it would be applicable to different scenarios and populations. It is known that prediction models may vary greatly in accuracy when used in different populations [69]. This is most likely due to small sample size for validation, inadequate methodology used for modeling and lack of external validation with different populations [69]. Thus, it is important to properly assess these characteristics both when designing a study or when learning from one. Separate studies, one done with a TBI cohort consisting of 517 patients and another being a secondary analysis of a TBI data registry including 3138 patients, both applied in LMIC populations, have reported similar results when compared to studies in higher-income populations [61, 69]. This shows that, most likely, properly designed studies will be appropriate for different populations, despite stark differences in demographics, social, economical and clinical settings.

Nonetheless, there are still some challenges to be overcome. Research with ML and its algorithms involves a key conceptual difference compared to what is done in traditional research. Traditional research is curated, with heavily selected data based on an investigator's design and plan [70]. It would be, for example, necessary to give up on causation for correlation, at least initially, in the hopes that, after a certain period of accumulating correlations, causation will eventually be found [70], which may lead to several biases, potentially new biases we may not even be aware of currently. The data harvested may also be confusing and most likely, incomplete. There is also a liability issue, that is, the concern regarding who is liable if ML software commits mistakes and, even more so, if such errors are detectable in the first place. Although early results are promising, we may need to endure a longer adaptation process to make use of ML's full potential.

12.4 Conclusion

In conclusion, ML thrives on the concept of software being able to learn autonomously and, in consequence, deliver responses that become more assertive and specific over time. In addition, ML, whenever placed in contact with new values, reprograms itself, updating the definitions and settings according to new data. Therefore, the technology is constantly evolving, as it can recognize patterns based on results from previous analyses and refine its own interpretation, frequently without the need for human interference.

As multimodality monitoring becomes more effective, both clinically and financially, with technological developments and advent of non-invasive equipment, more and more patients will be monitored with increasing precision, but at the cost of an enormous amount of data being constantly generated. Machine learning rises as a solution to this "data tsunami" turning a significant portion of the collected data into clinically relevant information that may be able to prognosticate outcomes, divide patients in more specific phenotypes and predict adverse events in a timely fashion, allowing for prompt treatment. As technologies for monitoring and machine learning evolve, they improve each other in a mutually beneficial manner, with each one serving as a substrate for the other's progress: monitoring provides data and ML digests and transforms that data into information. Clinicians can harness these technologies together as tools to deliver optimal care to patients and to continue to build upon the flourishing fields of neurocritical care and neurotraumatology.

References

1. Cifu DX, Cohen SI, Lew HL, Jaffee M, Sigford B. The history and evolution of traumatic brain injury rehabilitation in military service members and veterans. Am J Phys Med Rehabil. 2010;89(8):688–94. https://doi.org/10.1097/PHM.0b013e3181e722ad.
2. Wijdicks EFM. The history of neurocritical care. Handb Clin Neurol. 2017;140:3–14. https://doi.org/10.1016/B978-0-444-63600-3.00001-5.
3. Chaudhry F, Hunt RJ, Hariharan P, Anand SK, Sanjay S, Kjoller EE, et al. Machine learning applications in the neuro ICU: a solution to big data mayhem? Front Neurol. 2020;11:554633. https://doi.org/10.3389/fneur.2020.554633.
4. Yang MT. Multimodal neurocritical monitoring. Biom J. 2020;43(3):226–30. https://doi.org/10.1016/j.bj.2020.05.005.
5. Fantini S, Sassaroli A, Tgavalekos KT, Kornbluth J. Cerebral blood flow and autoregulation: current measurement techniques and prospects for noninvasive optical methods. Neurophotonics. 2016;3(3):031411. https://doi.org/10.1117/1.NPh.3.3.031411.
6. Venturini S, Bhatti F, Timofeev I, Carpenter KLH, Hutchinson PJ, Guilfoyle MR, et al. Microdialysis-based classifications of abnormal metabolic states following traumatic brain injury: a systematic review of the literature. J Neurotrauma. 2022. https://doi.org/10.1089/neu.2021.0502
7. Smith M. Multimodality neuromonitoring in adult traumatic brain injury: a narrative review. Anesthesiology. 2018;128(2):401–15. https://doi.org/10.1097/ALN.0000000000001885.
8. Robba C, Graziano F, Rebora P, Elli F, Giussani C, Oddo M, et al. Intracranial pressure monitoring in patients with acute brain injury in the intensive care unit (SYNAPSE-ICU): an international, prospective observational cohort study. Lancet Neurol. 2021;20(7):548–58. https://doi.org/10.1016/S1474-4422(21)00138-1.
9. Carney N, Totten AM, O'Reilly C, Ullman JS, Hawryluk GWJ, Bell MJ, Bratton SL, Chesnut R, Harris OA, Kissoon N, Rubiano AM, Shutter L, Tasker RC, Vavilala MS, Wilberger J, Wright DW, Ghajar J. Neurosurgery. 2017;80(1):6–15. https://doi.org/10.1227/NEU.0000000000001432.
10. Aiolfi A, Benjamin E, Khor D, Inaba K, Lam L, Demetriades D. Brain trauma foundation guidelines for intracranial pressure monitoring: compliance and effect on outcome. World J Surg. 2017;41(6):1543–9. https://doi.org/10.1007/s00268-017-3898-6.
11. Rønning P, Helseth E, Skaga NO, Stavem K, Langmoen IA. The effect of ICP monitoring in severe traumatic brain injury: a propensity score–weighted and adjusted regression approach. J Neurosurg. 2018;131(6):1896–904. https://thejns.org/view/journals/j-neurosurg/131/6/article-p1896.xml.

12. Ren J, Wu X, Huang J, Cao X, Yuan Q, Zhang D, et al. Intracranial pressure monitoring-aided management associated with favorable outcomes in patients with hypertension-related spontaneous intracerebral hemorrhage. Transl Stroke Res. 2020;11(6):1253–63. https://doi.org/10.1007/s12975-020-00798-w.
13. Sun Z, Liu J, Dong S, Duan X, Xue F, Miao X. Prognostic predictive value of intracranial pressure and cerebral oxygen metabolism monitoring in patients with spontaneous intracerebral hemorrhage. Acta Neurol Belg. 2022. https://doi.org/10.1007/s13760-022-02037-5.
14. Dallagiacoma S, Robba C, Graziano F, Rebora P, Hemphill JC, Galimberti S, et al. Intracranial pressure monitoring in patients with spontaneous intracerebral hemorrhage: insights from the SYNAPSE-ICU study. Neurology. 2022;99(2):98–108. https://doi.org/10.1212/WNL.0000000000200568.
15. Tavakoli S, Peitz G, Ares W, Hafeez S, Grandhi R. Complications of invasive intracranial pressure monitoring devices in neurocritical care. Neurosurg Focus. 2017;43(5):6. https://doi.org/10.3171/2017.8.FOCUS17450.
16. Battaglini D, Santori G, Chandraptham K, Iannuzzi F, Bastianello M, Tarantino F, et al. Neurological complications and noninvasive multimodal neuromonitoring in critically ill mechanically ventilated COVID-19 patients. Front Neurol. 2020;11:602114. https://doi.org/10.3389/fneur.2020.602114.
17. Rasulo FA, Togni T, Romagnoli S. Essential noninvasive multimodality neuromonitoring for the critically ill patient. Crit Care. 2020;24(1):100. https://doi.org/10.1186/s13054-020-2781-2.
18. Dong J, Li Q, Wang X, Fan Y. A review of the methods of non-invasive assessment of intracranial pressure through ocular measurement. Bioengineering. 2022;9(7):304. https://doi.org/10.3390/bioengineering9070304.
19. de Moraes FM, Rocha E, Barros FCD, Freitas FGR, Miranda M, Valiente RA, et al. Waveform morphology as a surrogate for ICP monitoring: a comparison between an invasive and a noninvasive method. Neurocrit Care. 2022;37(1):219–27. https://doi.org/10.1007/s12028-022-01477-4.
20. Hassett CE, Uysal SP, Butler R, Moore NZ, Cardim D, Gomes JA. Assessment of cerebral autoregulation using invasive and noninvasive methods of intracranial pressure monitoring. Neurocrit Care. 2022. https://doi.org/10.1007/s12028-022-01585-1.
21. Radolovich DK, Aries MJH, Castellani G, Corona A, Lavinio A, Smielewski P, et al. Pulsatile intracranial pressure and cerebral autoregulation after traumatic brain injury. Neurocrit Care. 2011;15(3):379–86. https://doi.org/10.1007/s12028-011-9553-4.
22. De Georgia MA. Brain tissue oxygen monitoring in neurocritical care. J Intensive Care Med. 2015;30(8):473–83. https://doi.org/10.1177/0885066614529254.
23. Gouvea Bogossian E, Diaferia D, Ndieugnou Djangang N, et al. Brain tissue oxygenation guided therapy and outcome in non-traumatic subarachnoid hemorrhage. Sci Rep. 2021;11:16235. https://doi.org/10.1038/s41598-021-95602-6.
24. Okonkwo DO, Shutter LA, Moore C, Temkin NR, Puccio AM, Madden CJ, Andaluz N, Chesnut RM, Bullock MR, Grant GA, McGregor J, Weaver M, Jallo J, LeRoux PD, Moberg D, Barber J, Lazaridis C, Diaz-Arrastia RR. Brain oxygen optimization in severe traumatic brain injury phase-II: a phase II randomized trial. Crit Care Med. 2017;45(11):1907–14. https://doi.org/10.1097/CCM.0000000000002619. PMID: 29028696; PMCID: PMC5679063.
25. Nangunoori R, Maloney-Wilensky E, Stiefel M, Park S, Andrew Kofke W, Levine JM, et al. Brain tissue oxygen-based therapy and outcome after severe traumatic brain injury: a systematic literature review. Neurocrit Care. 2012;17(1):131–8. https://doi.org/10.1007/s12028-011-9621-9.
26. Oddo M, Bösel J, Participants in the International Multidisciplinary Consensus Conference on Multimodality Monitoring. Monitoring of brain and systemic oxygenation in neurocritical care patients. Neurocrit Care. 2014;21(2):103–20. https://doi.org/10.1007/s12028-014-0024-6.
27. Gomez A, Sainbhi AS, Froese L, Batson C, Alizadeh A, Mendelson AA, et al. Near infrared spectroscopy for high-temporal resolution cerebral physiome characterization in TBI: a narrative review of techniques, applications, and future directions. Front Pharmacol. 2021;12:719501. https://doi.org/10.3389/fphar.2021.719501.

28. Zweifel C, Castellani G, Czosnyka M, Helmy A, Manktelow A, Carrera E, et al. Noninvasive monitoring of cerebrovascular reactivity with near infrared spectroscopy in head-injured patients. J Neurotrauma. 2010;27(11):1951–8. https://doi.org/10.1089/neu.2010.1388.
29. Kovacs M, Peluso L, Njimi H, De Witte O, Gouvêa Bogossian E, Quispe Cornejo A, et al. Optimal cerebral perfusion pressure guided by brain oxygen pressure measurement. Front Neurol. 2021;12:732830. https://doi.org/10.3389/fneur.2021.732830.
30. Tisdall MM, Smith M. Cerebral microdialysis: research technique or clinical tool. Br J Anaesth. 2006;97(1):18–25. https://doi.org/10.1093/bja/ael109. Epub 2006 May 12. PMID: 16698861.
31. Zimphango C, Alimagham FC, Carpenter KLH, Hutchinson PJ, Hutter T. Monitoring neurochemistry in traumatic brain injury patients using microdialysis integrated with biosensors: a review. Meta. 2022;12:393. https://doi.org/10.3390/metabo12050393.
32. Baldini F. Microdialysis-based sensing in clinical applications. Anal Bioanal Chem. 2010;397(3):909–16. https://doi.org/10.1007/s00216-010-3626-7. Epub 2010 Mar 17.
33. Vespa P, Bergsneider M, Hattori N, Wu HM, Huang SC, Martin NA, et al. Metabolic crisis without brain ischemia is common after traumatic brain injury: a combined microdialysis and positron emission tomography study. J Cereb Blood Flow Metab. 2005;25(6):763–74. https://doi.org/10.1038/sj.jcbfm.9600073.
34. Magnoni S, Tedesco C, Carbonara M, Pluderi M, Colombo A, Stocchetti N. Relationship between systemic glucose and cerebral glucose is preserved in patients with severe traumatic brain injury, but glucose delivery to the brain may become limited when oxidative metabolism is impaired. Crit Care Med. 2012;40:1785–91. https://doi.org/10.1097/ccm.0b013e318246bd45.
35. Guilfoyle MR, Helmy A, Donnelly J, Stovell MG, Timofeev I, Pickard JD, et al. Characterising the dynamics of cerebral metabolic dysfunction following traumatic brain injury: a microdialysis study in 619 patients. PLoS One. 2021;16(12):e0260291. https://doi.org/10.1371/journal.pone.0260291.
36. Larach DB, Kofke WA, Le Roux P. Potential non-hypoxic/ischemic causes of increased cerebral interstitial fluid lactate/pyruvate ratio: a review of available literature. Neurocrit Care. 2011;15(3):609–22. https://doi.org/10.1007/s12028-011-9517-8.
37. Timofeev I, Czosnyka M, Carpenter KLH, Nortje J, Kirkpatrick PJ, Al-Rawi PG, et al. Interaction between brain chemistry and physiology after traumatic brain injury: impact of autoregulation and microdialysis catheter location. J Neurotrauma. 2011;28:849–60. https://doi.org/10.1089/neu.2010.1656.
38. Hutchinson PJ, Jalloh I, Helmy A, et al. Consensus statement from the 2014 International Microdialysis Forum. Intensive Care Med. 2015;41:1517–28.
39. Nordström CH, Forsse A, Jakobsen RP, Mölström S, Nielsen TH, Toft P, et al. Bedside interpretation of cerebral energy metabolism utilizing microdialysis in neurosurgical and general intensive care. Front Neurol. 2022;13:968288. https://doi.org/10.3389/fneur.2022.968288.
40. Oddo M, Schmidt JM, Carrera E, Badjatia N, Connolly ES, Presciutti M, Ostapkovich ND, Levine JM, Le Roux P, Mayer SA. Impact of tight glycemic control on cerebral glucose metabolism after severe brain injury: a microdialysis study. Crit Care Med. 2008;36(12):3233–8. https://doi.org/10.1097/CCM.0b013e31818f4026.
41. Sarrafzadeh AS, Haux D, Lüdemann L, Amthauer H, Plotkin M, Küchler I, Unterberg AW. Cerebral ischemia in aneurysmal subarachnoid hemorrhage: a correlative microdialysis-PET study. Stroke. 2004;35(3):638–43. https://doi.org/10.1161/01.STR.0000116101.66624.F1. Epub 2004 Feb 12. PMID: 14963287.
42. Chamoun R, Suki D, Gopinath SP, Goodman JC, Robertson C. Role of extracellular glutamate measured by cerebral microdialysis in severe traumatic brain injury. J Neurosurg. 2010;113(3):564–70. https://doi.org/10.3171/2009.12.JNS09689.
43. Belli A, Sen J, Petzold A, Russo S, Kitchen N, Smith M. Metabolic failure precedes intracranial pressure rises in traumatic brain injury: a microdialysis study. Acta Neurochir. 2008;150(5):461–9; discussion 470. https://doi.org/10.1007/s00701-008-1580-3.
44. Carpenter KLH, Young AMH, Hutchinson PJ. Advanced monitoring in traumatic brain injury. Curr Opin Crit Care. 2017;23:103–9. https://doi.org/10.1097/mcc.0000000000000400.

45. Sonja M, Ioana G, Miaoqing Y, Anna K. Understanding value in health data ecosystems: a review of current evidence and ways forward. Rand Health Q. 2018;7(2):3. https://www.ncbi.nlm.nih.gov/pubmed/29416943.
46. Donald R, Howells T, Piper I, Enblad P, Nilsson P, Chambers I, Gregson B, Citerio G, Kiening K, Neumann J, Ragauskas A, Sahuquillo J, Sinnott R, Stell A, BrainIT Group. Forewarning of hypotensive events using a Bayesian artificial neural network in neurocritical care. J Clin Monit Comput. 2019;33(1):39–51. https://doi.org/10.1007/s10877-018-0139-y. Epub 2018 May 24.
47. Mitchell T. Machine learning. New York: McGraw Hill; 1997.
48. Arsenijevic U, Jovic M. Artificial intelligence marketing: chatbots. In: 2019 International Conference on Artificial Intelligence: Applications and Innovations (IC-AIAI); 2019, pp. 19–193. https://doi.org/10.1109/IC-AIAI48757.2019.00010.
49. Bessen J. Artificial intelligence and jobs: the role of demand. In: Agrawal A, Gans J, Goldfarb A, editors. The economics of artificial intelligence: an agenda. Chicago: National Bureau of Economic Research; 2019. p. 291–307.
50. Marr D. Artificial intelligence—a personal view. Artif Intell. 1977;9(1):37–48. https://doi.org/10.1016/0004-3702(77)90013-3.
51. Turing I. Computing machinery and intelligence. Mind. 1950;LIX(236):433–60. https://doi.org/10.1093/mind/LIX.236.433.
52. Weiss EA. Biographies: Eloge: Arthur Lee Samuel (1901-90). IEEE Ann History Comput. 1992;14(3):55–69. https://doi.org/10.1109/85.150082.
53. Candanedo IS, Nieves EH, González SR, Martín MTS, Briones AG. Machine learning predictive model for industry 4.0. In: Uden L, Hadzima B, Ting IH, editors. Knowledge management in organizations. KMO 2018. Communications in computer and information science, vol. 877. Cham: Springer; 2018. https://doi.org/10.1007/978-3-319-95204-8_42.
54. Daas P, Puts M. Big data as a source of statistical information. J Off Stat. 2014;31(2):249–62.
55. Essien AE, Petrounias I, Sampaio P, Sampaio S. Deep-PRESIMM: integrating deep learning with microsimulation for traffic prediction. In: 2019 IEEE international conference on systems, man and cybernetics (SMC). Piscataway: IEEE; 2019. p. 4257–62. https://doi.org/10.1109/SMC.2019.8914604.
56. Huie JR, Almeida CA, Ferguson AR. Neurotrauma as a big-data problem. Curr Opin Neurol. 2018;31(6):702–8. https://doi.org/10.1097/WCO.0000000000000614. PMID: 30379703; PMCID: PMC7075373.
57. Ambale-Venkatesh B, Yang X, Wu CO, Liu K, Hundley WG, McClelland R, Gomes AS, Folsom AR, Shea S, Guallar E, Bluemke DA, Lima JAC. Cardiovascular event prediction by machine learning: the multi-ethnic study of atherosclerosis. Circ Res. 2017;121(9):1092–101. https://doi.org/10.1161/CIRCRESAHA.117.311312. Epub 2017 Aug 9. PMID: 28794054; PMCID: PMC5640485.
58. Folweiler KA, Sandsmark DK, Diaz-Arrastia R, Cohen AS, Masino AJ. Unsupervised machine learning reveals novel traumatic brain injury patient phenotypes with distinct acute injury profiles and long-term outcomes. J Neurotrauma. 2020;37(12):1431–44. https://doi.org/10.1089/neu.2019.6705. Epub 2020 Mar 11. PMID: 32008422; PMCID: PMC7249479.
59. Boutet A, Madhavan R, Elias GJB, Joel SE, Gramer R, Ranjan M, Paramanandam V, Xu D, Germann J, Loh A, Kalia SK, Hodaie M, Li B, Prasad S, Coblentz A, Munhoz RP, Ashe J, Kucharczyk W, Fasano A, Lozano AM. Predicting optimal deep brain stimulation parameters for Parkinson's disease using functional MRI and machine learning. Nat Commun. 2021;12(1):3043. https://doi.org/10.1038/s41467-021-23311-9. PMID: 34031407; PMCID: PMC8144408.
60. Arbabshirani MR, Fornwalt BK, Mongelluzzo GJ, Suever JD, Geise BD, Patel AA, et al. Advanced machine learning in action: identification of intracranial hemorrhage on computed tomography scans of the head with clinical workflow integration. NPJ Digit Med. 2018;1:9. https://doi.org/10.1038/s41746-017-0015-z.
61. Hernandes Rocha TA, Elahi C, Cristina da Silva N, Sakita FM, Fuller A, Mmbaga BT, Green EP, Haglund MM, Staton CA, Nickenig Vissoci JR. A traumatic brain injury prognostic model

to support in-hospital triage in a low-income country: a machine learning-based approach. J Neurosurg. 2019;132(6):1961–9. https://doi.org/10.3171/2019.2.JNS182098.
62. Zhou Z, Huang C, Fu P, Huang H, Zhang Q, Wu X, Yu Q, Sun Y. Prediction of in-hospital hypokalemia using machine learning and first hospitalization day records in patients with traumatic brain injury. CNS Neurosci Ther. 2022. https://doi.org/10.1111/cns.13993.
63. Abujaber A, Fadlalla A, Gammoh D, Abdelrahman H, Mollazehi M, El-Menyar A. Prediction of in-hospital mortality in patients on mechanical ventilation post traumatic brain injury: machine learning approach. BMC Med Inform Decis Mak. 2020;20(1):336. https://doi.org/10.1186/s12911-020-01363-z. PMID: 33317528; PMCID: PMC7737377.
64. Raj R, Wennervirta JM, Tjerkaski J, Luoto TM, Posti JP, Nelson DW, Takala R, Bendel S, Thelin EP, Luostarinen T, Korja M. Dynamic prediction of mortality after traumatic brain injury using a machine learning algorithm. NPJ Digit Med. 2022;5(1):96. https://doi.org/10.1038/s41746-022-00652-3. PMID: 35851612; PMCID: PMC9293936.
65. Güiza F, Depreitere B, Piper I, Van den Berghe G, Meyfroidt G. Novel methods to predict increased intracranial pressure during intensive care and long-term neurologic outcome after traumatic brain injury: development and validation in a multicenter dataset. Crit Care Med. 2013;41(2):554–64. https://doi.org/10.1097/CCM.0b013e3182742d0a.
66. Feld SI, Hippe DS, Miljacic L, Polissar NL, Newman SF, Nair BG, Vavilala MS. A machine learning approach for predicting real-time risk of intraoperative hypotension in traumatic brain injury. J Neurosurg Anesthesiol. 2021. https://doi.org/10.1097/ANA.0000000000000819.
67. Shih YJ, Liu YL, Chen JH, Ho CH, Yang CC, Chen TY, Wu TC, Ko CC, Zhou JT, Zhang Y, Su MY. Prediction of intraparenchymal hemorrhage progression and neurologic outcome in traumatic brain injury patients using radiomics score and clinical parameters. Diagnostics. 2022;12(7):1677. https://doi.org/10.3390/diagnostics12071677. PMID: 35885581; PMCID: PMC9320220.
68. Wagner MW, Namdar K, Biswas A, Monah S, Khalvati F, Ertl-Wagner BB. Radiomics, machine learning, and artificial intelligence—what the neuroradiologist needs to know. Neuroradiology. 2021;63(12):1957–67. https://doi.org/10.1007/s00234-021-02813-9.
69. Amorim RL, Oliveira LM, Malbouisson LM, Nagumo MM, Simoes M, Miranda L, et al. Prediction of early TBI mortality using a machine learning approach in a LMIC population. Front Neurol. 2019;10:1366. https://doi.org/10.3389/fneur.2019.01366.
70. Agoston DV, Langford D. Big data in traumatic brain injury; promise and challenges. Concussion. 2017;2(4):CNC45. https://doi.org/10.2217/cnc-2016-0013. PMID: 30202589; PMCID: PMC6122694.

Out-of-Hospital Management of Traumatic Brain Injury

13

James M. Bradford, Marc D. Trust, James Kempema, and Carlos V. R. Brown

13.1 Introduction

Traumatic brain injury (TBI) accounts for approximately 61,000 deaths per year in the USA, with suicide surpassing motor vehicle accidents as the leading cause of TBI-related mortality [1]. Half of deaths from TBI happen within the first two hours after injury, which underscores the importance of out-of-hospital management in survival and recovery [2]. The goals during this out-of-hospital phase of care are to identify that brain injury has occurred, correct modifiable causes of secondary injury, and rapidly transport the patient to an appropriately equipped facility.

13.2 Initial Evaluation

The initial out-of-hospital evaluation of a patient with suspected head injury begins with assessing airway, breathing, and circulation [2–4]. Up to 55% of patients with TBI have coexisting hypoxemia which contributes to poor neurologic outcomes. Early hypotension also doubles mortality in patients with severe TBI [5–8]. For those reasons, frequent assessment with blood pressure measurement and continuous oxygen saturation monitoring are started immediately.

The next step in evaluation is to identify that a brain injury has occurred. The Glasgow Coma Scale (GCS) and pupillary examination are reliable out-of-hospital indicators of brain injury [4]. GCS is a standardized measurement of consciousness that assesses three domains: eye opening, motor response, and verbal response [2]. The severity of brain injury can be stratified by cumulative GCS score into mild

J. M. Bradford · M. D. Trust · J. Kempema · C. V. R. Brown (✉)
Department of Surgery and Perioperative Care, Dell Medical School, University of Texas at Austin, Austin, TX, USA
e-mail: James.Bradford@uchicagomedicine.org; mdtrust@ascension.org; jkempema@ascension.org; carlos.brown@austin.utexas.edu

E. Brogi et al. (eds.), *Traumatic Brain Injury*, Hot Topics in Acute Care Surgery and Trauma, https://doi.org/10.1007/978-3-031-50117-3_13

(13–15), moderate (9–12), or severe (3–8) which correlate with increasing mortality and neurologic morbidity [9, 10].

Intoxication and chemical sedation may complicate GCS assessments in patients with TBI. It is estimated that as many as 50% of patients with TBI present intoxicated; however, alcohol does not appear to significantly affect GCS scores among patients with true brain injury. Said differently, altered consciousness should be attributed to TBI, rather than intoxication, until proven otherwise [11, 12]. GCS should ideally be calculated on scene before attempting airway interventions or chemical sedation. If that cannot be done, though, the motor component of GCS can still be used to predict the severity of brain injury and overall appears to perform as well if not better than the cumulative GCS score in identifying brain injury [4, 10]. Finally, repeated assessment of GCS should be conducted frequently as decreases in GCS of two or more points are associated with the presence of an expanding intracranial bleed [10].

The pupillary examination consists of an evaluation of pupil size, symmetry, and reactivity to light. Like GCS, pupillary dysfunction predicts mortality and neurologic morbidity in TBI [13, 14]. Abnormal findings include acute pupillary dilation, asymmetry (>1 mm difference), or non-reactivity to light (<1 mm response to bright light). In the context of intracranial injury, acute pupillary dilation suggests brainstem ischemia or compression of the oculomotor nerve (CNIII) by herniated brain tissue [10]. However, damage to the cervical sympathetic chain or orbital trauma may also alter pupillary response but not be indicative of intracranial injury [2, 3].

The AVPU score is an additional tool that can quickly assess a patient's level of consciousness. The score categorizes a patient's level of consciousness into Alert (A), Verbally Responsive (V), Physically Responsive (P), or Unresponsive (U). Any score below (A) is considered abnormal and indicative of some type of injury. AVPU assessments successfully identify pediatric and geriatric patients who would benefit from transport to a trauma center [15–17].

13.3 Treatment

13.3.1 Airway

Patients suffering brain injury are at high risk for airway collapse, aspiration, or obstruction from surrounding facial trauma. Out-of-hospital airway management in TBI begins with an assessment of the patient's ability to oxygenate and ventilate. Patients who can do both should be started on supplemental oxygen and rapidly transported to a trauma center. For patients who cannot oxygenate and/or ventilate, airway management begins basic airway maneuvers: jaw thrust, oropharyngeal airway (OPA), or nasopharyngeal airway (NPA). The primary contraindications for OPA and NPA are an intact gag reflex and basilar skull fracture, respectively [18]. The Brain Trauma Foundation (BTF) prehospital TBI guidelines recommend escalating management to a definitive airway in patients with GCS $\leq$ 8 or persistent hypoxemia (oxygen saturations <90%) despite supplemental oxygen [2, 19, 20].

Supraglottic airway devices and endotracheal (ET) intubation are two options for advanced out-of-hospital airway management. An overwhelming number of observational studies argue that out-of-hospital ET intubation increases mortality in patients with TBI. The mechanisms hypothesized to underly this association are that out-of-hospital ET intubation prolongs time to the emergency department, causes iatrogenic oxygen desaturations, and mechanically stimulates a sympathetic response that increases intracerebral pressure (ICP) [21–28]. The most significant support for out-of-hospital ET intubation comes from a 2010 randomized control trial that reported improved 6-month functional neurologic outcomes in patients with severe TBI who underwent out-of-hospital ET intubation compared to those intubated by physicians in the emergency department [29]. However, patients in the RSI arm of this study did not have improvements in physiology known to mediate secondary brain injury, namely hypoxia and hypotension. There were no differences in PaO_2 on initial blood gas between groups, and there was a higher incidence of cardiopulmonary arrest in the RSI group [29, 30]. Taken together, out-of-hospital emergency systems should not prioritize ET intubation in TBI as it does not improve markers of secondary injury or survival for most brain injured patients. However, in cases where severely injured patients must be transported long distances, or where prehospital providers must be available to perform other life-sustaining interventions, ET intubation by experienced providers may be appropriate.

The decision to utilize induction and neuromuscular blocking agents when an advanced airway is attempted remains controversial as well. Induction and neuromuscular blockade improve the success rate of ET intubation by out-of-hospital providers; however, peri-intubation hypotension and cardiac arrest are well documented complications that occur in up to 21% and 5% of out-of-hospital rapid sequence intubation (RSI) attempts, respectively [23, 31]. Due to these concerns, etomidate and ketamine are popular choices for induction given their relatively mild effects on blood pressure [23, 32]. Push-dose epinephrine (10–20 μg) can also be utilized to increase mean arterial pressure before or immediately following RSI [33] for patients with pre-intubation hypotension or an elevated shock index. As for neuromuscular blocking agents, succinylcholine is rapidly metabolized and allows for more frequent assessments of mental status as the drug is metabolized [32]. However, in patients with severe TBI, succinylcholine has been associated with higher mortality when compared to rocuronium, perhaps by increasing intracranial pressure [34].

Supraglottic airway devices (SGA) (Laryngeal Mask Airway, I-Gel Supraglottic Airway, King LT) have emerged as popular alternatives to ET intubation in out-of-hospital airway management. These devices are positioned above the larynx and open the upper airway for ventilation. Compared with ET intubation, supraglottic airway devices require less training to successfully place and have demonstrated better first-pass success in patients with out-of-hospital cardiac arrest [7, 22, 33, 34]. However, no evidence has demonstrated SGA are better for neurologic outcomes than basic airway maneuvers or ET intubation in patients with TBI; however, their outcomes may be non-inferior [35].

13.3.2 Breathing

Cerebral hypoxia is well understood to be associated with worse outcomes in patients with TBI. Therefore, optimizing oxygenation is one of the key priorities in all phases of care in these patients. Continuous oxygen saturation monitoring should be used, and supplemental oxygen administered to achieve SpO_2 of ≥95% [36]. Ventilation rate is also a key driver of cerebral perfusion and is critical to the management of patients with TBI. Carbon dioxide (CO_2) and pH, driven by partial pressure of CO_2 ($PaCO_2$), regulate cerebral blood flow by controlling vasodilation and vasoconstriction in cerebral vasculature. As $PaCO_2$ increases, cerebral vessels dilate and cerebral blood flow increases. Out-of-hospital prophylactic hyperventilation ($PaCO_2 < 25$ mmHg) was traditionally employed to induce vasoconstriction and reduce intracerebral pressure (ICP) and the risk of brain herniation. However, cerebral vasoconstriction can exacerbate cerebral ischemia, which has also been identified early after TBI [19, 20, 37]. To minimize the risk of cerebral ischemia, out-of-hospital prophylactic hyperventilation is no longer recommended unless exam findings suggest active herniation (anisocoria, non-reactive pupil, posturing) [2, 38]. The goal for patients without signs of herniation should be normal ventilation rate and rapid transport to a trauma center where access to invasive monitoring can help further guide interventions. Continuous end-tidal CO_2 monitoring can assist prehospital providers in appropriate ventilatory rates.

13.3.3 Circulation

Out-of-hospital hypotension, defined as a systolic blood pressure <90 mmHg, is associated with poor outcomes in patients with TBI. Under normal circumstances, cerebral perfusion is tightly regulated by the cerebral vasculature across a wide range of systemic pressures. TBI causes these mechanisms of regulation to fail, at which point brain perfusion becomes dependent on systemic arterial pressure. Preventing systemic hypotension is thus an important tenet of management to avoid losing cerebral perfusion and causing ischemia. The optimal blood pressure target for out-of-hospital management is a topic of ongoing investigation and there have not been recently updated consensus guidelines on the topic. The literature that does exist, though, suggests that goals should likely be higher than the previously defined thresholds of 90 mmHg [39, 40]. In fact, a large observational study in Japan found mortality to increase at systolic pressures below 110 mmHg [40]. It is important that out-of-hospital providers recognize the acuity of blood pressures that may be acceptable for hemorrhaging patients as potentially fatal in TBI given the risk for cerebral ischemia.

The optimal fluid for out-of-hospital resuscitation in TBI has been isotonic rather than hypertonic crystalloid. Hyperosmolar solutions such as hypertonic saline, colloids, and mannitol cause free fluid to move from the interstitial to the intravascular space. Through this mechanism, they have been hypothesized to reduce intracerebral pressure (ICP) and increase systemic blood pressure. 7.5% hypertonic saline (HTS), with and without 6% dextran, are the two most extensively studied solutions in the out-of-hospital literature. It is known that hypertonic saline administered in the ICU either continuously or as a bolus has been shown to effectively reduce ICP, increase circulating blood volume, and improve mortality in patients with TBI [41]. However, studies that examined starting hyperosmolar fluid in the out-of-hospital phase have not found similarly impressive results [42–44]. Among both hypotensive and normotensive patients presenting with severe TBI, out-of-hospital resuscitation with bolus hyperosmolar solutions (HTS +/− Dextran) did not improve survival or neurologic outcomes compared with standard crystalloid solution. Interestingly, administration of hyperosmolar solutions did not decrease initial ICP measurements or increase arrival systolic blood pressure in these studies, either [42, 43]. The lack of effect may be due to the inability to infuse a clinically significant amount of fluid in the out-of-hospital period, but nonetheless these studies do not argue for its widespread use. Additionally, the use of albumin is also associated with worse outcomes in patients with TBI and should also be avoided.

The effect of blood transfusion in patients with isolated and non-isolated TBI has garnered more attention in recent years. It is well known that the optimal emergency resuscitation fluid in patients with hemorrhagic shock is whole blood or blood components in an equivalent ratio of plasma to platelets to packed red cells [45, 46]. Out-of-hospital blood transfusion has become feasible for some EMS systems and has demonstrated success, especially in military settings [47]. Blood products may also have an important role in patients with TBI. For one, many of these patients present with polytrauma and are at risk for concurrent hemorrhagic shock. Secondly, specific to intracranial physiology, blood products can increase oxygen carrying capacity, improve brain tissue oxygenation, and protect against coagulopathy and worsening intracranial bleeding [48]. A secondary analysis of the Prehospital Air Medical Plasma (PAMPer) trial demonstrated improved survival at 30 days for patients with TBI and risk for hemorrhagic shock who received 2 units of thawed plasma [49]. Similarly, animal studies have shown that early resuscitation with whole blood may improve brain tissue oxygenation at lower blood pressures than crystalloid solution, which could reduce aggressive out-of-hospital crystalloid resuscitation to achieve blood pressure goals in polytrauma patients [48]. As mechanisms for storing and carrying products become more economically and practically feasible, blood products may soon become the preferred out-of-hospital fluid in brain injured patients.

Finally, tranexamic acid (TXA) is an anti-fibrinolytic that has been shown to reduce mortality when administered early in trauma patients who are bleeding [50]. Early TXA administration within 3 h of injury also reduces mortality from head injury in patients with mild to moderate TBI [51]. Among patients with confirmed intracerebral hemorrhage (ICH), a 2 g out-of-hospital bolus of TXA reduced 28-day mortality as well [52]. These findings support the routine use of TXA, either as 2 g bolus or 1 g loading dose followed by a 1 g in-hospital maintenance dose, in the out-of-hospital phase of care.

13.3.4 Hypothermia

Therapeutic hypothermia (32C-35C) for TBI has been employed in select intensive care units. The physiologic basis for the treatment is that hypothermia mitigates hypoxic cellular injury, protects the blood–brain barrier, and reduces tissue metabolic demand [53, 54]. It has been shown that therapeutic hypothermia successfully reduces ICP after TBI [54]. However, its effect on survival and neurologic outcomes has been mixed over the years and largely dependent on the centers at which it is employed [53–55].

Prophylactic hypothermia, initiated during the prehospital phase or early in the emergency department, has also been hypothesized to reduce secondary brain injury by mitigating the early inflammatory response to TBI [56]. In four randomized control trials to date, early initiation of hypothermia after suspected brain injury has not been associated with improved neurologic outcomes [57–60]. The most recent and robust of those trials, the Prophylactic Hypothermia Trial to Lessen Traumatic Brain Injury–Randomized Clinical Trial (POLAR-RCT), randomized patients at a median of 1.9 h after injury (45% enrolled prehospital), targeted cooling temperatures of 33 °C–35 °C for greater than 72 h, and titrated rewarming at slow increments (<0.25 °C/h) based on ICP measurements. On top of finding no neurologic benefit at 6 months for prophylactic hypothermic, the trial demonstrated that prophylactic hypothermia did not reduce ICP while patients were maintained hypothermic or rewarmed.

Complications of prophylactic hypothermia are also not trivial. In the POLAR-RCT, the incidence of pneumonia was higher in patients treated with prophylactic hypothermia compared to normothermia [57]. Additionally, hypothermia can cause or worsen coagulopathy and should be avoided in the initial care of trauma patients. For these reasons prophylactic hypothermia has not been widely adopted, and this is supported by the Brain Trauma Foundation guidelines, which do not recommend early prophylactic hypothermia within 2.5 h of injury [20].

13.3.5 Spine Stabilization

Spinal motion restriction (SMR) is the attempt to maintain the spine in anatomic alignment and minimize movement with adjuncts such as cervical collar, backboard, scoop stretcher, vacuum mattress, or ambulance cot [61]. The purpose of SMR is to prevent iatrogenic spinal injury during transport, which has been quoted as occurring in up to 25% of spinal cord injuries, although the true incidence is difficult to quantify [62]. Because up to 20% of spinal injuries occur at multiple noncontinuous vertebral levels, motion restriction must take into account the whole spine with cervical collar plus a form of thoracic and lumbar alignment (backboard, scoop stretcher, vacuum mattress, or ambulance cot) [61, 63]. The ability to measure how significantly SMR reduces neurologic morbidity is also difficult to quantify, and the scientific basis for continuing current SMR practice has largely been supported by lower-quality evidence [62]. SMR does not come without risks, though. The most notable adverse effects of full SMR are increased ICP, more difficult airway access, pain, pressure ulcers, and more frequent radiological exams [62, 64].

In the emergency department, providers evaluate the need for cervical spine precautions using the NEXUS (National Emergency X-Radiography Utilization Study) or Canadian C-spine Rules. NEXUS and Canadian C-spine Rules have greater than 83% and 90% sensitivity to detect clinically important cervical spine fractures, respectively [65]. The American College of Emergency Physicians (ACEP) endorses utilizing similar risk factors in the evaluation of patients for SMR in the prehospital phase of care as well [66]. In a joint statement between the American College of Surgeons Committee on Trauma (ACS-COT), American College of Emergency Physicians (ACEP), and the National Association of EMS Physicians (NAEMSP), the following factors among patients with blunt trauma were identified as indications for prehospital SMR: acutely altered level of consciousness (GCS < 15, evidence of intoxication), midline neck or back pain and/or tenderness, focal neurologic signs and/or symptoms, anatomic deformity of the spine, or distracting circumstance or injury [61]. Further, patients with suspected severe blunt head trauma may be transported with the head at 30 degrees, rather than the standard SMR protocol of transporting patients flat and supine [67]. It is generally recommended that patients with isolated penetrating injury, including to the head or neck, not be treated with SMR [61, 63, 66–68].

13.4 Triage

13.4.1 Transport Destination

The 2021 National Guideline for the Field Triage of Injured Patients (FTIP) recommends that any patient unable to follow commands, defined as motor GCS ≤ 5, be transported to the highest-level trauma center available [69]. The motor GCS component replaced GCS ≤ 13 in the most recent FTIP guidelines due to the similarly predictive value of the two scores and easier application of one GCS domain. These guidelines also recommend transport to the highest-level trauma facility if the patient has a penetrating injury to the head, skull deformity, or new neurologic deficiency (Fig. 13.1). Level I trauma facilities provide immediate access to neurosurgical interventions, and survival is known to be better for TBI patients transported to Level I centers compared with Level II centers or patients first triaged in an ED then transported to another hospital for neurosurgical intervention [10].

Patients with mildly altered consciousness can be more difficult to triage than those with more obvious severe injuries. Mild TBI is broadly characterized by a GCS score of 13–15. As a more conceptual description of mild TBI, the CDC

Guideline	American College of Emergency Physicians and Centers of Disease Control and Prevention Clinical Policy: Neuroimaging and Decision making in Adult Mild Traumatic Brain Injury in the Acute Setting	National guidelines for the field triage of injured patients: Recommendations of the National Expert Panel on Field Triage, 2021	National guidelines for the field triage of injured patients: Recommendations of the National Expert Panel on Field Triage, 2021
Recommendation	Patients with mild TBI who should have a noncontrast CT scan in the emergency department	Red Criteria: Patients meeting any of the criteria should be transported to the highest-level trauma center available	Yellow Criteria: Patients meeting any of the criteria (and not a Red Criteria) should be preferentially transported to a trauma center, but not necessarily highest-level trauma center
Risk Factors	Loss of consciousness or posttraumatic amnesia PLUS one of the following Headache Vomiting Age >60 years old Drug or alcohol intoxication Deficits in short-term memory Physical evidence of trauma above the clavicle Posttraumatic seizure GCS<15 Focal neurologic deficit Coagulopathy	Red Criteria *Injury Patterns* Penetrating injuries to head, neck, torso, and proximal extremities Skull deformity, suspected skull fracture Suspected spinal injury with new motor or sensory loss Chest wall instability, deformity, or suspected flair chest Suspected pelvic fracture Suspected fracture of two or more proximal long bones Crushed, degloved, mangled, or pulseless extremity Amputation proximal to wrist or ankle Active bleeding requiring a tourniquet or wound packing with continuous pressure *Mental Status and Vital Signs* Unable to follow commands (motor GCS < 6)	Yellow Criteria High-Risk Auto Crash • Partial or complete ejection • Significant intrusion • Death in passenger compartment • Vehicle telemetry data consistent with severe injury Rider separated from transport vehicle with significant impact (e.g., motorcycle, ATV, horse, etc.) Pedestrian/bicycle rider thrown, run over, or with significant impact Fall from height (>10 feet) Low-level falls in young children (age<6 years) or older adults (>64 years) with significant head impact Anticoagulant use Suspicion of child abuse

Fig. 13.1 Transport destination recommendations based on evidenced-based risk factors. (Adapted from American College of Emergency Physicians and Centers of Disease Control and Prevention Clinical Policy: Neuroimaging and Decision making in Adult Mild Traumatic Brain Injury in the Acute Setting and National guidelines for the field triage of injured patients: Recommendations of the National Expert Panel on Field Triage, 2021 [69, 70])

developed the following definition: (1) any period of observed or self-reported transient confusion, disorientation, or impaired consciousness; (2) any period of observed or self-reported dysfunction of memory around the time of injury; (3) observed signs of other neurologic or neuropsychological dysfunction; or (4) any period of observed or self-reported loss of consciousness lasting 30 min or less [71]. The goal in prehospital triage for these injuries should be to identify patients who may require computed tomography (CT) scan or who, based on their mechanism of injury and comorbid conditions, are at higher risk for having intracranial pathology requiring neurosurgical intervention. On the whole, the literature reports that up to 15% of patients with GCS of 14 or 15 will have an intracranial injury on CT, while only 1% of that population will need neurosurgical intervention [70].

Consolidating risk factors identified by the studies underlying the Canadian Head CT Rule and the New Orleans Criteria, the 2008 American College of Emergency Physicians (ACEP), and US Centers for Disease Control and prevention (CDC) released the following criteria that should prompt a noncontrast head CT in the ED (Fig. 13.1) [70]. While the sensitivity and specificity of the criteria for intracranial injury or neurosurgical requirement may not be directly applicable in the prehospital phase, many of these factors can still be considered risk factors that should prompt transport to an emergency department with CT capabilities. The FTIP guidelines also laid out moderate risk criteria that should direct transport to a trauma center with such capabilities, although not necessarily the highest-level trauma center available (Fig. 13.1). Patients with any of these risk factors should at least be transferred to a facility with CT capabilities and ideally to a trauma center.

Guideline	American College of Emergency Physicians and Centers of Disease Control and Prevention Clinical Policy: Neuroimaging and Decision making in Adult Mild Traumatic Brain Injury in the Acute Setting	National guidelines for the field triage of injured patients: Recommendations of the National Expert Panel on Field Triage, 2021	National guidelines for the field triage of injured patients: Recommendations of the National Expert Panel on Field Triage, 2021
Recommendation	Patients with mild TBI who should have a noncontrast CT scan in the emergency department	Red Criteria: Patients meeting any of the criteria should be transported to the highest-level trauma center available	Yellow Criteria: Patients meeting any of the criteria (and not a Red Criteria) should be preferentially transported to a trauma center, but not necessarily highest-level trauma center

Risk factors	Loss of consciousness or posttraumatic amnesia <u>PLUS</u> one of the following: Headache Vomiting Age > 60 years old Drug or alcohol intoxication Deficits in short-term memory Physical evidence of trauma above the clavicle Posttraumatic seizure GCS < 15 Focal neurologic deficit Coagulopathy	Red Criteria *Injury patterns* Penetrating injuries to head, neck, torso, and proximal extremities Skull deformity, suspected skull fracture Suspected spinal injury with new motor or sensory loss Chest wall instability, deformity, or suspected flair chest Suspected pelvic fracture Suspected fracture of two or more proximal long bones Crushed, degloved, mangled, or pulseless extremity Amputation proximal to wrist or ankle Active bleeding requiring a tourniquet or wound packing with continuous pressure *Mental status and vital signs* Unable to follow commands (motor GCS < 6) RR <10 or >29 breaths/min Respiratory distress or need for respiratory support Room air pulse oximetry <90%	Yellow Criteria High-Risk Auto Crash • Partial or complete ejection • Significant intrusion • Death in passenger compartment • Vehicle telemetry data consistent with severe injury Rider separated from transport vehicle with significant impact (e.g., motorcycle, ATV, horse, etc.) Pedestrian/bicycle rider thrown, run over, or with significant impact Fall from height (>10 feet) Low-level falls in young children (age < 6 years) or older adults (>64 years) with significant head impact Anticoagulant use Suspicion of child abuse Special, high-resource healthcare needs[a] Pregnancy >20 weeks Burns in conjunction with trauma

[a] Ex: tracheostomy with ventilator dependence, cardiac assist devices, etc.

13.4.2 Transport Mode

There is a prevalent concept of the "Golden Hour" in trauma which historically has been applied to the care of patients with brain injuries [72]. The concept supports the idea that one of the most important components of out-of-hospital trauma care is rapidly transporting severely injured TBI patient to a trauma center, especially among patients with expanding lesions or who for other reasons are at risk for herniation [10]. In patients with severe TBI there may be some benefit to helicopter transport. However, this is most likely to be derived more from the higher quality of prehospital care by air medical crews rather than the mode of transport's effect on total prehospital time [10, 28, 69, 73, 74]. The most efficient method of transport largely depends on regional and geographic specific factors, such as distance to the nearest trauma center. Regardless of transport mode, the best outcomes happen when patients are transported rapidly to trauma centers with neurosurgical capabilities [5].

13.4.3 Summary

The out-of-hospital management of patients with suspected traumatic brain injury should focus on initial management of airway, breathing, and circulation and rapid transport to a trauma center. Adherence to these principles will help mitigate the secondary insults to brain tissue, specifically hypoxemia and hypotension. These patients should be triaged to the nearest trauma centers with neurosurgical capabilities as quickly as possible while minimizing the performance of all but the most necessary interventions to maintain oxygenation and blood pressure.

References

1. Daugherty J, Waltzman D, Sarmiento K, Xu L. Traumatic brain injury-related deaths by race/ethnicity, sex, intent, and mechanism of injury - United States, 2000-2017. MMWR Morb Mortal Wkly Rep. 2019;68(46):1050–6.
2. Badjatia N, Carney N, Crocco TJ, Fallat ME, Hennes HMA, Jagoda AS, et al. Guidelines for prehospital management of traumatic brain injury, 2nd edition. Prehosp Emerg Care. 2008;12(Suppl 1):S1–52.
3. Dewall J. The ABCs of TBI. Evidence-based guidelines for adult traumatic brain injury care. JEMS. 2010;35(4):54–61; quiz 63.
4. Schneider ALC, Ling GSF. Prehospital care of traumatic brain injury. In: Brain injury medicine; 2021. p. 77–83.
5. Geeraerts T, Velly L, Abdennour L, Asehnoune K, Audibert G, Bouzat P, et al. Management of severe traumatic brain injury (first 24 hours). Anaesth Crit Care Pain Med. 2018;37(2):171–86.
6. Maas AIR, Marmarou A, Murray GD, Teasdale SGM, Steyerberg EW. Prognosis and clinical trial design in traumatic brain injury: the IMPACT study. J Neurotrauma. 2007;24(2):232–8.
7. Stocchetti N, Furlan A, Volta F. Hypoxemia and arterial hypotension at the accident scene in head injury. J Trauma. 1996;40(5):764–7.
8. Chesnut RM, Marshall SB, Piek J, Blunt BA, Klauber MR, Marshall LF. Early and late systemic hypotension as a frequent and fundamental source of cerebral ischemia following severe brain injury in the traumatic coma data Bank. Acta Neurochir Suppl (Wien). 1993;59:121–5.
9. Davis DP, Serrano JA, Vilke GM, Sise MJ, Kennedy F, Eastman AB, et al. The predictive value of field versus arrival Glasgow coma scale score and TRISS calculations in moderate-to-severe traumatic brain injury. J Trauma. 2006;60(5):985–90.
10. Stiver SI, Manley GT. Prehospital management of traumatic brain injury. Neurosurg Focus. 2008;25(4):E5.
11. Sperry JL, Gentilello LM, Minei JP, Diaz-Arrastia RR, Friese RS, Shafi S. Waiting for the patient to "sober up": effect of alcohol intoxication on Glasgow coma scale score of brain injured patients. J Trauma. 2006;61(6):1305–11.

12. Stuke L, Diaz-Arrastia R, Gentilello LM, Shafi S. Effect of alcohol on Glasgow coma scale in head-injured patients. Ann Surg. 2007;245(4):651–5.
13. Stubbs JL, Thornton AE, Sevick JM, Silverberg ND, Barr AM, Honer WG, et al. Traumatic brain injury in homeless and marginally housed individuals: a systematic review and meta-analysis. Lancet Public Health. 2020;5(1):e19–32.
14. Majdan M, Steyerberg EW, Nieboer D, Mauritz W, Rusnak M, Lingsma HF. Glasgow coma scale motor score and pupillary reaction to predict six-month mortality in patients with traumatic brain injury: comparison of field and admission assessment. J Neurotrauma. 2015;32(2):101–8.
15. Haukoos JS, Gill MR, Rabon RE, Gravitz CS, Green SM. Validation of the simplified motor score for the prediction of brain injury outcomes after trauma. Ann Emerg Med. 2007;50(1):18–24.
16. Hoffmann F, Schmalhofer M, Lehner M, Zimatschek S, Grote V, Reiter K. Comparison of the AVPU scale and the pediatric GCS in prehospital setting. Prehosp Emerg Care. 2016;20(4):493–8.
17. Wasserman EB, Shah MN, Jones CMC, Cushman JT, Caterino JM, Bazarian JJ, et al. Identification of a neurologic scale that optimizes EMS detection of older adult traumatic brain injury patients who require transport to a trauma center. Prehosp Emerg Care. 2015;19(2):202–12.
18. Brown CVR, Inaba K, Shatz DV, Moore EE, Ciesla D, Sava JA, et al. Western trauma association critical decisions in trauma: airway management in adult trauma patients. Trauma Surg Acute Care Open. 2020;5(1):e000539.
19. Goldberg SA, Rojanasarntikul D, Jagoda A. The prehospital management of traumatic brain injury. Handb Clin Neurol. 2015;127:367–78.
20. Carney N, Totten AM, O'Reilly C, Ullman JS, Hawryluk GWJ, Bell MJ, et al. Guidelines for the management of severe traumatic brain injury, fourth edition. Neurosurgery. 2017;80(1):6–15.
21. Davis DP, Peay J, Sise MJ, Kennedy F, Simon F, Tominaga G, et al. Prehospital airway and ventilation management: a trauma score and injury severity score-based analysis. J Trauma. 2010;69(2):294–301.
22. Bossers SM, Schwarte LA, Loer SA, Twisk JWR, Boer C, Schober P. Experience in prehospital endotracheal intubation significantly influences mortality of patients with severe traumatic brain injury: a systematic review and meta-analysis. PloS One. 2015;10(10):e0141034.
23. Davis DP, Hoyt DB, Ochs M, Fortlage D, Holbrook T, Marshall LK, et al. The effect of paramedic rapid sequence intubation on outcome in patients with severe traumatic brain injury. J Trauma. 2003;54(3):444–53.
24. Helm M, Kremers G, Lampl L, Hossfeld B. Incidence of transient hypoxia during pre-hospital rapid sequence intubation by anaesthesiologists. Acta Anaesthesiol Scand. 2013;57(2):199–205.
25. Dunford JV, Davis DP, Ochs M, Doney M, Hoyt DB. Incidence of transient hypoxia and pulse rate reactivity during paramedic rapid sequence intubation. Ann Emerg Med. 2003;42(6):721–8.
26. Haltmeier T, Benjamin E, Siboni S, Dilektasli E, Inaba K, Demetriades D. Prehospital intubation for isolated severe blunt traumatic brain injury: worse outcomes and higher mortality. Eur J Trauma Emerg Surg. 2017;43(6):731–9.
27. Bukur M, Kurtovic S, Berry C, Tanios M, Margulies DR, Ley EJ, et al. Pre-hospital intubation is associated with increased mortality after traumatic brain injury. J Surg Res. 2011;170(1):e117–21.
28. Davis DP, Peay J, Sise MJ, Vilke GM, Kennedy F, Eastman AB, et al. The impact of prehospital endotracheal intubation on outcome in moderate to severe traumatic brain injury. J Trauma. 2005;58(5):933–9.
29. Bernard SA, Nguyen V, Cameron P, Masci K, Fitzgerald M, Cooper DJ, et al. Prehospital rapid sequence intubation improves functional outcome for patients with severe traumatic brain injury: a randomized controlled trial. Ann Surg. 2010;252(6):959–65.
30. Kingsbury D. Paramedic RSI remains difficult to advocate. Ann Surg. 2014;259(5):e80.
31. Elmer J, Brown F, Martin-Gill C, Guyette FX. Prevalence and predictors of post-intubation hypotension in prehospital trauma care. Prehosp Emerg Care. 2020;24(4):461–9.

32. Kramer N, Lebowitz D, Walsh M, Ganti L. Rapid sequence intubation in traumatic brain-injured adults. Cureus. 2018;10(4):e2530.
33. Bakhsh A, Alotaibi L. Push-dose pressors during peri-intubation hypotension in the emergency department: a case series. Clin Pract Cases Emerg Med. 2021;5(4):390–3.
34. Patanwala AE, Erstad BL, Roe DJ, Sakles JC. Succinylcholine is associated with increased mortality when used for rapid sequence intubation of severely brain injured patients in the emergency department. Pharmacotherapy. 2016;36(1):57–63.
35. Kempema J, Trust MD, Ali S, Cabanas JG, Hinchey PR, Brown LH, et al. Prehospital endotracheal intubation vs extraglottic airway device in blunt trauma. Am J Emerg Med. 2015;33(8):1080–3.
36. ACS TQIP Best Practices in the Management of Traumatic Brain Injury. American College of Surgeons Committee on Trauma; 2015.
37. Kinoshita K. Traumatic brain injury: pathophysiology for neurocritical care. J Intensive Care. 2016;4:29.
38. Carney N, Totten AM, Cheney T, Jungbauer R, Neth MR, Weeks C, et al. Prehospital airway management: a systematic review. Prehosp Emerg Care. 2022;26:716–27.
39. Spaite DW, Hu C, Bobrow BJ, Chikani V, Sherrill D, Barnhart B, et al. Mortality and prehospital blood pressure in patients with major traumatic brain injury: implications for the hypotension threshold. JAMA Surg. 2017;152(4):360–8.
40. Shibahashi K, Hoda H, Okura Y, Hamabe Y. Acceptable blood pressure levels in the prehospital setting for patients with traumatic brain injury: a multicenter observational study. World Neurosurg. 2021;149:e504–11.
41. Mekonnen M, Ong V, Florence TJ, Mozaffari K, Mahgerefteh N, Rana S, et al. Hypertonic saline treatment in traumatic brain injury: a systematic review. World Neurosurg. 2022;162:98–110.
42. Cooper DJ, Myles PS, McDermott FT, Murray LJ, Laidlaw J, Cooper G, et al. Prehospital hypertonic saline resuscitation of patients with hypotension and severe traumatic brain injury: a randomized controlled trial. JAMA. 2004;291(11):1350–7.
43. Bulger EM, May S, Brasel KJ, Schreiber M, Kerby JD, Tisherman SA, et al. Out-of-hospital hypertonic resuscitation following severe traumatic brain injury: a randomized controlled trial. JAMA. 2010;304(13):1455.
44. Bergmans SF, Schober P, Schwarte LA, Loer SA, Bossers SM. Prehospital fluid administration in patients with severe traumatic brain injury: a systematic review and meta-analysis. Injury. 2020;51(11):2356–67.
45. Holcomb JB, Tilley BC, Baraniuk S, Fox EE, Wade CE, Podbielski JM, et al. Transfusion of plasma, platelets, and red blood cells in a 1:1:1 vs a 1:1:2 ratio and mortality in patients with severe trauma: the PROPPR randomized clinical trial. JAMA. 2015;313(5):471.
46. Gallaher JR, Dixon A, Cockcroft A, Grey M, Dewey E, Goodman A, et al. Large volume transfusion with whole blood is safe compared with component therapy. J Trauma Acute Care Surg. 2020;89(1):238–45.
47. Brito AMP, Schreiber M. Prehospital resuscitation. Trauma Surg Acute Care Open. 2021;6(1):e000729.
48. Zusman BE, Kochanek PM, Bailey ZS, Leung LY, Vagni VA, Okonkwo DO, et al. Multifaceted benefit of whole blood versus lactated Ringer's resuscitation after traumatic brain injury and hemorrhagic shock in mice. Neurocrit Care. 2021;34(3):781–94.
49. Gruen DS, Guyette FX, Brown JB, Okonkwo DO, Puccio AM, Campwala IK, et al. Association of Prehospital Plasma with Survival in patients with traumatic brain injury: a secondary analysis of the PAMPer cluster randomized clinical trial. JAMA Netw Open. 2020;3(10):e2016869.
50. Roberts I, Shakur H, Coats T, Hunt B, Balogun E, Barnetson L, et al. The CRASH-2 trial: a randomised controlled trial and economic evaluation of the effects of tranexamic acid on death, vascular occlusive events and transfusion requirement in bleeding trauma patients. Health Technol Assess. 2013;17(10):1–79.
51. CRASH-3 Trial Collaborators. Effects of tranexamic acid on death, disability, vascular occlusive events and other morbidities in patients with acute traumatic brain injury (CRASH-3): a randomised, placebo-controlled trial. Lancet. 2019;394(10210):1713–23.

52. Rowell SE, Meier EN, McKnight B, Kannas D, May S, Sheehan K, et al. Effect of out-of-hospital tranexamic acid vs placebo on 6-month functional neurologic outcomes in patients with moderate or severe traumatic brain injury. JAMA. 2020;324(10):961.
53. Polderman KH. Induced hypothermia and fever control for prevention and treatment of neurological injuries. Lancet. 2008;371(9628):1955–69.
54. Ahmed A, Bullock MR, Dietrich WD. Hypothermia in traumatic brain injury. Neurosurg Clin N Am. 2016;27(4):489–97.
55. Andrews PJD, Sinclair HL, Rodriguez A, Harris BA, Battison CG, Rhodes JKJ, et al. Hypothermia for intracranial hypertension after traumatic brain injury. N Engl J Med. 2015;373(25):2403–12.
56. Polderman KH. Mechanisms of action, physiological effects, and complications of hypothermia. Crit Care Med. 2009;37(7 Suppl):S186–202.
57. Cooper DJ, Nichol AD, Bailey M, Bernard S, Cameron PA, Pili-Floury S, et al. Effect of early sustained prophylactic hypothermia on neurologic outcomes among patients with severe traumatic brain injury: the POLAR randomized clinical trial. JAMA. 2018;320(21):2211–20.
58. Clifton GL, Miller ER, Choi SC, Levin HS, McCauley S, Smith KR, et al. Lack of effect of induction of hypothermia after acute brain injury. N Engl J Med. 2001;344(8):556–63.
59. Clifton GL, Valadka A, Zygun D, Coffey CS, Drever P, Fourwinds S, et al. Very early hypothermia induction in patients with severe brain injury (the National Acute Brain Injury Study: hypothermia II): a randomised trial. Lancet Neurol. 2011;10(2):131–9.
60. Maekawa T, Yamashita S, Nagao S, Hayashi N, Ohashi Y, Brain-Hypothermia Study Group. Prolonged mild therapeutic hypothermia versus fever control with tight hemodynamic monitoring and slow rewarming in patients with severe traumatic brain injury: a randomized controlled trial. J Neurotrauma. 2015;32(7):422–9.
61. Fischer PE, Perina DG, Delbridge TR, Fallat ME, Salomone JP, Dodd J, et al. Spinal motion restriction in the trauma patient—a joint position statement. Prehosp Emerg Care. 2018;22(6):659–61.
62. Sundstrøm T, Asbjørnsen H, Habiba S, Sunde GA, Wester K. Prehospital use of cervical collars in trauma patients: a critical review. J Neurotrauma. 2014;31(6):531–40.
63. Theodore N, Hadley MN, Aarabi B, Dhall SS, Gelb DE, Hurlbert RJ, et al. Prehospital cervical spinal immobilization after trauma. Neurosurgery. 2013;72(Suppl 2):22–34.
64. Maschmann C, Jeppesen E, Rubin MA, Barfod C. New clinical guidelines on the spinal stabilisation of adult trauma patients – consensus and evidence based. Scand J Trauma Resusc Emerg Med. 2019;27(1):77.
65. Michaleff ZA, Maher CG, Verhagen AP, Rebbeck T, Lin CWC. Accuracy of the Canadian C-spine rule and NEXUS to screen for clinically important cervical spine injury in patients following blunt trauma: a systematic review. CMAJ. 2012;184(16):E867–76.
66. EMS management of patients with potential spinal injury. Ann Emerg Med. 2015;66(4):445.
67. Cunningham C, Kamin R. National Association of State EMS Officials (NASEMSO) National Model EMS Clinical Guidelines Version 3.0 [Internet]. 2022. https://nasemso.org/wp-content/uploads/National-Model-EMS-Clinical-Guidelines_2022.pdf.
68. Stuke LE, Pons PT, Guy JS, Chapleau WP, Butler FK, McSwain NE. Prehospital spine immobilization for penetrating trauma—review and recommendations from the Prehospital Trauma Life Support Executive Committee. J Trauma. 2011;71(3):763–9; discussion 769–770.
69. Newgard CD, Fischer PE, Gestring M, Michaels HN, Jurkovich GJ, Lerner EB, et al. National guideline for the field triage of injured patients: recommendations of the National Expert Panel on Field Triage, 2021. J Trauma Acute Care Surg. 2022;93:e49–60. https://doi.org/10.1097/TA.0000000000003627.
70. Jagoda AS, Bazarian JJ, Bruns JJ, Cantrill SV, Gean AD, Howard PK, et al. Clinical policy: neuroimaging and decision making in adult mild traumatic brain injury in the acute setting. Ann Emerg Med. 2008;52(6):714–48.
71. Report to congress on mild traumatic brain injury in the United States: steps to prevent a serious public health problem [internet]. Centers for Disease Control and Prevention; 2003. https://www.cdc.gov/traumaticbraininjury/pdf/mtbireport-a.pdf.

72. Seelig JM, Becker DP, Miller JD, Greenberg RP, Ward JD, Choi SC. Traumatic acute subdural hematoma: major mortality reduction in comatose patients treated within four hours. N Engl J Med. 1981;304(25):1511–8.
73. Gravesteijn BY, Sewalt CA, Stocchetti N, Citerio G, Ercole A, Lingsma HF, et al. Prehospital management of traumatic brain injury across Europe: a CENTER-TBI study. Prehosp Emerg Care. 2021;25(5):629–43.
74. Bekelis K, Missios S, Mackenzie TA. Prehospital helicopter transport and survival of patients with traumatic brain injury. Ann Surg. 2015;261(3):579–85.

14 Sedation, Pain, and Delirium in Patients with Traumatic Brain Injury

Jean-François Payen, Clotilde Schilte, and Alexandre Behouche

14.1 Introduction

Guidelines have recently been published regarding the general clinical management of pain, sedation, and delirium within the intensive care unit (ICU) [1] and others regarding the early management of patients with severe traumatic brain injury (TBI) [2–4]. However, neither set of guidelines gave much attention to the specific management of sedation and analgesia in brain-injured patients, probably due to the lack of evidence based on which recommendations can be made for these specific patients. There remains a paucity of literature reviews concerning the clinical management of pain, sedation, and delirium in brain-injured patients [5, 6]. This chapter will discuss objectives, drugs, strategies, pain monitoring, and termination of sedation and analgesia in adult patients with severe TBI.

14.2 Objectives of Sedation/Analgesia in Patients with TBI

The general goals of sedation and analgesia in the ICU are to provide comfort, prevent, and treat any sources of pain, facilitate mechanical ventilation, and improve tissue oxygenation. The level of sedation is adjusted to keep the patient calm and alert or in light sedation, i.e. with a Richmond Agitation-Sedation Scale (RASS) score of −2 to +1. In the case of severe acute respiratory failure, however, the level of sedation will be deeper to permit the use of permissive hypercapnia, i.e. RASS score of −4 to −5. In the neurointensive care unit (NICU), the objectives of sedation/analgesia are focused on preventing alterations in brain perfusion secondary to the injury, and restoring an optimal balance in supply and demand of oxygen to the brain. Indeed, in such patients the control of intracranial pressure (ICP) keeping it

J.-F. Payen (✉) · C. Schilte · A. Behouche
Pôle d'Anesthésie-Réanimation, Grenoble Alpes University Hospital, Grenoble, France
e-mail: jfpayen@univ-grenoble-alpes.fr

E. Brogi et al. (eds.), *Traumatic Brain Injury*, Hot Topics in Acute Care Surgery and Trauma, https://doi.org/10.1007/978-3-031-50117-3_14

below 20–25 mmHg via the maintenance of optimal cerebral perfusion pressure (CPP) is paramount to prevent brain ischemia [2–4]. This can be achieved through the correct management of sedation/analgesia that enables the removal of any source of nociception during nursing interventions, the maintenance of normocapnia during mechanical ventilation, the required reduction in brain oxygen consumption rate, the prevention of seizures, and potentially the limited development of cortical spreading depolarizations (CSD).

14.3 Sedative and Analgesic Drugs

One systematic review found no evidence of any one sedative or analgesic drug being more efficacious than another at improving outcomes of patients with TBI [7]. Apart from that concerning the treatment of refractory intracranial hypertension, i.e. barbiturates and high-dose propofol, no specific drugs are recommended, in either the French or US guidelines, for use in the sedation and analgesia of patients with TBI [2, 3]. However, it is possible to consider all known effects, potential advantages and side effects, in order to determine the optimal sedative and analgesic drugs for use in these patients [5, 6].

Propofol (1–4 mg/kg/h) is largely used for pain management, sedation, and the control of ICP in patients with TBI. At higher doses, propofol can induce EEG burst-suppression to treat status epilepticus and refractory intracranial hypertension. However, poor tolerance in patients with hemodynamic instability has been reported, and an increased risk of propofol-related infusion syndrome (PRIS) occurring at high doses (>5 mg/kg/h) following more than 48 h exposure was found in TBI patients [8].

Midazolam (1–15 mg/h) is also used in the NICU, in particular in cases of TBI with hemodynamic instability. However, this drug is associated with tissue accumulation of metabolites that delays awakening and reliable neurological examination. In addition, midazolam may result in withdrawal syndrome and tachyphylaxis at higher doses. Although propofol and midazolam appear equally effective in patients with controlled ICP, midazolam is less effective than propofol in the treatment of intracranial hypertension [7].

Ketamine (1–3 mg/kg/h) is well tolerated regarding systemic hemodynamics and respiratory drive and provides antihyperalgesic properties at low doses (<0.3 mg/kg/h). It can also be used safely in patients with TBI, showing no deleterious effect on ICP [9] and inhibition of CSD over a wide range of doses commonly used for sedation [10]. However, in view of psychomimetic adverse events and dose-dependent hepatic dysfunction [11], its use should be considered in adjunction to other sedatives rather than as a first-line therapy in patients with TBI. S-ketamine, which is twice as potent as the racemic mixture, might be associated with fewer side effects [12] and was found to significantly reduce CSD incidence in patients with aneurysmal subarachnoid hemorrhage (SAH) [13].

Dexmedetomidine (Dex) (0.3–1.4 μg/kg/h) is a short-term selective alpha-2 adrenergic agonist with moderate sedative and analgesic properties. Although data are limited regarding its use in patients with TBI, Dex has been associated with reduced agitation, reduced doses of opioids and other sedatives, and less rescue therapies for intracranial hypertension [14–16]. Due to its potential impact on hemodynamics, Dex should be used in stable patients, in particular to facilitate the cessation of sedation (see below).

The inhaled agent isoflurane is emerging as an alternative sedative for use in ICUs equipped with specific systems for delivery and expertise. Isoflurane sedation permitted a reduction in opioid dose intensity compared to propofol along with a faster wake-up time in ICU patients [17]. In patients with SAH but no intracranial hypertension, isoflurane allowed a greater increase in regional blood flow with no difference in ICP levels compared to propofol [18]. Isoflurane might therefore be considered in patients with TBI without high ICP in the event of tachyphylaxis or hemodynamic instability during intravenous sedation. The dose of isoflurane commonly used in the ICU corresponds to a minimal alveolar concentration (MAC) of 0.5–1. At higher doses (MAC >1), isoflurane exerts brain vasodilation that could alter CPP in brains with low compliance. It should be noted that sevoflurane should be abandoned in the ICU setting because of the risk of drug-induced nephrogenic diabetes insipidus [19, 20].

Barbiturates cannot be viewed as sedative agents in patients with TBI because of their numerous side effects, i.e. hemodynamic and immune depression. Barbiturates must be used as a third-tier therapy for refractory intracranial hypertension [3].

Alongside sedative agents, analgesics are mandatory in mechanically ventilated patients with TBI to remove any sources of nociception susceptible to increasing ICP. All opioids can be used through continuous intravenous infusion: fentanyl (0.7–10 μg/kg/h), sufentanil (0.1–1 μg/kg/h), and remifentanil (0.5–15 μg/kg/h). As with general ICU patients, non-opioid analgesics including acetaminophen, nefopam, gabapentin, pregabalin, and non-steroidal anti-inflammatory drugs should be considered as opioid-sparing agents in patients with TBI [1]. Of note was a practice survey from 6 NICUs showing discordance in both physicians self-reporting and objective analgesic delivery audits based on pharmacy database [21]. This suggests the continued suboptimal use of analgesics in the NICU.

14.4 Strategies of Sedation/Analgesia

Repeated clinical examination is essential in the clinical monitoring of patients with TBI. However, the neurological assessment of a sedated patient with brain lesions is unreliable due to the direct effects of sedation on brain function. Conversely, sedation is a prerequisite in the important control of ICP [22]. In this situation, the in-charge physician must decide between two equally undesirable alternatives: to interrupt the sedation despite the associated risks in order to obtain information about the neurological status, i.e. perform a neurological wake-up test (NWT), or to continue the sedation to control ICP and prevent secondary brain lesions despite disallowing the assessment of brain status.

14.4.1 The Neurological Wake-Up Test

Clinical situations in which an NWT is indicated include the discrepancy between severe clinical data and normal brain imaging on CT scan, or altered Glasgow Coma Scale (GCS) score due to hypothermia, alcohol intoxication, seizures, or metabolic disorders. An NWT may also be indicated after treating the cause of a neurological degradation, e.g. ruptured aneurysm or compressive subdural hematoma. In the absence of high ICP, an NWT can provide useful information for detecting changes in neurological status some of which may require more active management. The NWT may also reduce the duration of mechanical ventilation and the incidence of secondary complications including nosocomial infections and delirium. However, it can expose patients to a stress response with agitation, oxygen desaturation, increased ICP and cerebral hypoperfusion if the brain compliance is limited. Episodes of brain hypoxia do occur during inappropriate NWT procedures [23].

Therefore, the NWT should not be used in patients with ICP and/or CPP problems, or in patients with cardiorespiratory instability, status epilepticus, or marked hyperthermia [24]. However, it is not always easy to anticipate the ICP response and to detect patients at risk of elevated ICP secondary to sedation interruption. A midline shift >5 mm and/or absent or compressed basal cisterns are two reliable brain CT scan indicators of probable intracranial hypertension [25]. Patients with initial GCS <9, early neurological degradation, hemostasis disorders, or large cerebral hemorrhagic contusions are at risk of initial brain lesion enlargement and secondary intracranial hypertension. NWT is not appropriate in these situations.

When decided, the NWT includes sedative interruption, the maintenance of a low dose of opioid, and a careful monitoring of ICP and CPP. The patient is then assessed regarding signs of arousal and consciousness, the motor component of the GCS, pupillary reflexes, and focal neurological deficits. The more reliable neurological information permitted by performing an NWT may be useful in making an important clinical decision to consider cessation or maintenance of sedation, to indicate new imaging (e.g. MRI) or new brain monitoring (e.g. brain tissue oxygen pressure [$PbtO_2$]), to change therapies, or to discuss end-of-life procedure if the responses to clinical examination are very poor.

14.4.2 Continuing Sedation

If the conditions to interrupt sedation after severe brain injury are not met (see above), the sedation/analgesia must be continued and adjusted to prevent episodes of high ICP during nursing interventions and mobilization. An appropriate level of sedation along with other first-tier therapies, i.e. osmotherapy, cerebrospinal fluid (CSD) drainage, and mild hypocapnia, can be effective at controlling ICP in more than 60% of patients after severe TBI [26]. There exist two ICP-dependent clinical situations in sedated and mechanically ventilated patients (Fig. 14.1):

- For an ICP below 20 mmHg, sedation can be continued using low doses of sedatives and opioids until the patient meets all the criteria to terminate sedation (see

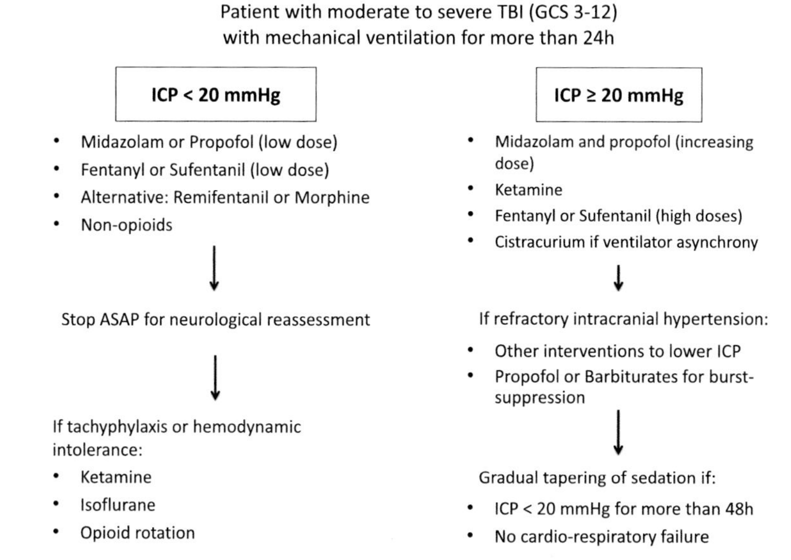

Fig. 14.1 A practical algorithm to use sedatives and analgesics in mechanically ventilated patients with acute brain damage. *GCS* Glasgow Coma Scale, *ICP* intracranial pressure

below). In case of tachyphylaxis or hemodynamical instability, the introduction of low-dose ketamine, isoflurane, or another opioid (opioid rotation) can be considered.

– For an ICP persistently above or equal to 20 mmHg, treatment should include increasing doses of midazolam and propofol, high doses of opioids, and the adjunction of ketamine and cisatracurium if adaptation of the patient to the ventilator is needed. The treatment of refractory intracranial hypertension requires third-tier therapies such as therapeutic hypothermia (34–35 °C), metabolic suppression with barbiturates or high-dose propofol, moderate hypocapnia ($PaCO_2$ 30–35 mmHg), and decompressive craniectomy.

Continuing sedation renders infeasible any reliable neurological clinical assessment. Cerebral homeostasis should be assessed using multimodal monitoring including continuous measurements of ICP and/or $PbtO_2$ measurements, repeated measurements of transcranial Doppler (TCD), and brain CT imaging.

14.5 Monitoring Pain in Patients with TBI

Assessing pain in the NICU is directly linked to the level of sedation that, in turn, is dictated by the need to control ICP (see above). Pain can be assessed in non-sedated patients with TBI who can communicate reliably, even if intubated, through the use of self-rate instruments such as the 0–10 Numeric Rating Scale (NRS) administered either verbally or visually.

Clinical and non-clinical tools are needed in patients unable to self-report pain yet in whom behaviors are observable. In such cases, the Behavioral Pain Scale (BPS), the BPS for non-intubated (BPS-NI) patients, and the Critical Care Pain Observation Tool (CPOT) have shown the best performances in monitoring pain [1]. In nonverbal brain-injured patients, the BPS and the CPOT have shown strong reliability [27–29], and NRS, BPS, and RASS have demonstrated excellent inter-rater reliability [30]. The Nociception Coma Scale (NCS) and its revised version (NCS-R) were designed to assess nociception in patients with severe disorders of consciousness, i.e. vegetative and minimally conscious state patients [31, 32]. The reliability of both of these clinical scales and the BPS in assessing pain in intubated brain-injured patients was recently validated [33]. However, atypical behaviors observed in patients with TBI, such as flushing, sudden eye opening, eye weeping, flexion of upper limb, may alter the performance of the above-cited clinical pain assessment tools [34]. The alternative is the use of non-clinical tools to assess nociception, i.e. the physiological processing of nociceptive stimuli.

Nociception is reflected by a shift in the sympathovagal balance toward a sympathetic stress response. This response can be assessed through measurements of changes in heart rate, increased peripheral vasoconstriction, pupillary dilation, and increased electrical skin conductance. However, there are confounding factors that strongly affect the sympathovagal balance such as age, beta-blockers, vasoactive agents, atropine, cardiac arrhythmia, pacemaker, intravascular fluid status, neuromuscular blocking agents, and level of sedation [35]. Changes in vital signs such as heart rate, blood pressure, and ICP during nursing interventions or mobilization are thus not valid indicators for nociception in patients with TBI. It should be noted that most of the commercialized devices were developed to assess intraoperative nociception [35], and studies concerning their use in patients with TBI are very limited. Current techniques include:

- Analgesia-nociception index (ANI): a 0–100 dimensionless score is calculated from the assessment of heart rate variability. High ANI values (>70) indicate anti-nociception. Studies about the use of ANI in the ICU are still inconclusive [36, 37].
- The electrical skin conductance based on the sympathetic control of the palmar sweat glands. Anti-nociception is defined by a number of skin conductance fluctuations <0.07/s. Due to many confounders in ICU patients, measurements of skin conductance have been found to poorly correlate with nociception [38].
- The measurement of pupillary diameter. Changes in diameter induced by a predefined noxious stimulus, i.e. 20 mA tetanic stimulation, were tested to predict a reaction to endotracheal suctioning in ICU patients [39]. To avoid uncomfortable painful stimulations in lightly sedated patients, the development of pupillary pain index (PPI) was derived from a stepwise increase from 10 to 60 mA until pupil size had increased by 13% compared to baseline. In sedated brain-injured patients, the determination of PPI score predicted the nociceptive response to

endotracheal suctioning [40]. Furthermore, by contrast with endotracheal suctioning, tetanic stimulation had no effect on ICP. Anti-nociception is reflected by a PPI score <5.

- The nociception level (NOL): A multiparametric test combining various sensors and including photoplethysmography, electrical skin conductance, temperature and heart rate variability. A NOL score <25 indicates anti-nociception. NOL values could discriminate between nociceptive and non-nociceptive procedures in the cardiac-ICU [41].

While other nociceptive monitors (Surgical Pleth Index, RIII reflex, qNOX) have been developed, none has yet been studied in the ICU setting. Although all devices appear to reflect nociception, further studies are warranted prior to their implementation for routine use in critically ill patients, in particular those with TBI.

14.6 Termination of Sedation/Analgesia

One challenging situation in the ICU is the weaning off from sedation/analgesia. This phase has almost never been discussed in reviews on acute brain-injured patients. A 30–50% increase in energy expenditure and global oxygen consumption (VO_2) compared to baseline following cessation of sedation [42] can be difficult to manage in patients with severe TBI. Before considering stopping sedation in patients with TBI, certain criteria must be fulfilled: no elevation in ICP over the last 48 h, no new findings or midline shift >10 mm on a recent brain CT scan, no TCD and $PbtO_2$ abnormalities, no cardiorespiratory failure, and no refractory status epilepticus. However, a possible rebound in the ICP during this phase should not indicate the need to restart sedation if the patient shows clinical signs of awakening. If unsuccessful, the cessation of sedation may result in one of the three unexpected scenarios in patients with TBI: persisting coma, severe agitation, and delirium.

14.6.1 Persisting Coma

The persistence of a poor response to clinical examination is not uncommon in the NICU. Specifically, elderly and/or obese patients, or those with renal/liver impairment can become over-sedated with sedatives and/or opioids; this complicates the neurological assessment of such "slow to wake" patients. However, this situation may also reflect a neurological complication such as hydrocephalus, new brain lesions, or non-convulsive seizures, and a brain CT scan and/or EEG recording should be considered if in doubt. Measuring the blood concentrations of midazolam and its glucuronide metabolites was found useful in distinguishing oversedation and neurological damage among patients for whom coma persisted after termination of sedation [43].

14.6.2 Agitated Patient

Agitation, defined as a RASS score of +2 or more, is common on awakening of patients with TBI, with an incidence of 11–70% in acute cases [44–46]. An agitated patient is exposed to the life-threatening risk of accidental device removal and the continued use of sedatives with prolonged duration of mechanical ventilation and ICU-related complications. Causes of agitation are numerous in the ICU and can be medical-related (sepsis, metabolic disturbances, respiratory dysfunction, hepatic encephalopathy, stroke, and non-convulsive seizures), or not (urinary retention, fecal impaction, pain, hyperactive delirium, withdrawal from drugs or substances, drug-induced agitation, and sleep deprivation) [47]. In addition, agitation in patients with TBI may also reflect hidden neurological complications such as cerebrospinal fluid infection, cerebral vasospasm, or extended or new intra-cerebral lesions. The use of amantadine may increase the risk of agitation in this population [45].

Once all treatable causes of agitation have been eliminated, pharmacological agents are often used, although there is no consensus on the most efficacious and safest therapeutic strategy in patients with TBI [46]. In a recent review on ICU patients, we proposed to arbitrarily distinguish between the treatment of withdrawal syndromes and that of agitation symptoms [47]. Clonidine, buprenorphine, methadone, and benzodiazepines are validated options for withdrawal syndromes [48–51]. The pharmacological treatment of agitation symptoms preferably comprises short-acting drugs to prevent any interference with the neurological assessment: neuroleptics (loxapine, tiapride, haloperidol, cyamemazine, risperidone), alpha-2 agonists (clonidine, Dex), and benzodiazepines (clorazepate, diazepam) [47]. Dex has been shown to reduce moderate agitation in recovering patients with TBI [14]. Using Dex to minimize the use of benzodiazepines and antipsychotic drugs was also suggested to reduce confusion, anamnestic effect, and impairment of motor recovery [15].

14.6.3 Patient with Delirium

Delirium is defined as a state of acute confusion with disturbance in attention, awareness, or cognition that develops over hours or days and that cannot be explained by sedation. It is associated with increased mortality and long-term cognitive impairment. There are numerous causes for the development of delirium in patients with TBI, including primary and secondary brain damage, hyperosmolar therapy, seizures, drugs, organ failure, sepsis, sleep deprivation, sensory deprivation, and pre-existing pathology [52]. The use of sedatives has been established as one cause of delirium with long-term cognitive impairment [53]. As with the general ICU population, brain-injured patients can be assessed for delirium using the Confusion Assessment Method for the ICU (CAM-ICU) or Intensive Care Delirium Screening Checklist (ICDSC) according to a systemic review of 7 studies including patients with stroke or TBI the pooled prevalence rate of which was 12–43% [54]. The ICDSC showed better diagnostic performance than CAM-ICU in detecting delirium in a cohort of assessable NICU patients, i.e. RASS score of −2 or above [55]. However, testing for delirium is not always possible in patients with TBI due to their decreased level of consciousness relating either to the primary injury itself or to the deep sedation (RASS of −3 or below) necessary for high ICP.

Among the general population of patients in the ICU, non-pharmacological approaches aimed at optimizing the patient's environment and improving levels of comfort, e.g. cognitive stimulation, minimizing light and noise, reducing sedation, reducing hearing and/or visual impairment, can be considered to reduce the occurrence of delirium [1]. Indeed, early passive and active mobilization combined with spontaneous awakening and breathing trials was shown to reduce the duration of mechanical ventilation and delirium [56]. Also, the routine use of physical restraint to prevent agitated patients from self-extubation was associated with a higher risk of delirium [57]. However, these multicomponent interventions are more difficult to implement in patients with TBI due to their presentation and/or requirement for deep sedation. In addition, there is no evidence that antipsychotics improve their clinical outcomes. Haloperidol can be used to treat delirium symptoms but it may increase the risk of seizures [58]. Prophylactic use of haloperidol failed to improve quality of life at 6 months post-ICU [59]. Beta-blockers, anticonvulsive drugs, or Dex can be considered to treat brain-injured patients with delirium [52, 60].

14.7 Conclusion

Sedation-analgesia plays a central role in preventing and treating episodes of intracranial hypertension in patients with TBI. Various drugs exist although none has shown superior performance over others. While analgesia should always be maintained, the levels of sedation required should be adapted depending on the need of the patient and the need to perform neurological clinical assessment. The most challenging issue for the in-charge physician is choosing the best strategy of sedation and when best to permit its cessation in patients with TBI.

References

1. Devlin JW, Skrobik Y, Gelinas C, Needham DM, Slooter AJC, Pandharipande PP, et al. Executive summary: clinical practice guidelines for the prevention and management of pain, agitation/sedation, delirium, immobility, and sleep disruption in adult patients in the ICU. Crit Care Med. 2018;46(9):1532–48.
2. Geeraerts T, Velly L, Abdennour L, Asehnoune K, Audibert G, Bouzat P, et al. Management of severe traumatic brain injury (first 24 hours). Anaesth Crit Care Pain Med. 2018;37(2):171–86.
3. Carney N, Totten AM, O'Reilly C, Ullman JS, Hawryluk GW, Bell MJ, et al. Guidelines for the management of severe traumatic brain injury, fourth edition. Neurosurgery. 2017;80(1):6–15.
4. Meyfroidt G, Bouzat P, Casaer MP, Chesnut R, Hamada SR, Helbok R, et al. Management of moderate to severe traumatic brain injury: an update for the intensivist. Intensive Care Med. 2022;48(6):649–66.
5. Oddo M, Crippa IA, Mehta S, Menon D, Payen JF, Taccone FS, et al. Optimizing sedation in patients with acute brain injury. Crit Care. 2016;20(1):128.

6. Opdenakker O, Vanstraelen A, De Sloovere V, Meyfroidt G. Sedatives in neurocritical care: an update on pharmacological agents and modes of sedation. Curr Opin Crit Care. 2019;25(2):97–104.
7. Roberts DJ, Hall RI, Kramer AH, Robertson HL, Gallagher CN, Zygun DA. Sedation for critically ill adults with severe traumatic brain injury: a systematic review of randomized controlled trials. Crit Care Med. 2011;39(12):2743–51.
8. Krajcova A, Waldauf P, Andel M, Duska F. Propofol infusion syndrome: a structured review of experimental studies and 153 published case reports. Crit Care. 2015;19:398.
9. Cohen L, Athaide V, Wickham ME, Doyle-Waters MM, Rose NG, Hohl CM. The effect of ketamine on intracranial and cerebral perfusion pressure and health outcomes: a systematic review. Ann Emerg Med. 2015;65(1):43–51 e2.
10. Carlson AP, Abbas M, Alunday RL, Qeadan F, Shuttleworth CW. Spreading depolarization in acute brain injury inhibited by ketamine: a prospective, randomized, multiple crossover trial. J Neurosurg. 2018;1-7:288.
11. Wendel-Garcia PD, Erlebach R, Hofmaenner DA, Camen G, Schuepbach RA, Jungst C, et al. Long-term ketamine infusion-induced cholestatic liver injury in COVID-19-associated acute respiratory distress syndrome. Crit Care. 2022;26(1):148.
12. Wang X, Lin C, Lan L, Liu J. Perioperative intravenous S-ketamine for acute postoperative pain in adults: a systematic review and meta-analysis. J Clin Anesth. 2021;68:110071.
13. Santos E, Olivares-Rivera A, Major S, Sanchez-Porras R, Uhlmann L, Kunzmann K, et al. Lasting s-ketamine block of spreading depolarizations in subarachnoid hemorrhage: a retrospective cohort study. Crit Care. 2019;23(1):427.
14. Bilodeau V, Saavedra-Mitjans M, Frenette AJ, Burry L, Albert M, Bernard F, et al. Safety of dexmedetomidine for the control of agitation in critically ill traumatic brain injury patients: a descriptive study. J Clin Pharm Ther. 2021;46(4):1020–6.
15. Humble SS, Wilson LD, Leath TC, Marshall MD, Sun DZ, Pandharipande PP, et al. ICU sedation with dexmedetomidine after severe traumatic brain injury. Brain Inj. 2016;30(10):1266–70.
16. Schomer KJ, Sebat CM, Adams JY, Duby JJ, Shahlaie K, Louie EL. Dexmedetomidine for refractory intracranial hypertension. J Intensive Care Med. 2019;34(1):62–6.
17. Meiser A, Volk T, Wallenborn J, Guenther U, Becher T, Bracht H, et al. Inhaled isoflurane via the anaesthetic conserving device versus propofol for sedation of invasively ventilated patients in intensive care units in Germany and Slovenia: an open-label, phase 3, randomised controlled, non-inferiority trial. Lancet Respir Med. 2021;9(11):1231–40.
18. Villa F, Iacca C, Molinari AF, Giussani C, Aletti G, Pesenti A, et al. Inhalation versus endovenous sedation in subarachnoid hemorrhage patients: effects on regional cerebral blood flow. Crit Care Med. 2012;40(10):2797–804.
19. Sneyd JR. Avoiding kidney damage in ICU sedation with sevoflurane: use isoflurane instead. Br J Anaesth. 2022;129(1):7–10.
20. Maussion E, Combaz S, Cuisinier A, Chapuis C, Payen JF. Renal dysfunction during sevoflurane sedation in the ICU: a case report. Eur J Anaesthesiol. 2019;36(5):377–9.
21. Zeiler FA, AlSubaie F, Zeiler K, Bernard F, Skrobik Y. Analgesia in Neurocritical care: an international survey and practice audit. Crit Care Med. 2016;44(5):973–80.
22. Stocchetti N, Maas AI. Traumatic intracranial hypertension. N Engl J Med. 2014;370(22):2121–30.
23. Helbok R, Kurtz P, Schmidt MJ, Stuart MR, Fernandez L, Connolly SE, et al. Effects of the neurological wake-up test on clinical examination, intracranial pressure, brain metabolism and brain tissue oxygenation in severely brain-injured patients. Crit Care. 2012;16(6):R226.
24. Marklund N. The neurological wake-up test—a role in neurocritical care monitoring of traumatic brain injury patients? Front Neurol. 2017;8:540.
25. Maas AI, Hukkelhoven CW, Marshall LF, Steyerberg EW. Prediction of outcome in traumatic brain injury with computed tomographic characteristics: a comparison between the computed tomographic classification and combinations of computed tomographic predictors. Neurosurgery. 2005;57(6):1173–82.

26. Stocchetti N, Zanaboni C, Colombo A, Citerio G, Beretta L, Ghisoni L, et al. Refractory intracranial hypertension and "second-tier" therapies in traumatic brain injury. Intensive Care Med. 2008;34(3):461–7.
27. Dehghani H, Tavangar H, Ghandehari A. Validity and reliability of behavioral pain scale in patients with low level of consciousness due to head trauma hospitalized in intensive care unit. Arch Trauma Res. 2014;3(1):e18608.
28. Joffe AM, McNulty B, Boitor M, Marsh R, Gelinas C. Validation of the critical-care pain observation tool in brain-injured critically ill adults. J Crit Care. 2016;36:76–80.
29. Gelinas C, Berube M, Puntillo KA, Boitor M, Richard-Lalonde M, Bernard F, et al. Validation of the critical-care pain observation tool-neuro in brain-injured adults in the intensive care unit: a prospective cohort study. Crit Care. 2021;25(1):142.
30. Yu A, Teitelbaum J, Scott J, Gesin G, Russell B, Huynh T, et al. Evaluating pain, sedation, and delirium in the neurologically critically ill-feasibility and reliability of standardized tools: a multi-institutional study. Crit Care Med. 2013;41(8):2002–7.
31. Schnakers C, Chatelle C, Vanhaudenhuyse A, Majerus S, Ledoux D, Boly M, et al. The nociception coma scale: a new tool to assess nociception in disorders of consciousness. Pain. 2010;148(2):215–9.
32. Chatelle C, Majerus S, Whyte J, Laureys S, Schnakers C. A sensitive scale to assess nociceptive pain in patients with disorders of consciousness. J Neurol Neurosurg Psychiatry. 2012;83(12):1233–7.
33. Bernard C, Delmas V, Duflos C, Molinari N, Garnier O, Chalard K, et al. Assessing pain in critically ill brain-injured patients: a psychometric comparison of 3 pain scales and videopupillometry. Pain. 2019;160(11):2535–43.
34. Arbour C, Choiniere M, Topolovec-Vranic J, Loiselle CG, Puntillo K, Gelinas C. Detecting pain in traumatic brain-injured patients with different levels of consciousness during common procedures in the ICU: typical or atypical behaviors? Clin J Pain. 2014;30(11):960–9.
35. Ledowski T. Objective monitoring of nociception: a review of current commercial solutions. Br J Anaesth. 2019;123(2):e312–e21.
36. Broucqsault-Dedrie C, De Jonckheere J, Jeanne M, Nseir S. Measurement of heart rate variability to assess pain in sedated critically ill patients: a prospective observational study. PloS One. 2016;11(1):e0147720.
37. Chanques G, Tarri T, Ride A, Prades A, De Jong A, Carr J, et al. Analgesia nociception index for the assessment of pain in critically ill patients: a diagnostic accuracy study. Br J Anaesth. 2017;119(4):812–20.
38. Fratino S, Peluso L, Talamonti M, Menozzi M, Costa Hirai LA, Lobo FA, et al. Evaluation of nociception using quantitative Pupillometry and skin conductance in critically ill unconscious patients: a pilot study. Brain Sci. 2021;11(1):109.
39. Paulus J, Roquilly A, Beloeil H, Theraud J, Asehnoune K, Lejus C. Pupillary reflex measurement predicts insufficient analgesia before endotracheal suctioning in critically ill patients. Crit Care. 2013;17(4):R161.
40. Vinclair M, Schilte C, Roudaud F, Lavolaine J, Francony G, Bouzat P, et al. Using pupillary pain index to assess nociception in sedated critically ill patients. Anesth Analg. 2019;129(6):1540–6.
41. Gelinas C, Shahiri TS, Richard-Lalonde M, Laporta D, Morin JF, Boitor M, et al. Exploration of a multi-parameter technology for pain assessment in postoperative patients after cardiac surgery in the intensive care unit: the nociception level index (NOL)(TM). J Pain Res. 2021;14:3723–31.
42. Bruder N, Lassegue D, Pelissier D, Graziani N, Francois G. Energy expenditure and withdrawal of sedation in severe head-injured patients. Crit Care Med. 1994;22(7):1114–9.
43. McKenzie CA, McKinnon W, Naughton DP, Treacher D, Davies G, Phillips GJ, et al. Differentiating midazolam over-sedation from neurological damage in the intensive care unit. Crit Care. 2005;9(1):R32–6.
44. McNett M, Sarver W, Wilczewski P. The prevalence, treatment and outcomes of agitation among patients with brain injury admitted to acute care units. Brain Inj. 2012;26(9):1155–62.

45. Gramish JA, Kopp BJ, Patanwala AE. Effect of amantadine on agitation in critically ill patients with traumatic brain injury. Clin Neuropharmacol. 2017;40(5):212–6.
46. Williamson DR, Frenette AJ, Burry L, Perreault MM, Charbonney E, Lamontagne F, et al. Pharmacological interventions for agitation in patients with traumatic brain injury: protocol for a systematic review and meta-analysis. Syst Rev. 2016;5(1):193.
47. Aubanel S, Bruiset F, Chapuis C, Chanques G, Payen JF. Therapeutic options for agitation in the intensive care unit. Anaesth Crit Care Pain Med. 2020;39(5):639–46.
48. Barr J, Fraser GL, Puntillo K, Ely EW, Gelinas C, Dasta JF, et al. Clinical practice guidelines for the management of pain, agitation, and delirium in adult patients in the intensive care unit. Crit Care Med. 2013;41(1):263–306.
49. Awissi DK, Lebrun G, Fagnan M, Skrobik Y. Regroupement de Soins critiques RdSRQ. Alcohol, nicotine, and iatrogenic withdrawals in the ICU. Crit Care Med. 2013;41(9 Suppl 1):S57–68.
50. Liatsi D, Tsapas B, Pampori S, Tsagourias M, Pneumatikos I, Matamis D. Respiratory, metabolic and hemodynamic effects of clonidine in ventilated patients presenting with withdrawal syndrome. Intensive Care Med. 2009;35(2):275–81.
51. Reynaud-Davin I, Francony G, Fauvage B, Canet C, Coppo F, Payen JF. Evaluation d'un protocole d'arrêt de la sédation chez le patient cérébrolésé. Ann Fr Anesth Reanim. 2012;31(2):109–13.
52. Roberson SW, Patel MB, Dabrowski W, Ely EW, Pakulski C, Kotfis K. Challenges of delirium management in patients with traumatic brain injury: from pathophysiology to clinical practice. Curr Neuropharmacol. 2021;19(9):1519–44.
53. Girard TD, Thompson JL, Pandharipande PP, Brummel NE, Jackson JC, Patel MB, et al. Clinical phenotypes of delirium during critical illness and severity of subsequent long-term cognitive impairment: a prospective cohort study. Lancet Respir Med. 2018;6(3):213–22.
54. Patel MB, Bednarik J, Lee P, Shehabi Y, Salluh JI, Slooter AJ, et al. Delirium monitoring in neurocritically ill patients: a systematic review. Crit Care Med. 2018;46(11):1832–41.
55. Larsen LK, Frokjaer VG, Nielsen JS, Skrobik Y, Winkler Y, Moller K, et al. Delirium assessment in neuro-critically ill patients: a validation study. Acta Anaesthesiol Scand. 2019;63(3):352–9.
56. Schweickert WD, Pohlman MC, Pohlman AS, Nigos C, Pawlik AJ, Esbrook CL, et al. Early physical and occupational therapy in mechanically ventilated, critically ill patients: a randomised controlled trial. Lancet. 2009;373(9678):1874–82.
57. Pan Y, Jiang Z, Yuan C, Wang L, Zhang J, Zhou J, et al. Influence of physical restraint on delirium of adult patients in ICU: a nested case-control study. J Clin Nurs. 2018;27(9–10):1950–7.
58. Page VJ, Ely EW, Gates S, Zhao XB, Alce T, Shintani A, et al. Effect of intravenous haloperidol on the duration of delirium and coma in critically ill patients (Hope-ICU): a randomised, double-blind, placebo-controlled trial. Lancet Respir Med. 2013;1(7):515–23.
59. Rood PJT, Zegers M, Slooter AJC, Beishuizen A, Simons KS, van der Voort PHJ, et al. Prophylactic haloperidol effects on long-term quality of life in critically ill patients at high risk for delirium: results of the REDUCE study. Anesthesiology. 2019;131(2):328–35.
60. Tang JF, Chen PL, Tang EJ, May TA, Stiver SI. Dexmedetomidine controls agitation and facilitates reliable, serial neurological examinations in a non-intubated patient with traumatic brain injury. Neurocrit Care. 2011;15(1):175–81.

15 Intracranial Pressure Management: The Stepwise Approach

Rachel D. Appelbaum, Jacqueline Kraft, and Aarti Sarwal

15.1 Introduction

Intracranial pressure (ICP) monitoring and interventions to decrease ICP are routinely used in patients with sTBI. The Brain Trauma Foundation (BTF), a non-profit organization, synthesizes available evidence on sTBI to develop recommendations for intervention, monitoring, and treatment and provides guidance on treatment protocols incorporating expert consensus and clinical judgment [1]. In this chapter, we describe the pathophysiology of intracranial pressure, current methods of intracranial pressure monitoring, and targets for current therapies guided by ICP monitoring with a stepwise approach to ICP management.

15.2 Pathophysiology of Intracranial Pressure

The cranial vault is made up of brain parenchyma, cerebrospinal fluid (CSF), and blood all held in a fixed box, the skull. The Monro-Kellie doctrine states an increase in one component within this fixed space must be accounted for by a decrease in one or both of the other two [2–4], Fig. 15.1. If cerebral edema or intracranial hemorrhage related to TBI adds to the cerebral volume, then one of the contents, blood or cerebrospinal fluid, must decrease to maintain ICP. This displacement is limited by

R. D. Appelbaum
Vanderbilt University Medical Center, Nashville, TN, USA
e-mail: rachel.appelbaum@vumc.org

J. Kraft
Neurology and Neurosurgery, Emory University Hospital, Atlanta, GA, USA
e-mail: jacqueline.kraft@emoryhealthcare.org

A. Sarwal (✉)
Neurology, Wake Forest University School of Medicine, Winston-Salem, NC, USA
e-mail: asarwal@wakehealth.edu

E. Brogi et al. (eds.), *Traumatic Brain Injury*, Hot Topics in Acute Care Surgery and Trauma, https://doi.org/10.1007/978-3-031-50117-3_15

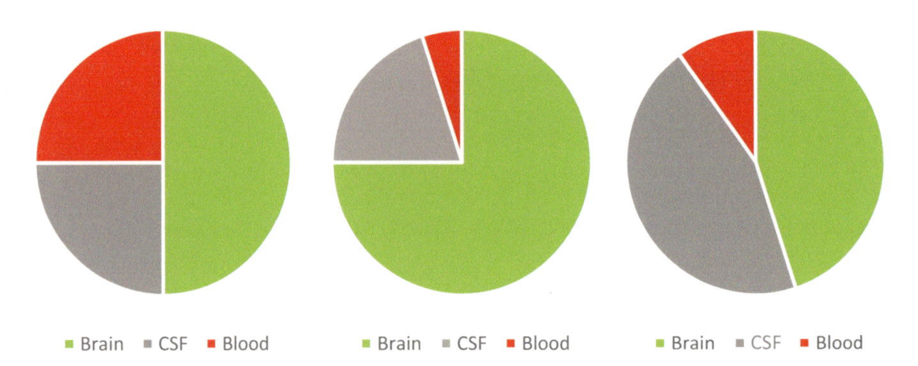

Fig. 15.1 Monro-Kellie doctrine. The Monro-Kellie doctrine describes the internal volume balance of the cranial compartment as incompressible, and its contents as brain parenchyma (green), cerebrospinal fluid (CSF, gray), and blood (red) (left panel). An increase in one component must be accounted for by a reduction in the other two. In most instances, cerebral edema caused by intracranial hematomas, contusions, or diffuse brain swelling leads to an increase in the "brain" compartment causing reduction in the CSF and blood compartments to keep the intracranial pressure within normal limits (middle panel). Further increase in swelling will exponentially increase intracranial pressure leading to herniation, global cerebral ischemia, and eventually brain death. In some instances, hydrocephalus may increase the CSF compartment causing compression of the brain and blood compartments which may need external ventricular drainage (right panel)

volume of the skull and after a certain threshold, ICP increases exponentially. Without intervention, this can lead to ischemia, brain herniation, and/or death. To better understand monitoring and intervening to prevent this process, we must better understand ICP, compliance, and ultimately, perfusion, discussed in more detail in Chap. 7.

Normal intracranial pressure inside the cranium is known to be 7–15 mmHg and is considered pathologic when it is greater than 20 mmHg [4]. ICP elevates when there is an increase in any of the three cranial components that alter intracranial compliance. Cerebral compliance is defined as the change in pressure in the cranium over a given change in intracranial volume and the cranial vault's adaptive ability to keep ICPs within normative range despite initial increase in cranial volume [5]. ICP and intracranial compliance correlate in a non-linear fashion. At lower ICPs, cerebral autoregulation compensates to allow appropriate cerebral perfusion, *the initial phase*. As the brain becomes less compliant due to increasing volume of brain tissue, blood, or CSF, intracranial pressure rises more sharply, the *transition phase*. With increasing intracranial volume, a critical volume threshold is crossed and beyond this critical point, compliance is too low, or non-existent, ICP rises exponentially, all autoregulatory mechanisms fail and eventually cerebral perfusion is lost, *the ascending phase* [5], Fig. 15.2.

In addition to assessing the transduced ICP quantitatively, it is valuable to monitor ICP waveforms, the graphical representation of cranial pulsation in response to cerebral blood flow (CBF) pulsations. These can provide information about change in brain compliance. ICP waveforms have three peaks which correlate to the ICP fluctuations along the cardiac cycle. *P1*, the first peak or percussion wave,

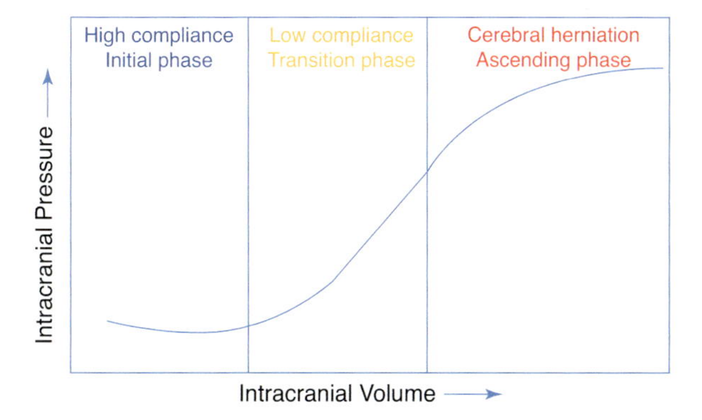

Fig. 15.2 Pressure–volume curve for changes in intracranial pressure. Blue represents the initial stage where the brain adjusts to allow adequate cerebral perfusion pressure despite increasing volume. Yellow is the transition phase where compliance decreases due to the sharp rise in volume and intracranial pressure. Red represents the ascending phase where compliance plummets and autoregulatory mechanisms in the brain fail leading to microvasculature collapse and herniation

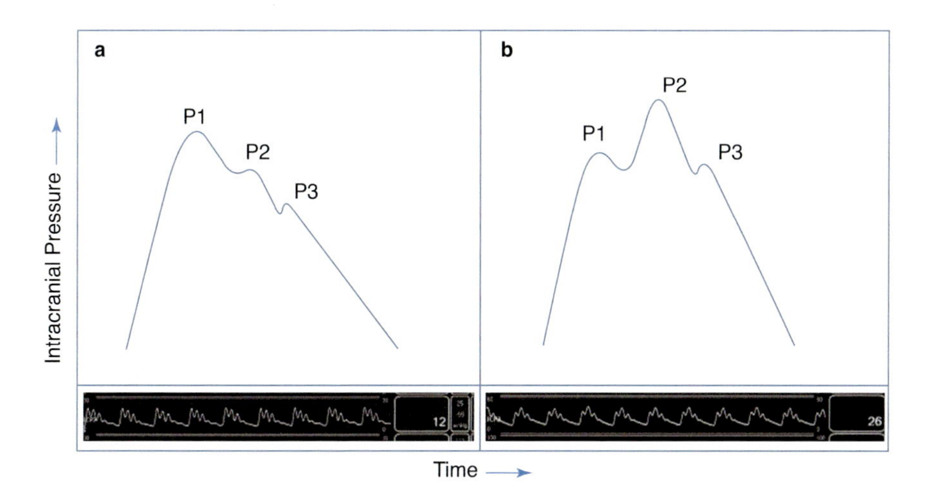

Fig. 15.3 Intracranial pressure waveforms. (**a**) Normal intracranial pressure waveform. The second peak should be lower than the first peak. (**b**) Waveform indicating increased intracranial pressure. The second peak is higher than the first peak

represents the arterial pulsation. *P2*, second peak or tidal wave, represents brain compliance. *P3*, dicrotic wave, represents aortic valve closure. A normal intracranial waveform has a rapid systolic upstroke followed by stepwise systolic deceleration hence *P1* is higher than *P2*, Fig. 15.3a. A waveform with *P2* higher in amplitude than *P1* indicates a decrease in intracranial compliance that heralds an increase in ICP, Fig. 15.3b. This may precede or succeed an episode of intracranial hypertension and denotes a brain at risk of losing perfusion at smaller increments on ICP because of right shifting of the pressure–volume curve in the transition phase, Fig. 15.2.

Intracranial pressure is a convenient metric to measure the progression of acute brain injury, but it truly serves as a surrogate for cerebral perfusion pressure (CPP) which is the core target for all therapeutic options aimed at reducing the impact of secondary brain injury. CPP is measured with the equation:

$$\text{Cerebral Perfusion Pressure (CPP)} = \text{Mean Arterial Pressure (MAP)} - \text{Intracranial Pressure (ICP)}$$

CPP directly affects the oxygen delivery going into brain tissue and should be kept between 60 and 80 mmHg, because cerebral autoregulation is intact within this range, Fig. 15.4. Autoregulation tends to maintain the CPPs normally within a physiological range of fluctuations in ICP and systemic parameters like systolic blood pressure (SBP). If CPP is too low or high, then the cerebral blood vessels will vasodilate or vasoconstrict, respectively. CPP below 60 mmHg can lead to cerebral ischemia, and CPP above 110 mmHg can lead to hyperperfusion and cerebral edema [5]. This autoregulation may shift to the right or the left in patients with acute brain injury highlighting the importance of measuring patient's autoregulatory status. In addition to lowering ICP, therapeutic strategies aimed at maintaining CPP with in a patient's autoregulatory zone are physiologically intuitive as CPP is the nidus to which the cerebral autoregulatory response of the vasculature occurs. In patients with abnormal intracranial compliance and ICP, close monitoring of CPP and MAP can ensure the brain has adequate blood flow and oxygen.

Early results using CPP targeted management in sTBI suggested superiority compared to traditional ICP focused management. Rosner et al. aimed to refine management techniques directed at CPP maintenance. Targeting high CPP allowed for better control of ICP without cerebral ischemia, but this approach has failed to show improvement in neurological outcome with some contribution of outcomes offset by increased incidence of acute lung injury related to the use of vasopressors and fluids required to maintain high CPP values in the high CPP group [6].

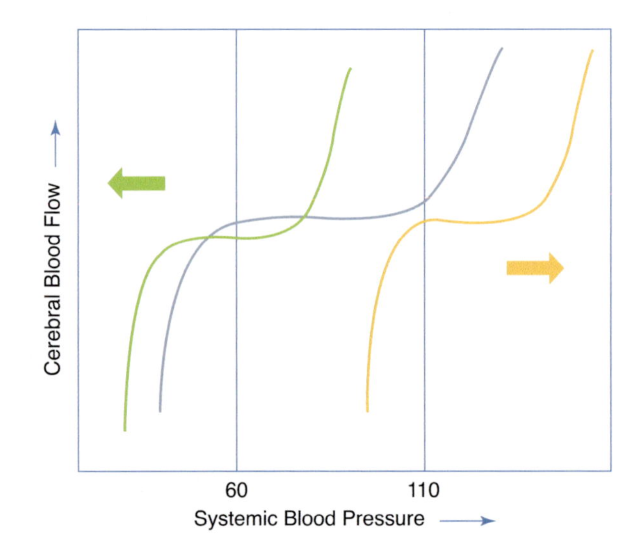

Fig. 15.4 Cerebral autoregulation. Cerebral autoregulation maintains cerebral blood flow within the physiological range of systemic blood pressures. Acute brain injury can result in the curve being shifted to the right causing cerebral ischemia at physiologically normal blood pressures or reperfusion injury if the curve is shifted to the left

Realization of leftwards shift of the autoregulation curve in sTBI patients with loss of autoregulation also raised concerns related to perfusion injury. This led to the BTF recommendations for targeting lower CPPs in patients with loss of autoregulation at physiological range of systemic pressures [1].

In addition to CPP, brain tissue oxygen ($PbtO_2$) monitoring was included in the Seattle International Severe Traumatic Brain Injury Conference's (SIBICC) updated consensus document, see Chap. 11 for additional details. The average $PbtO_2$ level for white matter, typical location of a $PbtO_2$ monitor, is 23 ± 7 [7], with values less than 20 mmHg representing brain hypoxia. $PbtO_2$ values less than 20, commonly seen following sTBI [8–10], are associated with worse outcomes [10, 11]. Additionally, observational studies suggest exploring the value of $PbtO_2$ directed therapy in combination with traditional CPP and ICP directed therapy [12, 13]. BOOST II validated the safety and feasibility of a tiered treatment regimen for $PbtO_2$ [14]. BOOST III trial is exploring the efficacy of sTBI clinical care informed by $PbtO_2$ measures.

15.3 Techniques for Intracranial Pressure Measurements

Physical exam and serial neuroimaging remain the cornerstone of clinical ICP monitoring in intensive care, but should prompt the use of more advanced intracranial monitoring techniques when a patient's exam is poor or limited by confounders such as impaired consciousness at presentation or sedatives. ICP can be monitored using non-invasive methods like ultrasound or transcranial Doppler and invasively using parenchymal ICP monitor or external ventricular drainage catheter (EVD). The choice of ICP monitoring modality in a given clinical setting depends on the patient, comorbidities, relative risk benefit profile of device related adverse events, and available neurosurgical expertise to insert invasive ICP monitors or EVD, Fig. 15.5. We describe a synopsis of the different modalities used to assess for increased ICPs including clinical and radiological signs of increased ICP, and the most commonly used ICP monitoring devices in clinical use.

15.3.1 History and Physical Examination

Frequent neurological assessments by trained providers are the cornerstone of ICP management in most ICUs across the world even in the most resourceful settings where additional neuromonitoring modalities are typically used as an adjunct to change in exam, or used when neurological exam is impaired or confounded by sedation [15]. The RESCUEicp trial showed no significant benefit of ICP guided clinical paradigms when compared with escalation of ICP lowering therapies guided by change in clinical examination in conjunction with radiological evaluation reinforcing focus on clinical monitoring [16].

Sudden severe headaches, vomiting, and changes in level of consciousness in a patient at risk of cerebral edema or hydrocephalus can indicate intracranial hypertension. Pupillary dilation and impairment of the pupillary reflex are common

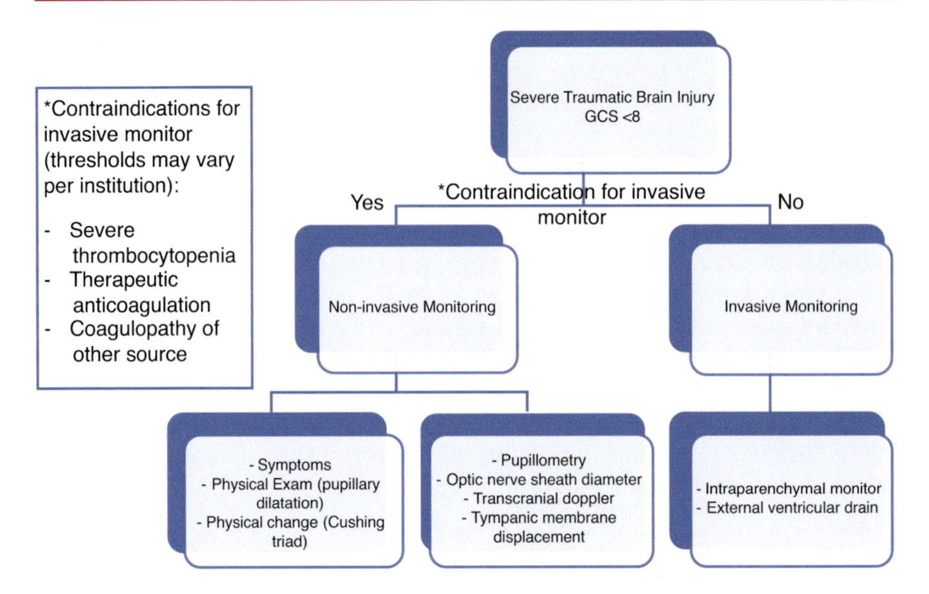

Fig. 15.5 Monitoring in severe traumatic brain injury. Algorithm for choice of non-invasive vs. invasive monitoring. Note this may be institution dependent as neurosurgery collaboration and resources will determine approach. Contraindications for invasive monitor placement include severe thrombocytopenia, therapeutic anticoagulation, and coagulopathy of other source

findings in evolving uncal herniation and are the basis of automated pupillometry. In addition, cranial VI or abducens nerve palsy, or impaired upgaze may be noted in patients with upward herniation or hydrocephalus, respectively. Despite being the most commonly used monitoring modality, the overall diagnostic accuracy of these clinical signs is not robust. Pupillary dilatation has a low sensitivity 28.2%, but high specificity 85.9% for detecting elevated ICP. Motor posturing and level of consciousness have 54.3% and 75.8% sensitivity and 63.6% and 39.9% specificity, respectively, in diagnosing intracranial hypertension [17]. Several standardized scales, such as GCS and FOUR score, have been used to detect changes in ICP, and decreased scores correspond to neurological decline associated with cerebral herniation. Clinical examination may have limited value or present challenges in patients presenting with poor examination or patients needing sedation for mechanical ventilation. Clinical exam based ICP detection care has a significant limitation in that clinical deterioration typically occurs at the far right of the pressure–volume curve and may miss early opportunities for intervention before intracranial hypertension impairs CPP.

15.3.2 Neuroimaging

Cerebral herniation is a shift of cerebral tissue from its normal location into an adjacent space and is the downstream effect of intracranial HTN (iHTN). Radiological stigmata of intracranial hypertension include subtle changes with cortical

Table 15.1 Cerebral herniation syndromes [18]

Herniation syndrome	Clinical signs	Radiological signs
Subfalcine	Anterior cerebral artery syndrome	Mass effect leading to midline shift
Transtentorial descending	Paralysis of third nerve, compression of PCA and choroidal arteries	Mass effect leading to downward herniation; occipital and medial temporal infarction
Transtentorial ascending	Brain stem, cerebellar, PCA, and SCA compression	Mass effect leading to upward herniation; occipital cerebral and superior cerebellar infarction
Tonsillar	Brain stem, cerebellar, and PICA compression	Inferior descent of the cerebellar tonsils below the foramen magnum >3 mm; posterior inferior cerebellum, inferior cerebellar vermis, and lateral medulla infarction

effacement, midline shift, and displacement of brain causing cisternal and ventricular effacement. Radiological hallmark of intracranial herniation includes: subfalcine herniation, transtentorial herniation, and tonsillar herniation [18]. Each type of herniation may be associated with a specific neurologic syndrome, Table 15.1. When untreated, cerebral herniation can progress to brain death, a clinical diagnosis characterized by the irreversible loss of neurologic function including the brain and brain stem [19].

15.3.3 Non-Invasive Monitors

Non-invasive techniques for measuring ICP include: pupillometry, optic nerve sheath diameter (ONSD), transcranial Doppler (TCD), and tympanic membrane displacement (TMD), discussed in more detail in Chaps. 8 and 9. These modalities are typically reserved for clinical settings where invasive techniques are not readily available or amenable due to clinical condition. Non-invasive monitors have the obvious advantage of lack of risk of intracranial infection or hemorrhage inherent in invasive techniques but lack accuracy with regard to non-invasive prediction of ICP. Serial assessments using patients own baseline have been clinically useful, but an easy to use, reliable non-invasive pressure monitor that is as accurate as invasive ICP catheters remains elusive.

15.3.4 Invasive Monitors

Invasive intracranial monitors remain the gold standard for accurate intracranial pressure monitoring. These devices include EVD and fiberoptic/strain gauge monitors, including epidural, subarachnoid, and intraparenchymal devices. Current BTF guidelines recommend intracranial pressure monitoring in sTBI without recommending a particular monitoring modality [1]. Invasive monitors come with increased risk of hemorrhage related to insertion and since they require access to the intracranial space, there is an associated risk of infection that can be abated by sterile insertion techniques. Invasive ICP monitors are typically placed in the right frontal region, but they can be placed in other regions safely, although pressures may be different when measured in different locations [20, 21].

15.3.4.1 Intraparenchymal Monitors (IPM)

Microsensor monitors were developed in the early 1990s and are either based on fiberoptic (Camino) or electrical impedance (Codman microsensor, Spiegelberg pressure sensor) based measurement of ICP. These monitors can be placed intraparenchymal or in the subarachnoid, subdural, or epidural spaces, Fig. 15.6. The common term "bolt" is erroneously used and represents the screw placed through the skull through which these sensors are inserted. Intraparenchymal monitors are considered less invasive compared to EVDs and provide reliable ICP monitoring for a few days after insertion. After 5–7 days, signal draft causes loss of accuracy in the range of 0.5–3.2 mmHg. Since calibration can only be done during insertion, prolonged need for ICP monitoring typically requires reinsertion of a new monitor after a week [22–24]. They are also preferred in patients with no imminent need for CSF sampling or drainage. IPMs in general have lower infection and symptomatic hemorrhage rates when compared to EVDs due to the small size and lack of external access to CSF [21, 22]. IPMs also allow continuous transduction of ICP waveforms which can be assessed alongside the systemic blood pressures to facilitate assessment of autoregulation.

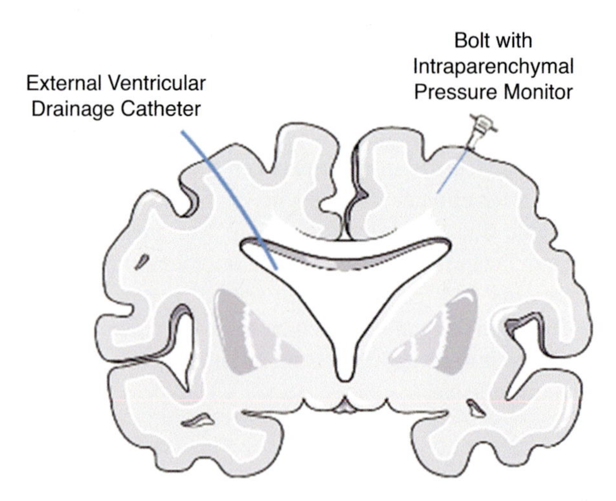

Fig. 15.6 Invasive monitors. This figure demonstrates two invasive monitors and the targets of placement. An external ventricular drain (EVD) enters through the parenchyma, often at Kocher's point, of the right frontal lobe given that in the majority of the population this is a non-dominant site and the target location of the ventricles. This monitor is diagnostic and therapeutic as it can drain off CSF. Bolts with intraparenchymal pressure monitors shown are monitors that terminate in the brain parenchyma. (Parts of the figure were drawn by using pictures from Servier Medical Art. Servier Medical Art by Servier is licensed under a Creative Commons Attribution 3.0 Unported License (https://creativecommons.org/licenses/by/3.0/))

15.3.4.2 External Ventricular Drains

The eighteenth century use of EVDs spurred after Nils Lundberg published the clinical applications in ICP monitoring in brain tumor patients in the 1960s [25]. EVDs are generally considered as the gold standard of ICP monitors, because of their longer history of use, and secondary benefit of CSF drainage. Studies comparing the rates of infection and hemorrhage of EVDs to IPM have found variable outcomes ranging from equal outcomes by Aiolfi et al. 2018, better outcomes with EVDs by Liu et al. 2015, or lower morality and functional outcomes by Bales et al. 2019 [26–28]. EVDs in general are more invasive given the technique of insertion and size of the catheter. In addition, measurements of ICP using an EVD require clamping to assess pressures using manometry, and that does not lend to a continuous transduction of ICP waveforms when continuous drainage of CSF is required. In such cases, ICP monitoring is either done at frequency, typically 15-min intervals or an EVD is inserted along with a fiberoptic ICP sensor that allows continuous ICP measurement as the EVD drains CSF. An EVD is calibrated at the tragus, though the practice of leveling the EVD at the left atrium is used by some to allow accurate measurement of CPP. It is also important to be consistent with units of measurement of ICP when using an EVD as it allows measurement in cm of CSF based on manometer as well as mmHg, both scales being present on the drainage system. In general, the consensus of the choice of device is based on patient factors depending on safety of accessing ventricles based on imaging, therapeutic needs for draining or sampling CSF, and preferences of the proceduralist.

15.4 Management Strategies

When a patient develops a clinical exam concerning for intracranial hypertension and neuroimaging is consistent with worsening cerebral edema, it is imperative to have a stepwise approach to treating the escalating ICP expeditiously to prevent a sustained decrease in CPP. The exact threshold of escalating treatment varies in different clinical settings, but the most common target endorsed by many studies showing impaired CPPs above these thresholds defines iHTN, as a sustained ICP elevation above 20–22 mmHg for 5–20 min. Different clinical approaches continue to exist across different regions using a clinical, radiological, brain tissue oxygen, autoregulation targeted approach including the RESCUEicp trial [16], the Chesnut study [15], the Lund concept [29], and then ultimately the BTF guidelines [1], but none has proven to be superior to the other. A tiered approach proposed by the SIBICC, to put forth a clinically applicable and provider friendly management algorithm, is presented here to provide a physiologically based clinical paradigm of ICP management, Fig. 15.7.

15.4.1 Tier 0

With any brain injury, the essential care targeted of reducing the impact of secondary brain injury is recommended. This care is considered tier zero and is not dependent on ICP or $PbtO_2$ [30, 31], though intracranial monitoring is recommended in

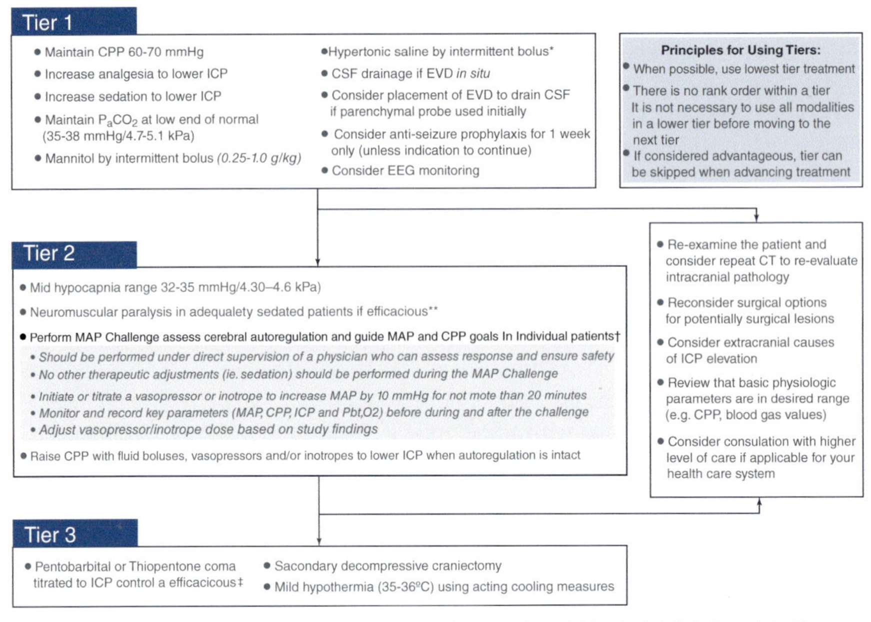

Fig. 15.7 Seattle International Severe Traumatic Brain Injury Consensus Conference (SIBICC) consensus-based algorithm. This consensus-based algorithm was created for the management of severe traumatic brain injury guided by intracranial pressure measurements. (This image was obtained from the 2019 publication by Hawryluk et al. "A Management Algorithm for Patients with Intracranial Pressure Monitoring: The Seattle International Severe Traumatic Brain Injury Consensus Conference (SIBICC)" and is licensed under a Creative Commons Attribution-NonCommercial 4.0 International License (http://creativecommons.org/licenses/by-nc/4.0/) [31]). *CPP* cerebral perfusion pressure, *EEG* electroencephalogram, *EVD* external ventricular drain, *ICP* intracranial pressure, *kPa* kiloPascals, *MAP* mean arterial pressure, $PaCO_2$ arterial partial pressure of carbon dioxide

patients with poor exam. The patient should be admitted to the ICU, intubated for airway protection and mechanical ventilation if the exam warrants. Proper patient positioning to help with venous return from the head should be done and includes elevation of patient's head of bed to 30–45°, midline head position, and ensuring the cervical collar is not too tight. Analgesia and sedation should be used to manage pain, agitation, and ventilator dys-synchrony. To help ensure adequate brain oxygenation and cerebral perfusion, SpO_2 should be maintained at or above 94%. The BTF recommends SBP 110 mmHg or above for patients 15–49 or >70 years old and 100 mmHg or above for patients 50–69 years old [1]. While modulating blood pressure, it is important to ensure CPP is maintained at 60 mmHg or above. Active temperature management should be in place to prevent fever, treating a core temperature above 38 °C [30, 31].

Frequent laboratory monitoring should target maintaining a hemoglobin >7 g/dL to ensure adequate oxygenation to the brain. Hyponatremia should be promptly treated to avoid exacerbation of cerebral edema and interstitial volume shifts. Blood pressure stabilization is crucial to prevent secondary brain injury, avoiding rapid fluctuations of both hypotension and hypertension in the acute phase, and can be facilitated by continuous hemodynamic monitoring with an arterial line [30, 31].

Anti-seizure medications should be considered for 1 week and continued longer if there are definitive clinical indication including recurrent seizures, epileptogenicity of electroencephalography (EEG) associated with fluctuating exam or concern for non-convulsive seizures [30, 31]. This recommendation is based on prevalence of early post-traumatic seizures (PTS) in sTBI, and the potential of seizures causing secondary brain injury. Clinical seizures can be seen in up to 12% of patients, while subclinical seizures are even more prevalent up to 25% patients monitored with continuous EEG. Patients at particular risk of early PTS include patients younger than 65 years, those with GCS less than 10, chronic alcoholism, seizures at onset of injury, linear or depressed skull fracture, penetrating skull injury, presence of intracranial hemorrhage (subdural, epidural, or intraparenchymal hematoma), or cortical contusion [32]. Both phenytoin and levetiracetam have been recommended as prophylactic agents without sufficient evidence of superiority of one agent over the other. Small studies have compared prophylaxis with a single agent, but large robust randomized control trials are lacking [33]. Prophylactic use of anti-seizure medications has not shown a reduction in incidence of late post-traumatic epilepsy. In addition, use of anti-seizure medications without definitive indications is associated with adverse neurocognitive outcomes after discharge, hence BTF guidelines recommend against the prophylactic use of anti-seizure medications after 7 days.

15.4.2 Tier 1

The next tier in management, Tier 1 is instituted when intracranial hypertension is noted despite attempts at normocarbia and maintain normal CPPs around 60–70 mmHg, Fig. 15.7. The goal of management includes prevention of secondary injury as well as progression of cerebral edema and focuses on CSF and cerebral volume management strategies.

15.4.2.1 Cerebrospinal Fluid Volume Management Strategies

Intracranial hypertension in sTBI may benefit from EVD to relieve obstruction of CSF outflow caused by intraventricular hemorrhage or mechanical obstruction of ventricular outflow from local cerebral edema. In addition, cautious drainage of CSF can help maintain CPPs in the case of progressive cerebral edema. Target ICP goals and drainage parameters are often established in collaboration with neurosurgery consultants and critical care providers based on patient parameters. An EVD system zeroed at the tragus (midbrain) with continuous drainage of CSF may be considered to lower the ICP burden more effectively than intermittent drainage and should be used in those with initial GCS <6 during the first 12 h after injury [1].

Drainage of a fixed volume of CSF per desired time, or as needed according to ICP elevations is the less preferred strategy [34].

15.4.2.2 Cerebral Volume Management Strategies

Cerebral edema results from the pathologic accumulation of excess water within the brain parenchyma. This edema may be vasogenic in origin from increased permeability due to disruption of the blood–brain barrier or cytotoxic edema due to disrupted brain parenchymal cells. Cerebral edema ultimately leads to increased intracranial volume, and thus increased ICP when the cerebral cavity is unable to further compensate [35]. The focus of this tier is to prevent the patient from crossing the critical threshold of ICP on the pressure–volume curve where increase in cerebral volume causes an irreversible loss of autoregulation and cerebral herniation, Fig. 15.2.

Osmotic Therapy

Osmotic therapy, mannitol and hypertonic saline, decreases intracranial pressure by causing an osmotic shift of fluids across the intact blood–brain barrier into interstitial and intravascular space and positive effects on rheology improving cerebral microvascular blood flow. Mannitol is an osmotic diuretic agent commonly administered as a 20% concentration, dose 0.25–1.5 g/kg IV as scheduled or as-needed bolus to maintain serum osmolarity around 300–320 mosm/L or osmolar gap less than 15 mosm/L [30, 31, 35]. Mannitol is a potent osmotic diuretic and can decrease a patient's intravascular volume suggesting caution in patients at risk of hypovolemic, hemorrhagic, or other forms of shock as this may exacerbate hypotension and possibly cause acute kidney injury. Mannitol must be injected with an in-line filter as it may crystallize at low temperatures [35]. The BTF suggests restricting the use of mannitol to patients with intracranial hypertension on ICP monitoring and patients with signs of transtentorial herniation or progressive neurologic deterioration not attributable to extracranial causes [1].

Hypertonic saline in concentrations of 2–23.4% is also a potent osmotic agent. Hypertonic 3% saline is generally given in 250–500 mL boluses over 30–60 min, while hypertonic 23.4% saline is typically administered in a 30 mL bolus over 10–15 min to avoid hypotension and bradycardia seen with faster infusions. Hyperchloremic metabolic acidosis associated with use of sodium-chloride solutions can be avoided by using buffered acetate which may also reduce the risk of acute kidney injury [36]. Serial basic metabolic panels every 4–6 h are typically monitored to guide the administration and address associated hypokalemia and hypomagnesemia. Hypertonic saline over 3% requires central line access to avoid peripheral vascular injury [35].

While robust evidence of superiority of one agent over the other is lacking there is general consensus that both 3% hypertonic saline and mannitol can effectively reduce ICP, but 3% hypertonic saline has a more sustained effect on ICP and can effectively increase CPP [37]. Hypertonic saline boluses may be superior to mannitol in reduction of the combined burden of intracranial hypertension and associated cerebral hypoperfusion [38]. With either therapy, it is important to maintain serum osmolarity at less than 320 mOsm to avoid adverse effects, such as hypovolemia, hyperosmolarity, and renal failure [39].

Analgesia and Sedative Agents

Analgesia and sedation are widely used to improve intracranial hypertension by decreasing cerebral metabolism and oxygen consumption utilizing neurovascular coupling [40, 41]. BTF recommends propofol for ICP given its ability to decrease cerebral metabolism and oxygen consumption; however, propofol does not decrease mortality or 6 month outcomes and should be used with cautions due to its adverse effects of hyperkalemia, metabolic acidosis, rhabdomyolysis, and renal failure when used at high doses over longer periods of time [42]. Other agents used for sedation include midazolam and fentanyl infusions. Dexmedetomidine, selective $\alpha 2$ adrenergic agonist used for anxiolysis without sedation has variable effects on ICPs and at this time is not recommended. The SIBICC consensus recommends using analgesia and sedatives to lower ICP, but do not further make recommendations as to how or what agents to use.

Since non-convulsive seizures have known prevalence in this population, and seizure induced increased metabolism can cause increased CBF and hence iHTN, continuous EEG monitoring should be considered to ensure that ictal hyperemia is not contributing to intracranial hypertension.

15.4.3 Tier 2

When intracranial hypertension persists despite CSF drainage, osmotic therapy, and appropriate sedation, escalation of management to tier 2 interventions should be considered. These include neuromuscular blockade, mild hypocapnia (CO_2 32–35), and correcting brain tissue hypoxia using invasive $PbtO_2$ monitoring to guide care, if available [30]. Any need for escalation in care should prompt repeat imaging to evaluate for a change in intracranial processes that may be amenable to surgical intervention, i.e., increasing hydrocephalus may warrant increasing CSF drainage or surgical hematoma evacuation may alleviate ICP crisis caused by an expanding parenchymal hemorrhage. Efforts to obtain imaging should focus on minimizing processes that cause ICP elevations including minimizing supine time and interruptions in ventilation for critical care transport.

15.4.3.1 Neuromuscular Blockade

The exact mechanism of neuromuscular (NMS) blockade in reducing ICP beyond minimizing the contribution of muscle activity by reducing energy expenditure, eliminating shivering during normothermia, and minimizing ventilator dyssynchrony are unclear [43, 44]. The positive effect of paralysis on ventilation and therefore optimizing oxygen and CO_2 levels may help improve CBF and thus ICP [45]. A systematic review evaluating neuromuscular blockade in sTBI found low level evidence with mixed data [46]. BTF does not make recommendations on neuromuscular blockade, but SIBICC recommends a trial of neuromuscular paralysis as a tier 2 intervention and continuation only if found to be effective [1, 30].

15.4.3.2 Controlled Hyperventilation

CBF is linearly determined by $PaCO_2$ levels. Hyperventilation associated with low CO_2 typically reduces CBF with risk of ischemia, if prolonged. Hypercarbia and high CO_2 can lead to hyperemia and elevations in ICP. Based on these physiological observations, BTF recommends normocarbia, keeping CO_2 in the range of 35–45 mmHg and use of brief hyperventilation to lower elevated ICP only as a temporizing measure. Routine hyperventilation is not recommended to prevent or treat intracranial hypertension and should be particularly avoided in the first 24 h post-sTBI since CBF is often more significantly reduced during this time [1]. The SIBICC recommends mild hypocapnia (CO_2 32–35 mmHg) in ICP crisis not responding to osmotic therapy with cautions against lowering CO_2 less than 30 [30].

15.4.3.3 Brain Tissue Oxygenation

Both BTF and SIBICC recommend brain tissue oxygen monitoring ($PbtO_2$), when available, to guide hyperventilation. Patients may present with four clinical scenarios based on results of ICP and brain oxygen monitors, these have been phenotyped as types A, B, C, and D by SIBICC. Type A patients have normal ICP with normal $PbtO_2$ and require no further interventions beyond supportive care of tier zero. Type B patients have elevated ICP with normal $PbtO_2$ and should be managed with ICP lowering strategies in Tier 1 and 2. Type C patients with normal ICP with low $PbtO_2$; and type D patients with elevated ICP and low $PbtO_2$, both should have augment ventilation to get $PaO_2 > 150$ mmHg/20 kPa when $PbtO_2$ is less than 20. Neuromuscular blockade, sedation, and blood transfusion can be used to improve oxygenation, as needed, if initial trial is effective. It is important to note that augmentation of oxygenation has potential benefits but can also result in hyperoxia related toxicity. There is also criticism that higher $PbtO_2$ monitor readings may not parallel improved oxygen availability [30, 31], so it is important to make changes on a patient-by-patient basis.

A trial of induced hypertension in controlled settings may be performed to assess for autoregulation induced cerebral vasoconstriction in reducing ICP crisis. This may also help distinguish oligemic intracranial hypertension benefitting from induced hypertension to augment CPP from hyperemic intracranial hypertension where patients may benefit from lower CPP [47].

15.4.4 Tier 3

Persistent ICP elevations with appropriate rapid escalation of ICP lowering or persistent hypoperfusion suspected due to CPP < 60 should prompt escalation to Tier 3 interventions. These include hypothermia, surgical decompression, and barbiturates, Fig. 15.7.

15.4.4.1 Mild Hypothermia

Despite observed lowering of ICP with induced hypothermia, there is significant paucity of data surrounding the impact of hypothermia on clinical outcomes hence SIBICC recommends moderate hypothermia (35–36 °C) only as a third tier intervention. Coagulopathy and immunosuppression are risks of hypothermia and accidental deep hypothermia (<32 °C) may predispose the patient to cardiac arrhythmias and cardiac arrest [48]. The BTF does not endorse prophylactic hypothermia due to lack of association with outcomes and possible increase in mortality [49, 50].

15.4.4.2 Surgical Intervention

Decompressive craniectomy (DC) involves removing a section of the skull and opening the underlying dura mater to relieve ICPs. Primary DC refers to leaving a large bone flap out after evacuation of an intracranial hematoma in the acute phase after a sTBI with planned replacement once the acute phase of cerebral edema has passed. Secondary DC is used as part of tiered therapeutic protocols in ICUs to control refractory ICP as a last tier intervention to ensure adequate CPP [16]. DC can be done unilaterally to decompress one side of the cerebrum or bifrontally to decompress both hemispheres when edema is more diffuse. Most data on DC comes from the DECRA and RESCUEicp trials. The DECRA trial analyzed patients with ICP greater than 20 mmHg for more than 15 min (continuously or intermittently) within a 1-h period, despite optimized first-tier interventions and randomly assigned patients to early bifrontal DC versus standard care alone. Prophylactic bifrontal DC was associated with more unfavorable outcomes than standard care alone despite increased ICP and decrease in ICU length of stay [1, 51]. The BTF does not recommend bifrontal craniotomy based on this data.

Further studies investigating DC versus medical management alone have not yielded better outcomes [52, 53]. Studies assessing the size of DC which impacts ICPs have shown better outcomes in the large DC group though data is low evidence. These have informed BTF recommendations that a large frontotemporoparietal DC (not less than 12 × 15 cm or 15 cm diameter) is recommended over a small frontotemporoparietal DC for reduced mortality and improved neurologic outcomes in patients with severe TBI when DC is pursued [1, 54, 55].

The RESCUEicp trial evaluated the effect of DC on clinical outcomes in patients with refractory traumatic intracranial hypertension with large unilateral DC for patients with unilateral edema and bifrontal DC for patients with diffuse brain swelling. Patients were randomized to DC or usual care only if they had refractory elevated ICP >25 mmHg for 1–12 h despite tier 1 and 2 treatments. The study found that DC in patients with sTBI and refractory iHTN resulted in lower mortality but higher rates of vegetative state and severe disability compared to medical care without increasing chances of good recovery [16]. In combination with data from the DECRA trial, it would seem that while DC is a lifesaving therapy, but may lead to poor functional outcomes. In deciding if this procedure is right for a patient who has failed standard therapies for refractory iHTN, a shared decision making model by sharing the limited but available data factors may guide discussions with family.

15.4.4.3 Metabolic Suppression

After Eisenberg et al. demonstrated the efficacy of pentobarbital coma (PBC) in lowering ICP for sTBI patients with refractory intracranial hypertension and emerging studies explored the neuroprotective effects of pentobarbital, barbiturate coma gained popularity as advanced therapy for refractory iHTN when other measures have failed.

BTF and SIBICC have both incorporated pentobarbital into the last tier of tiered algorithm for ICP crisis. Pentobarbital has been demonstrated to reduce CBF and cerebral metabolic rate of oxygen ($CMRO_2$) in a dose-dependent fashion and thus reduces ICP. There is no significant evidence of decrease in death or disability with its use. Additionally, barbiturate use in critically ill patients has significant adverse effects including the need for prolonged ventilator support, nutrition support with the need for tracheostomy, percutaneous endoscopic gastrostomy tube, and prolonged nursing care [30, 31, 56]. The role of barbiturates is limited to potential salvage therapy for patients with refractory ICP and care should be taken in initiating this treatment given the significant adverse effects that come with it.

15.5 Target for ICP Lowering Therapy

Though the tiers represent escalating therapies targeted at lowering ICPs with higher risk therapies reserved for higher tiers, the framework should not be used in a waterfall design. The choice of therapies in a given tier and escalation to the next tier should be tailored to the patient's pathology and physiology driving increasing ICPs. A patient with non-convulsive refractory status may need earlier escalation to therapeutic coma and a patient with an enlarging hematoma amenable to therapy may need earlier escalation to surgical decompression.

As more investigations evaluate the management strategies for improving cerebral perfusion hence outcomes in sTBI, more focus is being shifted from the traditional paradigm of an ICP lowering focus to precision medicine approach and patient centric goals for ICP, CPP, and other physiological parameters assessed using multimodality monitoring. One area of interest is to focus on pressure time dose measurement of intracranial pressure rather than ICP elevation as a singular targets or biomarker with emerging evidence that higher ICP time dose may have association with mortality and poor outcomes, an association not consistently seen with episodic increases in ICP [57]. Another focus is to assess if ICP lowering therapies should be tailored to the physiological subsets of intracranial hypertension distinguishing oligemic intracranial hypertension from hyperemic intracranial hypertension [47]. BOOST III is evaluating the efficacy of utilizing both a $PbtO_2$ targeting approach with ICP compared to a strategy guided by treatment goals based on ICP monitoring alone in sTBI. COGiTATE trial recently showed the feasibility and safety of targeting an individualized and dynamic autoregulation-based CPP target for therapy in sTBI [58].

15.6 Conclusion

Severe traumatic brain injury management needs a personalized approach to cerebral hemodynamic management, and understanding the pathophysiology of sTBI and iHTN pertinent to patients' presentation is crucial to determining the targets of therapy and recommendations for management.

References

1. Carney N, et al. Guidelines for the management of severe traumatic brain injury, fourth edition. Neurosurgery. 2017;80(1):6–15.
2. Kellie G. An account of the appearances observed in the dissection of two of three individuals presumed to have perished in the storm of the 3d, and whose bodies were discovered in the vicinity of Leith on the morning of the 4th, November 1821; with some reflections on the pathology of the Brain: part I. Trans Med Chir Soc Edinb. 1824;1:84–122.
3. Monro A. Observations on the structure and functions of the nervous system. Edinburgh: Printed for, and Sold by, W. Creech; 1783. 176 p.
4. Mokri B. The Monro-Kellie hypothesis: applications in CSF volume depletion. Neurology. 2001;56(12):1746–8.
5. Harper AM, et al. Proceedings: the upper limit of 'autoregulation' of cerebral blood flow in the baboon. J Physiol. 1973;234(2):61P–2P.
6. Donnelly J, Aries MJ, Czosnyka M. Further understanding of cerebral autoregulation at the bedside: possible implications for future therapy. Expert Rev Neurother. 2015;15(2):169–85.
7. Pennings FA, et al. Brain tissue oxygen pressure monitoring in awake patients during functional neurosurgery: the assessment of normal values. J Neurotrauma. 2008;25(10):1173–7.
8. Asil T, et al. Monitoring of increased intracranial pressure resulting from cerebral edema with transcranial Doppler sonography in patients with middle cerebral artery infarction. J Ultrasound Med. 2003;22(10):1049–53.
9. Valadka AB, et al. Relationship of brain tissue PO2 to outcome after severe head injury. Crit Care Med. 1998;26(9):1576–81.
10. van Santbrink H, Maas AI, Avezaat CJ. Continuous monitoring of partial pressure of brain tissue oxygen in patients with severe head injury. Neurosurgery. 1996;38(1):21–31.
11. van den Brink WA, et al. Brain oxygen tension in severe head injury. Neurosurgery. 2000;46(4):868–76; discussion 876–8.
12. Bohman LE, et al. Medical management of compromised brain oxygen in patients with severe traumatic brain injury. Neurocrit Care. 2011;14(3):361–9.
13. Nangunoori R, et al. Brain tissue oxygen-based therapy and outcome after severe traumatic brain injury: a systematic literature review. Neurocrit Care. 2012;17(1):131–8.
14. Okonkwo DO, et al. Brain oxygen optimization in severe traumatic brain injury phase-II: a phase II randomized trial. Crit Care Med. 2017;45(11):1907–14.
15. Chesnut RM, et al. A trial of intracranial-pressure monitoring in traumatic brain injury. N Engl J Med. 2012;367(26):2471–81.
16. Hutchinson PJ, et al. Trial of decompressive craniectomy for traumatic intracranial hypertension. N Engl J Med. 2016;375(12):1119–30.
17. Fernando SM, et al. Diagnosis of elevated intracranial pressure in critically ill adults: systematic review and meta-analysis. BMJ. 2019;366:l4225.
18. Riveros Gilardi B, et al. Types of cerebral herniation and their imaging features. Radiographics. 2019;39(6):1598–610.
19. Gastala J, et al. Brain death: radiologic signs of a non-radiologic diagnosis. Clin Neurol Neurosurg. 2019;185:105465.
20. Gambardella G, d'Avella D, Tomasello F. Monitoring of brain tissue pressure with a fiberoptic device. Neurosurgery. 1992;31(5):918–21; discussion 921–2.
21. Poca MA, et al. Fiberoptic intraparenchymal brain pressure monitoring with the Camino V420 monitor: reflections on our experience in 163 severely head-injured patients. J Neurotrauma. 2002;19(4):439–48.
22. Gelabert-Gonzalez M, et al. The Camino intracranial pressure device in clinical practice. Assessment in a 1000 cases. Acta Neurochir. 2006;148(4):435–41.
23. Munch E, et al. The Camino intracranial pressure device in clinical practice: reliability, handling characteristics and complications. Acta Neurochir. 1998;140(11):1113–9; discussion 1119-20.

24. Shapiro S, et al. The fiberoptic intraparenchymal cerebral pressure monitor in 244 patients. Surg Neurol. 1996;45(3):278–82.
25. Srinivasan VM, et al. The history of external ventricular drainage. J Neurosurg. 2014;120(1):228–36.
26. Aiolfi A, et al. Intracranial pressure monitoring in severe blunt head trauma: does the type of monitoring device matter? J Neurosurg. 2018;128(3):828–33.
27. Bales JW, et al. Primary external ventricular drainage catheter versus Intraparenchymal ICP monitoring: outcome analysis. Neurocrit Care. 2019;31(1):11–21.
28. Liu H, et al. External ventricular drains versus Intraparenchymal intracranial pressure monitors in traumatic Brain injury: a prospective observational study. World Neurosurg. 2015;83(5):794–800.
29. Koskinen LO, Olivecrona M, Grande PO. Severe traumatic brain injury management and clinical outcome using the Lund concept. Neuroscience. 2014;283:245–55.
30. Chesnut R, et al. A management algorithm for adult patients with both brain oxygen and intracranial pressure monitoring: the Seattle international severe traumatic Brain injury consensus conference (SIBICC). Intensive Care Med. 2020;46(5):919–29.
31. Hawryluk GWJ, et al. A management algorithm for patients with intracranial pressure monitoring: the Seattle international severe traumatic brain injury consensus conference (SIBICC). Intensive Care Med. 2019;45(12):1783–94.
32. Torbic H, et al. Use of antiepileptics for seizure prophylaxis after traumatic brain injury. Am J Health Syst Pharm. 2013;70(9):759–66.
33. Hazama A, et al. The effect of Keppra prophylaxis on the incidence of early onset, post-traumatic brain injury seizures. Cureus. 2018;10(5):e2674.
34. Muralidharan R. External ventricular drains: management and complications. Surg Neurol Int. 2015;6(Suppl 6):S271–4.
35. Koenig MA. Cerebral edema and elevated intracranial pressure. Continuum (Minneap Minn). 2018;24(6):1588–602.
36. Sadan O, et al. Correction to: low-chloride- versus high-chloride-containing hypertonic solution for the treatment of subarachnoid hemorrhage-related complications: the ACETatE (a low ChloriE hyperTonic solution for brain edema) randomized trial. J Intensive Care. 2020;8:66.
37. Shi J, et al. Hypertonic saline and mannitol in patients with traumatic brain injury: a systematic and meta-analysis. Medicine (Baltimore). 2020;99(35):e21655.
38. Mangat HS, et al. Hypertonic saline is superior to mannitol for the combined effect on intracranial pressure and cerebral perfusion pressure burdens in patients with severe traumatic Brain injury. Neurosurgery. 2020;86(2):221–30.
39. Rangel-Castilla L, Gopinath S, Robertson CS. Management of intracranial hypertension. Neurol Clin. 2008;26(2):521–41, x.
40. Bar-Joseph G, et al. Effectiveness of ketamine in decreasing intracranial pressure in children with intracranial hypertension. J Neurosurg Pediatr. 2009;4(1):40–6.
41. Roberts I, Sydenham E. Barbiturates for acute traumatic brain injury. Cochrane Database Syst Rev. 2012;12(12):CD000033.
42. Kelly DF, et al. Propofol in the treatment of moderate and severe head injury: a randomized, prospective double-blinded pilot trial. J Neurosurg. 1999;90(6):1042–52.
43. Kerr ME, et al. Effect of neuromuscular blockers and opiates on the cerebrovascular response to endotracheal suctioning in adults with severe head injuries. Am J Crit Care. 1998;7(3):205–17.
44. McCall M, et al. Effect of neuromuscular blockade on energy expenditure in patients with severe head injury. JPEN J Parenter Enteral Nutr. 2003;27(1):27–35.
45. Papazian L, et al. Neuromuscular blockers in early acute respiratory distress syndrome. N Engl J Med. 2010;363(12):1107–16.
46. Sanfilippo F, et al. The role of neuromuscular blockade in patients with traumatic brain injury: a systematic review. Neurocrit Care. 2015;22(2):325–34.
47. Kofke WA, et al. Defining a taxonomy of intracranial hypertension: is ICP more than just a number? J Neurosurg Anesthesiol. 2020;32(2):120–31.

48. Brain Trauma F, et al. Guidelines for the management of severe traumatic brain injury. XV Steroids. J Neurotrauma. 2007;24(Suppl 1):S91–5.
49. Adelson PD, et al. Comparison of hypothermia and normothermia after severe traumatic brain injury in children (cool kids): a phase 3, randomised controlled trial. Lancet Neurol. 2013;12(6):546–53.
50. Hutchison JS, et al. Hypothermia therapy after traumatic brain injury in children. N Engl J Med. 2008;358(23):2447–56.
51. Cooper DJ, et al. Decompressive craniectomy in diffuse traumatic brain injury. N Engl J Med. 2011;364(16):1493–502.
52. Olivecrona M, et al. Effective ICP reduction by decompressive craniectomy in patients with severe traumatic brain injury treated by an ICP-targeted therapy. J Neurotrauma. 2007;24(6):927–35.
53. Soustiel JF, et al. Cerebral blood flow and metabolism following decompressive craniectomy for control of increased intracranial pressure. Neurosurgery. 2010;67(1):65–72; discussion 72.
54. Jiang JY, et al. Efficacy of standard trauma craniectomy for refractory intracranial hypertension with severe traumatic brain injury: a multicenter, prospective, randomized controlled study. J Neurotrauma. 2005;22(6):623–8.
55. Qiu W, et al. Effects of unilateral decompressive craniectomy on patients with unilateral acute post-traumatic brain swelling after severe traumatic brain injury. Crit Care. 2009;13(6):R185.
56. Downar J, et al. Guidelines for the withdrawal of life-sustaining measures. Intensive Care Med. 2016;42(6):1003–17.
57. Sheth KN, et al. Intracranial pressure dose and outcome in traumatic brain injury. Neurocrit Care. 2013;18(1):26–32.
58. Tas J, et al. Targeting autoregulation-guided cerebral perfusion pressure after traumatic Brain injury (COGiTATE): a feasibility randomized controlled clinical trial. J Neurotrauma. 2021;38(20):2790–800.

Ventilation Strategy and the Time of Tracheotomy: A Different Approach in Trauma?

16

Bianca Maria Mainini, Marco Di Lecce, Chiara Robba,
Luca Cattani, Vito Montanaro, Massimo Petranca,
and Edoardo Picetti

16.1 Introduction

Traumatic brain injury (TBI) is a leading cause of mortality and disability worldwide, with devastating effects on patients and their families [1]. The pathophysiology of TBI is characterized by two distinct and closely related events: primary and secondary brain injury [2–4]. Primary brain injury occurs at the time of the trauma. The underlying mechanisms are direct impact, rapid acceleration or deceleration, penetrating injuries and shock waves. Resulting damage can include focal contusions and hematomas [epidural hematomas (EDHs), subdural hematomas (SDHs), subarachnoid hemorrhage (SAH), etc.], diffuse axonal injury (DAI), and cerebral edema. Secondary brain injury occurs after the initial event and is potentially amenable of treatment. It results from a cascade of molecular mechanisms that begin at the time of trauma and last for hours or days. These mechanisms include: excitotoxicity, free-radical injury to cell membranes, altered blood–brain barrier (BBB) permeability, mitochondrial dysfunction, etc. The main goal of neurocritical care is to prevent secondary insults (such as hypotension, hypoxia, intracranial hypertension, etc.) to the injured brain [3–5]. These events, increasing and strengthening secondary brain injury, are associated with unfavorable neurological outcomes [3–5]. Endotracheal intubation and mechanical ventilation are often required in severe TBI with the aim to protect the airways from aspiration and to prevent the above-mentioned secondary insults, in particular hypoxemia and hypercapnia [6–8].

B. M. Mainini · M. Di Lecce · L. Cattani · V. Montanaro · M. Petranca · E. Picetti (✉)
Department of Anesthesia and Intensive Care, Parma University Hospital, Parma, Italy

C. Robba
Anesthesia and Intensive Care, San Martino Policlinico Hospital, IRCCS for Oncology and Neurosciences, Genoa, Italy

Department of Surgical Sciences and Integrated Diagnostics, University of Genoa, Genoa, Italy

E. Brogi et al. (eds.), *Traumatic Brain Injury*, Hot Topics in Acute Care Surgery and Trauma, https://doi.org/10.1007/978-3-031-50117-3_16

Invasive mechanical ventilation is also required in case of extracranial injuries and/or to manipulate the arterial partial pressure of carbon dioxide ($PaCO_2$) for intracranial pressure (ICP) management [5–8]. Moreover, during ICU stay, brain injured patients can develop severe respiratory failure and acute respiratory distress syndrome (ARDS) [9]. TBI may be a risk factor for ventilator-induced lung injury (VILI) [10]. In particular, brain injury is associated with an increase in pulmonary vascular hydrostatic pressure and endothelial permeability and triggers inflammatory mechanisms able to make the lung more susceptible to a mechanical injury induced by artificial ventilation [10, 11]. Pulmonary complications reported in TBI patients are associated with unfavorable neurological outcomes [9–11]. A lung-protective ventilation (LPV) strategy, with low tidal volumes (TVs) and moderate-to-high positive end-expiratory pressure (PEEP), has been shown to be associated with improved outcomes in patients with and without ARDS [12]. This approach, considering the potential adverse cerebrovascular effects, is challenging to be applied in TBI patients [6–8, 13]. Indeed, acute brain injured (ABI) patients have been excluded from studies exploring lung-protective ventilation strategies in ARDS [13]. However, a recent worldwide survey, from the European Society of Intensive Care Medicine (ESICM), showed a wide variability regarding the ventilatory management of TBI patients [14]. Recent guidelines for the management of mechanical ventilation in this population have demonstrated a low level of evidence on literature regarding this topic, and most recommendations are based on the experts' opinion [7].

This chapter focuses, in a practical way, on the setting of invasive mechanical ventilation and tracheotomy in TBI patients with and without concurrent respiratory failure.

16.2 Invasive Mechanical Ventilation in TBI Without Concomitant Respiratory Failure (Lung Injury)

After a brain injury, hypoventilation and aspiration can be a consequence of impaired consciousness and altered brainstem reflexes [6]. Current TBI management recommendations consider endotracheal intubation as mandatory when Glasgow Coma Score (GCS) is ≤ 8 [5, 7]. This maneuver should be considered also in case of loss of airway protective reflexes, severe agitation, and intracranial hypertension (Fig. 16.1) [7]. Techniques for tracheal intubation in TBI patients are beyond the scope of this chapter. We suggest readers to refer to several published reviews, guidelines, and textbooks on this topic.

Optimal settings of mechanical ventilation in TBI may contribute to secondary brain injury, due to interactions between cerebral and respiratory dynamics, affecting cerebral perfusion pressure (CPP), venous return, vasomotor tonus, and oxygen delivery [15]. LPV strategies have shown to have a beneficial impact on outcome in patients with and without ARDS [12]. In particular, the utilization of low TVs is

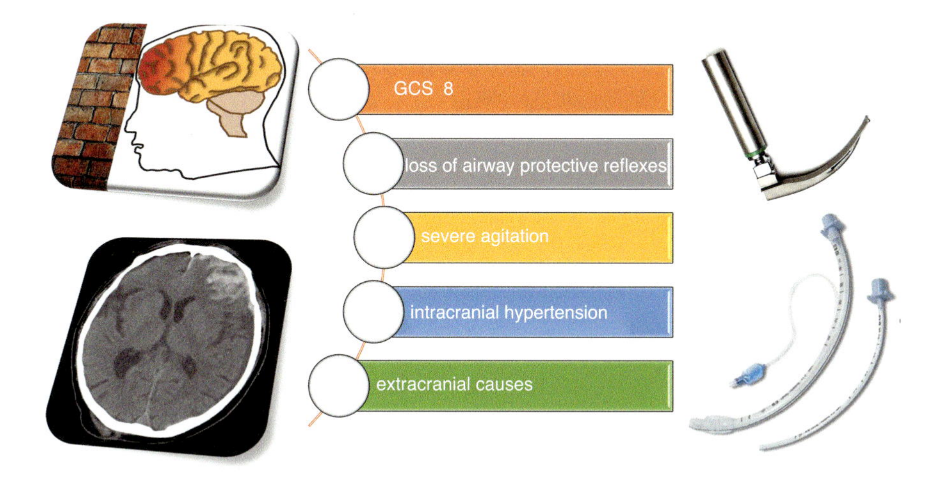

Fig. 16.1 Indications for endotracheal intubation in TBI patients. *GCS* Glasgow Coma Scale

associated with a reduced mortality in ARDS patients [16]. However, this approach can potentially cause hypercapnia, and in TBI patients the consequent intracranial cerebral vessel vasodilation can result in an increase in cerebral blood volume (CBV) and ICP [15].

Recently, literature suggest that the use of high TV [>9 mL/kg predicted body weight (PBW)] in TBI patients, with normal lung at ICU admission, is associated with the development of ARDS [17]. In a multicenter observational study, ABI patients had a comparable mean tidal volume compared to non-neurologic patients [18]. However, a significantly lower proportion of patients with intracranial hemorrhage received low TV probably because of the fear of hypercapnia [18]. Considering the above, prospective studies regarding low TVs are lacking in TBI and the optimal TV value still needs to be established in this setting. However, literature suggest that protective TV with the aim to maintain plateau pressure (Pplat) < 25–27 cmH_2O should be applied even in TBI patients in order to avoid VILI [7].

The application of PEEP is also an important component of LPV. PEEP reduces atelectasis and improves the arterial partial pressure of oxygen (PaO_2) and lung compliance. Traditionally, low PEEP levels (≤5 mmHg) have been utilized in ABI patients because of the potential risks on cerebral circulation and ICP; in particular, the effect of PEEP on ICP seems to be related to both hemodynamic factors and respiratory system compliance [6, 15]. Elevated PEEP levels may reduce systemic venous return, mean arterial pressure (MAP), and consequently CPP with detrimental consequences on cerebral blood flow (CBF), especially in cases of altered cerebral autoregulation [6, 15, 19]. Conversely, respiratory system compliance influences the effect of PEEP on ICP and brain circulation [20]. In patients with low compliance, a PEEP increase (up to 10–12 cmH_2O) is not associated with ICP increase; in contrast, in patients with normal compliance, PEEP induces lung overdistension, reduction in cerebral venous return, and ICP increases. In patients without lung injury, an initial PEEP of 5 cmH_2O set on respiratory mechanics and hemodynamics should be used, and ZEEP should be avoided [7].

Mechanical power, defined as the amount of energy transferred from the ventilator to the respiratory system per unit time (joules/minute), can be calculated utilizing an equation which takes into account TV, respiratory rate, PEEP, airway resistance, and inspiratory-to-expiratory time ratio [21]. A higher mechanical power has been associated with increased ICU mortality in patients with and without brain injury [22–24]. Further investigations in this field are needed.

Driving pressure (ΔP) is the difference between Pplat and PEEP. Higher values of ΔP (>15 cmH_2O) are associated with an increase in mortality in patients with ARDS independent of TV [25–27]. Increments in ΔP are associated with the development of ARDS in TBI patients [28, 29]. Additional studies are needed to confirm these findings.

Hyperoxia and hypoxia, being associated with poor outcome after ABI, should be avoided [7, 30]. A recent ESICM consensus conference recommends maintaining PaO_2 80–120 mmHg in TBI patients with or without intracranial hypertension [7]. These ranges are higher compared to those generally targeted in patients without ABI (PaO_2 55–80 mmHg) [16]. Future well powered studies are necessary to identify the optimal oxygenation targets in this setting. Moreover, the availability of brain oxygen monitoring can help to individualize the optimal PaO_2 [31]. Hypercapnia and hypocapnia are also dangerous for the injured brain and should be avoided [5, 7]. The above-mentioned consensus conference recommends maintaining $PaCO_2$ 35–45 mmHg in TBI patients without intracranial hypertension; no recommendations are provided in case of elevated ICP [7]. Short-term hyperventilation should be considered only in case of life-threatening brain herniation [7]. This last temporary maneuver might make sense especially while waiting for an emergent neurosurgical procedure. The Seattle International Severe Traumatic Brain Injury Consensus Conference (SIBICC) recommends mild hypocapnia ($PaCO_2$ 32–35 mmHg) as second tier treatment for intracranial hypertension in TBI [32]. Also in this case the availability of brain oxygen monitoring can help to personalize the $PaCO_2$ target [31].

Suggested ventilatory and respiratory targets are reported in Fig. 16.2.

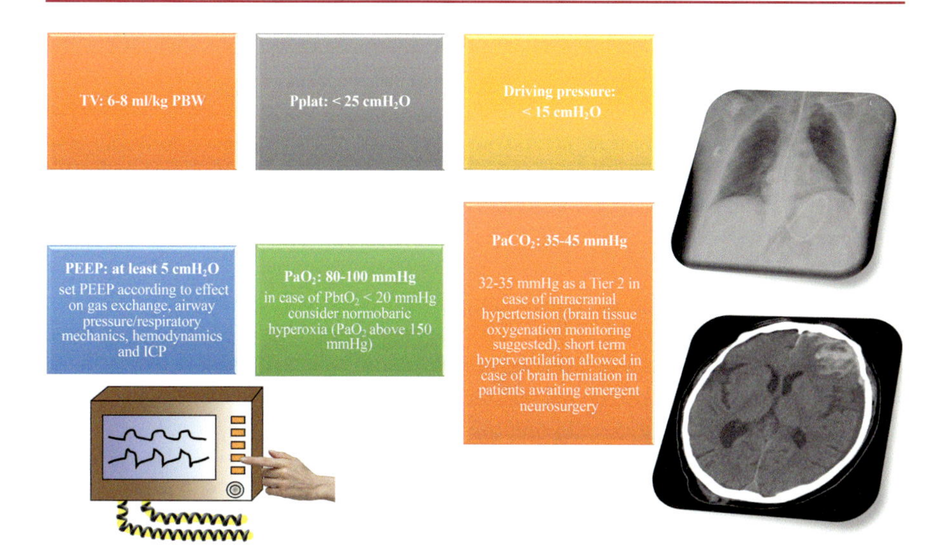

Fig. 16.2 Suggested ventilatory and respiratory targets in severe TBI patients without concomitant respiratory failure. *TV* tidal volume, *PBW* predicted body weight, *Pplat* plateau pressure, *PEEP* positive end-expiratory pressure, *ICP* intracranial pressure, PaO_2 arterial partial pressure of oxygen, $PbtO_2$ brain tissue oxygenation, $PaCO_2$ arterial partial pressure of carbon dioxide

16.3 Invasive Mechanical Ventilation in TBI With Concomitant Respiratory Failure (Lung Injury)

The management of patients with concurrent TBI and acute respiratory failure is a challenging scenario requiring an adequate pathophysiological knowledge. ABI patients are at increased risk of development of ARDS [10, 15]. This condition has been associated with higher mortality and worse neurological outcome [9]. The mechanism of TBI-associated ARDS is multifactorial [10, 11]. Brain injury causes the activation of the sympathoadrenal axis and a systemic inflammation response, especially during ICP crisis. The sympathetic surge, driven by hypothalamic pituitary pathway, causes vasoconstriction of peripheral vessels, leading to elevated systemic arterial pressure and pulmonary hydrostatic pressure resulting in pulmonary edema. The inflammatory response following TBI leads to increased inflammatory mediators causing end-organ damage, including ultrastructural changes in the type II pneumocytes in the lung and increased vascular permeability, which worsens pulmonary edema and ARDS [10, 11].

The ventilatory management of TBI (with or without polytrauma) can be difficult, as brain-specific ventilatory targets may be in conflict with lung-specific priorities [7, 13, 33]. TV/Pplat limitation and PEEP optimization are interventions utilized in ARDS patients to minimize additional lung injury and to improve outcomes [34]. Moreover, rescue therapies [neuromuscular blocking agents (NMBAs), recruitment maneuvers, prone positioning, inhaled nitric oxide (iNO), and extracorporeal membrane oxygenation (ECMO)] are increasingly used in severe ARDS as part of a stepwise algorithm for refractory hypoxemia [34].

The main target for clinicians managing TBI patients is to ensure that the chosen ventilatory strategy minimizes the risk of secondary brain injury, avoiding hypoxemia with a PaO_2 target 80–120 mmHg, higher compared to the range commonly targeted in the general ICU population (55–80 mmHg) [7]. Low TVs (4–6 mL/kg PBW), utilized in case of severe ARDS, may require the tolerance of higher $PaCO_2$ values than those preferable in case of intracranial hypertension, and the level of PEEP needed for clinically significant pulmonary benefits may lead to a reduction in MAP and CPP [6, 15, 33]. In addition, a significant subset of TBI patients have concurrent spinal injuries and prone positioning might be unsafe, the use of NMBA may delay neurologic examination, and ECMO can be difficult to apply since it usually requires systemic anticoagulation that may have catastrophic consequences in patients who have suffered a recent injury [7]. Data supporting the efficacy of these measures are limited in patients with TBI. Where ARDS and TBI coexist, a fine balance must be found between $PaCO_2$ control and lungs protection. Considering the mortality benefits of LPV in ARDS [16], recent data shows that clinicians feel increasingly comfortable applying LPV in patients with ABI [14]. Although low TVs can potentially cause hypercapnia and consequent intracranial cerebral vessel vasodilation, especially in those with low baseline intracranial compliance, the use of high TVs in TBI patients (>9 mL/kg PBW) with normal lung at ICU admission is associated with the development of ARDS [17]. Prospective studies regarding low TVs are lacking in TBI and the optimal TV value still needs to be established in this setting. Balancing the risks and benefits of LPV, a recent ESICM consensus strongly recommends to use an LPV in TBI patients with ARDS without simultaneous concerns for raised ICP [7]. As a practical starting point, clinicians should aim to maintain TV at 4–8 mL/kg PBW and Pplat <30 cmH_2O [5]. The same consensus weakly recommends to consider an LPV in TBI patients without ARDS and elevated ICP [7]. In case of concurrent clinically significant ICP elevation and ARDS, ventilatory parameters should be individualized (with an adequate neuro- and respiratory monitoring) with the goal to reduce ICP while minimizing the potential for VILI [5, 7].

Proper use of PEEP in the ARDS can improve oxygenation and lung compliance, reduce intrapulmonary shunting, and prevent alveolar derecruitment [34, 35]. However, the incorrect setting of higher levels of PEEP can lead to barotrauma and alveolar overdistension with increased dead space resulting in higher $PaCO_2$ levels [34, 35]. Elevated PEEP levels may also reduce systemic venous return, MAP, and consequently CPP with detrimental consequences on CBF [6, 15, 19, 33]. In TBI patients with ARDS, the effects of PEEP on brain circulation may differ depending on respiratory system compliance: in patients with low compliance, increased PEEP may result in alveolar recruitment (with a direct benefit on PaO_2 and $PbtO_2$) without ICP increases [20, 36]; in contrast, in patients with normal compliance, PEEP may lead to lung overdistension, hypotension, reduced cerebral venous return, and increased ICP [20]. Patients with greater lung recruitment have an improvement in

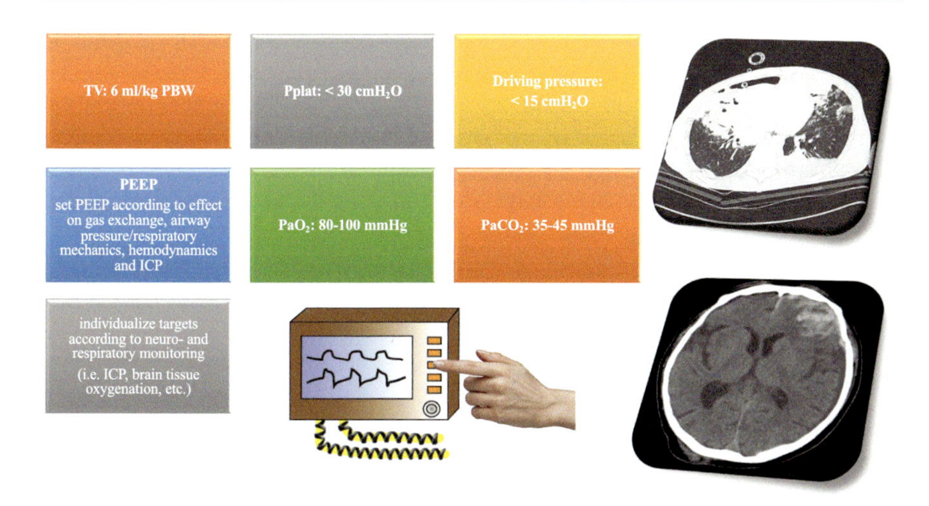

Fig. 16.3 Suggested ventilatory and respiratory targets in severe TBI patients with concomitant respiratory failure. *TV* tidal volume, *PBW* predicted body weight, *Pplat* plateau pressure, *PEEP* positive end-expiratory pressure, *ICP* intracranial pressure, PaO_2 arterial partial pressure of oxygen, $PaCO_2$ arterial partial pressure of carbon dioxide

the lung gas distribution not resulting in ICP increase, while non-recruiters have an over-inflation of already aerated areas with a negative impact on dead space and possibly on venous return [37]. PEEP may have a detrimental effect on ICP only when it causes alveolar hyperinflation leading to a significant increase in $PaCO_2$, whereas when PEEP leads to alveolar recruitment, ICP does not change [37]. In the VENTILO (VENTILatOry strategies in patients with severe traumatic brain injury) survey, the most utilized highest PEEP target among patients without intracranial hypertension was 15 cmH_2O, regardless of oxygenation [PaO_2/fraction of inspired oxygen (FiO_2) >300, PaO_2/FiO_2 300–150, $PaO_2/FiO_2 < 150$]. Conversely, in patients with intracranial hypertension, the most widely used PEEP was 5 cmH_2O for $PaO_2/FiO_2 > 300$ and 10 cmH_2O for PaO_2/FiO_2 150–300 and < 150 [14]. If intracranial hypertension and ARDS coexist, PEEP should be used to improve cerebral oxygenation. In this case, the response to PEEP should always be assessed by monitoring Pplat, PaO_2, $PaCO_2$, MAP, CPP, and ICP [15, 33].

Suggested ventilatory and respiratory targets in patients with concomitant lung and brain injury are reported in Fig. 16.3.

16.3.1 Rescue Therapies

In refractory respiratory failure, several rescue maneuvers are generally employed as adjuncts to invasive mechanical ventilation [14, 34, 35]. According to the VENTILO survey, neuromuscular blockade is the most commonly used rescue strategy [14]. This may be related also to its potential beneficial effect on intracranial hypertension control [32, 38]. Studies on the use of NMBAs as rescue therapy for patients with concurrent TBI and ARDS are not available. In this setting, based on evidence suggesting beneficial effects in severe ARDS [38], the short-term use of NMBAs, in combination with appropriate sedation, may be considered if targets (primarily $PaCO_2$ and ICP) cannot be achieved with sedation only [7, 33].

Recruitment maneuvers, being short and controlled increases in airway pressure with the goal of restoring ventilation in collapsed alveolar spaces, may improve pulmonary gas exchange and respiratory mechanics in respiratory failure [34, 35]. Available guidelines are controversial regarding their routinely utilization in the care of ARDS [34, 35]. The limited data available in ABI patients have demonstrated that RMs can harm cerebral oxygenation reducing venous return and CPP and causing elevation in ICP [33]. Hence, RMs should be considered on a case-by-case basis and with an appropriate neuromonitoring (i.e. ICP). In this regard, no recommendations were provided from the ESICM consensus [7].

Prone position is frequently used in ARDS patients because of its ability to improve ventilation/perfusion ratio, to increase end-expiratory lung volume, and to decrease VILI by ameliorating the distribution of the TV [35, 39]. This maneuver can improve mortality in ARDS if applied for more than 16 h/day and in patients with a $PaO_2/FiO_2 < 150$ [35, 39]. Small studies have been published so far in ABI patients: in this situation, despite an improvement in systemic/brain oxygenation, an increase in ICP was observed in case of impairment of cerebral venous drainage caused by the head and neck positioning [26, 40–42]. In addition, in this setting, the risk of removal/dislodgement of ICP bolts/drains is elevated; therefore, the maneuver should be carried out with great care. Considering the beneficial effect on gas exchange and on brain oxygenation, the prone position could be reasonably considered in mechanically ventilated patients with concomitant moderate or severe ARDS (PaO_2/FiO_2 ratio < 150) when ICP is not increased and under strict multimodal neuromonitoring [7]. ICP monitoring can be used to facilitate the positioning avoiding the above-mentioned adverse effects. The recommended position is a 30° head-up tilt combined with a straight head position [13]. Among patients with intracranial hypertension, no recommendations were provided from the ESICM consensus [7].

Considering its pulmonary vasodilative effect (in ventilated alveoli), iNO has been utilized in case of ARDS-refractory hypoxemia to optimize the ventilation perfusion matching [35]. However, the use of iNO in TBI patients with intracranial hypertension and ARDS has been reported only in a few case reports [27, 43, 44]. In these scenarios, iNO improved oxygenation without significant adverse effects on ICP and CPP, suggesting a benefit through improved oxygenation and a reduction in biochemical markers of inflammation and brain injury. Nevertheless, further studies of the effects of iNO in this setting are necessary and there are currently no recommendations on its use in TBI patients [7].

Extracorporeal oxygenation techniques, such as venovenous ECMO (VV-ECMO), are useful temporary lifesaving strategies applied in severe ARDS

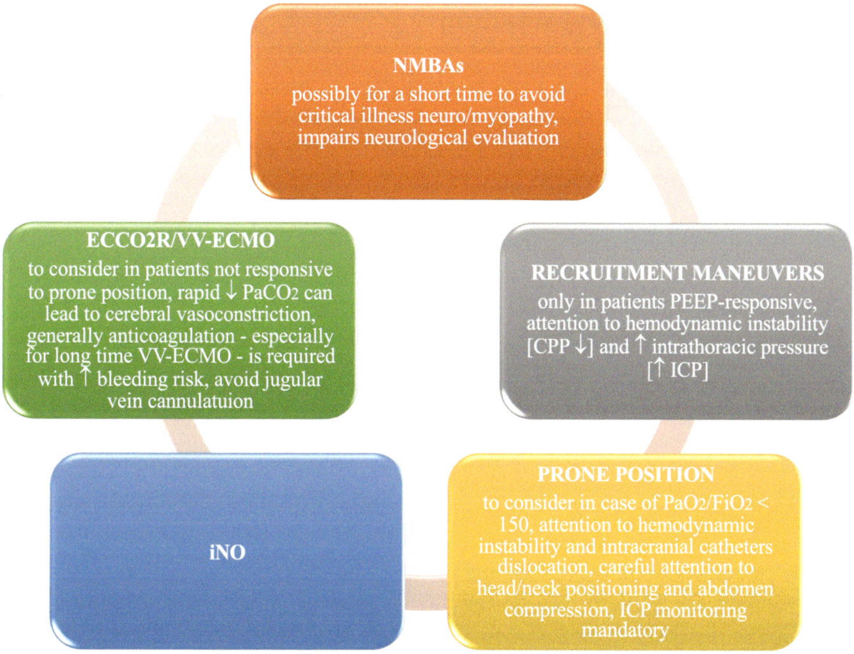

NMBAs
possibly for a short time to avoid critical illness neuro/myopathy, impairs neurological evaluation

RECRUITMENT MANEUVERS
only in patients PEEP-responsive, attention to hemodynamic instability [CPP ↓] and ↑ intrathoracic pressure [↑ ICP]

PRONE POSITION
to consider in case of PaO2/FiO2 < 150, attention to hemodynamic instability and intracranial catheters dislocation, careful attention to head/neck positioning and abdomen compression, ICP monitoring mandatory

iNO

ECCO2R/VV-ECMO
to consider in patients not responsive to prone position, rapid ↓ PaCO2 can lead to cerebral vasoconstriction, generally anticoagulation - especially for long time VV-ECMO - is required with ↑ bleeding risk, avoid jugular vein cannulatuion

Fig. 16.4 Suggested rescue (respiratory) therapies in severe TBI patients with concomitant respiratory failure. *NMBAs* neuromuscular blocking agents, *PEEP* positive end-expiratory pressure, *CPP* cerebral perfusion pressure, *ICP* intracranial pressure, PaO_2 arterial partial pressure of oxygen, FiO_2 inspired oxygen fraction, *iNO* inhaled nitric oxide, *ECCO2R* extracorporeal carbon dioxide removal, *VV-ECMO* venovenous extracorporeal membrane oxygenation, $PaCO_2$ arterial partial pressure of carbon dioxide

patients when conventional strategies have failed [35]. The experience with ECMO and extracorporeal CO_2 removal ($ECCO_2R$) in TBI patients with severe respiratory failure is limited due to serious hemorrhagic concerns related to the consequences of these techniques [45–48]. Moreover, improvements in ECMO technology, including the use of centrifugal pumps and heparin-coated circuits, are progressively reducing the amount of heparin required, with studies showing that short durations of heparin-free ECMO are feasible and not accompanied by increased circuit clotting or oxygenator dysfunction [33, 49]. Despite the large number of complications associated with this treatment, the decision to start VV-ECMO in TBI patients should be considered in case of refractory respiratory failure: patient selection, timing, as well as a multidisciplinary approach, are crucial for achieving success. For this reason, no consensus or guidelines are currently available on the use of these techniques in this population [7].

Suggestions about rescue respiratory therapies are reported in Fig. 16.4.

16.4 Extubation and Weaning

Liberation from invasive mechanical ventilation at the earliest possible time is a widely accepted principle in the ICU and is composed of two successive phases: weaning of pressure support (ventilator) and removal of endotracheal tube [50]. Classic extubation criteria have been established in the general critical care setting, targeting pulmonary function and cooperativeness of the patient [50]. First, readiness to breathe unsupported by the ventilator is gauged by a spontaneous breathing trial (SBT) [50]. ABI patients can successfully pass SBT but fail the extubation (or delay it) due to neurological and respiratory impairment [51, 52]. Particularly, the anatomical site of the injury may affect central respiratory centers and their connections, with impaired respiratory drive, impaired swallowing reflex, and airway control [34, 53, 54]. Before to start weaning, clinicians must ensure that patients do not require ongoing sedation for management of ICP, seizures or for precise regulation of $PaCO_2$ and PaO_2 because these will become less predictable in assisted modes. Appropriate candidates for initiation of ventilator liberation include patients who can tolerate sedation interruption, who have a sufficient respiratory drive, and who are expected to continue on a trajectory of clinical improvement [34].

It is not easy to identify clinical parameters predicting a possible extubation failure or success; it is also unclear the patient who can directly benefit from tracheostomy without an extubation attempt [55]. ABI patients have not been considered in international guidelines regarding the weaning from invasive mechanical ventilation [8], and the latest guidelines in neurocritical care patients highlight the poor level of evidence for extubation management or the use of tracheostomy [7]. Extubation failure is defined as the need for reintubation after the first planned or accidental extubation attempt [56], and even if there is no consensus about its time frame, current trends tend to extend the time definition to 5–7 days to better differentiate early failure from cardiorespiratory incompetency to a real neurologic and airway impairment [8, 52]. In neurocritical care patients, extubation failure rates are higher than that of the general ICU population, ranging from 17 to 40%, with a negative burden in terms of outcome and mortality [8, 51]. Conversely, delaying extubation increases the risk of ventilator-associated pneumonia (VAP) with longer ICU-length of stay (LOS) and higher healthcare costs, without giving a guarantee of success in the extubation attempt [6, 51]. Previous studies have identified various clinical features compatible with successful extubation, and specific scores were developed [52, 57, 58]. While some authors suggested the use of GCS score to find the correct timing [59, 60], others observed no association between GCS and extubation [51, 52, 57]. Asehnoune et al. performed a multicentric study including 437 severely brain-damaged patients and identified several factors predicting successful extubation such as: GCS >10 on the day of extubation, age <40 years old, visual pursuit, and attempts of swallowing [58]. These items composed the VISAGE score which is, at present, one of the most appropriate tests for predicting extubation readiness (90% extubation success for 3 points) [58]. Other factors associated with successful extubation identified in observational studies were: preserved upper airway reflexes, younger age, and negative fluid balance [52, 57]. However, all these

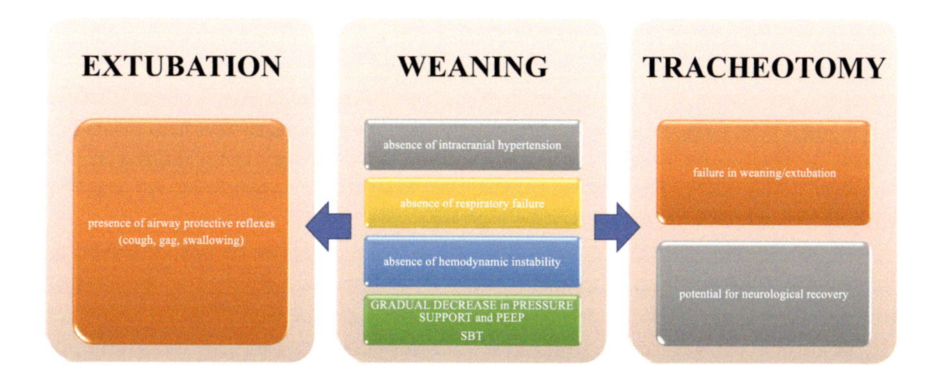

Early Tracheotomy

- to consider in case of good ICP control
- brain CT features (i.e. intracranial hemorrhage, posterior fossa involvement compatible with long time of mechanical ventilation and impairment of airway protective reflexes)
- possible ↓: invasive mechanical ventilation time, VAP, ICU/hospital LOS

Fig. 16.5 Suggestions for respiratory weaning, extubation, and tracheotomy in severe TBI patients. *PEEP* positive end-expiratory pressure, *SBT* spontaneous breathing trial, *ICP* intracranial pressure, *CT* computed tomography, *VAP* ventilator-associated pneumonia, *ICU* intensive care unit, *LOS* length of stay

studies are often monocentric [52, 61] and have methodological limitations which preclude definite conclusions [62]. Recently, the "Extubation Strategies in Neuro-Intensive Care Unit Patients and Associations with Outcomes" (ENIO) study was performed to describe the current management of weaning from invasive ventilation, focusing on decisions on timing of extubation and tracheostomy in ABI patients admitted to the ICU [55]. This international multicenter observational study showed that extubation failure is common and associated with unfavorable outcomes in neurocritical care patients and the authors created a score, combining the level of arousal, upper airway function, and general ICU features which could predict extubation success in this population with good accuracy [55, 63]. In conclusion, as stated also by the ESICM consensus [7], the evaluation of airway protective reflexes (cough, gag, swallowing) and the level of consciousness should be taken into account prior to extubation.

Suggestions for weaning and extubation are reported in Fig. 16.5.

16.5 Tracheotomy

The choice to perform a tracheotomy in patients with severe TBI is influenced by several neurological and non-neurological factors. The indication and the timing of this maneuver are controversial, with great variability among different centers [64]. A recent European multicenter study, involving 1358 TBI patients, showed that brain injured patients underwent tracheostomy more frequently than the general ICU population (31.8% vs. 10%, respectively) [64]. Among the 433 tracheostomized brain injured patients, age, GCS ≤ 8, unreactive pupils and the presence of early secondary insults (hypoxemia e/o thoracic trauma) were the main predictive factors for need of tracheostomy [64]. In patients at higher risk of extubation failure (i.e. difficulties in the management of secretions, absence of protective airway reflexes) tracheotomy can facilitate weaning, potentially shortening the duration of MV/ICU LOS and reducing complications from prolonged tracheal intubation such as VAP or tracheal lesions [8].

Conventionally, tracheostomies performed in the first week are classified as early, while tracheostomies performed later than 7 days are defined as late [65]. In some patients with TBI for whom prolonged mechanical ventilation is expected, primary tracheostomy without an extubation attempt is a frequent consideration; rates of primary tracheostomy of 18–21% have been reported among mechanically ventilated patients with brain injury [55, 66]. Observational studies and systematic review involving TBI patients suggest that performing early tracheostomy may reduce the duration of mechanical ventilation, with lower incidence of pneumonia, ICU, and hospital LOS. However, no differences in mortality have been identified between early and late tracheostomy so far [61, 67]. In patients with TBI for whom the expected duration of mechanical ventilation is uncertain, there are no clear data regarding when tracheostomy should be performed. The current recommendation is to consider tracheostomy in patients failing one or more extubation attempts and in whom there is a persistent decrease in the level of consciousness with an expected acceptable quality of life [7].

Suggestions for tracheotomy are reported in Fig. 16.5.

16.6 Conclusions

The respiratory management of TBI patient require in-depth knowledge of the "brain-lung crosstalk." The monitoring of brain and lung function is essential to provide the best possible care in this challenging scenario.

References

1. Maas AI, Menon DK, Manley GT, Abrams M, Åkerlund C, Andelic N, Aries M, Bashford T, Bell MJ, Bodien YG, Brett BL, Büki A, Chesnut RM, Citerio G, Clark D, Clasby B, Cooper DJ, Czeiter E, Czosnyka M, Dams-O'Connor K, De Keyser V, Diaz-Arrastia R, Ercole A, van Essen TA, Falvey É, Ferguson AR, Figaji A, Fitzgerald M, Foreman B, Gantner D, Gao G, Giacino J, Gravesteijn B, Guiza F, Gupta D, Gurnell M, Haagsma JA, Hammond FM, Hawryluk G, Hutchinson P, van der Jagt M, Jain S, Jain S, Jiang JY, Kent H, Kolias A, Kompanje EJO, Lecky F, Lingsma HF, Maegele M, Majdan M, Markowitz A, McCrea M, Meyfroidt G, Mikolić A, Mondello S, Mukherjee P, Nelson D, Nelson LD, Newcombe V, Okonkwo D, Orešič M, Peul W, Pisică D, Polinder S, Ponsford J, Puybasset L, Raj R, Robba C, Røe C, Rosand J, Schueler P, Sharp DJ, Smielewski P, Stein MB, von Steinbüchel N, Stewart W, Steyerberg EW, Stocchetti N, Temkin N, Tenovuo O, Theadom A, Thomas I, Espin AT, Turgeon AF, Unterberg A, Van Praag D, van Veen E, Verheyden J, Vyvere TV, Wang KKW, Wiegers EJA, Williams WH, Wilson L, Wisniewski SR, Younsi A, Yue JK, Yuh EL,

Zeiler FA, Zeldovich M, Zemek R, InTBIR Participants and Investigators. Traumatic brain injury: progress and challenges in prevention, clinical care, and research. Lancet Neurol. 2022;21(11):1004–60. Epub 2022 Sep 29. Erratum in: Lancet Neurol. 2022 Oct 7;: PMID: 36183712. https://doi.org/10.1016/S1474-4422(22)00309-X.

2. Marshall LF. Head injury: recent past, present, and future. Neurosurgery. 2000;47(3):546–61. PMID: 10981741. https://doi.org/10.1097/00006123-200009000-00002.
3. Stocchetti N, Carbonara M, Citerio G, Ercole A, Skrifvars MB, Smielewski P, Zoerle T, Menon DK. Severe traumatic brain injury: targeted management in the intensive care unit. Lancet Neurol. 2017;16(6):452–64. PMID: 28504109. https://doi.org/10.1016/S1474-4422(17)30118-7.
4. Picetti E, Rossi S, Ottochian M, Stein DM. Brain injury in the ACS patient: nuts and bolts of neuromonitoring and management. In: Picetti E, Pereira B, Razek T, Narayan M, Kashuk J, editors. Intensive Care for Emergency Surgeons. Hot topics in acute care surgery and trauma. Cham: Springer; 2019. https://doi.org/10.1007/978-3-030-11830-3_6.
5. Meyfroidt G, Bouzat P, Casaer MP, Chesnut R, Hamada SR, Helbok R, Hutchinson P, Maas AIR, Manley G, Menon DK, Newcombe VFJ, Oddo M, Robba C, Shutter L, Smith M, Steyerberg EW, Stocchetti N, Taccone FS, Wilson L, Zanier ER, Citerio G. Management of moderate to severe traumatic brain injury: an update for the intensivist. Intensive Care Med. 2022;48(6):649–66. https://doi.org/10.1007/s00134-022-06702-4.
6. Asehnoune K, Roquilly A, Cinotti R. Respiratory management in patients with severe brain injury. Crit Care. 2018;22(1):76. PMID: 29558976; PMCID: PMC5861645. https://doi.org/10.1186/s13054-018-1994-0.
7. Robba C, Poole D, McNett M, Asehnoune K, Bösel J, Bruder N, Chieregato A, Cinotti R, Duranteau J, Einav S, Ercole A, Ferguson N, Guerin C, Siempos II, Kurtz P, Juffermans NP, Mancebo J, Mascia L, McCredie V, Nin N, Oddo M, Pelosi P, Rabinstein AA, Neto AS, Seder DB, Skrifvars MB, Suarez JI, Taccone FS, van der Jagt M, Citerio G, Stevens RD. Mechanical ventilation in patients with acute brain injury: recommendations of the European Society of Intensive Care Medicine consensus. Intensive Care Med. 2020;46(12):2397–410. https://doi.org/10.1007/s00134-020-06283-0.
8. Cinotti R, Bouras M, Roquilly A, Asehnoune K. Management and weaning from mechanical ventilation in neurologic patients. Ann Transl Med. 2018;6(19):381. PMID: 30460255; PMCID: PMC6212362. https://doi.org/10.21037/atm.2018.08.16.
9. Rincon F, Ghosh S, Dey S, Maltenfort M, Vibbert M, Urtecho J, McBride W, Moussouttas M, Bell R, Ratliff JK, Jallo J. Impact of acute lung injury and acute respiratory distress syndrome after traumatic brain injury in the United States. Neurosurgery. 2012;71(4):795–803. PMID: 22855028. https://doi.org/10.1227/NEU.0b013e3182672ae5.
10. Blanch L, Quintel M. Lung-brain cross talk in the critically ill. Intensive Care Med. 2017;43(4):557–9. Epub 2016 Oct 6. PMID: 27714405. https://doi.org/10.1007/s00134-016-4583-1.
11. Pelosi P, Rocco PR. The lung and the brain: a dangerous cross-talk. Crit Care. 2011;15(3):168. Epub 2011 Jun 30. PMID: 21722336; PMCID: PMC3219008. https://doi.org/10.1186/cc10259.
12. Serpa Neto A, Hemmes SN, Barbas CS, Beiderlinden M, Biehl M, Binnekade JM, Canet J, Fernandez-Bustamante A, Futier E, Gajic O, Hedenstierna G, Hollmann MW, Jaber S, Kozian A, Licker M, Lin WQ, Maslow AD, Memtsoudis SG, Reis Miranda D, Moine P, Ng T, Paparella D, Putensen C, Ranieri M, Scavonetto F, Schilling T, Schmid W, Selmo G, Severgnini P, Sprung J, Sundar S, Talmor D, Treschan T, Unzueta C, Weingarten TN, Wolthuis EK, Wrigge H, Gama de Abreu M, Pelosi P, Schultz MJ, PROVE Network Investigators. Protective versus conventional ventilation for surgery: a systematic review and individual patient data meta-analysis. Anesthesiology. 2015;123(1):66–78. PMID: 25978326. https://doi.org/10.1097/ALN.0000000000000706.
13. Della Torre V, Badenes R, Corradi F, Racca F, Lavinio A, Matta B, Bilotta F, Robba C. Acute respiratory distress syndrome in traumatic brain injury: how do we manage it? J Thorac Dis.

2017;9(12):5368–81. PMID: 29312748; PMCID: PMC5756968. https://doi.org/10.21037/jtd.2017.11.03.
14. Picetti E, Pelosi P, Taccone FS, Citerio G, Mancebo J, Robba C, on the behalf of the ESICM NIC/ARF Sections. VENTILatOry strategies in patients with severe traumatic brain injury: the VENTILO Survey of the European Society of Intensive Care Medicine (ESICM). Crit Care. 2020;24(1):158. PMID: 32303255; PMCID: PMC7165367. https://doi.org/10.1186/s13054-020-02875-w.
15. Oddo M, Citerio G. ARDS in the brain-injured patient: what's different? Intensive Care Med. 2016;42(5):790–3. Epub 2016 Mar 11. PMID: 26969670. https://doi.org/10.1007/s00134-016-4298-3.
16. Network ARDS, Brower RG, Matthay MA, Morris A, Schoenfeld D, Thompson BT, Wheeler A. Ventilation with lower tidal volumes as compared with traditional tidal volumes for acute lung injury and the acute respiratory distress syndrome. N Engl J Med. 2000;342(18):1301–8. PMID: 10793162. https://doi.org/10.1056/NEJM200005043421801.
17. Mascia L, Zavala E, Bosma K, Pasero D, Decaroli D, Andrews P, Isnardi D, Davi A, Arguis MJ, Berardino M, Ducati A, Brain IT Group. High tidal volume is associated with the development of acute lung injury after severe brain injury: an international observational study. Crit Care Med. 2007;35(8):1815–20. PMID: 17568331. https://doi.org/10.1097/01.CCM.0000275269.77467.DF.
18. Pelosi P, Ferguson ND, Frutos-Vivar F, Anzueto A, Putensen C, Raymondos K, Apezteguia C, Desmery P, Hurtado J, Abroug F, Elizalde J, Tomicic V, Cakar N, Gonzalez M, Arabi Y, Moreno R, Esteban A, Ventila Study Group. Management and outcome of mechanically ventilated neurologic patients. Crit Care Med. 2011;39(6):1482–92. PMID: 21378554. https://doi.org/10.1097/CCM.0b013e31821209a8.
19. Muench E, Bauhuf C, Roth H, Horn P, Phillips M, Marquetant N, Quintel M, Vajkoczy P. Effects of positive end-expiratory pressure on regional cerebral blood flow, intracranial pressure, and brain tissue oxygenation. Crit Care Med. 2005;33(10):2367–72. PMID: 16215394. https://doi.org/10.1097/01.ccm.0000181732.37319.df.
20. Caricato A, Conti G, Della Corte F, Mancino A, Santilli F, Sandroni C, Proietti R, Antonelli M. Effects of PEEP on the intracranial system of patients with head injury and subarachnoid hemorrhage: the role of respiratory system compliance. J Trauma. 2005;58(3):571–6. PMID: 15761353. https://doi.org/10.1097/01.ta.0000152806.19198.db.
21. Gattinoni L, Tonetti T, Cressoni M, Cadringher P, Herrmann P, Moerer O, Protti A, Gotti M, Chiurazzi C, Carlesso E, Chiumello D, Quintel M. Ventilator-related causes of lung injury: the mechanical power. Intensive Care Med. 2016;42(10):1567–75. PMID: 27620287. https://doi.org/10.1007/s00134-016-4505-2.
22. Serpa Neto A, Deliberato RO, Johnson AEW, Bos LD, Amorim P, Pereira SM, Cazati DC, Cordioli RL, Correa TD, Pollard TJ, Schettino GPP, Timenetsky KT, Celi LA, Pelosi P, Gama de Abreu M, Schultz MJ, PROVE Network Investigators. Mechanical power of ventilation is associated with mortality in critically ill patients: an analysis of patients in two observational cohorts. Intensive Care Med. 2018;44(11):1914–22. PMID: 30291378. https://doi.org/10.1007/s00134-018-5375-6.
23. Zhang Z, Zheng B, Liu N, Ge H, Hong Y. Mechanical power normalized to predicted body weight as a predictor of mortality in patients with acute respiratory distress syndrome. Intensive Care Med. 2019;45(6):856–64. PMID: 31062050. https://doi.org/10.1007/s00134-019-05627-9.
24. Jiang X, Zhu Y, Zhen S, Wang L. Mechanical power of ventilation is associated with mortality in neurocritical patients: a cohort study. J Clin Monit Comput. 2022;36(6):1621–8. PMID: 35059914; PMCID: PMC9637601. https://doi.org/10.1007/s10877-022-00805-5.
25. Amato MB, Meade MO, Slutsky AS, Brochard L, Costa EL, Schoenfeld DA, Stewart TE, Briel M, Talmor D, Mercat A, Richard JC, Carvalho CR, Brower RG. Driving pressure and survival in the acute respiratory distress syndrome. N Engl J Med. 2015;372(8):747–55. PMID: 25693014. https://doi.org/10.1056/NEJMsa1410639.

26. Nekludov M, Bellander BM, Mure M. Oxygenation and cerebral perfusion pressure improved in the prone position. Acta Anaesthesiol Scand. 2006;50(8):932–6. PMID: 16923086. https://doi.org/10.1111/j.1399-6576.2006.01099.x.
27. Vavilala MS, Roberts JS, Moore AE, Newell DW, Lam AM. The influence of inhaled nitric oxide on cerebral blood flow and metabolism in a child with traumatic brain injury. Anesth Analg. 2001;93(2):351–3. PMID: 11473859. https://doi.org/10.1097/00000539-200108000-00023.
28. Thiara S, Griesdale DE, Henderson WR, Sekhon MS. Effect of cerebral perfusion pressure on acute respiratory distress syndrome. Can J Neurol Sci. 2018;45(3):313–9. PMID: 29455690. https://doi.org/10.1017/cjn.2017.292.
29. Tejerina E, Pelosi P, Muriel A, Peñuelas O, Sutherasan Y, Frutos-Vivar F, Nin N, Davies AR, Rios F, Violi DA, Raymondos K, Hurtado J, González M, Du B, Amin P, Maggiore SM, Thille AW, Soares MA, Jibaja M, Villagomez AJ, Kuiper MA, Koh Y, Moreno RP, Zeggwagh AA, Matamis D, Anzueto A, Ferguson ND, Esteban A, for VENTILA Group. Association between ventilatory settings and development of acute respiratory distress syndrome in mechanically ventilated patients due to brain injury. J Crit Care. 2017;38:341–5. PMID: 27914908. https://doi.org/10.1016/j.jcrc.2016.11.010.
30. Davis DP, Meade W, Sise MJ, Kennedy F, Simon F, Tominaga G, Steele J, Coimbra R. Both hypoxemia and extreme hyperoxemia may be detrimental in patients with severe traumatic brain injury. J Neurotrauma. 2009;26(12):2217–23. PMID: 19811093. https://doi.org/10.1089/neu.2009.0940.
31. Chesnut R, Aguilera S, Buki A, Bulger E, Citerio G, Cooper DJ, Arrastia RD, Diringer M, Figaji A, Gao G, Geocadin R, Ghajar J, Harris O, Hoffer A, Hutchinson P, Joseph M, Kitagawa R, Manley G, Mayer S, Menon DK, Meyfroidt G, Michael DB, Oddo M, Okonkwo D, Patel M, Robertson C, Rosenfeld JV, Rubiano AM, Sahuquillo J, Servadei F, Shutter L, Stein D, Stocchetti N, Taccone FS, Timmons S, Tsai E, Ullman JS, Vespa P, Videtta W, Wright DW, Zammit C, Hawryluk GWJ. A management algorithm for adult patients with both brain oxygen and intracranial pressure monitoring: the Seattle International Severe Traumatic Brain Injury Consensus Conference (SIBICC). Intensive Care Med. 2020;46(5):919–29. Epub 2020 Jan 21. PMID: 31965267; PMCID: PMC7210240. https://doi.org/10.1007/s00134-019-05900-x.
32. Hawryluk GWJ, Aguilera S, Buki A, Bulger E, Citerio G, Cooper DJ, Arrastia RD, Diringer M, Figaji A, Gao G, Geocadin R, Ghajar J, Harris O, Hoffer A, Hutchinson P, Joseph M, Kitagawa R, Manley G, Mayer S, Menon DK, Meyfroidt G, Michael DB, Oddo M, Okonkwo D, Patel M, Robertson C, Rosenfeld JV, Rubiano AM, Sahuquillo J, Servadei F, Shutter L, Stein D, Stocchetti N, Taccone FS, Timmons S, Tsai E, Ullman JS, Vespa P, Videtta W, Wright DW, Zammit C, Chesnut RM. A management algorithm for patients with intracranial pressure monitoring: the Seattle International Severe Traumatic Brain Injury Consensus Conference (SIBICC). Intensive Care Med. 2019;45(12):1783–94. Epub 2019 Oct 28. PMID: 31659383; PMCID: PMC6863785. https://doi.org/10.1007/s00134-019-05805-9.
33. Taran S, Cho SM, Stevens RD. Mechanical ventilation in patients with traumatic brain injury: is it so different? Neurocrit Care. 2022;38:178. Epub ahead of print. PMID: 36071333. https://doi.org/10.1007/s12028-022-01593-1.
34. Fan E, Del Sorbo L, Goligher EC, Hodgson CL, Munshi L, Walkey AJ, Adhikari NKJ, Amato MBP, Branson R, Brower RG, Ferguson ND, Gajic O, Gattinoni L, Hess D, Mancebo J, Meade MO, McAuley DF, Pesenti A, Ranieri VM, Rubenfeld GD, Rubin E, Seckel M, Slutsky AS, Talmor D, Thompson BT, Wunsch H, Uleryk E, Brozek J, Brochard LJ, American Thoracic Society, European Society of Intensive Care Medicine, and Society of Critical Care Medicine. An Official American Thoracic Society/European Society of Intensive Care Medicine/Society of Critical Care Medicine Clinical Practice Guideline: Mechanical Ventilation in Adult Patients with Acute Respiratory Distress Syndrome. Am J Respir Crit Care Med. 2017;195(9):1253–63. Erratum in: Am J Respir Crit Care Med. 2017 Jun 1;195(11):1540. PMID: 28459336. https://doi.org/10.1164/rccm.201703-0548ST.
35. Fan E, Brodie D, Slutsky AS. Acute respiratory distress syndrome: advances in diagnosis and treatment. JAMA. 2018;319(7):698–710. PMID: 29466596. https://doi.org/10.1001/jama.2017.21907.

36. Nemer SN, Caldeira JB, Santos RG, Guimarães BL, Garcia JM, Prado D, Silva RT, Azeredo LM, Faria ER, Souza PC. Effects of positive end-expiratory pressure on brain tissue oxygen pressure of severe traumatic brain injury patients with acute respiratory distress syndrome: a pilot study. J Crit Care. 2015;30(6):1263–6. Epub 2015 Jul 26. PMID: 26307004. https://doi.org/10.1016/j.jcrc.2015.07.019.
37. Robba C, Ball L, Nogas S, Battaglini D, Messina A, Brunetti I, Minetti G, Castellan L, Rocco PRM, Pelosi P. Effects of positive end-expiratory pressure on lung recruitment, respiratory mechanics, and intracranial pressure in mechanically ventilated brain-injured patients. Front Physiol. 2021;12:711273. PMID: 34733173; PMCID: PMC8558243. https://doi.org/10.3389/fphys.2021.711273.
38. deBacker J, Hart N, Fan E. Neuromuscular blockade in the 21st century management of the critically ill patient. Chest. 2017;151(3):697–706. Epub 2016 Nov 3. PMID: 27818334. https://doi.org/10.1016/j.chest.2016.10.040.
39. Guérin C, Albert RK, Beitler J, Gattinoni L, Jaber S, Marini JJ, Munshi L, Papazian L, Pesenti A, Vieillard-Baron A, Mancebo J. Prone position in ARDS patients: why, when, how and for whom. Intensive Care Med. 2020;46(12):2385–96. Epub 2020 Nov 10. PMID: 33169218; PMCID: PMC7652705. https://doi.org/10.1007/s00134-020-06306-w.
40. Beuret P, Carton MJ, Nourdine K, Kaaki M, Tramoni G, Ducreux JC. Prone position as prevention of lung injury in comatose patients: a prospective, randomized, controlled study. Intensive Care Med. 2002;28(5):564–9. Epub 2002 Apr 9. PMID: 12029403. https://doi.org/10.1007/s00134-002-1266-x.
41. Reinprecht A, Greher M, Wolfsberger S, Dietrich W, Illievich UM, Gruber A. Prone position in subarachnoid hemorrhage patients with acute respiratory distress syndrome: effects on cerebral tissue oxygenation and intracranial pressure. Crit Care Med. 2003;31(6):1831–8. PMID: 12794427. https://doi.org/10.1097/01.CCM.0000063453.93855.0A.
42. Thelandersson A, Cider A, Nellgård B. Prone position in mechanically ventilated patients with reduced intracranial compliance. Acta Anaesthesiol Scand. 2006;50(8):937–41. PMID: 16923087. https://doi.org/10.1111/j.1399-6576.2006.01037.x.
43. Papadimos TJ, Medhkour A, Yermal S. Successful use of inhaled nitric oxide to decrease intracranial pressure in a patient with severe traumatic brain injury complicated by acute respiratory distress syndrome: a role for an anti-inflammatory mechanism? Scand J Trauma Resusc Emerg Med. 2009;17:5. PMID: 19222848; PMCID: PMC2657771. https://doi.org/10.1186/1757-7241-17-5.
44. Gritti P, Lanterna LA, Re M, Martchenko S, Olivotto P, Brembilla C, Agostinis C, Paganoni G, Lorini FL. The use of inhaled nitric oxide and prone position in an ARDS patient with severe traumatic brain injury during spine stabilization. J Anesth. 2013;27(2):293–7. Epub 2012 Oct 13. PMID: 23065049. https://doi.org/10.1007/s00540-012-1495-2.
45. Bein T, Scherer MN, Philipp A, Weber F, Woertgen C. Pumpless extracorporeal lung assist (pECLA) in patients with acute respiratory distress syndrome and severe brain injury. J Trauma. 2005;58(6):1294–7. PMID: 15995487. https://doi.org/10.1097/01.ta.0000173275.06947.5c.
46. Bruzek AK, Vega RA, Mathern BE. Extracorporeal membrane oxygenation support as a life-saving measure for acute respiratory distress syndrome after craniectomy. J Neurosurg Anesthesiol. 2014;26(3):259–60. PMID: 24064715. https://doi.org/10.1097/ANA.0b013e3182a5d0fd.
47. Biscotti M, Gannon WD, Abrams D, Agerstrand C, Claassen J, Brodie D, Bacchetta M. Extracorporeal membrane oxygenation use in patients with traumatic brain injury. Perfusion. 2015;30(5):407–9. Epub 2014 Oct 13. PMID: 25313096. https://doi.org/10.1177/0267659114554327.
48. Robba C, Ortu A, Bilotta F, Lombardo A, Sekhon MS, Gallo F, Matta BF. Extracorporeal membrane oxygenation for adult respiratory distress syndrome in trauma patients: a case series and systematic literature review. J Trauma Acute Care Surg. 2017;82(1):165–73. PMID: 27779577. https://doi.org/10.1097/TA.0000000000001276.
49. Kurihara C, Walter JM, Karim A, Thakkar S, Saine M, Odell DD, Kim S, Tomic R, Wunderink RG, Budinger GRS, Bharat A. Feasibility of venovenous extracorporeal membrane oxygenation

without systemic anticoagulation. Ann Thorac Surg. 2020;110(4):1209–15. Epub 2020 Mar 12. PMID: 32173339; PMCID: PMC7486253. https://doi.org/10.1016/j.athoracsur.2020.02.011.
50. Thille AW, Cortés-Puch I, Esteban A. Weaning from the ventilator and extubation in ICU. Curr Opin Crit Care. 2013;19(1):57–64. PMID: 23235542. https://doi.org/10.1097/MCC.0b013e32835c5095.
51. Coplin WM, Pierson DJ, Cooley KD, Newell DW, Rubenfeld GD. Implications of extubation delay in brain-injured patients meeting standard weaning criteria. Am J Respir Crit Care Med. 2000;161(5):1530–6. PMID: 10806150. https://doi.org/10.1164/ajrccm.161.5.9905102.
52. Godet T, Chabanne R, Marin J, Kauffmann S, Futier E, Pereira B, Constantin JM. Extubation failure in Brain-injured patients: risk factors and development of a prediction score in a preliminary prospective cohort study. Anesthesiology. 2017;126(1):104–14. PMID: 27749290. https://doi.org/10.1097/ALN.0000000000001379.
53. Bösel J. Who is safe to extubate in the neuroscience intensive care unit? Semin Respir Crit Care Med. 2017;38(6):830–9. Epub 2017 Dec 20. PMID: 29262440. https://doi.org/10.1055/s-0037-1608773.
54. Battaglini D, Siwicka Gieroba D, Brunetti I, Patroniti N, Bonatti G, Rocco PRM, Pelosi P, Robba C. Mechanical ventilation in neurocritical care setting: a clinical approach. Best Pract Res Clin Anaesthesiol. 2021;35(2):207–20. Epub 2020 Sep 18. PMID: 34030805. https://doi.org/10.1016/j.bpa.2020.09.001.
55. Cinotti R, Mijangos JC, Pelosi P, Haenggi M, Gurjar M, Schultz MJ, Kaye C, Godoy DA, Alvarez P, Ioakeimidou A, Ueno Y, Badenes R, Suei Elbuzidi AA, Piagnerelli M, Elhadi M, Reza ST, Azab MA, McCredie V, Stevens RD, Digitale JC, Fong N, Asehnoune K, ENIO Study Group, the PROtective VENTilation network, the European Society of Intensive Care Medicine, the Colegio Mexicano de Medicina Critica, the Atlanréa group and the Société Française d'Anesthésie-Réanimation–SFAR research network. Extubation in neurocritical care patients: the ENIO international prospective study. Intensive Care Med. 2022;48(11):1539–50. Epub 2022 Aug 29. PMID: 36038713. https://doi.org/10.1007/s00134-022-06825-8.
56. Boles JM, Bion J, Connors A, Herridge M, Marsh B, Melot C, Pearl R, Silverman H, Stanchina M, Vieillard-Baron A, Welte T. Weaning from mechanical ventilation. Eur Respir J. 2007;29(5):1033–56. PMID: 17470624. https://doi.org/10.1183/09031936.00010206.
57. McCredie VA, Ferguson ND, Pinto RL, Adhikari NK, Fowler RA, Chapman MG, Burrell A, Baker AJ, Cook DJ, Meade MO, Scales DC, Canadian Critical Care Trials Group. Airway management strategies for Brain-injured patients meeting standard criteria to consider Extubation. A prospective cohort study. Ann Am Thorac Soc. 2017;14(1):85–93. PMID: 27870576. https://doi.org/10.1513/AnnalsATS.201608-620OC.
58. Asehnoune K, Seguin P, Lasocki S, Roquilly A, Delater A, Gros A, Denou F, Mahé PJ, Nesseler N, Demeure-Dit-Latte D, Launey Y, Lakhal K, Rozec B, Mallédant Y, Sébille V, Jaber S, Le Thuaut A, Feuillet F, Cinotti R, ATLANREA Group. Extubation success prediction in a multicentric cohort of patients with severe brain injury. Anesthesiology. 2017;127(2):338–46. PMID: 28640020. https://doi.org/10.1097/ALN.0000000000001725.
59. Namen AM, Ely EW, Tatter SB, Case LD, Lucia MA, Smith A, Landry S, Wilson JA, Glazier SS, Branch CL, Kelly DL, Bowton DL, Haponik EF. Predictors of successful extubation in neurosurgical patients. Am J Respir Crit Care Med. 2001;163(3 Pt 1):658–64. PMID: 11254520. https://doi.org/10.1164/ajrccm.163.3.2003060.
60. Navalesi P, Frigerio P, Moretti MP, Sommariva M, Vesconi S, Baiardi P, Levati A. Rate of reintubation in mechanically ventilated neurosurgical and neurologic patients: evaluation of a systematic approach to weaning and extubation. Crit Care Med. 2008;36(11):2986–92. PMID: 18824909. https://doi.org/10.1097/CCM.0b013e31818b35f2.
61. Lu Q, Xie Y, Qi X, Li X, Yang S, Wang Y. Is early tracheostomy better for severe traumatic brain injury? A meta-analysis. World Neurosurg. 2018;112:e324–30. Epub 2018 Jan 11. PMID: 29337171. https://doi.org/10.1016/j.wneu.2018.01.043.
62. Cinotti R, Pelosi P, Schultz MJ, Aikaterini I, Alvarez P, Badenes R, McCredie V, Elbuzidi AS, Elhadi M, Godoy DA, Gurjar M, Haenggi M, Kaye C, Mijangos-Méndez JC, Piagnerelli M, Piracchio R, Reza ST, Stevens RD, Yoshitoyo U, Asehnoune K, ENIO Study Group.

Extubation strategies in neuro-intensive care unit patients and associations with outcomes: the ENIO multicentre international observational study. Ann Transl Med. 2020;8(7):503. PMID: 32395547; PMCID: PMC7210208. https://doi.org/10.21037/atm.2020.03.160.
63. Cinotti R, Citerio G, Asehnoune K. Extubation in neurocritical care patients: lesson learned. Intensive Care Med. 2022;49:230. Epub ahead of print. PMID: 36253548. https://doi.org/10.1007/s00134-022-06907-7.
64. Robba C, Galimberti S, Graziano F, Wiegers EJA, Lingsma HF, Iaquaniello C, Stocchetti N, Menon D, Citerio G, CENTER-TBI ICU participants and Investigators. Tracheostomy practice and timing in traumatic brain-injured patients: a CENTER-TBI study. Intensive Care Med. 2020;46(5):983–94. Epub 2020 Feb 5. PMID: 32025780; PMCID: PMC7223805. https://doi.org/10.1007/s00134-020-05935-5.
65. Andriolo BN, Andriolo RB, Saconato H, Atallah ÁN, Valente O. Early versus late tracheostomy for critically ill patients. Cochrane Database Syst Rev. 2015;1(1):CD007271. PMID: 25581416; PMCID: PMC6517297. https://doi.org/10.1002/14651858.CD007271.pub3.
66. Dos Reis HFC, Gomes-Neto M, Almeida MLO, da Silva MF, Guedes LBA, Martinez BP, de Seixas RM. Development of a risk score to predict extubation failure in patients with traumatic brain injury. J Crit Care. 2017;42:218–22. Epub 2017 Jul 31. PMID: 28780488. https://doi.org/10.1016/j.jcrc.2017.07.051.
67. McCredie VA, Alali AS, Scales DC, Adhikari NK, Rubenfeld GD, Cuthbertson BH, Nathens AB. Effect of early versus late tracheostomy or prolonged intubation in critically ill patients with acute brain injury: a systematic review and meta-analysis. Neurocrit Care. 2017;26(1):14–25. PMID: 27601069. https://doi.org/10.1007/s12028-016-0297-z.

17 Systemic Hemodynamic Monitoring and Blood Pressure Target During Acute Brain Injury

Sanjeev Sivakumar

17.1 Introduction

Critically ill acute brain injury patients often receive hemodynamic monitoring in addition to brain-physiology specific monitoring in order to optimize cerebral blood flow, cerebral perfusion, and oxygen delivery. Hemodynamic monitoring is essential during blood pressure flow augmentation and volume status manipulation that are commonly employed in the setting of intracranial pressure (ICP) and cerebral perfusion pressures (CPP) targeted therapies in severe traumatic brain injury (TBI). Systolic blood pressure (SBP) levels have long been identified to play a key role in the secondary injury cascade after severe traumatic brain injury. Continuous monitoring and data interpretation are necessary for the control and adjustment of mean arterial pressure, cardiac output (CO), systemic filling pressures and volumes, and dynamic markers of fluid responsiveness. While the traditional invasive hemodynamic monitoring employs the use of the Swan-Ganz or pulmonary artery catheter, its usage recently has declined lately, with increased implementation of several less invasive methods of hemodynamic monitoring for patients with acute brain injury and TBI [1, 2].

This chapter provides an overview of cerebral autoregulation, and blood pressure targets in patients with acute traumatic brain injury. We review hemodynamic monitoring modalities and methods to assess volume responsiveness such as single indicator transpulmonary thermodilution, arterial waveform and pulse contour analysis, and bedside cardiorespiratory sonography in critically ill patients, followed by goal directed hemodynamic therapy in patients with brain injury.

S. Sivakumar (✉)
Neurology, Neurocritical Care, Prisma Health-Upstate, University of South Carolina-Greenville School of Medicine, Greenville, SC, USA

Center for Neurology, Greer, SC, USA
e-mail: Sanjeev.sivakumar@prismahealth.org

E. Brogi et al. (eds.), *Traumatic Brain Injury*, Hot Topics in Acute Care Surgery and Trauma, https://doi.org/10.1007/978-3-031-50117-3_17

17.2 Cerebral Autoregulation: A Brief Overview

Cerebral autoregulation refers to the ability of cerebral arterioles to maintain steady cerebral blood flow (CBF) over varying ranges of mean arterial pressures (MAP) [3]. This is termed as cerebral pressure autoregulation and is classically described using the Lassen curve [4]. In this curve on cerebral autoregulation, MAP on the x-axis is plotted against CBF on the y-axis. A steady CBF is achieved by vasodilation and vasoconstriction of cerebral arterioles which in turn are influenced by neurogenic, myogenic, and metabolic mechanisms that respond to changes in MAP [5]. Neurogenic regulation is thought to be influenced via sympathetic and cholinergic pathways [6], whereas myogenic regulation is via the smooth muscle cells in the cerebral vessels that are responsible for myogenic tone and subsequently cerebral vascular resistance [7]. Metabolic regulation is related to changes in perineuronal concentrations of CO_2, O_2, K+, Ca2+, H+, and adenosine [8–12].

Segmental and regional heterogeneity, however, exists between the pial and parenchymal arteries and arterioles and their response to the above regulatory factors. This may result in varying levels of CBF over the same range of CPP in different regions of the brain [7, 13, 14]. Traumatic brain injury resulting in impaired cerebral autoregulation is a well-established concept. In TBI, disturbed cerebral autoregulation even within "normal" ranges of CPP and CBF has been demonstrated [15, 16]. The loss of autoregulation can result in cerebral edema, ischemia, or hemorrhage even with slight changes in CPP, due to a combination of impaired neurogenic, myogenic, metabolic, and pressure dependent mechanisms [17]. Lassen curve of cerebral autoregulation is shown in Fig. 17.1 [18].

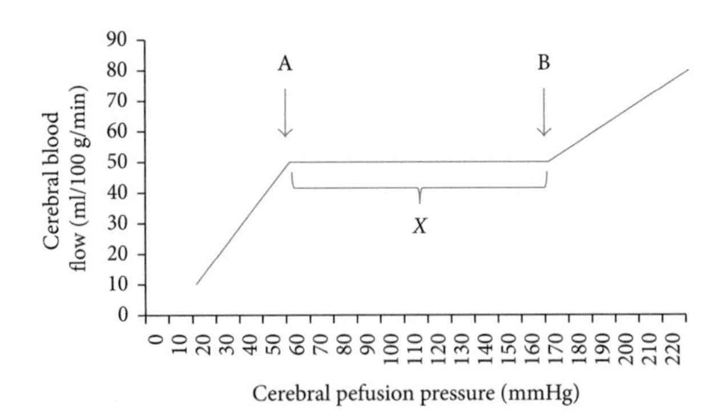

Fig. 17.1 Lassen curve of autoregulation depicting variations of cerebral blood flow (CBF) over a range of cerebral perfusion pressures (CPP). Point A is the lower limit of autoregulation (LLA) after which a decrease in CPP will lead to reductions in CBF. Point B is the higher limit of autoregulation (HLA) after which an increase in CPP with increase CBF. The range of CPP depicted by *X* is the zone of autoregulation where the CBF remains constant over changes in CPP. This is regulated by vasoconstriction and vasodilation of cerebral arterioles. (Reprinted with permission. From Kazmi SO, Sivakumar S, Karakitsos D, Alharthy A, Lazaridis C. Cerebral Pathophysiology in Extracorporeal Membrane Oxygenation: Pitfalls in Daily Clinical Management. *Crit Care Res Pract*. 2018; 2018:3237810. Published 2018 Mar 18. doi: 10.1155/2018/3237810)

17.3 Blood Pressure Targets in Acute Brain Injury

Blood pressure plays a major role and is closely associated with secondary brain injury after TBI. Early studies in the 1980s demonstrated a mortality rate of 35% among TBI patients admitted with a SBP < 85 mmHg, compared with 6% mortality in patients with higher SBP [19]. Hypotensive patients with severe TBI have a higher incidence of diffuse brain swelling [20]. The cerebral autoregulatory cascade plays an important role in secondary brain injury, or its lack thereof. Optimizing capillary hydrostatic pressure via blood pressure control has long been suggested for reducing cerebral edema in severe TBI [21]. In patients with intact autoregulation, a drop in SBP triggers autoregulatory vasodilation which aims to maintain cerebral perfusion. This results in increased cerebral blood volume, however, which can in turn elevate intracranial pressure. In patients with TBI where autoregulation is not intact, there is dependency on SBP to prevent cerebral ischemia. Secondary brain injury due to ischemia is among the most important factors that determine neurological outcomes in TBI [22].

For patients with an ICP monitor, blood pressure should be titrated based on the cerebral perfusion pressure. Among patients with severe TBI, a CPP >70 was associated with unfavorable outcomes among patients thought to have impaired cerebral autoregulation based on analysis of ICP and MAP data, whereas CPP <60 was associated with favorable outcomes in these same impaired patients [23]. As a result, the Brain Trauma Foundation (BTF) now issues Level IIB recommendations to maintain CPPs between 60 and 70, but note that the minimum threshold may depend on the autoregulatory function of the patient. The guidelines maintain prior Level III recommendations that aggressive treatment to maintain CPP >70 should be avoided. Guidelines issue a level IIB recommendation on treating ICP above 22 mmHg.

In its first iteration, the BTF guidelines defined hypotension as SBP <90 mmHg in TBI, and therapies typically targeted this endpoint. Blood pressure targets have been updated in subsequent iterations, informed by data from numerous cohorts. As one considers the below threshold recommendations from the guidelines, the interrelationships between SBP, MAP, and CPP should be considered. While there was insufficient evidence to support a Level I or II recommendation, the fourth iteration of the BTF guidelines issued a Level III recommendation for management of BP (low quality of evidence) to decrease mortality and improve outcomes [24]. Guideline-recommended blood pressure targets in acute traumatic brain injury are provided in Table 17.1 [24].

With regard to prehospital blood pressure goals, a prospective study of 717 patients from the Traumatic Coma Databank suggested that SBP <90 mmHg is an independent predictor of mortality [25]. In this study, even a single episode of

Table 17.1 Guideline-recommended blood pressure targets in acute traumatic brain injury

Patient age	Recommended blood pressure targets
15–49 years	SBP ≥110 mmHg
50–69 years	SBP ≥100 mmHg
>70 years	SBP ≥110 mmHg

hypotension from the time of injury to resuscitation doubled mortality and increased morbidity. In a more recent multicenter cohort among 5057 patients with TBI from the European trauma registry, an admission of SBP even below 120 mmHg was associated with increased mortality rates [26]. In this study, the adjusted odds of death were 1.5 times greater at SBP <120 mmHg, 2 times greater at SBP <100 mmHg, three times at SBP <90 mmHg, and six times greater at SBP < 70 mmHg. Management strategies that prevent or minimize hypotension in the prehospital phase improve outcomes in severe TBI [27]. Odds for mortality increased from 2 to 8 with repeated episodes of hypotension during initial resuscitative efforts for TBI in a prospective cohort [28].

In a retrospective cohort of adult trauma patients across Los Angeles County, the authors predefined three age categories (15–49, 50–69, and 70 or older), and for each category, the probability of death was estimated for SBP cutoffs from 60 to 150 mmHg in increments of 10 mmHg. This study concluded that hypotension be defined as SBP below 90 mmHg, based on their identification of 100 mmHg and 110 mmHg as thresholds associated with lower mortality [29]. Evidence from this class 2 study was incorporated into the updated recommendations on blood pressure thresholds (Table 17.1).

In the early phase of hospital management within the first 48 hours after injury, Brenner et al. studied the correlations between SBP thresholds and outcome. In this single center study, SBP <110 mmHg and < 120 mmHg within the first 48 hours were thresholds to avoid, to minimize morality, and improve 12-month outcomes [30]. Analysis from the IMPACT database of individual patient level data from 8 RCTs showed that SBP ranges from 120 mmHg and 150 mmHg, and MAP ranges from 85 mmHg and 110 mmHg are threshold to target, to improve outcomes [31]. Several prospective and retrospective studies have evaluated BP targets, as an in-hospital predictor of outcome in severe TBI patients. Hypotension, defined as SBP ≤80 mm Hg [32], SBP <90 mmHg [33], and < 95 mmHg [34, 35], are independent predictors of increased morbidity and mortality. The duration of hypotension is a predictor of morbidity and mortality [36].

Intraoperative hypotension during early surgery after severe TBI is also associated with increased mortality. A mortality rate of about 80% was seen in patients with hypotension, compared to 25% in the normotensive group, and the duration of intraoperative hypotension inversely correlated with Glasgow Outcome Scale score [37].

17.4 Systemic Hemodynamic Monitoring in TBI

Patients with severe traumatic brain injury require close hemodynamic monitoring, in order to optimize CBF, cerebral perfusion, and oxygen delivery. The management and manipulation of MAP, cardiac output (CO), systemic filling pressures and volumes, and dynamic markers of fluid responsiveness require continuous monitoring and interpretation of acquired data. While the traditional invasive hemodynamic monitoring employs the use of the Swan-Ganz or pulmonary artery catheter, less invasive modalities are more frequently in current use. The modalities include single indicator transpulmonary thermodilution, arterial waveform and pulse contour analysis, and bedside ultrasonography. They are reviewed below and categorized into monitoring of cardiac output derivatives, and volume status assessment with measures of fluid responsiveness.

17.4.1 Monitoring Cardiac Output Derivatives

17.4.1.1 Transpulmonary Thermodilution Devices

Traditional invasive hemodynamic monitoring is synonymous with use of the Swan-Ganz catheter or pulmonary artery catheter (PAC). Swan-Ganz catheter usage has recently decreased, due to a lack of evidence demonstrating improvement in patient outcomes in randomized controlled trials [1, 2, 38], and due to the limited performance of filling pressures as indicators of fluid responsiveness [39]. The estimation of cardiac output by use of the PAC employs a temperature-time curve, that is derived from measurements obtained in the pulmonary artery after injection of cold saline. In the single indicator (thermal) transpulmonary thermodilution (TPT), CO measurements are based on cold saline injection through a central venous catheter placed in the subclavian or internal jugular veins. The thermistor is located at an arterial site (radial, axillary or femoral artery) which contains a 4–5 Fr catheter. The Stewart-Hamilton principle is then used to calculate the CO, and a temperature-time curve is constructed [40]. Such TPT based CO estimations when compared with PAC have shown a high degree of correlation in both experimental [41] and clinical settings [42, 43]. Several transpulmonary thermodilution devices are available that use different algorithms, like PiCCO, LiDCCO (uses lithium to measure CO) and noninvasive cardiac output (NICO).

The detection of global end-diastolic volume index (GEDVI), intrathoracic blood volume index (ITBVI), and extravascular lung water index (EVLWI) through an advanced transpulmonary thermodilution device is known as the pulse index continuous cardiac output (PiCCO) (Pulsion Medical Systems, Munich, Germany and Philips Medical Systems). This system uses the arterial pulse contour analysis for continuous display and monitoring of CO. The GEDV (normal: 600–800 cc/m^2) is the volume of blood in all 4 cardiac chambers at the end of diastole, which can be used as a marker of cardiac preload. Extravascular lung water (EVLW) calculates the amount of water outside the pulmonary blood system, giving an idea of the water in the interstitial tissue of the lung. A detailed overview of methodology used for extravascular lung water measurements is beyond the scope of this chapter and can be found elsewhere [40]. The principles involved in calculation of filling volumes and EVLW are graphically demonstrated in Fig. 17.2 [44]. PiCCO has been shown to successfully differentiate between hydrostatic and permeable types of pulmonary edema. A flow-time curve is created based on a given arterial trace, by mathematical modeling of vascular resistance, impedance, and capacitance [45–47]. Thermodilution generated CO measurements are used to calibrate pulse contour analysis of continuous CO at scheduled time intervals. By recalibrating when

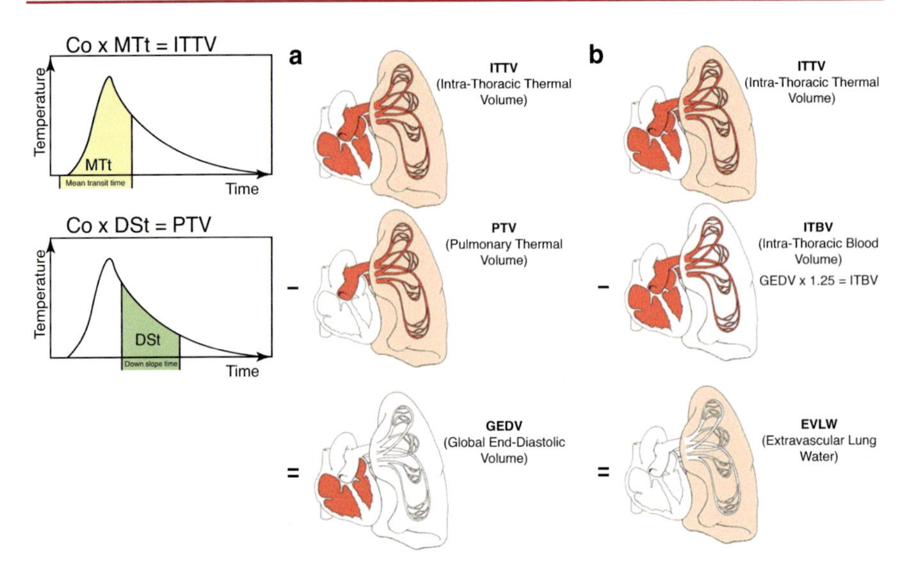

Fig. 17.2 Transpulmonary thermodilution—calculation of filling volumes and extravascular lung water. (Reprinted with permission, from Lazaridis C. Advanced hemodynamic monitoring: principles and practice in neurocritical care. *Neurocrit Care*. 2012;16(1):163–169. doi:10.1007/s12028-011-9568-x. With permission from Springer Nature)

the hemodynamic and physiological vascular state of a patient changes, CO can be accurately monitored [48].

Pulmonary artery catheter based measurements of CO have been compared with transpulmonary thermodilution using PiCCO based derivation of CO in the neurocritical care population [49]. A high correlation and agreement between PAC based assessment of cardiac index, TPCI, and transpulmonary thermodilution calibrated pulse contour CI were found, in a pooled analysis of CI values. A cardiac function index (CFI; normal: 4.5–6.5 L/min) can be calculated via TPT that is supplementary to CO measurements for the assessment of left ventricular contractility. This is the ratio of CO over the blood volume contained in the four chambers of the heart at end-diastole (global end-diastolic volume GEDV and index-GEDI) [50]. In a prospective study, a CFI of <3.2 min-1 predicted LVEF of <35% with a sensitivity of 81% and specificity of 88% [51]. PiCCO monitoring has been successfully used in the integrated management of neurogenic pulmonary edema in patients with TBI [52].

17.4.1.2 Pulse Contour Analysis

Arterial waveform analysis presents another method of deriving continuous CO that does not require thermodilution. This principle is used by FloTrac®/Vigileo (Edwards Lifesciences, Irvine, CA) [53]. In this method, a self-calibrating algorithm is used that incorporates a proprietary equation taking into account biometric variables such as age and sex that are related to arterial compliance and geometric variables describing the arterial pressure waveform [54, 55]. The equation was developed and validated from a database of arterial pressure tracings and thermodilution based CO reference values. In trauma patients, pulse contour analysis has been demonstrated to complement echocardiography in evaluating hemodynamics [56].

17.4.1.3 Bioimpedance and Bioreactance Devices

Employing thoracic electrical bioimpedance/reactance for deriving hemodynamic variables assumes that changes in intrathoracic blood volume, during the cardiac cycle, induce changes in the electrical conductivity of the thorax that are mainly related to changes in aortic volume. In this method, a noninvasive CO measurement signal is determined separately from each side of the body, and the final noninvasive CO measurement signal is obtained as an average [57]. Noninvasive bioreactance CO monitoring system (NICOM; Cheetah Medical, Newton Center, MA) is used as a reference standard for bioreactance derived CO. This system has shown acceptable agreement with other CO monitoring systems that use arterial waveform [58], pulse contour analysis [59], and with continuous pulmonary artery thermodilution in ICU patients and those undergoing off-pump coronary artery bypass surgery [60–62]. Bioreactance-based CO monitoring and assessments of fluid responsiveness by PLR were successfully evaluated in a small cohort of patients with aneurysmal subarachnoid hemorrhage [63].

17.4.1.4 Cardiac Output Estimation Based on Fick Principle Applied to Carbon Dioxide

The NICO® Cardiopulmonary Management System is a noninvasive modality that provides continual cardiac output monitoring. With this method, the cardiac output is computed on breath-by-breath measurements of carbon dioxide (CO_2) elimination, typically in sedated and mechanically ventilated patients. This is conducted through a proprietary disposable rebreathing loop attached to the ventilatory circuit. The ratio of the change in end-tidal carbon dioxide and CO2 elimination after a brief period of partial rebreathing (usually 50 s) provides a noninvasive estimate of the CO [64]. It is important to note that validation studies were performed in deeply sedated and mechanically ventilated patients [65].

17.4.1.5 Esophageal Doppler

Esophageal Doppler monitoring is a partially invasive technique that can also be used to measure CO, as a monitor of global cardiac performance and fluid response. With the help of a Doppler transducer (4-MHz continuous wave or 5-MHz pulsed wave), the esophageal Doppler technique assesses the blood flow velocity in the descending aorta. A characteristic aortic velocity signal is obtained after the probe is inserted into the esophagus of sedated, mechanically ventilated patients, and then rotated so the transducer faces the descending aorta. The distribution of the CO to the descending aorta, the measured blood flow velocity in the aorta, and the diameter of the aorta (measured or approximated) are used to determine the CO [65].

Studies have shown a good correlation between esophageal doppler and thermodilution techniques [66, 67]. The end expiratory occlusion test described in the section below can be used to assess volume responsiveness.

A systematic review and meta-analysis studied 1543 patients from 37 studies that compared CO measured using bolus thermodilution with noninvasive techniques including noninvasive pulse contour analysis, thoracic electrical bioimpedance/bioreactance and CO2 rebreathing. This study showed high heterogeneity with wide percentage error, implying that noninvasive CO devices are not completely interchangeable with thermodilution [68].

17.4.2 Volume Status and Assessment of Fluid Responsiveness

Hemodynamic augmentation to improve cerebral perfusion is frequently employed to prevent secondary brain injury among patients with severe TBI and intracranial hypertension. Since the goal is to optimize forward flow toward the brain, preload and fluid responsiveness assessments need to be routinely performed in acute brain injury. The decision to administer fluids is not without complications, due to harmful consequences of positive fluid balance among critically ill patients and those with acute brain injury [69–71]. A prospective, multicenter study performed across 18 countries among patients with traumatic brain injury, the CENTER-TBI cohort in Europe and OzENTER-TBI in Australia, found significant variability in fluid management [72]. In this study, more positive fluid balances were associated with higher ICU mortality and worse functional outcome. Positive fluid balance in the early phase of TBI has also been associated with increased ICP [73].

Several static and dynamic markers of fluid responsiveness are widely used to aid management of volume status in acute brain injury. Static preload filling-pressure markers such as central venous pressure (CVP) and pulmonary artery occlusion pressure (PAOP) have been shown to correlate poorly with ventricular filling volumes and fluid responsiveness, both in healthy volunteers [39] and critically ill patients [74, 75]. In the 2018 ESICM consensus and clinical practice recommendations, CVP as a standalone metric was not recommended as a target or safety endpoint, for guiding fluid management in neurocritically ill patients [76]. On the contrary, the use of static markers and clinical assessment of volume status remains the most commonly employed variables by intensivists treating acute brain injury [77]. Daily fluid balances as a marker of euvolemia, while frequently utilized, have been demonstrated to correlate poorly with direct measures of circulating blood volume [78]. The end expiratory occlusion test (EEO) together with ultrasonography is a static hemodynamic monitoring method that can be used to measure fluid responsiveness [79]. Here, interruption to the respiratory cycle at the end of expiration averts the expected cyclical changes in venous return and cardiac output. The EEO cannot be used in non-intubated patients and in patients who interrupt a 15 s inspiratory hold.

The goal of volume expansion in TBI is to achieve augmentation of stroke volume requiring biventricular preload dependence. With the use of dynamic arterial waveform variability that is based on the principle of heart-lung interactions during positive pressure ventilation, our ability to predict ventricular performance on the Frank-Starling curve has improved [80, 81]. This allows for estimation as to whether volume expansion will increase the stroke volume. Such interactions result from effects of transpulmonary and pleural pressures, on cardiac chambers and blood vessels. Main components on the right heart include decreased venous return, increased RV afterload leading to reduced LV preload [82]. For the left heart, increase in pleural pressures reduces afterload [82, 83]. The direct relationship between these effects and the variance in LV stroke volume depends on chamber compliance, contractility, and intravascular volume. This stroke volume variation (SVV) has been shown to be an accurate predictor of fluid responsiveness [84]. Pulse pressure variation (PPV), systolic pressure variation (SPV), and SVV can all be derived by analysis of the arterial blood pressure waveform that is routinely obtained using arterial catheter. This can be quantified, continuously monitored, and displayed. PPV has been shown to perform superiorly to SPV, thus reflecting the property of pulse pressure as a surrogate of stroke volume. Among mechanically ventilated patients, a PPV >13% has been shown to predict a positive response in cardiac index (defined as a 15% increase in CI) to a 500 mL fluid bolus with a positive predictive value of 94%, whereas a PPV <13% has a negative predictive value of 96% [80]. In the same study, CVP and PAOP were found to be less reliable as predictors of fluid responsiveness.

There are limitations of dynamic markers of fluid responsiveness. Limitations include open-chest conditions (e.g., cardiac surgery), less reliability with spontaneous breathing activity and while on small tidal volumes, and sustained cardiac arrhythmia [84]. The use of low tidal volume positive pressure ventilation within a protective ventilation strategy is now routine practice in the general ICU population with ARDS and is associated with improved outcomes [85]. Low tidal volume lung protective ventilation is frequently used in patients with severe TBI, and this may not induce stroke volume variations in an otherwise volume responsive patient. Studies validating SVV, did so in heavily sedated, and at times paralyzed patients, that were mechanically ventilated with tidal volumes of 8–10 mg/Kg ideal body weight. SVV has demonstrated reliability at tidal volumes of at least 8 mL/kg [86]. Among patients with ARDS ventilated with a mean tidal volume of 6.5 mL/kg, a PPV cut-off of 12% had a specificity of 100% in discriminating fluid responders from non-responders, albeit with a sensitivity of 68% [87]. These shortcomings may be overcome by transiently increasing tidal volume to 8 mL/kg, or using a short acting paralytic to ensure ventilator synchrony. It is important to consider and maintain the PaCO2 goals suggested by TBI guidelines while manipulating ventilation settings in brain injured patients [24]. For patients in sustained arrhythmia or atrial fibrillation, it is important to consider that observed beat-to-beat SVV is due to altered cardiac filling times.

The passive leg raise test (PLR) is a useful bedside tool that assesses fluid responsiveness without the need to administer IV fluids. In PLR, the patient's legs are raised to 45 degrees, leading to an autotransfusion of volume pooled in the lower extremities and pelvic veins. Detection of an increased CI immediately following this maneuver has been shown to be an accurate predictor of fluid responsiveness [88–90]. Limitations for use in patients with severe TBI include the possibility that sudden changes to body position in patients with impaired intracranial compliance could lead to ICP crises in a minority of extremely position sensitive patients. Bioreactance-based noninvasive cardiac output monitoring has also been used and validated in the assessment of fluid responsiveness by using PLR [91–93].

Point-of-care bedside ultrasound has found a place in hemodynamic assessments and is complementary to above modalities. On transthoracic parasternal short axis view, systolic obliteration of left ventricular cross-sectional area is a marker for severe hypovolemia [94]. Quantification of respiratory variations in inferior vena cava diameter (dIVC) is an accurate marker for fluid responsiveness among mechanically ventilated patients. A cutoff between 12% and 18% for respiratory variation in dIVC among mechanically ventilated patients discriminates fluid responders from non-responders with a high sensitivity and specificity [95, 96]. The normal ranges and goals for markers of volume responsiveness are shown in Table 17.2 [97, 98].

17.4.3 Goal-Directed Hemodynamic Management in Acute Brain Injury

Monitoring strategies outlined above can aid in optimizing hemodynamic variables to target parameters such as CBF, metabolic data from cerebral microdialysis, and tissue parameters such as brain tissue oxygen saturation. The normal range for advanced hemodynamic monitoring modalities is given in Table 17.2. Treatments aimed at reduction of ICP and augmenting CPP with close monitoring of volume status are key factors in the management of patients with severe TBI. Taking into account the pressure autoregulation, brain oxygenation and tissue metabolic parameters allow for individualization of CPP targets. The recommended target CPP for survival and favorable outcomes is between 60 and 70 mmHg [24]. Avoidance of aggressive attempts at maintaining CPP above 70 mmHg with fluids and vasopressors is recommended, due to the increased risk for acute lung injury and ARDS [99]. Both hypovolemia and hypervolemia are associated with adverse outcomes in patients with brain injury, with significant negative fluid balances found to be associated with adverse outcomes independent of its relationship to MAP, ICP, and CPP [100]. Similarly, induced hypertension in patients with severe injury has been associated with development of symptomatic ARDS [99]. There is evidence in support of normovolemic hypertension in achieving CBF augmentation without affecting brain oxygenation in other forms of severe brain injury such as aneurysmal subarachnoid hemorrhage [101].

For volume resuscitation, crystalloids and balanced salt solutions are generally preferred. Hypertonic fluids play a critical role in the medical management of patients with intracranial hypertension and can restore cerebral perfusion with potential effects on modulation of inflammatory response. In the prehospital setting and early management of TBI, randomized trials show that hypertonic crystalloids

Table 17.2 Advanced hemodynamic monitoring: Variables and normal range

Hemodynamic variables and normal ranges
Preload
GEDI = 680–800 mL/m^2
– Volume of all 4 cardiac chambers at end-diastole
– Index of cardiac preload
TTE = LV CSA obliteration indicates hyperdynamic-hypovolemic ventricle
LV performance
CI = 3.0–5.0 L/min/m^2
CFI = 4.5–6.5 min −1 (<3.2 predictive of EF <35%)
TTE = visual inspection of LV/RV size and contractility
Fluid responsiveness: Markers for positive response to fluid challenge
SVV > 10%
PPV > 13%
dIVC >16%
Caveats: Patients on controlled mechanical ventilation, no open lung, synchronous with ventilator, tidal volume ~ 8 cc/kg, no arrhythmia
Pulmonary edema
ELWI = 3.0–10.0 mL/kg (<10 mL/kg)
– Increases in hydrostatic pulmonary edema and ARDS
– Quantified the volume of pulmonary edema
PVPI = <3
– Differentiate hydrostatic pulmonary edema and ARDS
– Indicates the risk for pulmonary edema
Lung ultrasound
– B-line predominance suggests subpleural interstitial edema
Hemodynamic augmentation
Recommended CPP target: Between 60 and 70 mmHg (level IIB)
Avoid CPP above 70 mmHg with fluids and pressors (level III)
Normovolemic hypertension:
– Vasopressors: Norepinephrine/phenylephrine/dopamine
– Primary CO augmentation: Dobutamine/milrinone
– Monitor preload, markers of fluid responsiveness

GEDI global end-diastolic volume index, *TTE* transthoracic echocardiography, *LV* left ventricle, *RV* right ventricle, *CSA* cross-sectional area, *CI* cardiac index, *CFI* cardiac function index, *SVV* stroke volume variability, *PPV* pulse pressure variation. *dIVC* inferior vena cava diameter, *ELWI* extravascular lung water index, *PVPI* pulmonary vascular permeability index, *CPP* cerebral perfusion pressure

and colloid solutions compared to isotonic saline did not have a favorable effect on long term outcomes [102, 103]. Early fluid resuscitation with albumin compared to normal saline was associated with higher mortality rates in the SAFE trial [104]. Thus, crystalloid resuscitation targeting avoidance of both extremes of overt hypovolemia and fluid overload should be the goal. Red blood cell transfusions are generally safe, but have a small risk of immune, hemolytic, or infectious complications. The hemoglobin thresholds to administer transfusion remain controversial and should be based on individual systemic and cerebral physiological targets, targeted to multimodal monitoring [105].

In clinical scenarios such as TBI patients with ICP crises, vasopressors are typically used to augment CPP. While randomized evidence to inform vasopressor choice in these clinical settings are lacking, norepinephrine appears to be the most used in practice, compared to other inotropes such as phenylephrine and dopamine [106, 107]. Dopamine produces less predictable CPP augmentation than norepinephrine [108]. Vasopressin and analogues (such as terlipressin) should be used with caution because of risk of hyponatremia and subsequent cerebral edema. For primary cardiac output augmentation, dobutamine and milrinone are agents that are considered and titrated to CI goals. The level at which MAP is referenced (mid-axillary line versus external auditory meatus), a fundamental aspect of CPP management, remains under debate and is inconsistently applied, both in reported studies and in clinical practice [109]. For appropriate CPP calculation, both MAP and ICP should be calibrated at the level of the foramen of Monro which corresponds to the external auditory meatus.

Continuous monitoring of MAP and CI is imperative in patients with ICP crisis, and indirect reconstruction of Frank-Starling curves can assist in titration of fluids, inotropes, diuretics, or vasopressors. Using transpulmonary thermodilution, filling volumes [the global end-diastolic volume index (GEDI)] can be measured, and quantification of pulmonary edema and extravascular lung water (EVLW) is possible. An increase in EVLW index is associated with increased mortality and poor outcomes in ICU patients with ARDS [110, 111]. Hydrostatic and high permeability edema formation are believed to have a role in the pathophysiology of neurogenic pulmonary edema [112]. In mechanically ventilated patients with severe lung injury, Monnet et al. studied two indices of pulmonary permeability estimated by transpulmonary thermodilution that may be useful for determining the mechanism of pulmonary edema [113]. Using TPT, the ratios EVLW/pulmonary blood volume (PVPI) and EVLWI/GEDI were calculated. A PVPI ≥ 3 and an EVLWI/GEDI $\geq 1.8 \times 10{-}2$ were successful in diagnosing ALI/ARDS with a sensitivity of 85% and specificity of 100%. Bedside point-of-care ultrasonography and echocardiography are useful tools to inform the intensivist caring for severe acute brain injury. In severe TBI patients with neurogenic stress cardiomyopathy, bedside ultrasound can detect a severely reduced cardiac output. Interstitial edema can be assessed for by the identification of "B-lines": a comet-tail ultrasonographic artifact generated by edematous subpleural interlobular septa that are surrounded by air filled alveoli [114]. By implementing protocols to obtain and closely monitor these variables, one can individualization hemodynamic goals for patients with severe acute brain injury.

17.5 Conclusion

Caring for patients with acute severe brain injury often requires monitoring and management of multiple organ systems. Blood pressure management in the acute phase of brain injury is critical for the preservation of cerebral perfusion and averting the secondary injury cascade. SBP ≥ 110 mm Hg among patients 15–49 years and > 70 years and SBP ≥ 100 mmHg among patients aged 50–69 years are guideline-recommended blood pressure targets following acute traumatic brain injury. While individualization of cerebral perfusion pressure goals has found a place in the treatment protocols for TBI, a CPP value to target for favorable outcomes is between 60 and 70 mmHg. Systemic hemodynamic monitoring using invasive and noninvasive means, such as pulmonary artery catheter, transpulmonary thermodilution, arterial pulse contour and waveform analyses, bedside point-of-care ultrasonography can better inform volume status and flow augmentation strategies and help minimize volume overload, lung injury, and adverse clinical outcomes.

References

1. Harvey S, Harrison DA, Singer M, Ashcroft J, Jones CM, Elbourne D, et al. Assessment of the clinical effectiveness of pulmonary artery catheters in management of patients in intensive care (PAC-man): a randomised controlled trial. Lancet. 2005;366(9484):472–7.
2. Wiener RS, Welch HG. Trends in the use of the pulmonary artery catheter in the United States, 1993-2004. JAMA. 2007;298(4):423–9.
3. Paulson OB, Strandgaard S, Edvinsson L. Cerebral autoregulation. Cerebrovasc Brain Metab Rev. 1990;2(2):161–92.
4. Lassen NA. Cerebral blood flow and oxygen consumption in man. Physiol Rev. 1959;39(2):183–238.
5. Xiong L, Liu X, Shang T, Smielewski P, Donnelly J, Guo ZN, et al. Impaired cerebral autoregulation: measurement and application to stroke. J Neurol Neurosurg Psychiatry. 2017;88(6):520–31.
6. Hamel E. Perivascular nerves and the regulation of cerebrovascular tone. J Appl Physiol. 2006;100(3):1059–64.
7. Cipolla MJ, Li R, Vitullo L. Perivascular innervation of penetrating brain parenchymal arterioles. J Cardiovasc Pharmacol. 2004;44(1):1–8.
8. Lassen NA, Christensen MS. Physiology of cerebral blood flow. Br J Anaesth. 1976;48(8):719–34.
9. Kuschinsky W, Wahl M. Local chemical and neurogenic regulation of cerebral vascular resistance. Physiol Rev. 1978;58(3):656–89.
10. Winn HR, Welsh JE, Rubio R, Berne RM. Brain adenosine production in rat during sustained alteration in systemic blood pressure. Am J Phys. 1980;239(5):H636–41.
11. Kontos HA, George E. Brown memorial lecture. Oxygen radicals in cerebral vascular injury. Circ Res. 1985;57(4):508–16.
12. Wei EP, Kontos HA. Increased venous pressure causes myogenic constriction of cerebral arterioles during local hyperoxia. Circ Res. 1984;55(2):249–52.
13. Iadecola C. Neurovascular regulation in the normal brain and in Alzheimer's disease. Nat Rev Neurosci. 2004;5(5):347–60.
14. Faraci FM, Mayhan WG, Heistad DD. Segmental vascular responses to acute hypertension in cerebrum and brain stem. Am J Phys. 1987;252(4 Pt 2):H738–42.
15. Bouma GJ, Muizelaar JP, Bandoh K, Marmarou A. Blood pressure and intracranial pressure-volume dynamics in severe head injury: relationship with cerebral blood flow. J Neurosurg. 1992;77(1):15–9.
16. Czosnyka M, Smielewski P, Piechnik S, Steiner LA, Pickard JD. Cerebral autoregulation following head injury. J Neurosurg. 2001;95(5):756–63.
17. Rangel-Castilla L, Gasco J, Nauta HJ, Okonkwo DO, Robertson CS. Cerebral pressure autoregulation in traumatic brain injury. Neurosurg Focus. 2008;25(4):E7.
18. Kazmi SO, Sivakumar S, Karakitsos D, Alharthy A, Lazaridis C. Cerebral pathophysiology in extracorporeal membrane oxygenation: pitfalls in daily clinical management. Crit Care Res Pract. 2018;2018:3237810.

19. Klauber MR, Marshall LF, Luerssen TG, Frankowski R, Tabaddor K, Eisenberg HM. Determinants of head injury mortality: importance of the low risk patient. Neurosurgery. 1989;24(1):31–6.
20. Eisenberg HM, Gary HE Jr, Aldrich EF, Saydjari C, Turner B, Foulkes MA, et al. Initial CT findings in 753 patients with severe head injury. A report from the NIH traumatic coma data Bank. J Neurosurg. 1990;73(5):688–98.
21. Eker C, Asgeirsson B, Grande PO, Schalen W, Nordstrom CH. Improved outcome after severe head injury with a new therapy based on principles for brain volume regulation and preserved microcirculation. Crit Care Med. 1998;26(11):1881–6.
22. Bouma GJ, Muizelaar JP, Choi SC, Newlon PG, Young HF. Cerebral circulation and metabolism after severe traumatic brain injury: the elusive role of ischemia. J Neurosurg. 1991;75(5):685–93.
23. Johnson U, Nilsson P, Ronne-Engstrom E, Howells T, Enblad P. Favorable outcome in traumatic brain injury patients with impaired cerebral pressure autoregulation when treated at low cerebral perfusion pressure levels. Neurosurgery. 2011;68(3):714–21; discussion 21–2.
24. Carney N, Totten AM, O'Reilly C, Ullman JS, Hawryluk GW, Bell MJ, et al. Guidelines for the management of severe traumatic brain injury, fourth edition. Neurosurgery. 2017;80(1):6–15.
25. Chesnut RM, Marshall SB, Piek J, Blunt BA, Klauber MR, Marshall LF. Early and late systemic hypotension as a frequent and fundamental source of cerebral ischemia following severe brain injury in the traumatic coma data Bank. Acta Neurochir Suppl (Wien). 1993;59:121–5.
26. Fuller G, Hasler RM, Mealing N, Lawrence T, Woodford M, Juni P, et al. The association between admission systolic blood pressure and mortality in significant traumatic brain injury: a multi-Centre cohort study. Injury. 2014;45(3):612–7.
27. Gentleman D. Causes and effects of systemic complications among severely head injured patients transferred to a neurosurgical unit. Int Surg. 1992;77(4):297–302.
28. Manley G, Knudson MM, Morabito D, Damron S, Erickson V, Pitts L. Hypotension, hypoxia, and head injury: frequency, duration, and consequences. Arch Surg. 2001;136(10):1118–23.
29. Berry C, Ley EJ, Bukur M, Malinoski D, Margulies DR, Mirocha J, et al. Redefining hypotension in traumatic brain injury. Injury. 2012;43(11):1833–7.
30. Brenner M, Stein DM, Hu PF, Aarabi B, Sheth K, Scalea TM. Traditional systolic blood pressure targets underestimate hypotension-induced secondary brain injury. J Trauma Acute Care Surg. 2012;72(5):1135–9.
31. Murray GD, Butcher I, McHugh GS, Lu J, Mushkudiani NA, Maas AI, et al. Multivariable prognostic analysis in traumatic brain injury: results from the IMPACT study. J Neurotrauma. 2007;24(2):329–37.
32. Marmarou A, Anderson RL, Ward JD, Choi SC, Young HF, Eisenberg HM, et al. Impact of ICP instability and hypotension on outcome in patients with severe head trauma. J Neurosurg. 1991;75:S59.
33. Fearnside MR, Cook RJ, McDougall P, McNeil RJ. The Westmead head injury project outcome in severe head injury. A comparative analysis of pre-hospital, clinical and CT variables. Br J Neurosurg. 1993;7(3):267–79.
34. Miller JD, Becker DP. Secondary insults to the injured brain. J R Coll Surg Edinb. 1982;27(5):292–8.
35. Miller JD, Sweet RC, Narayan R, Becker DP. Early insults to the injured brain. JAMA. 1978;240(5):439–42.
36. Jones PA, Andrews PJ, Midgley S, Anderson SI, Piper IR, Tocher JL, et al. Measuring the burden of secondary insults in head-injured patients during intensive care. J Neurosurg Anesthesiol. 1994;6(1):4–14.
37. Pietropaoli JA, Rogers FB, Shackford SR, Wald SL, Schmoker JD, Zhuang J. The deleterious effects of intraoperative hypotension on outcome in patients with severe head injuries. J Trauma. 1992;33(3):403–7.

38. National Heart L, Blood Institute Acute Respiratory Distress Syndrome Clinical Trials N, Wheeler AP, Bernard GR, Thompson BT, Schoenfeld D, et al. Pulmonary-artery versus central venous catheter to guide treatment of acute lung injury. N Engl J Med. 2006;354(21):2213–24.
39. Kumar A, Anel R, Bunnell E, Habet K, Zanotti S, Marshall S, et al. Pulmonary artery occlusion pressure and central venous pressure fail to predict ventricular filling volume, cardiac performance, or the response to volume infusion in normal subjects. Crit Care Med. 2004;32(3):691–9.
40. Isakow W, Schuster DP. Extravascular lung water measurements and hemodynamic monitoring in the critically ill: bedside alternatives to the pulmonary artery catheter. Am J Physiol Lung Cell Mol Physiol. 2006;291(6):L1118–31.
41. Friedman Z, Berkenstadt H, Margalit N, Sega E, Perel A. Cardiac output assessed by arterial thermodilution during exsanguination and fluid resuscitation: experimental validation against a reference technique. Eur J Anaesthesiol. 2002;19(5):337–40.
42. Sakka SG, Reinhart K, Meier-Hellmann A. Comparison of pulmonary artery and arterial thermodilution cardiac output in critically ill patients. Intensive Care Med. 1999;25(8):843–6.
43. Della Rocca G, Costa MG, Pompei L, Coccia C, Pietropaoli P. Continuous and intermittent cardiac output measurement: pulmonary artery catheter versus aortic transpulmonary technique. Br J Anaesth. 2002;88(3):350–6.
44. Lazaridis C. Advanced hemodynamic monitoring: principles and practice in neurocritical care. Neurocrit Care. 2012;16(1):163–9.
45. Wesseling KH, Purschke R, Smith NT, Wust HJ, de Wit B, Weber HA. A computer module for the continuous monitoring of cardiac output in the operating theatre and the ICU. Acta Anaesthesiol Belg. 1976;27(suppl):327–41.
46. Wesseling KH, Jansen JR, Settels JJ, Schreuder JJ. Computation of aortic flow from pressure in humans using a nonlinear, three-element model. J Appl Physiol. 1993;74(5):2566–73.
47. Benington S, Ferris P, Nirmalan M. Emerging trends in minimally invasive haemodynamic monitoring and optimization of fluid therapy. Eur J Anaesthesiol. 2009;26(11):893–905.
48. Hamzaoui O, Monnet X, Richard C, Osman D, Chemla D, Teboul JL. Effects of changes in vascular tone on the agreement between pulse contour and transpulmonary thermodilution cardiac output measurements within an up to 6-hour calibration-free period. Crit Care Med. 2008;36(2):434–40.
49. Mutoh T, Kazumata K, Ishikawa T, Terasaka S. Performance of bedside transpulmonary thermodilution monitoring for goal-directed hemodynamic management after subarachnoid hemorrhage. Stroke. 2009;40(7):2368–74.
50. Combes A, Berneau JB, Luyt CE, Trouillet JL. Estimation of left ventricular systolic function by single transpulmonary thermodilution. Intensive Care Med. 2004;30(7):1377–83.
51. Jabot J, Monnet X, Bouchra L, Chemla D, Richard C, Teboul JL. Cardiac function index provided by transpulmonary thermodilution behaves as an indicator of left ventricular systolic function. Crit Care Med. 2009;37(11):2913–8.
52. Lin X, Xu Z, Wang P, Xu Y, Zhang G. Role of PiCCO monitoring for the integrated management of neurogenic pulmonary edema following traumatic brain injury: a case report and literature review. Exp Ther Med. 2016;12(4):2341–7.
53. Pratt B, Roteliuk L, Hatib F, Frazier J, Wallen RD. Calculating arterial pressure-based cardiac output using a novel measurement and analysis method. Biomed Instrum Technol. 2007;41(5):403–11.
54. Langewouters GJ, Wesseling KH, Goedhard WJ. The pressure dependent dynamic elasticity of 35 thoracic and 16 abdominal human aortas in vitro described by a five component model. J Biomech. 1985;18(8):613–20.
55. Langewouters GJ, Wesseling KH, Goedhard WJ. The static elastic properties of 45 human thoracic and 20 abdominal aortas in vitro and the parameters of a new model. J Biomech. 1984;17(6):425–35.
56. Franchi F, Falciani E, Donadello K, Zaca V, Silvestri R, Taccone FS, et al. Echocardiography and pulse contour analysis to assess cardiac output in trauma patients. Minerva Anestesiol. 2013;79(2):137–46.

57. Keren H, Burkhoff D, Squara P. Evaluation of a noninvasive continuous cardiac output monitoring system based on thoracic bioreactance. Am J Physiol Heart Circ Physiol. 2007;293(1):H583–9.
58. Marque S, Cariou A, Chiche JD, Squara P. Comparison between Flotrac-Vigileo and bioreactance, a totally noninvasive method for cardiac output monitoring. Crit Care. 2009;13(3):R73.
59. Squara P, Rotcajg D, Denjean D, Estagnasie P, Brusset A. Comparison of monitoring performance of bioreactance vs. pulse contour during lung recruitment maneuvers. Crit Care. 2009;13:R125.
60. Raval NY, Squara P, Cleman M, Yalamanchili K, Winklmaier M, Burkhoff D. Multicenter evaluation of noninvasive cardiac output measurement by bioreactance technique. J Clin Monit Comput. 2008;22(2):113–9.
61. Cheung H, Dong Q, Dong R, Yu B. Correlation of cardiac output measured by non-invasive continuous cardiac output monitoring (NICOM) and thermodilution in patients undergoing off-pump coronary artery bypass surgery. J Anesth. 2015;29(3):416–20.
62. Berlin DA, Peprah-Mensah H, Manoach S, Heerdt PM. Agreement of bioreactance cardiac output monitoring with Thermodilution during hemorrhagic shock and resuscitation in adult swine. Crit Care Med. 2017;45(2):e195–201.
63. Sivakumar S, Lazaridis C. Bioreactance-based noninvasive fluid responsiveness and cardiac output monitoring: a pilot study in patients with aneurysmal subarachnoid hemorrhage and literature review. Crit Care Res Pract. 2020;2020:2748181.
64. Kobe J, Mishra N, Arya VK, Al-Moustadi W, Nates W, Kumar B. Cardiac output monitoring: technology and choice. Ann Card Anaesth. 2019;22(1):6–17.
65. Marik PE. Noninvasive cardiac output monitors: a state-of the-art review. J Cardiothorac Vasc Anesth. 2013;27(1):121–34.
66. Cholley BP, Singer M. Esophageal Doppler: noninvasive cardiac output monitor. Echocardiography. 2003;20(8):763–9.
67. Nowack T, Christie DB 3rd. Ultrasound in trauma resuscitation and critical care with hemodynamic transesophageal echocardiography guidance. J Trauma Acute Care Surg. 2019;87(1):234–9.
68. Joosten A, Desebbe O, Suehiro K, Murphy LS, Essiet M, Alexander B, et al. Accuracy and precision of non-invasive cardiac output monitoring devices in perioperative medicine: a systematic review and meta-analysis dagger. Br J Anaesth. 2017;118(3):298–310.
69. Mascia L, Sakr Y, Pasero D, Payen D, Reinhart K, Vincent JL, et al. Extracranial complications in patients with acute brain injury: a post-hoc analysis of the SOAP study. Intensive Care Med. 2008;34(4):720–7.
70. Vincent JL, Sakr Y, Sprung CL, Ranieri VM, Reinhart K, Gerlach H, et al. Sepsis in European intensive care units: results of the SOAP study. Crit Care Med. 2006;34(2):344–53.
71. Boyd JH, Forbes J, Nakada TA, Walley KR, Russell JA. Fluid resuscitation in septic shock: a positive fluid balance and elevated central venous pressure are associated with increased mortality. Crit Care Med. 2011;39(2):259–65.
72. Wiegers EJA, Lingsma HF, Huijben JA, Cooper DJ, Citerio G, Frisvold S, et al. Fluid balance and outcome in critically ill patients with traumatic brain injury (CENTER-TBI and OzENTER-TBI): a prospective, multicentre, comparative effectiveness study. Lancet Neurol. 2021;20(8):627–38.
73. Moore E, Saxby ER, Wang J, Pilcher M, Bailey D, Heritier S, et al. The impact of fluid balance on intracranial pressure in patients with traumatic brain injury. Intensive Care Med Exp. 2015;3(Suppl 1):A439.
74. Osman D, Ridel C, Ray P, Monnet X, Anguel N, Richard C, et al. Cardiac filling pressures are not appropriate to predict hemodynamic response to volume challenge. Crit Care Med. 2007;35(1):64–8.
75. Marik PE, Baram M, Vahid B. Does central venous pressure predict fluid responsiveness? A systematic review of the literature and the tale of seven mares. Chest. 2008;134(1):172–8.

76. Oddo M, Poole D, Helbok R, Meyfroidt G, Stocchetti N, Bouzat P, et al. Fluid therapy in neurointensive care patients: ESICM consensus and clinical practice recommendations. Intensive Care Med. 2018;44(4):449–63.
77. Sivakumar S, Taccone FS, Rehman M, Hinson H, Naval N, Lazaridis C. Hemodynamic and neuro-monitoring for neurocritically ill patients: an international survey of intensivists. J Crit Care. 2017;39:40–7.
78. Hoff RG, van Dijk GW, Algra A, Kalkman CJ, Rinkel GJ. Fluid balance and blood volume measurement after aneurysmal subarachnoid hemorrhage. Neurocrit Care. 2008;8(3):391–7.
79. Depret F, Jozwiak M, Teboul JL, Alphonsine JE, Richard C, Monnet X. Esophageal Doppler can predict fluid responsiveness through end-expiratory and end-inspiratory occlusion tests. Crit Care Med. 2019;47(2):e96–e102.
80. Michard F, Boussat S, Chemla D, Anguel N, Mercat A, Lecarpentier Y, et al. Relation between respiratory changes in arterial pulse pressure and fluid responsiveness in septic patients with acute circulatory failure. Am J Respir Crit Care Med. 2000;162(1):134–8.
81. Michard F, Teboul JL. Predicting fluid responsiveness in ICU patients: a critical analysis of the evidence. Chest. 2002;121(6):2000–8.
82. Michard F, Teboul JL. Using heart-lung interactions to assess fluid responsiveness during mechanical ventilation. Crit Care. 2000;4(5):282–9.
83. Fessler HE, Brower RG, Wise RA, Permutt S. Mechanism of reduced LV afterload by systolic and diastolic positive pleural pressure. J Appl Physiol. 1988;65(3):1244–50.
84. Michard F. Stroke volume variation: from applied physiology to improved outcomes. Crit Care Med. 2011;39(2):402–3.
85. Bellani G, Laffey JG, Pham T, Fan E, Brochard L, Esteban A, et al. Epidemiology, patterns of care, and mortality for patients with acute respiratory distress syndrome in intensive care units in 50 countries. JAMA. 2016;315(8):788–800.
86. De Backer D, Heenen S, Piagnerelli M, Koch M, Vincent JL. Pulse pressure variations to predict fluid responsiveness: influence of tidal volume. Intensive Care Med. 2005;31(4):517–23.
87. von Werder K. Bromocriptine and puerperal seizures. Zentralbl Gynakol. 1996;118(7):395–6.
88. Boulain T, Achard JM, Teboul JL, Richard C, Perrotin D, Ginies G. Changes in BP induced by passive leg raising predict response to fluid loading in critically ill patients. Chest. 2002;121(4):1245–52.
89. Monnet X, Rienzo M, Osman D, Anguel N, Richard C, Pinsky MR, et al. Passive leg raising predicts fluid responsiveness in the critically ill. Crit Care Med. 2006;34(5):1402–7.
90. Monnet X, Teboul JL. Passive leg raising. Intensive Care Med. 2008;34(4):659–63.
91. Benomar B, Ouattara A, Estagnasie P, Brusset A, Squara P. Fluid responsiveness predicted by noninvasive bioreactance-based passive leg raise test. Intensive Care Med. 2010;36(11):1875–81.
92. Marik PE, Levitov A, Young A, Andrews L. The use of bioreactance and carotid Doppler to determine volume responsiveness and blood flow redistribution following passive leg raising in hemodynamically unstable patients. Chest. 2013;143(2):364–70.
93. Duus N, Shogilev DJ, Skibsted S, Zijlstra HW, Fish E, Oren-Grinberg A, et al. The reliability and validity of passive leg raise and fluid bolus to assess fluid responsiveness in spontaneously breathing emergency department patients. J Crit Care. 2015;30:e1–5.
94. Beaulieu Y, Marik PE. Bedside ultrasonography in the ICU: part 1. Chest. 2005;128(2):881–95.
95. Feissel M, Michard F, Faller JP, Teboul JL. The respiratory variation in inferior vena cava diameter as a guide to fluid therapy. Intensive Care Med. 2004;30(9):1834–7.
96. Barbier C, Loubieres Y, Schmit C, Hayon J, Ricome JL, Jardin F, et al. Respiratory changes in inferior vena cava diameter are helpful in predicting fluid responsiveness in ventilated septic patients. Intensive Care Med. 2004;30(9):1740–6.
97. Monnet X, Teboul JL. Transpulmonary thermodilution: advantages and limits. Crit Care. 2017;21(1):147.
98. Beurton A, Teboul JL, Monnet X. Transpulmonary thermodilution techniques in the haemodynamically unstable patient. Curr Opin Crit Care. 2019;25(3):273–9.

99. Contant CF, Valadka AB, Gopinath SP, Hannay HJ, Robertson CS. Adult respiratory distress syndrome: a complication of induced hypertension after severe head injury. J Neurosurg. 2001;95(4):560–8.
100. Clifton GL, Miller ER, Choi SC, Levin HS. Fluid thresholds and outcome from severe brain injury. Crit Care Med. 2002;30(4):739–45.
101. Muench E, Horn P, Bauhuf C, Roth H, Philipps M, Hermann P, et al. Effects of hypervolemia and hypertension on regional cerebral blood flow, intracranial pressure, and brain tissue oxygenation after subarachnoid hemorrhage. Crit Care Med. 2007;35(8):1844–51. quiz 52
102. Rosenfeld JV, Maas AI, Bragge P, Morganti-Kossmann MC, Manley GT, Gruen RL. Early management of severe traumatic brain injury. Lancet. 2012;380(9847):1088–98.
103. Bulger EM, May S, Brasel KJ, Schreiber M, Kerby JD, Tisherman SA, et al. Out-of-hospital hypertonic resuscitation following severe traumatic brain injury: a randomized controlled trial. JAMA. 2010;304(13):1455–64.
104. Investigators SS, Australian, New Zealand Intensive Care Society Clinical Trials G, Australian red cross blood S, George Institute for International H, Myburgh J, et al. Saline or albumin for fluid resuscitation in patients with traumatic brain injury. N Engl J Med. 2007;357(9):874–84.
105. Hawryluk GWJ, Aguilera S, Buki A, Bulger E, Citerio G, Cooper DJ, et al. A management algorithm for patients with intracranial pressure monitoring: the Seattle international severe traumatic brain injury consensus conference (SIBICC). Intensive Care Med. 2019;45(12):1783–94.
106. Thorup L, Koch KU, Upton RN, Ostergaard L, Rasmussen M. Effects of vasopressors on cerebral circulation and oxygenation: a narrative review of pharmacodynamics in health and traumatic brain injury. J Neurosurg Anesthesiol. 2020;32(1):18–28.
107. Huijben JA, Volovici V, Cnossen MC, Haitsma IK, Stocchetti N, Maas AIR, et al. Variation in general supportive and preventive intensive care management of traumatic brain injury: a survey in 66 neurotrauma centers participating in the collaborative European NeuroTrauma effectiveness research in traumatic brain injury (CENTER-TBI) study. Crit Care. 2018;22(1):90.
108. Steiner LA, Johnston AJ, Czosnyka M, Chatfield DA, Salvador R, Coles JP, et al. Direct comparison of cerebrovascular effects of norepinephrine and dopamine in head-injured patients. Crit Care Med. 2004;32(4):1049–54.
109. Depreitere B, Meyfroidt G, Guiza F. What do we mean by cerebral perfusion pressure? Acta Neurochir Suppl. 2018;126:201–3.
110. Craig TR, Duffy MJ, Shyamsundar M, McDowell C, McLaughlin B, Elborn JS, et al. Extravascular lung water indexed to predicted body weight is a novel predictor of intensive care unit mortality in patients with acute lung injury. Crit Care Med. 2010;38(1):114–20.
111. Phillips CR, Chesnutt MS, Smith SM. Extravascular lung water in sepsis-associated acute respiratory distress syndrome: indexing with predicted body weight improves correlation with severity of illness and survival. Crit Care Med. 2008;36(1):69–73.
112. Mascia L. Acute lung injury in patients with severe brain injury: a double hit model. Neurocrit Care. 2009;11(3):417–26.
113. Monnet X, Anguel N, Osman D, Hamzaoui O, Richard C, Teboul JL. Assessing pulmonary permeability by transpulmonary thermodilution allows differentiation of hydrostatic pulmonary edema from ALI/ARDS. Intensive Care Med. 2007;33(3):448–53.
114. Lichtenstein DA, Meziere GA, Lagoueyte JF, Biderman P, Goldstein I, Gepner A. A-lines and B-lines: lung ultrasound as a bedside tool for predicting pulmonary artery occlusion pressure in the critically ill. Chest. 2009;136(4):1014–20.

Temperature Control and the Role of Therapeutic Hypothermia in Traumatic Brain Injury

18

W. Dalton Dietrich and Helen M. Bramlett

18.1 Introduction

Traumatic brain injury (TBI) is a serious life threatening condition that can lead to impairments in psychosocial and cognitive function caused by a variety of insults [1, 2]. Traffic accidents, military incidents, falls, construction accidents, violent crimes, and gunshots are some of the initiators of TBI injury. According to the Center for Disease Control and Prevention, there is an estimated 1.7 million TBIs in the USA annually with a trimodal distribution of incidence being 0–4 years, 15–19 years, and greater than 16 years at highest risks [3–6]. The majority of TBIs are considered mild and recent emphasis has been placed on single or multiple episodes of concussion in sports-related injuries as well as in the military and other situations. More than 20 million people around the globe are living with the consequences of TBI related disabilities [7] with many individuals unable to return to normal life. Recent studies from the World Health Organization estimate that more than 100 billion dollars of expenditures are annually lost in income due to TBI related insults [8]. Over the past decade TBI related emergency department visits have increased >70%. Together this has led to a greater awareness of the importance of TBI in our society and the need for increased funding for preclinical and clinical studies targeting this serious medical problem [9].

W. D. Dietrich (✉)
Department of Neurological Surgery, Miami Project to Cure Paralysis, University of Miami Miller School of Medicine, Miami, FL, USA
e-mail: ddietrich@med.miami.edu

H. M. Bramlett
Department of Neurological Surgery, Miami Project to Cure Paralysis, University of Miami Miller School of Medicine, Miami, FL, USA

Bruce W. Carter Department of Veterans, Affairs Medical Center, Miami, FL, USA

E. Brogi et al. (eds.), *Traumatic Brain Injury*, Hot Topics in Acute Care Surgery and Trauma, https://doi.org/10.1007/978-3-031-50117-3_18

Profound levels of hypothermia have been known for years to be potentially effective in reducing brain edema and improving functional outcomes in models of TBI as well as other clinical conditions [10–13]. The benefits of hypothermia were noted 5000 years ago by the Egyptians and in the 1800s, local head cooling was used by Phelps for the treatment of head injury. In the 1940s, case reports and uncontrolled studies reported the benefits of induced hypothermia on neurological outcomes after cardiac arrest and TBI [14–17]. In these early investigations, studies were hampered by the potential side effects of profound hypothermia that produced difficulties due to lack of modern intensive care practices with patients commonly treated without ventilatory or circulatory support [12, 18]. Another aspect of those early studies was that it was assumed that the body temperature needed to be lowered as much as possible to achieve optimal therapeutic benefits. This assumption was made since it was presumed that the mechanisms of hypothermia primarily targeted metabolism and oxygen demand thereby necessitating profound levels of hypothermia [19]. Eventually, the risk factors associated with profound hypothermia as well as the discovery of new pharmacological interventions including novel neuroprotective compounds limited the testing of profound level of hypothermia in large-scale clinical trials [20].

In the 1980s and early 1990s, animal studies using large and small animal models of brain injury including cerebral ischemia and TBI were clarifying the pathophysiology of secondary injury mechanisms and searching for novel targets to provide neuroprotection [21, 22]. In a model of hypoxic/ischemic damage, **Berntman and colleagues** [23] reported improved biochemical markers of brain damage with 36 °C versus 37 °C in rodents. In models of transient forebrain global ischemia in rodents, investigations were being conducted to reproduce the injury mechanisms, neuropathology, and behavioral consequences of cardiac arrest and to identify pharmacological and molecular targets for neuroprotection [24–26]. In these models, evidence that relatively small variations in intra-ischemic brain temperature critically determined the severity of histopathological injury and subsequent functional outcomes in rodent models was first demonstrated. For example, **Busto and colleagues** [27] reported the importance of monitoring measurements of brain temperature during a period of transient global ischemia in determining the vulnerability of CA1 hippocampal neuropathology. In that study, data were presented showing that body and brain temperature differed during the anesthetized period of cerebral ischemia and that while mild-to-moderate reductions in brain temperature significantly reduced neuropathological damage, small elevations in intra-ischemic brain temperature significantly increased CA1 pathology compared to normothermic animals. These early investigations emphasized the need to closely monitor and maintain temperature at normothermic levels in all models of acute neurological injury such as focal ischemia, TBI, and spinal cord injury (SCI). This was specifically important for studies evaluating novel therapeutic agents to improve consistency and reproducibility of published findings.

The findings that mild variations in intra-ischemic brain temperature could have dramatic effects on histopathological outcomes helped stimulate new interest in the use of mild-to-moderate hypothermia in the postinjury period in multiple animal models [28]. Additional studies were conducted by research groups mostly replicating these initial findings and reporting the benefits of therapeutic hypothermia (TH) on clinically relevant outcomes [29–33]. In these studies, reports of postinjury cooling of relatively restricted durations and survival periods were published showing significant levels of protection compared to normothermic animals. However, subsequent studies that included longer survival periods showed that although restricted durations of hypothermia were protective compared to normothermic ischemic animals, this protection was lost if the animals were allowed to survive for longer periods [34, 35]. Taken together, these studies helped lead to the appreciation of the importance of more extended periods of cooling to provide longer lasting periods of neuroprotection [36, 37].

In parallel with these studies, other investigations emphasized the potentially detrimental effects of mild elevations in temperature during or after the insult [38]. For example, in models of global and focal ischemia and TBI, delayed increases in brain temperature to 39 °C resulted in worsening of neuropathological and behavioral outcomes [39, 40]. Subsequent clinical studies began to evaluate the frequency of periods of fever and reactive hyperthermia in severe brain injured patients and relate these physiological events to long-term outcomes [41–47]. These clinical studies provided important data showing that patients experiencing fevers in some cases demonstrated worsening of outcome measures [44–47]. Together these clinical and preclinical studies were critical in understanding the importance of targeted temperature management (TTM) in providing conditions to limit secondary insults. These investigations also provided support for the clinical translation of standardized intensive care strategies to induce mild-to-moderate hypothermia and to prevent periods of fever and reactive hyperthermia in severely injured patients.

18.2 Use of Moderate Hypothermia in Experimental TBI

In the clinical setting, the depth of hypothermia is stratified into mild (34–32 °C), moderate (31–28 °C), deep (27–11 °C), and profound (<10 °C) [13]. In terms of mild hypothermia following TBI, Clifton and colleagues [48] first reported that moderate hypothermia in a model of lateral fluid percussion brain injury in rats improved motor recovery if initiated before or after TBI. Animals treated 5 min after TBI with hypothermia (30 °C) for 1 h. displayed significantly less beam-walking, beam-balance, and body weight loss deficits compared to normothermia (38 °C). In subsequent TBI studies using a similar model, posttraumatic moderate hypothermia was reported to significantly reduce contusion volume and improve neuronal survival in cortical and hippocampal brain regions compared to normothermic conditions including chronic histopathological damage [49, 50]. Beneficial results with moderate hypothermia were also shown in multiple laboratories using other models of both focal and diffuse TBI showing that early hypothermia reduced histopathological damage including diffused axonal injury (DAI) and alterations in blood–brain barrier (BBB) [51–56]. Although most studies reported positive effects of therapeutic hypothermia on specific outcome measures, reported limitations of hypothermia indicated the need to further clarify questions regarding optimal treatment factors critical for long-term protection including therapeutic window, levels of hypothermia, duration of cooling as well as other issues [56, 57]. In terms of therapeutic window for posttraumatic cooling, **Markgraf and colleagues** [58] reported that hypothermia (3 h at 30 °C) induced immediately or 60 min after TBI significantly reduced increases in edema at 24 h and early neurological deficits. However, delaying the initiation of hypothermia by 90 or 120 min did not result in neurological protection. Importantly, some of the limitations for the successful use of TH that were first realized in these preclinical studies such as therapeutic window remain unanswered and have been recognized in clinical investigations [59, 60].

In a recent systematic review and meta-analysis of hypothermia in experimental TBI, 90 publications reporting 272 experiments testing hypothermia were examined [61]. In this preclinical literature review, limitations of the published literature including the quality of experimental designs were noted that could influence results including behavioral outcomes commonly reported in the clinical literature. Fortunately, research is still being conducted and high-quality preclinical studies are addressing specific questions that will enhance successful clinical translation by clarifying best practices for the use of TH and TTM. Most importantly, conditions that may allow researchers to predict TBI responders and non-responders to TH in very heterogeneous populations need to be addressed.

18.3 Mechanisms Underlying Temperature Effects

The pathophysiology of TBI is multifactorial and involves multiple injury mechanisms where each may have a major impact on determining the long-term outcomes in both experimental and clinical conditions [62, 63]. Following TBI, the temporal profile of these injury mechanisms has been reported using multiple techniques including immunocytochemical, biochemical, and molecular approaches to identify novel targets for therapeutic interventions. There is a growing list of injury processes that are sensitive to small variations in brain temperature and hypothermia including excitotoxicity, free radical generation, programmed cell death, and neural inflammation [33, 64–74]. In addition to alterations in neuronal injury, secondary injury pathways targeting blood–brain barrier breakdown and the activation and survival of glial cells have also been demonstrated [52, 75].

Over the past 20 years, preclinical studies have consistently reported the benefits of small reductions in core and head temperature on various posttraumatic pathophysiological mechanisms. Indeed, in terms of animal studies, therapeutic hypothermia is the most effective neuroprotective strategy demonstrated in the laboratory when applied early after injury and maintained for specific durations [76]. In addition to alterations in metabolism and cerebral blood flow, temperature sensitive changes in free radical generation, excitotoxicity, inflammation, and a variety of molecular events have been emphasized. Posttraumatic inflammatory processes have been implicated in the pathophysiology of TBI and different levels of therapeutic hypothermia have been shown to attenuate proinflammatory mediators including reduced levels of cytokines and chemokines detected in the injured tissues and blood biomarkers [77–80]. For example, **Truettner and colleagues** [81] first determined the effects of TH on subsets of proinflammatory or anti-inflammatory mediators. This study provided a link between temperature sensitive alterations and macrophage and microglia activation including the phenotypic polarization permissive for cell survival and repair. Hypothermia has also been reported to target various cell signaling cascades that are important in several intracellular processes involved in the maintenance of cytoskeletal components, synaptic function as well as cognitive deficits [28, 71, 76, 82, 83]. In one recent study, **Yan and colleagues** [84] reported using a closed cortical injury model that hypothermia treatment enhanced the activity of the antioxidant enzyme superoxide dismutase and glutathione peroxidase and upregulated the nuclear factor erythroid 2-related factor 2- antioxidant response element pathway (Nrf2-ARE). Recently, a role of the cold stress pathway and the induction of cold stress proteins that normally increase during cold stress as potential applications for neuroprotection have also recently been introduced into the TH literature [13]. Other studies reported that hypothermia may target reperfusion brain injury, posttraumatic reparative processes such as hippocampal neurogenesis and wound healing events with chronic posttraumatic cellular molecular events [72, 85].

The ability of small temperature variations to impact multiple secondary injury mechanisms following cerebral ischemia and neurotrauma makes this a very powerful experimental tool by which to manipulate the severity of secondary injuries as well as protect against long-term structural and functional outcomes. This is an important point since many pharmaceutical approaches target more selective pathways believed to play an important role in neuronal cell death. However, focusing on a single mechanism of action may have disadvantages because of the complexity of the pathophysiology of TBI and the possible need to target multiple injury cascades. Taken together these preclinical findings generated by many laboratories in different countries emphasize the importance of brain temperature in significantly influencing the short- and long-term consequences of acute CNS injury.

18.4 Early Clinical Studies with Hypothermia

Based on a wealth of preclinical data, clinical application was initiated to successfully translate this experimental treatment into the clinical arena. An important event that allowed TH to be critically investigated was standard protocol improvements in neuro-intensive care units where the side effects of hypothermia treatment could be assessed and treated. Also, new technologies were developed that improved the efficiency and convenience of inducing periods of TH and TTM in acutely injured patients including surface and intravascular cooling strategies. These advances were critical for rapidly reaching target temperatures and maintaining precise levels of cooling for extended periods of time. Additionally, controlled rewarming protocols are also implemented after TH with a positive effect in preventing rebound effects of returning to normothermia too quickly.

To date, TH and TTM have been tested in several neurological emergencies with some studies providing clear evidence for the beneficial effects while others having shown mixed or conflicting results [28]. Over the years, single institution clinical studies have assessed the efficacy of hypothermia in severe TBI in both adult and pediatric patient populations [12]. **Marion and colleagues** [86] first reported encouraging findings showing that posttraumatic hypothermia improved patient survival and functional outcomes when compared to normothermic levels. Other single institutional studies with relatively small numbers of severe TBI patients also reported positive findings including hypothermia-induced reductions in elevated intracranial pressure [12]. It is important to note that early clinical studies commonly utilized clinical protocols that differed from one institution to another. Also, some studies may not have been properly randomized between temperature groups which may have presented bias in the reported results. It is also important to note that early single institution studies were done in neurotrauma centers that specialized in the management of severe TBI patients. In these optimal conditions, available clinical personnel could properly manage potential side effects associated with the use of hypothermia in these severely injured patients.

In addition to the therapeutic window and duration of hypothermia, levels of hypothermia as well as rewarming phases are felt to be important factors in determining whether the treatment has a significant effect on neurological outcomes. More recently in the cardiac arrest and neonatal hypoxia literature where hypothermia is being utilized routinely, it has become clear that injury severity can play an important role in determining the benefits of hypothermia including levels of cooling [87–89]. In addition, evidence indicating that fever can also adversely affect neurological outcome in various types of neurological injury has led to standardized recommendations that call for limiting temperature elevations above 37.5 °C or maintain cooling at normothermia. Thus, in contrast to widespread use of cooling in many situations of critical care, randomized controlled studies indicate that fever prevention and the rigorous control of patients' temperature in the normothermic range may be effective in improving long-term neurological outcomes [90–95].

Unfortunately, although early hypothermia TBI studies provided support for hypothermia after clinical TBI, several multicenter trials failed to show similar benefits on neurological outcomes [96–98]. Three early multicenter trials reported either no difference or worse mortality rates in the hypothermia group compared to normothermia. For the initial National Acute Brain Injury Study Hypothermia (NABISH) [99], differences in critical care protocols across recruiting sites were mentioned as contributing to the lack of positive effects with hypothermia. Several other problems were appreciated in this rather large clinical trial including a delayed initiation of cooling and issues with hypotension, hypovolemia, electrolytes, and hypoglycemia. Also, it was noted that some of the centers that participated in this large TBI study had limited previous experience using hypothermia. Also noted was a substantial inter-center variance in outcomes between hospitals indicating that optimal use of TH in these severely traumatized patients may have varied between recruitment sites. However, in the second NABISH study as well as the Japanese Brain Hypothermia (B-HYPO) trial, no difference between severe TBI patients treated with hypothermia and normothermia was again reported [92, 100]. Interestingly, in the **Maekawa trial**, fever control management was reported to significantly reduce TBI-mediated mortality compared to the mild hypothermia group [101].

The Japanese Brain Hypothermia (B-HYPO) trial was a prospective multicenter randomized control trial where patients were assigned either to fever control (35.5 °C–37.0 °C) or mild TH (32.0 °C–34.0 °C) [92]. In that study where cooling was initiated within 2 h of TBI and maintained for at least 72 h, hypothermia treatment was not shown to be effective. In contrast to hypothermia, fever control management was reported to reduce TBI-mediated mortality compared to the mild hypothermia group [101]. Importantly, this result is consistent with systematic reviews indicating that controlled normothermia improves surrogate outcomes of severe TBI again suggesting a beneficial effect of limiting the potentially detrimental effects of periods of hyperthermia [102]. Another post-hoc analysis of the B-HYPO study reported that a proportion of patients with evacuated hematoma showed improvement if the slow rewarming period was prolonged over 48 h [103]. Also, using the CT database from the B-HYPO trial, **Kobata and colleagues** [104] reported a trend toward favorable outcomes when 35.5 °C was reached earlier in young patients with acute subdural hematoma.

The European **Eurotherm3235 Trial** represented a pragmatic trial examining the effectiveness of reducing ICP and morbidity and mortality at 6 months after TBI [105–107]. Subject enrollment for this trial was 385 patients enrolled in 47 centers in 18 countries and were randomized to receive either TH in addition to standard of care or only standard of care. The Eurotherm3235 trial reported that in patients with an ICP of more than 20 mmHg, hypothermia with standard of care successfully reduced ICP but led to a higher mortality rate and worse functional outcome. In this study, the ability to blind treatment allocations may have led to the biased recordings of serious adverse events indicating the need for accurately powered clinical trials for therapies used to reduce ICP.

Based on these studies, the duration of hypothermia necessary to target both early and late occurring secondary injury mechanisms that may remain active for extended posttraumatic periods was considered in additional clinical trials. Several studies have utilized extended cooling procedures including both early and prolonged cooling that in some cases included the period where ICP was elevated [93, 108, 109]. In the study by **Jiang and colleagues** [108], for example, extending the cooling period up to 5 days was reported to provide better neurological outcomes compared to a 2-day cooling protocol.

Several meta-analysis studies have been published based on systematic literature reviews for hypothermia therapy [102, 110–113]. In this regard, a Cochrane metanalysis of all clinical trials of hypothermia has not shown an overall benefit in severe TBI [114]. Thus, despite the widespread use of cooling in neuro-intensive care units, recent randomized control studies indicate that inhibiting periods of fever may be most beneficial for improving outcomes. Strategies using mild periods of TH or other TTM protocols to maintain rigorous control of patient temperature at 37 °C may be equally effective versus moderate therapeutic hypothermia to 33 °C on long-term neurological outcomes on adults/children with brain injury [92–97].

18.5 Recent Post-Hoc Analyses and Clinical Studies

As a follow-up to the Eurotherm3235 trial, **Abu-Arafeh and colleagues** [115] investigated whether increased temperature variability during the first 48 h or during the seven-day post randomization period were modifiable risk factors associated with poor outcome. This group reported that high levels of temperature variability within the first 48 h were associated with poor Glasgow Outcome Scale scores at 6 months post-randomization indicating that temperature variability may have been a significant variable in this trial.

In 2018 the POLAR trial that represented a high-quality international study reported that early and sustained TH did not improve mortality or neurological recovery in severe TBI patients [95, 116]. Thus, the use of early prophylactic hypothermia for this patient population was not recommended. Interestingly a subsequent meta-analysis of the POLAR study evaluated the extent of cooling using a cooling index (COIN) and reported that TH was beneficial in those TBI patients where the cooling index was significantly high [117]. In that study, deviations from the protocol in terms of achieving predetermined cooling levels were suggested to have possibly masked the benefits of TH.

In another recent study by **Hui and colleagues** [118], the safety and efficacy of long-term hypothermia for severe TBI with refractory intracranial hypotension were evaluated in a multicenter randomized control trial [118]. In this study, hypothermia 34–35 °C for 5 days compared to the normothermic group showed no difference on favorable outcomes between the groups. However, in select patients with an initial ICP of greater than 30 mmHg, hypothermia treatment significantly increased favorable outcomes over the normothermic group and did not increase the incidence of complications. These data indicate that TH may be a potential option in severe TBI patients with a specific range of initial ICP readings. Additional studies are currently being conducted to test this hypothesis.

A more recent meta-analysis by **Wu and colleagues** [119] used several electronic databases including Cochrane CENTRAL, PubMed, MedLine, and other sources of information to evaluate TH in severe TBI studies. This group also found no statistically significant differences in several studies testing the benefits of TH with complications being reported to be significantly higher in the hypothermia group. However, owing to the limited number of studies that met their inclusion criteria for evaluation, more randomized controlled trials are required to establish the true effects of early cooling in adult TBI using this method of analysis.

Recent clinical studies have also been directed at attempting to clarify factors that may differentiate severe TBI patients as responders and non-responders to TH and TTM. In a recent multicenter randomized clinical trial in patients with traumatic subdural hematoma, **Hergenroeder and colleagues** [120] assessed the effects of early induction and maintenance of hypothermia including assessing several blood biomarkers as potential diagnostic strategies. Interestingly, although the Data and Safety Monitoring Board recommended the early termination of the study because of futility, plasma levels of glial fibrillary acidic protein but not ubiquitin C-terminal hydrolase L1 were lower in patients with favorable outcomes compared to those with unfavorable outcomes. In the future, blood and other surrogate biomarker evaluations may provide guidance for treating physicians regarding which severe TBI patients may best benefit from extended cooling strategies including cooling levels.

A recent post-hoc analysis of a randomized controlled study of mild therapeutic hypothermia in evacuated hematoma patients with severe TBI reported that a proportion of hypothermic patients with good neurological outcomes were significantly different when divided into subgroups by a cutoff value of the rewarming time [103]. Indeed, slow rewarming periods greater than 48 h appeared to potentially improve the neurological outcomes of the patients undergoing prolonged mild therapeutic hypothermia. Another post-hoc analysis for the B-HYPO study reported that mild decreases in heart rate during the early phase of TH following tachycardia on admission were associated with unfavorable neurological outcomes after severe TBI [121].

18.6 Additional Variables Impacting the Use of TH and TTM

Age may be an important variable in determining the effects of any therapeutic intervention including brain hypothermia. In a recent study, **Kobata and colleagues** [104] investigated individual CT findings of severe TBI patients that were treated with TH from the B-HYPO study. Interestingly, potential benefits of early hypothermia in young patients with acute subdural hematoma were shown despite no difference between CT findings in the different groups. However, the use of TH and TTM in children with TBI remains controversial [96, 97, 122–125]. The Cool Kids Trial was a multi-national randomized controlled trial examining the effect of hypothermia and normothermia on mortality in children with severe TBI [90]. The trial randomly allocated patients stratified by recruitment site and age including <6 years, 6–15 years, and 16–17 years to either hypothermia (32–33 °C) or normothermia (36.5–37.5 °C) for 48–72 h. This trial was halted early for futility. In a recent study by **Rosario and colleagues** [126], secondary analysis of the Cool Kids Trial emphasized that severe TBI is a clinically heterogeneous disease that can be accompanied by a range of neurological impairments in a variety of injury patterns. This secondary analysis identified several characteristics associated with outcome among TBI with severe TBI that require better characterization in terms of multiple phenotypes within this population. A phase II randomized control clinical trial on hypothermia for TBI in children was also conducted by **Beca and colleagues** [97]. In this pilot study, early TH in children with severe TBI did not show improved outcome and therefore the reviewers concluded that it should not be used outside the clinical trial. A recent meta-analysis that searched six online databases including 8 randomized control trials indicated that hypothermia may increase the Glasgow Outcome Scores [125]. However, there were no significant differences in improving rates of complications, intracranial pressure, mortality, cerebral perfusion pressure, or length of stay in both hospital and pediatric ICUs. In a 2021 study that analyzed cerebrospinal fluid samples from the Cool Kids trial, **Zusman and colleagues** [127] reported that levels of sulfonylurea receptor-1 (SUR1), a key contributor to cerebral edema and hemorrhagic progression and possibly cell death were associated with intracranial pressure and outcomes in the Cool Kids Trial. These data indicate that SUR1 may be a therapeutic target in a subclass of pediatric TBI patients.

Finally, an important area of continued research in the areas of TH and TTM involves the continued development and testing of new temperature modulating devices to be used to actively cool patients. Currently there are no uniform targeted temperature management guidelines for this patient population [128]. In a recent study by **Bachatti and colleagues** [128], temperature management was discussed to determine whether a new esophageal temperature management (ETM) control device was effective in controlling core temperature in TBI cases. In a single site study, 12 patients received TTM protocol using ETM and reported that 11 out of 12 patients reached temperature during the first 10 h of treatment. In another study, **Ferreira and colleagues** [129], in a prospective nonrandomized interventional clinical trial of 5 patients with severe TBI evaluated the safety and efficacy of a nasal pharyngeal catheter for selective brain cooling. In this study nasal pharyngeal cooling through a catheter reduced temperature greater than ≥2 °C with the intervention appearing to be well tolerated with no significant changes observed in hemodynamic parameters. Because a recent meta-analysis found that therapeutic hypothermia can be initiated in patients with severe TBI as an optional treatment, strategies leading to reductions of temperature of the entire body versus more selective head or brain cooling is an area of continued research.

18.7 Summary and Final Comments

Traumatic brain injury is a complex and highly heterogenous neurological disorder that results in life long serious issues related to functional abnormalities and various quality of life issues. The pathophysiology of TBI is also complicated which has provided challenges for successfully translating neuroprotective and reparative treatments to the clinic. The fact that TH and TTM target many important secondary injury mechanisms supports the translation of this experimental therapy to the clinic. However, multiple factors including issues concerning patient heterogeneity, variations in temperature management as well as unknowns regarding the optimal duration or level of hypothermia remain to be determined.

Taken together, current clinical findings indicate that the injured adult human brain appears to be less protected by TH compared with the injured rodent brain based on preclinical data [13, 130]. As previously discussed, factors such as age-related differences, time to initiate cooling, duration of cooling, and depth of cooling remain critical questions for this field. It should also be noted that differences exist in cooling strategies where reaching the desired hypothermic level rapidly in small animal studies is much easier compared to the clinical situation. Other possible differences in standard of care, rates of rewarming, and managing multiorgan and adverse side effects in severely injured patients contribute to the complexity of using TH or TTM in the clinic [13]. Also, it should be stressed that over the last century, critical care has dramatically decreased mortality and increased the lifespan of the TBI population. These advances have potentially raised the bar to detect significant benefits of cooling after severe TBI when improvements in medical care are considered.

As we continue to evaluate this experimental therapy for severe TBI, there may be lessons learned from other neurological fields that could help identify strategies moving forward. For example, in clinical areas where TH has been successful in patients recovering from out-of-hospital cardiac arrest and neonatal hypoxic encephalopathy, recent studies are clarifying several factors relevant to TBI [131–133]. In the area of cardiac arrest, for example, it is now clear that patient heterogeneity and strategies for cooling are important factors in the success of the therapy. Indeed, cardiac arrest patients with mild, moderate, and severe insults may respond positively to different levels of hypothermia. Thus, the stratification of patients using clinical assessments or other biomarker signatures may be used to guide therapies [133, 134]. Likewise, the importance of initiating cooling strategies as soon as possible using the most effective cooling devices allowing for rapid targeted temperature and precise maintenance for extended times is critical. Influence of Cooling duration on Efficacy in Cardiac Arrest Patients (ICECAP) aims to answer how long to maintain hypothermic temperature control using an adaptive design and machine learning for patients to preferentially randomize to duration based on previous enrollees [133]. The use of combination approaches where targeted temperature is combined with a neuroprotective or reparative therapy might also be an important strategy especially in the most severely injured patient. Continued development of new effective technologies to better induce hypothermia rapidly that decrease temperature variability and that can be used effectively in the emergency vehicle or at the bedside represent continued areas of investigation. There is no doubt that more clinical studies will be conducted on the use of TH and TTM in this growing patient population. Hopefully in the coming years we can clarify specific patient populations that would benefit most from this experimental but powerful therapeutic intervention.

References

1. Faul MXL, Wald MM, Coronado VG. Traumatic brain injury in the United States: emergency department visits, hospitalizations, and deaths. Atlanta, GA: Centers for Disease Control and Prevention, National Center for Injury Prevention and Control; 2010.
2. Dewan MC, Rattani A, Gupta S, Baticulon RE, Hung YC, Punchak M, Agrawal A, Adeleye AO, Shrime MG, Rubiano AM, Rosenfeld JV, Park KB. Estimating the global incidence of traumatic brain injury. J Neurosurg. 2018;130:1080–97. Advance online publication.
3. Corrigan JD, Selassie AW, Orman JA. The epidemiology of traumatic brain injury. J Head Trauma Rehabil. 2010;25:72–80.
4. Langlois JA, Rutland-Brown W, Wald MM. The epidemiology and impact of traumatic brain injury: a brief overview. J Head Trauma Rehabil. 2006;21:375–8.
5. CDC. Traumatic Brain Injury in the United States, emergency department visits, hospitalizations, and deaths. 2016. http://www.cdc.gov/traumaticbraininjury/pdf/blue_book.pdf.

6. Sarnaik A, Ferguson NM, O'Meara A, Agrawal S, Deep A, Buttram S, Bell MJ, Wisniewski SR, Luther JF, Hartman AL, Vavilala MS, Investigators of the ADAPT Trial. Age and mortality in pediatric severe traumatic Brain Injury: results from an international study. Neurocrit Care. 2018;28(3):302–13.
7. Capizzi A, Woo J, Verduzco-Gutierrez M. Traumatic Brain Injury: an overview of epidemiology, pathophysiology, and medical management. Med Clin North Am. 2020;104(2):213–38.
8. Tarvonen-Schröder S, Tenovuo O, Kaljonen A, Laimi K. Usability of World Health Organization disability assessment schedule in chronic traumatic brain injury. J Rehabil Med. 2018;50(6):514–8.
9. Thurman DJ, Alverson C, Dunn KA, Guerrero J, Sniezek JE. Traumatic brain injury in the United States: a public health perspective. J Head Trauma Rehabil. 1999;14:602–15.
10. Rosomoff HL, Safar P. Management of the comatose patient. Clin Anesth. 1965;1:244–58.
11. Polderman KH, Tjong Tjin Joe R, Peerdeman SM, Vandertop WP, Girbes AR. Effects of therapeutic hypothermia on intracranial pressure and outcome in patients with severe head injury. Intensive Care Med. 2002;28:1563–73.
12. Polderman KH. Induced hypothermia and fever control for prevention and treatment of neurological injuries. Lancet (London, England). 2008;371(9628):1955–69.
13. Jackson TC, Kochanek PM. A new vision for therapeutic hypothermia in the era of targeted temperature management: a speculative synthesis. Ther Hypothermia Temp Manag. 2019;9(1):13–47.
14. Fay T. Observations on generalized refrigeration in cases of severe cerebral trauma. Assoc Res Nerv Ment Dis Proc. 1943;24:611–9.
15. Williams GR Jr, Spencer FC. The clinical use of hypothermia following cardiac arrest. Ann Surg. 1958;148:462–8.
16. Benson DW, Williams GR, Spencer FC. The use of hypothermia following cardiac arrest. Anesth Analg. 1959;38:423–8.
17. Alzaga AG, Salazar GA, Varon J. Resuscitation great. Breaking the thermal barrier: Dr. Temple Fay. Resuscitation. 2006;69:359–64.
18. Brain Trauma F, American Association of Neurological, S., Congress of Neurological, S. Guidelines for the management of severe traumatic brain injury. J Neurotrauma. 2007;24(Suppl 1):S1–106.
19. Rosomoff HL, Holaday DA. Cerebral blood flow and cerebral oxygen consumption during hypothermia. Am J Phys. 1954;179:85–8.
20. Karnatovskaia LV, Wartenberg KE, Freeman WD. Therapeutic hypothermia for neuroprotection: history, mechanisms, risks, and clinical applications. Neurohospitalist. 2014;4:153–63.
21. Dietrich WD, Busto R, Globus MY, Ginsberg MD. Brain damage and temperature: cellular and molecular mechanisms. Adv Neurol. 1996;71:177–97.
22. Polderman KH, Andrews PJ. Hypothermia in patients with brain injury: the way forward? Lancet Neurol. 2011;10:404–5. author reply 1180.0.
23. Berntman L, Welsh FA, Harp JR. Cerebral protective effect of low-grade hypothermia. Anesthesiology. 1981;55:495–8.
24. Pulsinelli WA, Brierley JB. A new model of bilateral hemispheric ischemia in the unanesthetized rat. Stroke. 1979;10:267–72.
25. Furlow TW Jr. Cerebral ischemia produced by four-vessel occlusion in the rat: a quantitative evaluation of cerebral blood flow. Stroke. 1982;13(6):852–5.
26. Blomgvist P, Mabe H, Ingvar M, Siesjo BK. Models for studying long-term recovery following forebrain ischemia in the rat.1. Circulatory and functional effects of 4-vessel occlusion. Acta Neurol Scand. 1984;69:376–84.
27. Busto R, Dietrich WD, Globus MY, Valdes I, Scheinberg P, Ginsberg MD. Small differences in intra ischemic brain temperature critically determine the extent of ischemic neuronal injury. J Cereb Blood Flow Metab. 1987;7:729–38.
28. Dietrich WD, Bramlett HM. Therapeutic hypothermia and targeted temperature management for traumatic brain injury: experimental and clinical experience. Brain Circ. 2017;3(4):186–98.

29. Leonov Y, Sterz F, Safar P, Radovsky A, Oku K, Tisherman S, Stezoski SW. Mild cerebral hypothermia during and after cardiac arrest improves neurologic outcome in dogs. J Cereb Blood Flow Metab. 1990;10:57–70.
30. Welsh FA, Sims RE, Harris VA. Mild hypothermia prevents ischemic injury in gerbil hippocampus. J Cereb Blood Flow Metab. 1990;10(4):557–63.
31. Onesti ST, Baker CJ, Sun PP, Solomon RA. Transient hypothermia reduces focal ischemic brain injury in the rat. Neurosurgery. 1991;29(3):369–73.
32. Bramlett HM, Green EJ, Dietrich WD, Busto R, Globus MY, Ginsberg MD. Posttraumatic brain hypothermia provides protection from sensorimotor and cognitive behavioral deficits. J Neurotrauma. 1995;12:289–98.
33. Dietrich WD, Atkins CM, Bramlett HM. Protection in animal models of brain and spinal cord injury with mild to moderate hypothermia. J Neurotrauma. 2009;26:301–12.
34. Dietrich WD, Busto R, Alonso O, Globus MY, Ginsberg MD. Intraischemic but not postischemic brain hypothermia protects chronically following global forebrain ischemia in rats. J Cereb Blood Flow Metab. 1993;13(4):541–9.
35. Colbourne F, Li H, Buchan AM. Indefatigable CA1 sector neuroprotection with mild hypothermia induced 6 hours after severe forebrain ischemia in rats. J Cereb Blood Flow Metab. 1999;19(7):742–9.
36. Corbett D, Hamilton M, Colbourne F. Persistent neuroprotection with prolonged postischemic hypothermia in adult rats subjected to transient middle cerebral artery occlusion. Exp Neurol. 2000;163(1):200–6.
37. Lu XC, Shear DA, Deng-Bryant Y, Leung LY, Wei G, Chen Z, Tortella FC. Comprehensive evaluation of neuroprotection achieved by extended selective brain cooling therapy in a rat model of penetrating ballistic-like brain injury. Ther Hypothermia Temp Manag. 2016;6(1):30–9.
38. Dietrich WD, Bramlett HM. Hyperthermia and central nervous system injury. Prog Brain Res. 2007;162:201–17.
39. Dietrich WD, Alonso O, Halley M, Busto R. Delayed posttraumatic brain hyperthermia worsens outcome after fluid percussion brain injury: a light and electron microscopic study in rats. Neurosurgery. 1996;38:533–41; discussion 541.
40. Yu CG, Jagid J, Ruenes G, Dietrich WD, Marcillo AE, Yezierski RP. Detrimental effects of systemic hyperthermia on locomotor function and histopathological outcome after traumatic spinal cord injury in the rat. Neurosurgery. 2001;49:152–8; discussion 158-9.
41. Kilpatrick MM, Lowry DW, Firlik AD, Yonas H, Marion DW. Hyperthermia in the neurosurgical intensive care unit. Neurosurgery. 2000;47:850–5; discussion 855-6.
42. Natale JE, Joseph JG, Helfaer MA, Shaffner DH. Early hyperthermia after traumatic brain injury in children: risk factors, influence on length of stay, and effect on short-term neurologic status. Crit Care Med. 2000;28:2608–15.
43. Thompson HJ, Pinto-Martin J, Bullock MR. Neurogenic fever after traumatic brain injury: an epidemiological study. J Neurol Neurosurg Psychiatry. 2003;74:614–9.
44. Diringer MN, Neurocritical Care Fever Reduction Trial, G. Treatment of fever in the neurologic intensive care unit with a catheter-based heat exchange system. Crit Care Med. 2004;32:559–64.
45. Todd MM, Hindman BJ, Clarke WR, Torner JC, Weeks JB, Bayman EO, Shi Q, Spofford CM, Investigators I. Perioperative fever and outcome in surgical patients with aneurysmal subarachnoid hemorrhage. Neurosurgery. 2009;64:897–908; discussion 908.
46. Li J, Jiang JY. Chinese head trauma data bank: effect of hyperthermia on the outcome of acute head trauma patients. J Neurotrauma. 2012;29:96–100.
47. Hifumi T, Kuroda Y, Kawakita K, Yamashita S, Oda Y, Dohi K, Maekawa T. Fever control management is preferable to mild therapeutic hypothermia in traumatic Brain Injury patients with abbreviated Injury scale 3-4: a multi-center, randomized controlled Trial. J Neurotrauma. 2016;33(11):1047–53.

48. Clifton GL, Jiang JY, Lyeth BG, Jenkins LW, Hamm RJ, Hayes RL. Marked protection by moderate hypothermia after experimental traumatic brain injury. J Cereb Blood Flow Metab. 1991;11:114–21.
49. Dietrich WD, Alonso O, Busto R, Globus MY, Ginsberg MD. Post-traumatic brain hypothermia reduces histopathological damage following concussive brain injury in the rat. Acta Neuropathol. 1994;87:250–8.
50. Bramlett HM, Dietrich WD, Green EJ, Busto R. Chronic histopathological consequences of fluid-percussion brain injury in rats: effects of post-traumatic hypothermia. Acta Neuropathol (Berl). 1997;93:190–9.
51. Lyeth BG, Jiang JY, Liu S. Behavioral protection by moderate hypothermia initiated after experimental traumatic brain injury. J Neurotrauma. 1993;10:57–64.
52. Smith SL, Hall ED. Mild pre- and posttraumatic hypothermia attenuates blood-brain barrier damage following controlled cortical impact injury in the rat. J Neurotrauma. 1996;13:1–9.
53. Dixon CE, Markgraf CG, Angileri F, Pike BR, Wolfson B, Newcomb JK, Bismar MM, Blanco AJ, Clifton GL, Hayes RL. Protective effects of moderate hypothermia on behavioral deficits but not necrotic cavitation following cortical impact injury in the rat. J Neurotrauma. 1998;15:95–103.
54. Matsushita Y, Bramlett HM, Alonso O, Dietrich WD. Posttraumatic hypothermia is neuroprotective in a model of traumatic brain injury complicated by a secondary hypoxic insult. Crit Care Med. 2001;29:2060–6.
55. Ma M, Matthews BT, Lampe JW, Meaney DF, Shofer FS, Neumar RW. Immediate short-duration hypothermia provides long-term protection in an in vivo model of traumatic axonal injury. Exp Neurol. 2009;215:119–27.
56. Bramlett HM, Dietrich WD. The effects of posttraumatic hypothermia on diffuse axonal Injury following Parasagittal fluid percussion brain injury in rats. Ther Hypothermia Temp Manag. 2012;2:14–23.
57. Bramlett H, Dietrich WD. Long-term consequences of traumatic brain injury: current status of potential mechanisms of Injury and neurologic outcomes. J Neurotrauma. 2014;32:1834.
58. Markgraf CG, Clifton GL, Moody MR. Treatment window for hypothermia in brain injury. J Neurosurg. 2001;95:979–83.
59. Suzuki T, Bramlett HM, Dietrich WD. The importance of gender on the beneficial effects of posttraumatic hypothermia. Exp Neurol. 2003;184:1017–26.
60. Suzuki T, Bramlett HM, Ruenes G, Dietrich WD. The effects of early post-traumatic hyperthermia in female and ovariectomized rats. J Neurotrauma. 2004;21:842–53.
61. Hirst TC, Klasen MG, Rhodes JK, Macleod MR, Andrews P. A systematic review and meta-analysis of hypothermia in experimental traumatic brain injury: why have promising animal studies not been replicated in pragmatic clinical trials? J Neurotrauma. 2020;37(19):2057–68.
62. Chesnut RM, Marshall LF, Klauber MR, Blunt BA, Baldwin N, Eisenberg HM, Jane JA, Marmarou A, Foulkes MA. The role of secondary brain injury in determining outcome from severe head injury. J Trauma. 1993a;34:216–22.
63. Robertson CS, Valadka AB, Hannay HJ, Contant CF, Gopinath SP, Cormio M, Uzura M, Grossman RG. Prevention of secondary ischemic insults after severe head injury. Crit Care Med. 1999;27:2086–95.
64. Dietrich WD. The importance of brain temperature in cerebral injury. J Neurotrauma. 1992;9(Suppl 2):S475–85.
65. Globus MY, Alonso O, Dietrich WD, Busto R, Ginsberg MD. Glutamate release and free radical production following brain injury: effects of posttraumatic hypothermia. J Neurochem. 1995;65:1704–11.
66. Kinoshita K, Chatzipanteli IK, Vitarbo E, Truettner JS, Alonso OF, Dietrich WD. Interleukin-1beta messenger ribonucleic acid and protein levels after fluid-percussion brain injury in rats: importance of injury severity and brain temperature. Neurosurgery. 2002a;51:195–203. discussion 203.

67. Truettner JS, Suzuki T, Dietrich WD. The effect of therapeutic hypothermia on the expression of inflammatory response genes following moderate traumatic brain injury in the rat. Brain Res Mol Brain Res. 2005;138:124–34.
68. Lotocki G, de Rivero Vaccari JP, Perez ER, Sanchez-Molano J, Furones-Alonso O, Bramlett HM, Dietrich WD. Alterations in blood-brain barrier permeability to large and small molecules and leukocyte accumulation after traumatic brain injury: effects of post-traumatic hypothermia. J Neurotrauma. 2009;26:1123–34.
69. Dietrich WD, Bramlett HM. The evidence for hypothermia as a neuroprotectant in traumatic brain injury. Neurotherapeutics. 2010;7:43–50.
70. Lotocki G, de Rivero Vaccari JP, Alonso O, Molano JS, Nixon R, Safavi P, Dietrich WD, Bramlett HM. Oligodendrocyte vulnerability following traumatic brain injury in rats. Neurosci Lett. 2011;499:143–8.
71. Yenari MA, Han HS. Neuroprotective mechanisms of hypothermia in brain ischaemia. Nat Rev Neurosci. 2012;13:267–78.
72. Yenari MA, Han HS. Influence of therapeutic hypothermia on regeneration after cerebral ischemia. Front Neurol Neurosci. 2013;32:122–8.
73. Han Z, Liu X, Luo Y, Ji X. Therapeutic hypothermia for stroke: where to go? Exp Neurol. 2015;272:67.
74. Li YH, Zhang CL, Zhang XY, Zhou HX, Meng LL. Effects of mild induced hypothermia on hippocampal connexin 43 and glutamate transporter 1 expression following traumatic brain injury in rats. Mol Med Rep. 2015;11:1991–6.
75. Jiang JY, Lyeth BG, Kapasi MZ, Jenkins LW, Povlishock JT. Moderate hypothermia reduces blood-brain barrier disruption following traumatic brain injury in the rat. Acta Neuropathol. 1992;84:495–500.
76. Dietrich WD, Bramlett HM. Therapeutic hypothermia and targeted temperature management in traumatic brain injury: clinical challenges for successful translation. Brain Res. 2016;1640(Pt A):94–103.
77. Chatzipanteli K, Wada K, Busto R, Dietrich WD. Effects of moderate hypothermia on constitutive and inducible nitric oxide synthase activities after traumatic brain injury in the rat. J Neurochem. 1999;72:2047–52.
78. Chatzipanteli K, Alonso OF, Kraydieh S, Dietrich WD. Importance of posttraumatic hypothermia and hyperthermia on the inflammatory response after fluid percussion brain injury: biochemical and immunocytochemical studies. J Cereb Blood Flow Metab. 2000;20:531–42.
79. Kinoshita K, Chatzipanteli K, Alonso OF, Howard M, Dietrich WD. The effect of brain temperature on hemoglobin extravasation after traumatic brain injury. J Neurosurg. 2002b;97:945–53.
80. Vitarbo EA, Chatzipanteli K, Kinoshita K, Truettner JS, Alonso OF, Dietrich WD. Tumor necrosis factor alpha expression and protein levels after fluid percussion injury in rats: the effect of injury severity and brain temperature. Neurosurgery. 2004;55:416–24; discussion 424-5.
81. Truettner JS, Bramlett HM, Dietrich WD. Posttraumatic therapeutic hypothermia alters microglial and macrophage polarization toward a beneficial phenotype. J Cereb Blood Flow Metab. 2017;37(8):2952–62.
82. Atkins CM, Oliva AA Jr, Alonso OF, Chen S, Bramlett HM, Hu BR, Dietrich WD. Hypothermia treatment potentiates ERK1/2 activation after traumatic brain injury. Eur J Neurosci. 2007;26:810–9.
83. Atkins CM, Truettner JS, Lotocki G, Sanchez-Molano J, Kang Y, Alonso OF, Sick TJ, Dietrich WD, Bramlett HM. Post-traumatic seizure susceptibility is attenuated by hypothermia therapy. Eur J Neurosci. 2010;32:1912–20.
84. Yan C, Mao J, Yao C, Liu Y, Yan H, Jin W. Neuroprotective effects of mild hypothermia against traumatic brain injury by the involvement of the Nrf2/ARE pathway. Brain Behav. 2022;12(8):e2686.

85. Bregy A, Nixon R, Lotocki G, Alonso OF, Atkins CM, Tsoulfas P, Bramlett HM, Dietrich WD. Posttraumatic hypothermia increases doublecortin expressing neurons in the dentate gyrus after traumatic brain injury in the rat. Exp Neurol. 2012;233:821–8.
86. Marion DW, Penrod LE, Kelsey SF, Obrist WD, Kochanek PM, Palmer AM, Wisniewski SR, DeKosky ST. Treatment of traumatic brain injury with moderate hypothermia. N Engl J Med. 1997;336:540–6.
87. Callaway CW, Donnino MW, Fink EL, Geocadin RG, Golan E, Kern KB, Leary M, Meurer WJ, Peberdy MA, Thompson TM, Zimmerman JL. Part 8: post-cardiac arrest care: 2015 American Heart Association guidelines update for cardiopulmonary resuscitation and emergency cardiovascular care. Circulation. 2015;132(18 Suppl 2):S465–82.
88. Suehiro E, Koizumi H, Fujisawa H, Fujita M, Kaneko T, Oda Y, Yamashita S, Tsuruta R, Maekawa T, Suzuki M. Diverse effects of hypothermia therapy in patients with severe traumatic brain injury based on the computed tomography classification of the traumatic coma data bank. J Neurotrauma. 2015;32:353–8.
89. Martinello K, Hart AR, Yap S, Mitra S, Robertson NJ. Management and investigation of neonatal encephalopathy: 2017 update. Arch Dis Child Fetal Neonatal Ed. 2017;102(4):F346–58.
90. Adelson PD, Wisniewski SR, Beca J, Brown SD, Bell M, Muizelaar JP, Okada P, Beers SR, Balasubramani GK, Hirtz D, Paediatric Traumatic Brain Injury C. Comparison of hypothermia and normothermia after severe traumatic brain injury in children (cool kids): a phase 3, randomised controlled trial. Lancet Neurol. 2013;12:546–53.
91. Nielsen N, Wettersley J, Cronberg T, Erlinge D, Gasche Y, Hassager C, Horn J, Hovdenes J, Kjaergaard J, Kuiper M, Pellis T, Stammet P, Wanscher M, Wise MP, Aneman A, AlSubaie N, Boesgaard S, Bro-Jeppesen J, Brunetti I, Bugge JF, Hingston CD, Juffermans NP, Koopmans M, Kober L, Langorgen J, Lilja G, Moller JE, Rundgren M, Rylander C, Smid O, Werer C, Winkel P, Friberg H. TTM Trial Investigators. Targeted temperature management at 33 degrees c versus 36 degrees c after cardia arrest. N Engl J Med. 2013;369:2197–206.
92. Maekawa T, Yamashita S, Nagao S, Hayashi N, Ohashi Y, Brain-Hypothermia Study G. Prolonged mild therapeutic hypothermia versus fever control with tight hemodynamic monitoring and slow rewarming in patients with severe traumatic brain injury: a randomized controlled trial. J Neurotrauma. 2015;32:422–9.
93. Moler FW, Silverstein FS, Holubkov R, Slomine BS, Christensen JR, Nadkarni VM, Meert KL, Clark AE, Browning B, Pemberton VL, Page K, Shankaran S, Hutchison JS, Newth CJ, Bennett KS, Berger JT, Topjian A, Pineda JA, Koch JD, Schleien CL, Dalton HJ, Ofori-Amanfo G, Goodman DM, Fink EL, McQuillen P, Zimmerman JJ, Thomas NJ, van der Jagt EW, Porter MB, Meyer MT, Harrison R, Pham N, Schwarz AJ, Nowak JE, Alten J, Wheeler DS, Bhalala US, Lidsky K, Lloyd E, Mathur M, Shah S, Wu T, Theodorou AA, Sanders RC Jr, Dean JM. THAPCA Trial Investigators. Therapeutic hypothermia after out-of-hospital cardiac arrest in children. N Engl J Med. 2015;372:1898–908.
94. Moler FW, Silverstein FS, Holubkov R, Slomine BS, Christensen JR, Nadkarni VM, Meert KL, Browning B, Pemberton VL, Page K, Gildea MR, Scholefield BR, Shankaran S, Hutchison JS, Berger JT, Ofori-Amanfo G, Newth CJ, Topjian A, Bennett KS, Koch JD, Pham N, Chanani NK, Pineda JA, Harrison R, Dalton HJ, Alten J, Schleien CL, Goodman DM, Zimmerman JJ, Bhalala US, Schwarz AJ, Porter MB, Shah S, Fink EL, McQuillen P, Wu T, Skellett S, Thomas NJ, Nowak JE, Baines PB, Pappachan J, Mathur M, Lloyd E, Vander Jagt EW, Dobyns EL, Meyer MT, Sanders RC Jr, Clark AE, Dean JM. THAPCA Trial Investigators. Therapeutic hypothermia after in hospital cardiac arrest in children. N Engl J Med. 2017;376:318–29.
95. Cooper DJ, Nichol AD, Bailey M, Bernard S, Cameron PA, Pili-Floury S, Forbes A, Gantner D, Higgins AM, Huet O, Kasza J, Murray L, Newby L, Presneill JJ, Rashford S, Rosenfeld JV, Stephenson M, Vallance S, Varma D, Webb S, POLAR Trial Investigators and the ANZICS Clinical Trials Group. Effect of early sustained prophylactic hypothermia on neurologic outcomes among patients with severe traumatic Brain Injury: the POLAR randomized clinical Trial. JAMA. 2018;320(21):2211–20.

96. Adelson PD, Wisniewski SR, Beca J, Brown SD, Bell M, Muizelaar JP, Okada P, Beers SR, Balasubramani GK, Hirtz D, Paediatric Traumatic Brain Injury Consortium. Comparison of hypothermia and normothermia after severe traumatic brain injury in children (cool kids): a phase 3, randomised controlled trial. Lancet Neurol. 2013;12(6):546–53.
97. Beca J, McSharry B, Erickson S, Yung M, Schibler A, Slater A, Wilkins B, Singhal A, Williams G, Sherring C, Butt W, Pediatric Study Group of the Australia and New Zealand Intensive Care Society Clinical Trials Group. Hypothermia for traumatic brain injury in children-a phase II randomized controlled Trial. Crit Care Med. 2015;43(7):1458–66.
98. Clifton GL, Valadka A, Zygun D, Coffey CS, Drever P, Fourwinds S, Janis LS, Wilde E, Taylor P, Harshman K, Conley A, Puccio A, Levin HS, McCauley SR, Bucholz RD, Smith KR, Schmidt JH, Scott JN, Yonas H, Okonkwo DO. Very early hypothermia induction in patients with severe brain injury (the National Acute Brain Injury Study: hypothermia II): a randomized trial. Lancet Neurol. 2011;10:131–9.
99. Clifton GL, Choi SC, Miller ER, Levin HS, Smith KR Jr, Muizelaar JP, Wagner FC Jr, Marion DW, Luerssen TG. Intercenter variance in clinical trials of head trauma—experience of the National Acute Brain Injury Study: hypothermia. J Neurosurg. 2001a;95:751–5.
100. Clifton GL, Miller ER, Choi SC, Levin HS, McCauley S, Smith KR Jr, Muizelaar JP, Wagner FC Jr, Marion DW, Luerssen TG, Chesnut RM, Schwartz M. Lack of effect of induction of hypothermia after acute brain injury. N Engl J Med. 2001b;344:556–63.
101. Hifumi T, Kuroda Y, Kawakita K, Yamashita S, Oda Y, Dohi K, Maekawa T. Fever control management is preferable to mild therapeutic hypothermia in traumatic brain injury patients with abbreviated Injury scale 3–4: a multi-center, randomized controlled TRIAL. J Neurotrauma. 2015;33:1047.
102. Madden LK, DeVon HA. A systematic review of the effects of body temperature on outcome after adult traumatic Brain Injury. J Neurosci Nurs. 2015;47:190–203.
103. Kaneko T, Fujita M, Yamashita S, Oda Y, Suehiro E, Dohi K, Kasaoka S, Kuroda Y, Kobata H, Maekawa T. Slow rewarming improved the neurological outcomes of prolonged mild therapeutic hypothermia in patients with severe traumatic brain injury and an evacuated hematoma. Sci Rep. 2018;8(1):11630.
104. Kobata H, Kuroda Y, Suehiro E, Kaneko T, Fujita M, Bunya N, Miyata K, Inoue A, Hifumi T, Oda Y, Dohi K, Yamashita S, Maekawa T. Benefits of hypothermia for young patients with acute subdural hematoma: a computed tomography analysis of the brain hypothermia study. Neurotrauma Rep. 2022;3(1):250–60.
105. Andrews PJ, Sinclair HL, Battison CG, Polderman KH, Citerio G, Mascia L, Harris BA, Murray GD, Stocchetti N, Menon DK, Shakur H, De Backer D, Eurotherm Trial, c. European society of intensive care medicine study of therapeutic hypothermia (32-35 degrees C) for intracranial pressure reduction after traumatic brain injury (the Eurotherm3235Trial). Trials. 2011;12:8.
106. Andrews PJ, Sinclair HL, Rodriguez A, Harris BA, Battison CG, Rhodes JK, Murray GD, Eurotherm3235 Trial Collaborators. Hypothermia for intracranial hypertension after traumatic brain injury. N Engl J Med. 2015;373(25):2403–12.
107. Andrews P, Rodriguez A, Suter P, Battison CG, Rhodes J, Puddu I, Harris BA. Mortality risk stratification after traumatic Brain Injury and Hazard of death with titrated hypothermia in the Eurotherm3235Trial. Crit Care Med. 2017;45(5):883–90.
108. Jiang JY, Xu W, Li WP, Gao GY, Bao YH, Liang YM, Luo QZ. Effect of long-term mild hypothermia or short-term mild hypothermia on outcome of patients with severe traumatic brain injury. J Cereb Blood Flow Metab. 2006;26(6):771–6.
109. Lei J, Gao G, Mao Q, Feng J, Wang L, You W, Jiang J, Collaborators, L.T.H.t. Rationale, methodology, and implementation of a nationwide multicenter randomized controlled trial of long-term mild hypothermia for severe traumatic brain injury (the LTH-1 trial). Contemp Clin Trials. 2015;40:9–14.
110. Crossley S, Reid J, McLatchie R, Hayton J, Clark C, MacDougall M, Andrews PJ. A systematic review of therapeutic hypothermia for adult patients following traumatic brain injury. Crit Care. 2014;18:R75.

111. Li P, Yang C. Moderate hypothermia treatment in adult patients with severe traumatic brain injury: a meta-analysis. Brain Inj. 2014;28:1036–41.
112. Zhang BF, Wang J, Liu ZW, Zhao YL, Li DD, Huang TQ, Gu H, Song JN. Meta-analysis of the efficacy and safety of therapeutic hypothermia in children with acute traumatic brain injury. World Neurosurg. 2015;83:567–73.
113. Thakur K, Kaur H, Dhandapani M, Xavier T, Srinivasan G, Gopichandran L, Dhandapani S. Systematic review exploring the effect of therapeutic hypothermia on patients with intracranial hypertension. Surg Neurol Int. 2022;13:237.
114. Marion DW, Regasa LE. Revisiting therapeutic hypothermia for severe traumatic brain injury again. Crit Care (London, England). 2014;18(3):160.
115. Abu-Arafeh A, Rodriguez A, Paterson RL, Andrews P. Temperature variability in a modern targeted temperature management Trial. Crit Care Med. 2018;46(2):223–8.
116. Nichol A, Gantner D, Presneill J, Murray L, Trapani T, Bernard S, Cameron P, Capellier G, Forbes A, McArthur C, Newby L, Rashford S, Rosenfeld JV, Smith T, Stephenson M, Varma D, Walker T, Webb S, Cooper DJ. Protocol for a multicentre randomised controlled trial of early and sustained prophylactic hypothermia in the management of traumatic brain injury. Crit Care Resusc. 2015;17:92–100.
117. Olah E, Poto L, Rumbus Z, Pakai E, Romanovsky AA, Hegyi P, Garami A. POLAR study revisited: therapeutic hypothermia in severe Brain Trauma should not be abandoned. J Neurotrauma. 2021;38(19):2772–6.
118. Hui J, Feng J, Tu Y, Zhang W, Zhong C, Liu M, Wang Y, Long L, Chen L, Liu J, Mou C, Qiu B, Huang X, Huang Q, Zhang N, Yang X, Yang C, Li L, Ma R, Wu X, LTH-1 Trial collaborators. Safety and efficacy of long-term mild hypothermia for severe traumatic brain injury with refractory intracranial hypertension (LTH-1): a multicenter randomized controlled trial. EClinicalMedicine. 2021;32:100732.
119. Wu X, Tao Y, Marsons L, Dee P, Yu D, Guan Y, Zhou X. The effectiveness of early prophylactic hypothermia in adult patients with traumatic brain injury: a systematic review and meta-analysis. Aust Crit Care. 2021;34(1):83–91.
120. Hergenroeder GW, Yokobori S, Choi HA, Schmitt K, Detry MA, Schmitt LH, McGlothlin A, Puccio AM, Jagid J, Kuroda Y, Nakamura Y, Suehiro E, Ahmad F, Viele K, Wilde EA, McCauley SR, Kitagawa RS, Temkin NR, Timmons SD, Diringer MN, Kim DH. Hypothermia for patients requiring evacuation of subdural hematoma: a multicenter randomized clinical Trial. Neurocrit Care. 2022;36(2):560–72.
121. Inoue A, Hifumi T, Kuroda Y, Nishimoto N, Kawakita K, Yamashita S, Oda Y, Dohi K, Kobata H, Suehiro E, Maekawa T, Brain Hypothermia (B-HYPO) Study Group in Japan. Mild decrease in heart rate during early phase of targeted temperature management following tachycardia on admission is associated with unfavorable neurological outcomes after severe traumatic brain injury: a post hoc analysis of a multicenter randomized controlled trial. Crit Care. 2018;22(1):352.
122. Hutchison, J.S., Ward, R.E., Lacroix, J., Hebert, P.C., Barnes, M.A., Bohn, D.J., Dirks, P.B., Doucette, S., Fergusson, D., Gottesman, R., Joffe, A.R., Kirpalani, H.M., Meyer, P.G., Morris, K.P., Moher, D., Singh, R.N., Skippen, P.W., (2008) Hypothermia pediatric head injury trial I. the Canadian critical Care Trials, G. hypothermia therapy after traumatic brain injury in children. N Engl J Med 358, 2447–2456.
123. Newmyer R, Mendelson J, Pang D, Fink EL. Targeted temperature management in pediatric central nervous system disease. Curr Treat Options Pediatr. 2015;1:38–47.
124. Lewis SR, Baker PE, Andrews PJ, Cheng A, Deol K, Hammond N, Saxena M. Interventions to reduce body temperature to 35 °C to 37 °C in adults and children with traumatic brain injury. Cochrane Database Syst Rev. 2020;10(10):CD006811.
125. Du Q, Liu Y, Chen X, Li K. Effect of hypothermia therapy on children with traumatic Brain Injury: a meta-analysis of randomized controlled trials. Brain Sci. 2022;12(8):1009.
126. Rosario BL, Horvat CM, Wisniewski SR, Bell MJ, Panigrahy A, Zuccoli G, Narayanan S, Balasubramani GK, Beers SR, Adelson PD, Investigators of the Cool Kids Trial. Presenting characteristics associated with outcome in children with severe traumatic Brain Injury: a

secondary analysis from a randomized, controlled Trial of therapeutic hypothermia. Pediatric Crit Care Med. 2018;19(10):957–64.
127. Zusman BE, Kochanek PM, Bell MJ, Adelson PD, Wisniewski SR, Au AK, Clark R, Bayır H, Janesko-Feldman K, Jha RM. Cerebrospinal fluid sulfonylurea Receptor-1 is associated with intracranial pressure and outcome after pediatric TBI: an exploratory analysis of the cool kids Trial. J Neurotrauma. 2021;38(12):1615–9.
128. Bhatti F, Naiman M, Tsarev A, Kulstad E. Esophageal temperature management in patients suffering from traumatic brain injury. Ther Hypothermia Temp Manag. 2019;9(4):238–42.
129. Ferreira R, de Paiva B, de Freitas F, Machado FR, Silva GS, Raposo RM, Silveira CF, Centeno RS. Efficacy and safety of a nasopharyngeal catheter for selective Brain cooling in patients with traumatic brain injury: a prospective, non-randomized pilot study. Neurocrit Care. 2021;34(2):581–92.
130. van der Worp HB, Sena ES, Donnan GA, Howells DW, Macleod MR. Hypothermia in animal models of acute ischaemic stroke: a systematic review and meta-analysis. Brain. 2007;130:3063–74.
131. Callaway CW, Coppler PJ, Faro J, Puyana JS, Solanki P, Dezfulian C, Doshi AA, Elmer J, Frisch A, Guyette FX, Okubo M, Rittenberger JC, Weissman A. Association of initial illness severity and outcomes after cardiac arrest with targeted temperature management at 36 °C or 33 °C. JAMA Netw Open. 2020;3(7):e208215.
132. Geocadin RG. Moving beyond one-size-fits-all treatment for patients after cardiac arrest. JAMA Netw Open. 2020;3(7):e208809.
133. Elmer J, He Z, May T, Osborn E, Moberg R, Kemp S, Stover J, Moyer E, Geocadin RG, Hirsch KG, PRECICECAP Study Team. Precision care in cardiac arrest: ICECAP (PRECICECAP) study protocol and informatics approach. Neurocrit Care. 2022;37(Suppl 2):237–47.
134. Yokobori S, Gajavelli S, Mondello S, Mo-Seaney J, Bramlett HM, Dietrich WD, Bullock MR. Neuroprotective effect of preoperatively induced mild hypothermia as determined by biomarkers and histopathological estimation in a rat subdural hematoma decompression model. J Neurosurg. 2013b;118:370–80.

19 Coagulopathy and Prophylaxis of Venous Thromboembolism in Traumatic Brain Injury

Charlotte Lindsay, Laura Green, Jack Henry, Philip J. O'Halloran, and Ross Davenport

19.1 Introduction

Older patients represent the largest demographic for traumatic brain injury (TBI) often complicated by co-morbidity and polypharmacy including antiplatelet and anticoagulant medications [1]. Outcomes for individuals of all ages with TBI have changed very little in the past 20 years, despite significant improvements overall trauma care [2]. This chapter will discuss our current understanding of TBI associated coagulopathy, diagnostics and treatment options for endogenous or pharmacological coagulopathy, and prophylaxis for venous thromboembolism (VTE) in TBI patients.

19.2 Coagulopathy and Clinical Course of TBI

Coagulation abnormalities in TBI were first described in the 1960s but the condition remains poorly defined, both for timing and type of abnormality with one systematic review finding 23 different combinations of coagulation tests [3, 4]. Most studies use definitions derived from polytrauma patients with trauma induced coagulopathy (TIC) and are based on conventional coagulation tests (CCTs), e.g. prothrombin time or INR. Even where definitions use the same tests, the threshold for diagnosis varies considerably, e.g. INR >1.1 to >1.5 [3]. CCTs provide a snapshot of haemostasis, may be normal even when systemic coagulation is abnormal, and the time taken to process the test limits their use in emergency settings [5]. For

C. Lindsay · L. Green · J. Henry · P. J. O'Halloran · R. Davenport (✉)
Centre for Trauma Sciences, Blizard Institute, Queen Mary University of London, London, UK
e-mail: ross.davenport@qmul.ac.uk

E. Brogi et al. (eds.), *Traumatic Brain Injury*, Hot Topics in Acute Care Surgery and Trauma, https://doi.org/10.1007/978-3-031-50117-3_19

anticoagulated patients, the use of point of care INR testing can shorten time to administration of reversal agents [6].

Viscoelastic haemostatic assays provide a more global functional characterisation of coagulation and give actionable results within a few minutes of sampling [7]. Both ROTEM and TEG are sensitive and specific measures of TIC and can guide management of coagulation during resuscitation [8, 9]. These assays are the only point of care test able to diagnosis fibrinolysis, but are relatively insensitivity, i.e. artificially low lytic parameters despite grossly elevated laboratory markers of fibrinolysis such as plasmin–antiplasmin complexes [10, 11].

The reported patterns of coagulopathy in TBI are varied with both hyper- and hypocoagulable states as well as hypo- and hyper-fibrinolytic activation [12, 13]. Wide temporal sampling confounds these descriptions as TBI coagulopathy is dynamic in the first 24 h and likely mirrors to phenotypic changes in TIC, e.g. early hypocoagulable state with bleeding transitions to hypercoagulability with VTE complications [13, 14]. Without consensus it is difficult to determine the significance of these abnormalities or evaluate the impact of therapeutic intervention. However, there is a clear association between admission coagulopathy and poor outcomes in TBI with progression of intracranial haemorrhage, a nine-fold increase in mortality, and worse disability in survivors [15–17]. Similarly, there are worse clinical and radiological outcomes for TBI patients taking anticoagulant medication [18].

19.3 Potential Mechanisms of Coagulopathy in TBI

The mechanisms of coagulopathy in TBI remain poorly understood but there are three main hypotheses.

19.3.1 Endothelial Injury and Protein C Activation

In polytrauma, endothelial injury occurs after tissue injury and shock, but patients with TBI often are not systemically hypoperfused [19]. Direct injury to the brain tissue and vessels, as well as catecholamine release has been linked to endothelial injury and inflammation [20]. In bleeding trauma patients, endothelial injury releases thrombomodulin into the circulation to form thrombin–thrombomodulin complexes and activate Protein C (aPC) [21]. The net result of increased aPC is depletion of plasminogen activator inhibitor 1 with massive fibrinolytic activation and hypocoagulability through cleavage of factor Va and VIIIa [7, 21, 22]. A similar pattern has been observed in patients with TBI, both with and without shock [23, 24]. Studies have found a similar pattern of endothelial activation in TBI and an association between markers of endothelial injury, coagulopathy, and adverse clinical outcomes [20, 25].

19.3.2 Predominance of Fibrinolysis in TBI

Several studies have described a close relationship between fibrinolytic activation and severity of TBI [23, 24, 26]. Fibrinolytic activation may occur via increased activation of protein C, tissue factor release or through direct release of plasminogen activators from the brain itself, e.g. tPA and uPA, with tPA peaking early before falling sharply and uPA rising more slowly to a prolonged peak around 8 h after injury [13, 27]. Release of other fibrinolytic mediators, e.g. membrane bound plasminogen receptor S100A10 which is widely expressed in the brain is associated with TBI coagulopathy. When expressed it catalyses tPA mediated activation of plasmin, and in trauma correlates with hyperfibrinolysis independent of tPA levels [10].

19.3.3 Tissue Factor Hypothesis

The brain is rich in tissue factor that is normally isolated from the vascular space by an intact blood–brain barrier (BBB) [28]. Following injury, disruption to vasculature exposes brain tissue factor to circulating VIIa resulting in thrombin generation and platelet activation [29, 30]. At the same time, tissue factor drives platelet and endothelial derived microvesicle release to cause further amplification, resulting in coagulation factor and platelet depletion [31].

19.4 Treatment of TBI Coagulopathy

Focusing on acute coagulation management to reduce bleeding may improve outcomes in TBI given the association between the size of intracranial bleeding and mortality risk [32, 33]. Bleeding continues after patients arrive at hospital and the risk of progression is higher in TBI with active haemorrhage on admission imaging [34, 35]. Fibrinogen, thrombin, and haemoglobin are directly toxic to the brain resulting in neuroinflammation and cytotoxic oedema which drives secondary injury and further increases in intracranial pressure [36]. Furthermore, the plasminogen system is central to BBB maintenance and the immune response, with evidence from animal studies suggesting modulation of this pathway improves outcomes [37].

There is limited evidence to guide the management of TBI coagulopathy. Recommendations to test coagulation outside of anticoagulant use are only briefly described in most TBI guidelines [38, 39]. While there are no specific guidelines for the management of TBI coagulopathy, there are four main therapeutic strategies: blood component transfusion, reversal of hyperfibrinolysis, clotting factor replacement, and anticoagulant reversal.

19.5 Blood Component Transfusion

Advances in understanding of TIC in trauma haemorrhage have shifted treatment to empiric resuscitation with blood components in balanced ratios, e.g. 1:1:1 red blood cells (RBC):fresh frozen plasma (FFP):platelets before switching to goal directed therapy using coagulation tests when available [2]. Evidence for similar approaches in TBI is limited, with many studies specifically excluding TBI patients. The ITACTIC trial compared VHAs with CCTs and found a small subgroup of bleeding patients with TBI were significantly less likely to die if they received haemostatic therapy guided by ROTEM or TEG [40]. Given the potential benefits, further research is needed to explore this finding with a view to developing and trialling treatment algorithms specific for TBI coagulopathy.

19.5.1 RBC Transfusion

Maintenance of adequate cerebral oxygenation is a central element of post-TBI care and may be compromised by anaemia [38]. Several studies have shown no difference in outcomes with restrictive versus liberal transfusion strategies, while others have suggested higher transfusion thresholds may be associated with worse neurological outcomes and increased VTE [41]. The HEMOTION study due to be completed this year aims to answer this question [42].

19.5.2 Fresh Frozen Plasma

There is limited and conflicting evidence for the role of FFP in TBI coagulopathy. A small RCT found early empiric FFP was associated with a significant increase in mortality in patients with TBI [43]. In contrast, a secondary analysis of the PAMPer RCT found prehospital plasma administration was associated with a 45% reduction in 30-day mortality in a subgroup of patients with isolated TBI and a 50% reduction in those with TBI and extracranial injuries [44].

19.5.3 Platelet Concentrates

A small observational study of patients with severe TBI and TEG-defined platelet dysfunction found administration of platelet concentrates was associated with reduced mortality [45]. Interestingly, high ratios of RBC:platelets but not RBC:FFP were associated with improved survival in massively transfused trauma patients with TBI [45, 46].

19.5.4 Fibrinogen

A single small RCT of fibrinogen in TBI found maintaining fibrinogen >2 g/L for the first 72 h after injury was associated with less progression of intracranial haemorrhage, reduced neurosurgical intervention, and improved GCS at discharge with no increase in adverse outcomes [47]. In addition, two observational studies have found improved survival in patients who maintained normal fibrinogen values, and in those who received early rather than late fibrinogen replacement [48, 49].

19.5.5 Reversal of Hyperfibrinolysis

Tranexamic acid (TXA) is a lysine analogue that blocks plasmin generation and subsequent fibrinolysis with a large evidence base in trauma haemorrhage and two recent RCTs reporting clinical benefit in TBI. The CRASH-3 trial found 1 g bolus +1 g infusion within 3 h of injury reduced mortality in patients with mild to moderate TBI, while later administration was associated with harm [50]. A second study trialled prehospital TXA for patients suspected of having TBI at two different doses, a 1 g bolus +1 g infusion vs 2 g bolus vs placebo. Patients with moderate to severe TBI with ICH who received 2 g TXA had improved survival and 6-month disability scores compared to those who received placebo [51]. In addition, administration of TXA within 45 min of injury was associated with reductions in DVT and cerebral vasospasm compared to those treated late [52]. Despite these benefits, neither study found reductions in the size or progression of intracranial haemorrhage [51, 53]. The plasminogen activator system has important functions in the brain unrelated to haemostasis including maintenance of the BBB and immunomodulation [54]. In animal studies, TXA has been shown to improve BBB integrity and oedema as well as increase reparative immune cells, suggesting the observed benefits may be more to do with reductions in oedema and secondary injury than bleeding specifically [37].

19.6 Factor Replacement

19.6.1 Recombinant Factor VIIa

One RCT trial found a reduction in haematoma progression who received recombinant factor VIIa though the overall rate of progression remained high. The study reported an increase in VTE for the rFVIIa arm, though the clinical significance of this is unclear as patients underwent asymptomatic screening [55]. Two small retrospective reviews of patients who received rFVIIa prior to emergency craniotomy found it was effective in correcting coagulopathy with one study reporting improved functional neurological outcomes for survivors, though it should be noted that both studies included patients with pre-injury anticoagulant use. Neither study identified an increase in VTE [56, 57]. A third, larger retrospective study found no benefit to rFVIIa in patients with TBI [58].

19.6.2 Factor XIII

Factor XIII stabilises forming fibrin clot and increases clot resistance to fibrinolysis [59]. Deficiency of factor XIII has been described in coagulopathic patients with TBI with factor activity reduced by 15–20% and has been linked to increased bleeding following neurosurgical procedures [24, 60]. In vitro studies of factor XIII supplementation have been found to improve clot formation and firmness in surgical patients and healthy volunteers [61, 62]. Despite the theoretical benefits of factor XIII it remains unstudied in TBI.

19.6.3 Prothrombin Complex Concentrate (PCC)

PCC contains vitamin K dependent clotting factors II, VII, IX, and X and is the reversal agent of choice for warfarinised patients with intracranial haemorrhage. INR prolongation and depletion of vitamin K dependent clotting factors have been described in non-anticoagulated TBI patients so in theory PCC may be of therapeutic value [3, 24, 63]. Limited evidence from small retrospective studies have found administration of PCC alone or in combination with FFP provided faster correction of coagulopathy and reduced time to craniotomy and transfusion requirements [64, 65].

19.7 Reversal of Anticoagulation

The most important aspects of the management of anticoagulated TBI patients are a) individualised assessment of the risks of arterial or venous thromboembolism when anticoagulation is reversed, and the potential risk of intracranial bleeding, and b) understanding the pharmacokinetics and pharmacodynamics of each anticoagulant, and how these can be reversed (Table 19.1). There are few large RCTs on the reversal of anticoagulants in TBI, hence, most of the evidence has come from studies of reversing the vitamin K antagonists [66]. The emerging of direct oral anticoagulants (DOACs) in the last two decades has further complicated the management of TBI for patients who are taking these drugs as the evidence for reversing DOACs in TBI is even poorer. Existing guidelines are based on limited studies of small sample sizes and more importantly, on theoretical knowledge of the pharmacokinetics and pharmacodynamics of each anticoagulant [67].

19.7.1 Risk Assessment

To minimise the devastating consequences of TBI normal haemostasis must be obtained as soon as possible. For patients who are already on anticoagulants, this may come at a cost as reversal, together with thromboembolic risks associated with trauma, could put these patients at very high risk of venous and/or arterial

Table 19.1 Mode of action and pharmacokinetic properties of oral anticoagulant agents

	Warfarin	Dabigatran	Rivaroxaban	Apixaban	Edoxaban	UFH	LMWH
Target	II, VII, IX, X, protein S/C	Factor IIa	Factor Xa	Factor Xa	Factor Xa	Potentiation of antithrombin and targets IIa, Xa, IXa, XIa	Potentiation of antithrombin and targets Xa, IIa, TFPI
T-max (hrs)	8	0.5–2	2–4	1–4	1–2		
Half-life (hrs)	40–70	12–17	5–9	9–14	7–11	30 mins–4 h	3–6 h
Excretion	–	Renal (80%)	65% renal (33% unchanged) and gut	Renal 25% and faeces 75%	Renal 1/3 and faeces 2/3	Low dose via RE system High dose: Renal	Renal
Laboratory measurements	INR	TT, ECT, and hemoclot	PT/APTT and anti-Xa	PT/APTT and anti-Xa	PT/APTT and anti-Xa	APTT	Anti-Xa
Reversal	Vitamin K (5–10 mg, iv) PLUS PCC (25 IU/kg) OR FFP (15–20 mL/kg)	Activated charcoal (50 g) within 2 h of ingestion and idarucizumab 5 g IV (in two 2.5 g/50 mL vials) Consider haemodialysis for refractory bleeding	Activated charcoal (50 g) within 2 h of ingestion and andexanet alfa Low-dose regimen: 400-mg IV bolus given at a rate of 30 mg per minute, followed by a 2-h IV infusion at a rate of 4 mg per minute High dose: 800-mg IV bolus given at a rate of 30 mg per minute, followed by a two-hour IV infusion given at a rate of 8 mg per minute PCC (25 IU/kg IV) if andexanet alpha not available			Protamine 1 mg IV for every 100 units of heparin administered in the previous 2–3 h *Up to 50 mg in a single dose*	Dosed within 8 h: protamine 1 mg IV per 1 mg unit of LMWH Dosed within 8–12 h: Protamine 0.5 mg IV per 1 mg LMWH *Up to 50 mg in a single dose*

UFH unfractionated heparin, *LMWH* low molecular weight heparin, *TFPI* tissue factor pathway inhibitor, *RE* reticuloendothelial, *INR* international normalised ratio, *PT* prothrombin time, *APTT* activated partial thromboplastin time, *TT* thrombin time, *ECT* ecarin clotting time, *PCC* prothrombin complex concentrate thrombosis, resulting in mortality, serious long-term morbidity, and impaired quality of life.

Similarly, TBI is associated with high rates of morbidity and mortality and the intake of oral anticoagulants will further exacerbate the risk of ICH following trauma [68]. The risk–benefit ratio of reversing anticoagulants in TBI must be assessed carefully. Age, medical and drug history, neurological examination, and CT findings in combination should be used to categorise patients into low-, medium-, and high-risk categories for clinically significant TBI. For patients in the high-risk category, anticoagulants should be reversed, while for those in low-risk groups, a temporary cessation of anticoagulants might suffice [67].

19.7.2 Warfarin

The rate of ICH with warfarin use has been found to be higher than with DOACs; however, the outcome of major bleeding including ICH has been reported to be the same, despite the latter not having antidotes when these studies were performed [69]. Reversal of warfarin can be achieved with vitamin K plus PCC or FFP [70]. Vitamin K alone is not sufficient to reverse the anticoagulant activity of warfarin quickly enough in TBI, taking up to 24 h to reduce the INR to a safe level (<1.4), while most intracranial haemorrhages expand within the first few hours [66]. However, vitamin K (either as 5 mg or 10 mg, intravenously) should be given in combination with PCC or FFP to ensure a sustained and durable reversal of anticoagulant activity of warfarin [70].

PCC is available as four-factor vitamin K dependent clotting factors or three-factor products (the latter does not include the Factor VII). The benefits of PCC over FFP are the rapid reversal of INR, lower volumes, and lower risk of infections as PCC is pathogen inactivated. RCTs comparing FFP vs PCC have found that PCC is superior to FFP for rapid INR correction [71]. Observational studies have shown that PCC vs FFP might be associated with a lower risk of death and better neurological recovery; however, these results have not been confirmed by other studies [72, 73]. Warfarin reversal should reduce the INR <1.5, as this is associated with better outcomes and INR checked within 15–60 min of administration of PCC to determine the need for repeat dosing [74].

FFP contains all coagulation factors inactivated by warfarin and therefore is a suitable reversal agent for all Vitamin K antagonists, particularly if PCC is not available. Compared to no reversal, FFP normalises the INR and reduces mortality rates associated with major bleeding from warfarin [72, 75]. The recommended FFP doses for treatment of major bleeding range from 10 to 20 mL/kg but this should be adjusted to account for the INR level at the time of the bleed as higher doses may be needed to correct the INR to a safe level [76].

19.7.3 Direct Oral Anticoagulants (DOACs)

Dabigatran etexilate is an oral direct thrombin inhibitor that is rapidly converted to its active form dabigatran. Unlike heparins, dabigatran inhibits not only the free thrombin but also the fibrin-bound thrombin [77]. Understanding the pharmacokinetics of DOACs and knowing when the last dose was taken are key to deciding on whether reversal agents is needed (Table 19.1). If dabigatran is administered more than 3–5 half-lives before presentation (and renal function test is normal), stopping dabigatran should be sufficient. For patients who have renal impairment, dabigatran is cleared more slowly and therefore the anticoagulant effect of dabigatran is likely to last longer. Idarucizumab is the specific reversal agent with the recommended dose being 2 × 2.5 g but there is no evidence base in TBI [67, 78]. If idarucizumab is not available, administration of activated oral charcoal (50 g) can be used to remove dabigatran (if last dose <2 h). PCC has been reported for the reversal of dabigatran in mainly observational studies [66].

19.7.4 Factor Xa Inhibitors

Rivaroxaban, apixaban, and edoxaban are the main oral direct FXa inhibitors in clinical practice. The FXa inhibitors have a shorter half-life than vitamin K antagonists and stopping these agents may be sufficient if the timing of the last dose is known as for DOACs. The specific reversal agent for FXa inhibitors is andexanet alpha but it is very costly and the RCTs on its efficacy and safety in major bleeding are non-existent [79]. The most commonly used reversal agent for FXa inhibitors remains the four-factor PCC with several observational studies showing good results [80].

19.8 VTE Risk and Prophylaxis

VTE is common following TBI, reported in up to 30% of severe TBI patients [81] and associated with worse outcomes [82]. Recent evidence has demonstrated that early initiation of chemoprophylaxis appears to be safe and effective in TBI, even after surgical evacuation of an intracranial haematoma [83].

Mechanical prophylaxis is a mainstay of treatment in all trauma patients, including those with TBI given its efficacy, low cost, extremely low risks, and few contraindications [84]. In one RCT mechanical prophylaxis alone appeared to be similarly effective to low-dose heparin; however, a second study has suggested the addition of mechanical prophylaxis to patients receiving chemoprophylaxis may confer little additional benefit [85, 86].

Historically, prophylaxis has been relatively contraindicated in TBI for perceived risk of intracranial haematoma expansion or blossoming of haemorrhagic contusions. However, recent evidence has demonstrated early prophylaxis to be safe and efficacious, and that therapeutic-dose anticoagulation is relatively safe when initiated as treatment for known VTE [83, 87]. In general, the risk of VTE appears to increase with delays in prophylaxis, with multiple meta-analyses demonstrating risks as low as 2–5% when initiated within 48 h, compared with up to 20% when initiated after 1 week [88, 89]. In a recent large prospective study, the initiation of anticoagulation was associated with a large reduction in VTE risk and was found to be safe when initiated at least 3 days following surgery [83]. However, initiation within 72 h appeared to be mildly associated with need for further surgery suggesting increased bleeding events [83]. In general, the risk of expansion of intracranial haematomata or haemorrhagic contusions in patients receiving chemoprophylaxis is 1–3% [83, 88, 90]. However, causality is not proven and is at least partially explained by the natural history of these injuries; therefore, the risk of expansion can be considered very low.

Uncertainties remain around patient selection, timing and choice of agent, and so the use of chemoprophylaxis has not been formally adopted in guidelines, with VTE prevention focused mainly on mechanical prophylaxis [38]. Institutions that have adopted formal chemoprophylaxis protocols for TBI have typically incorporated risk stratification based upon specific intracranial injuries. Therapy is generally low molecular weight heparins and only initiated upon documentation of injury stability but this approach has been found to be safe and effective [88].

Traditionally, inferior vena cava (IVC) filters are considered in patients too high risk for chemoprophylaxis. While specific evidence in TBI is lacking, many authors have identified the general lack of evidence supporting the use of IVC filters, and the potential for significant harm [91, 92]. Conversely, many complications of IVC filter usage occur in the longer term and may be mitigated by newer retrievable filters [93]. Given a lack of evidence of benefit, the potential for significant harm, and mounting evidence that early chemoprophylaxis is safe and effective, the role of IVC filters remains limited.

19.9 Conclusion

Admission coagulopathy is common in TBI patients and is associated with poor outcomes. There is limited evidence to guide management of coagulopathy in these patients despite the potential for haemostatic therapies to improve outcomes, highlighting a need for future research.

References

1. Lawrence T, Helmy A, Bouamra O, Woodford M, Lecky F, Hutchinson PJ. Traumatic brain injury in England and Wales: prospective audit of epidemiology, complications and standardised mortality. BMJ Open. 2016;6(11):1–8.
2. Cole E, Weaver A, Gall L, West A, Nevin D, Tallach R, et al. A decade of damage control resuscitation: new transfusion practice, new survivors, new directions. Ann Surg. 2021;273(6):1215–20.

3. Epstein DS, Mitra B, O'Reilly G, Rosenfeld JV, Cameron PA. Acute traumatic coagulopathy in the setting of isolated traumatic brain injury: a systematic review and meta-analysis. Injury [Internet]. 2014;45(5):819–24. https://doi.org/10.1016/j.injury.2014.01.011.
4. Sforza M, Pozzi N. Hematic fibrinolysis in cranial traumatisms. Biol Lat. 1960;13:93–9.
5. Davenport R, Manson J, De'Ath H, Platton S, Fibms C, Coates A, et al. Functional definition and characterisation of acute traumatic coagulopathy. Crit Care Med. 2012;39(12):2652–8.
6. Parry-Jones A. Cutting delays in reversing anticoagulation after intracerebral haemorrhage: three key changes at a UK comprehensive stroke centre. BMJ Qual Improv Rep. 2015;4(1):u208763.w3521.
7. Moore EE, Moore HB, Kornblith LZ, Neal MD, Hoffman M, Mutch NJ, et al. Trauma-induced coagulopathy. Nat Rev Dis Primers. 2021;7(1):30.
8. Baksaas-Aasen K, van Dieren S, Balvers K, Juffermans NP, Næss PA, Rourke C, et al. Data-driven development of ROTEM and TEG algorithms for the management of trauma hemorrhage: a prospective observational multicenter study. Ann Surg. 2019;270(6):1178–85.
9. Holcomb JB, Minei KM, Scerbo ML, Radwan ZA, Wade CE, Kozar RA, et al. Admission rapid thrombelastography can replace conventional coagulation tests in the emergency department: experience with 1974 consecutive trauma patients. Ann Surg. 2012;256(3):476–86.
10. Gall LS, Vulliamy P, Gillespie S, Jones TF, Pierre RSJ, Breukers SE, et al. The S100A10 pathway mediates an occult hyperfibrinolytic subtype in trauma patients. Ann Surg. 2019;269(6):1184–91.
11. Raza I, Davenport R, Rourke C, Platton S, Manson J, Spoors C, et al. The incidence and magnitude of fibrinolytic activation in trauma patients. J Thromb Haemost. 2013;11(2):307–14.
12. Leeper CM, Strotmeyer SJ, Neal MD, Gaines BA. Window of opportunity to mitigate trauma-induced coagulopathy: fibrinolysis shutdown not prevalent until 1 hour post-injury. Ann Surg. 2019;270(3):528–34. https://ovidsp.ovid.com/ovidweb.cgi?T=JS&PAGE=fulltext&D=ovft&CSC=Y&NEWS=N&SEARCH=0003-4932.is+and+%22270%22.vo+and+%223%22.ip+and+%22528%22.pg+or+%2210.1097/SLA.0000000000003464%22.di.
13. Maegele M, Schöchl H, Menovsky T, Maréchal H, Marklund N, Buki A, et al. Coagulopathy and haemorrhagic progression in traumatic brain injury: advances in mechanisms, diagnosis, and management. Lancet Neurol. 2017;16(8):630–47.
14. Nakae R, Takayama Y, Kuwamoto K, Naoe Y, Sato H, Yokota H. Time course of coagulation and fibrinolytic parameters in patients with traumatic brain injury. J Neurotrauma. 2016;33(7):688–95.
15. Oertel M, Kelly DF, McArthur D, John Boscardin W, Glenn TC, Jae HL, et al. Progressive hemorrhage after head trauma: predictors and consequences of the evolving injury. J Neurosurg. 2002;96(1):109–16.
16. Zhang D, Gong S, Jin H, Wang J, Sheng P, Zou W, et al. Coagulation parameters and risk of progressive hemorrhagic injury after traumatic brain injury: a systematic review and meta-analysis. Biomed Res Int. 2015;2015:1.
17. Talving P, Benfield R, Hadjizacharia P, Inaba K, Chan LS, Demetriades D. Coagulopathy in severe traumatic brain injury: a prospective study. J Trauma. 2009;66(1):55–61.
18. Gaonkar VB, Garg K, Agrawal D, Chandra PS, Kale SS. Risk factors for progression of conservatively managed acute traumatic subdural hematoma: a systematic review and meta-analysis. World Neurosurg. 2021;146:332–41. https://doi.org/10.1016/j.wneu.2020.11.031.
19. Johansson PI, Stensballe J, Ostrowski SR. Shock induced endotheliopathy (SHINE) in acute critical illness—a unifying pathophysiologic mechanism. Crit Care. 2017;21(1):1–7. https://doi.org/10.1186/s13054-017-1605-5.
20. di Battista AP, Rizoli SB, Lejnieks B, Min A, Shiu MY, Peng HT, et al. Sympathoadrenal activation is associated with acute traumatic coagulopathy and endotheliopathy in isolated brain injury. Shock. 2016;46(3S):96–103.
21. Brohi K, Cohen MJ, Ganter MT. Acute coagulopathy of trauma: hypoperfusion induces systemic anticoagulation and hyperfibrinolysis. J Trauma. 2008;64(5):1211–7.
22. Esmon CT. The protein C pathway*. Chest. 2003;124(3):26S–32S. https://doi.org/10.1378/chest.124.3_suppl.26S.

23. Cohen MJ, Brohi K, Ganter MT, Manley GT, Mackersie RC, Pittet JF. Early coagulopathy after traumatic brain injury: the role of hypoperfusion and the protein c pathway. J Trauma. 2007;63(6):1254–62.
24. Böhm JK, Schaeben V, Schäfer N, Güting H, Lefering R, Thorn S, et al. Extended coagulation profiling in isolated traumatic brain injury: a CENTER-TBI analysis. Neurocrit Care. 2021;36:927.
25. di Battista AP, Rhind SG, Hutchison MG, Hassan S, Shiu MY, Inaba K, et al. Inflammatory cytokine and chemokine profiles are associated with patient outcome and the hyperadrenergic state following acute brain injury. J Neuroinflammation. 2016;13(1):1–14. https://doi.org/10.1186/s12974-016-0500-3.
26. Nakae R, Murai Y, Wada T, Fujiki Y, Kanaya T, Takayama Y, et al. Hyperfibrinolysis and fibrinolysis shutdown in patients with traumatic brain injury. Sci Rep. 2022;12(1):1–10. https://doi.org/10.1038/s41598-022-23912-4.
27. Hijazi N, Fanne RA, Abramovitch R, Yarovoi S, Higazi M, Abdeen S, et al. Endogenous plasminogen activators mediate progressive intracerebral hemorrhage after traumatic brain injury in mice. Blood. 2015;125(16):2558–67.
28. MacKman N. The role of tissue factor and factor VIIa in hemostasis. Anesth Analg. 2009;108(5):1447–52.
29. Monroe DM, Hoffman M, Allen GA, Roberts HR. The factor VII-platelet interplay: effectiveness of recombinant factor VIIa in the treatment of bleeding in severe thrombocytopathia. Semin Thromb Hemost. 2000;26(4):373–7.
30. Hoffman M, Monroe DM. Tissue factor in brain is not saturated with factor VIIa: implications for factor VIIa dosing in intracerebral hemorrhage. Stroke. 2009;40(8):2882–4.
31. Nekludov M, Mobarrez F, Gryth D, Bellander BM, Wallen H. Formation of microparticles in the injured brain of patients with severe isolated traumatic brain injury. J Neurotrauma. 2014;31(23):1927–33.
32. Adatia K, Newcombe VFJ, Menon DK. Contusion progression following traumatic brain injury: a review of clinical and radiological predictors, and influence on outcome. Neurocrit Care. 2021;34(1):312–24. https://doi.org/10.1007/s12028-020-00994-4.
33. Perel P, Roberts I, Bouamra O, Woodford M, Mooney J, Lecky F. Intracranial bleeding in patients with traumatic brain injury: a prognostic study. BMC Emerg Med. 2009;9:1–8.
34. Letourneau-Guillon L, Huynh T, Jakobovic R, Milwid R, Symons SP, Aviv RI. Traumatic intracranial hematomas: prognostic value of contrast extravasation. Am J Neuroradiol. 2013;34(4):773–9.
35. Amoo M, Henry J, Alabi PO, Husien M, ben. The 'swirl sign' as a marker for haematoma expansion and outcome in intra-cranial haemorrhage: a meta-analysis. J Clin Neurosci. 2021;87:103–11. https://doi.org/10.1016/j.jocn.2021.02.028.
36. Stokum JA, Cannarsa GJ, Wessell AP, Shea P, Wenger N, Simard JM. When the blood hits your brain: the neurotoxicity of extravasated blood. Int J Mol Sci. 2021;22(10):5132.
37. Daglas M, Galle A, Draxler DF, Ho H, Liu Z, Sashindranath M, et al. Sex-dependent effects of tranexamic acid on blood-brain barrier permeability and the immune response following traumatic brain injury in mice. J Thromb Haemost. 2020;18(10):2658–71.
38. Carney N, Totten AM, O'Reilly C, Ullman JS, Hawryluk GWJ, Bell MJ, et al. Guidelines for the management of severe traumatic brain injury, fourth edition. Neurosurgery. 2017;80(1):6–15.
39. Kochanek PM, Tasker RC, Bell MJ, Adelson PD, Carney N, Vavilala MS, et al. Management of pediatric severe traumatic brain injury: 2019 consensus and guidelines-based algorithm for first and second tier therapies. Pediatr Crit Care Med. 2019;20(3):269–79.
40. Baksaas-Aasen K, Gall LS, Stensballe J, Juffermans NP, Curry N, Maegele M, et al. Viscoelastic haemostatic assay augmented protocols for major trauma haemorrhage (ITACTIC): a randomized, controlled trial. Intensive Care Med. 2021;47(1):49–59. https://doi.org/10.1007/s00134-020-06266-1.
41. Boutin A, Chassé M, Shemilt M, Lauzier F, Moore L, Zarychanski R, et al. Red blood cell transfusion in patients with traumatic brain injury: a systematic review and meta-analysis. Transfus Med Rev. 2016;30(1):15–24.

42. Turgeon AF, Fergusson DA, Clayton L, Patton MP, Zarychanski R, English S, et al. Haemoglobin transfusion threshold in traumatic brain injury optimisation (HEMOTION): a multicentre, randomised, clinical trial protocol. BMJ Open. 2022;12(10):e067117.
43. Etemadrezaie H, Baharvahdat H, Shariati Z, Lari SM, Shakeri MT, Ganjeifar B. The effect of fresh frozen plasma in severe closed head injury. Clin Neurol Neurosurg. 2007;109(2):166–71.
44. Gruen DS, Guyette FX, Brown JB, Okonkwo DO, Puccio AM, Campwala IK, et al. Association of Prehospital Plasma with survival in patients with traumatic brain injury: a secondary analysis of the PAMPer cluster randomized clinical trial. JAMA Netw Open. 2020;3(10):1–15.
45. Furay E, Daley M, Teixeira PG, Coopwood TB, Aydelotte JD, Malesa N, et al. Goal-directed platelet transfusions correct platelet dysfunction and may improve survival in patients with severe traumatic brain injury. J Trauma Acute Care Surg. 2018;85(5):881–7.
46. Spinella PC, Wade CE, Blackbourne LH, Borgman MA, Zarzabal LA, Du F, et al. The association of blood component use ratios with the survival of massively transfused trauma patients with and without severe brain injury. J Trauma. 2011;71(2 SUPPL. 3):343–52.
47. Sabouri M, Vahidian M, Sourani A, Mahdavi SB, Tehrani DS, Shafiei E. Efficacy and safety of fibrinogen administration in acute post-traumatic hypofibrinogenemia in isolated severe traumatic brain injury: a randomized clinical trial. J Clin Neurosci. 2022;101:204–11. https://doi.org/10.1016/j.jocn.2022.05.016.
48. Sugiyama K, Fujita H, Nishimura S. Effects of in-house cryoprecipitate on transfusion usage and mortality in patients with multiple trauma with severe traumatic brain injury: a retrospective cohort study. Blood Transfus. 2020;18(1):6–12.
49. Lv K, Yuan Q, Fu P, Wu G, Wu X, Du Z, et al. Impact of fibrinogen level on the prognosis of patients with traumatic brain injury: a single-center analysis of 2570 patients. World J Emerg Surg. 2020;15(1):1–9.
50. Roberts I, Shakur-Still H, Aeron-Thomas A, Belli A, Brenner A, Chaudary MA, et al. Effects of tranexamic acid on death, disability, vascular occlusive events and other morbidities in patients with acute traumatic brain injury (CRASH-3): a randomised, placebo-controlled trial. Lancet. 2019;394(10210):1713–23. https://doi.org/10.1016/S0140-6736(19)32233-0.
51. Rowell SE, Meier EN, McKnight B, Kannas D, May S, Sheehan K, et al. Effect of out-of-hospital tranexamic acid vs placebo on 6-month functional neurologic outcomes in patients with moderate or severe traumatic brain injury. JAMA. 2020;324(10):961–74.
52. Brito AMP, Schreiber MA, el Haddi J, Meier EN, Rowell SE. The effects of timing of prehospital tranexamic acid on outcomes after traumatic brain injury; sub analysis of a randomized controlled trial. J Trauma Acute Care Surg. 2022;94:86.
53. Mahmood A, Needham K, Shakur-Still H, Harris T, Jamaluddin SF, Davies D, et al. Effect of tranexamic acid on intracranial haemorrhage and infarction in patients with traumatic brain injury: a pre-planned substudy in a sample of CRASH-3 trial patients. Emerg Med J. 2021;38(4):270–8.
54. Medcalf RL. Fibrinolysis: from blood to the brain. J Thromb Haemost. 2017;15(11):2089–98.
55. Narayan RK, Maas AIR, Marshall LF, Servadei F, Skolnick BE, Tillinger MN. Recombinant factor viia in traumatic intracerebral hemorrhage: results of a dose-escalation clinical trial. Neurosurgery. 2008;62(4):776–86.
56. Brown CVR, Foulkrod KH, Lopez D, Stokes J, Villareal J, Foarde K, et al. Recombinant factor VIIa for the correction of coagulopathy before emergent craniotomy in blunt trauma patients. J Trauma. 2010;68(2):348–52.
57. McQuay N, Cipolla J, Franges EZ, Thompson GE. The use of recombinant activated factor VIIa in coagulopathic traumatic brain injuries requiring emergent craniotomy: is it beneficial? J Neurosurg. 2009;111(4):666–71.
58. Lombardo S, Millar D, Jurkovich GJ, Coimbra R, Nirula R. Factor VIIa administration in traumatic brain injury: an AAST-MITC propensity score analysis. Trauma Surg Acute Care Open. 2018;3(1):1–7.
59. Lorand L, Losowsky MS, Miloszewski KJ. Human factor XIII: fibrin-stabilizing factor. Prog Hemost Thromb. 1980;5:245–90.

60. Vrettou CS, Stavrinou LC, Halikias S, Kyriakopoulou M, Kollias S, Stranjalis G, et al. Factor XIII deficiency as a potential cause of supratentorial haemorrhage after posterior fossa surgery. Acta Neurochir. 2010;152(3):529–32.
61. Theusinger OM, Baulig W, Asmis LM, Seifert B, Spahn DR. In vitro factor XIII supplementation increases clot firmness in rotation thromboelastometry (ROTEM®). Thromb Haemost. 2010;104(2):385–91.
62. Dirkmann D, Görlinger K, Gisbertz C, Dusse F, Peters J. Factor XIII and tranexamic acid but not recombinant factor VIIa attenuate tissue plasminogen activator-induced hyperfibrinolysis in human whole blood. Anesth Analg. 2012;114(6):1182–8.
63. Böhm JK, Güting H, Thorn S, Schäfer N, Rambach V, Schöchl H, et al. Global characterisation of coagulopathy in isolated traumatic brain injury (iTBI): a CENTER-TBI analysis. Neurocrit Care. 2021;35(1):184–96.
64. Joseph B, Hadjizacharia P, Aziz H, Kulvatunyou N, Tang A, Pandit V, et al. Prothrombin complex concentrate: an effective therapy in reversing the coagulopathy of traumatic brain injury. J Trauma Acute Care Surg. 2013;74(1):248–53.
65. Joseph B, Pandit V, Khalil M, Kulvatunyou N, Aziz H, Tang A, et al. Use of prothrombin complex concentrate as an adjunct to fresh frozen plasma shortens time to craniotomy in traumatic brain injury patients. Neurosurgery. 2015;76(5):601–7.
66. Frontera JA, Lewin JJ 3rd, Rabinstein AA, Aisiku IP, Alexandrov AW, Cook AM, et al. Guideline for reversal of antithrombotics in intracranial hemorrhage: a statement for healthcare professionals from the neurocritical care society and Society of Critical Care Medicine. Neurocrit Care. 2016;24(1):6–46.
67. Wiegele M, Schöchl H, Haushofer A, Ortler M, Leitgeb J, Kwasny O, et al. Diagnostic and therapeutic approach in adult patients with traumatic brain injury receiving oral anticoagulant therapy: an Austrian interdisciplinary consensus statement. Crit Care. 2019;23(1):62.
68. Herou E, Romner B, Tomasevic G. Acute traumatic brain injury: mortality in the elderly. World Neurosurg. 2015;83(6):996–1001.
69. Green L, Tan J, Morris JK, Alikhan R, Curry N, Everington T, et al. A three-year prospective study of the presentation and clinical outcomes of major bleeding episodes associated with oral anticoagulant use in the UK (ORANGE study). Haematologica. 2018;103(4):738–45.
70. Keeling D, Baglin T, Tait C, Watson H, Perry D, Baglin C, et al. Guidelines on oral anticoagulation with warfarin—fourth edition. Br J Haematol. 2011;154(3):311–24.
71. Goldstein JN, Refaai MA, Milling TJJ, Lewis B, Goldberg-Alberts R, Hug BA, et al. Four-factor prothrombin complex concentrate versus plasma for rapid vitamin K antagonist reversal in patients needing urgent surgical or invasive interventions: a phase 3b, open-label, non-inferiority, randomised trial. Lancet. 2015;385(9982):2077–87.
72. Parry-Jones AR, di Napoli M, Goldstein JN, Schreuder FHBM, Tetri S, Tatlisumak T, et al. Reversal strategies for vitamin K antagonists in acute intracerebral hemorrhage. Ann Neurol. 2015;78(1):54–62.
73. Huttner HB, Schellinger PD, Hartmann M, Köhrmann M, Juettler E, Wikner J, et al. Hematoma growth and outcome in treated neurocritical care patients with intracerebral hemorrhage related to oral anticoagulant therapy: comparison of acute treatment strategies using vitamin K, fresh frozen plasma, and prothrombin complex concentrates. Stroke. 2006;37(6):1465–70.
74. Tan J, MacCallum P, Curry N, Stanworth S, Tait C, Morris JK, et al. Correction of international normalised ratio in major bleeding related to vitamin K antagonists is associated with better survival: a UK study. Thromb Res. 2021;197:153–9.
75. Sarode R, Milling TJJ, Refaai MA, Mangione A, Schneider A, Durn BL, et al. Efficacy and safety of a 4-factor prothrombin complex concentrate in patients on vitamin K antagonists presenting with major bleeding: a randomized, plasma-controlled, phase IIIb study. Circulation. 2013;128(11):1234–43.
76. Stanworth SJ, Dowling K, Curry N, Doughty H, Hunt BJ, Fraser L, et al. Haematological management of major haemorrhage: a British Society for haematology guideline. Br J Haematol. 2022;198:654–67.

77. Levy JH, Ageno W, Chan NC, Crowther M, Verhamme P, Weitz JI. When and how to use antidotes for the reversal of direct oral anticoagulants: guidance from the SSC of the ISTH. J Thromb Haemost. 2016;14(3):623–7.
78. Pollack CVJ, Reilly PA, Eikelboom J, Glund S, Verhamme P, Bernstein RA, et al. Idarucizumab for dabigatran reversal. N Engl J Med. 2015;373(6):511–20.
79. Cohen AT, Lewis M, Connor A, Connolly SJ, Yue P, Curnutte J, et al. Thirty-day mortality with andexanet alfa compared with prothrombin complex concentrate therapy for life-threatening direct oral anticoagulant-related bleeding. J Am Coll Emerg Physicians Open. 2022;3(2):e12655.
80. Green L, Tan J, Antoniou S, Alikhan R, Curry N, Everington T, et al. Haematological management of major bleeding associated with direct oral anticoagulants—UK experience. Br J Haematol. 2019;185(3):514–22.
81. Ekeh AP, Dominguez KM, Markert RJ, McCarthy MC. Incidence and risk factors for deep venous thrombosis after moderate and severe brain injury. J Trauma. 2010;68(4):912. https://journals.lww.com/jtrauma/Fulltext/2010/04000/Incidence_and_Risk_Factors_for_Deep_Venous.25.aspx.
82. Ali AB, Khawaja AM, Reilly A, Tahir Z, Rao SS, Bernstock JD, et al. Venous thromboembolism risk and outcomes following decompressive craniectomy in severe traumatic brain injury: an analysis of the Nationwide inpatient sample database. World Neurosurg. 2022;161:e531–45. https://www.sciencedirect.com/science/article/pii/S1878875022002169.
83. Byrne JP, Witiw CD, Schuster JM, Pascual JL, Cannon JW, Martin ND, et al. Association of venous thromboembolism prophylaxis after neurosurgical intervention for traumatic brain injury with thromboembolic complications, repeated neurosurgery, and mortality. JAMA Surg. 2022;157(3):–e215794. https://doi.org/10.1001/jamasurg.2021.5794.
84. Barrera LM, Perel P, Ker K, Cirocchi R, Farinella E, Morales Uribe CH. Thromboprophylaxis for trauma patients. Cochrane Database Syst Rev. 2013;(3):CD008303.
85. Kurtoglu M, Yanar H, Bilsel Y, Guloglu R, Kizilirmak S, Buyukkurt D, et al. Venous thromboembolism prophylaxis after head and spinal trauma: intermittent pneumatic compression devices versus low molecular weight heparin. World J Surg. 2004;28(8):807–11.
86. Arabi YM, Al-Hameed F, Burns KEA, Mehta S, Alsolamy SJ, Alshahrani MS, et al. Adjunctive intermittent pneumatic compression for venous thromboprophylaxis. N Engl J Med. 2019;380(14):1305–15. https://doi.org/10.1056/NEJMoa1816150.
87. Chipman AM, Radowsky J, Vesselinov R, Chow D, Schwartzbauer G, Tesoriero R, et al. Therapeutic anticoagulation in patients with traumatic brain injuries and pulmonary emboli. J Trauma Acute Care Surg. 2020;89(3):529–35.
88. Lu VM, Alvi MA, Rovin RA, Kasper EM. Clinical outcomes following early versus late pharmacologic thromboprophylaxis in patients with traumatic intracranial hemorrhage: a systematic review and meta-analysis. Neurosurg Rev. 2020;43(3):861–72.
89. Abdel-Aziz H, Dunham CM, Malik RJ, Hileman BM. Timing for deep vein thrombosis chemoprophylaxis in traumatic brain injury: an evidence-based review. Crit Care. 2015;19(1):96.
90. Bahloul M, Chelly H, Regaieg K, Rekik N, Bellil S, Chaari A, et al. Pulmonary embolism following severe traumatic brain injury: incidence, risk factors and impact outcome. Intensive Care Med. 2017;43:1433–5.
91. Ho KM, Rao S, Honeybul S, Zellweger R, Wibrow B, Lipman J, et al. A multicenter trial of vena cava filters in severely injured patients. N Engl J Med. 2019;381(4):328–37.
92. Sarosiek S, Rybin D, Weinberg J, Burke PA, Kasotakis G, Sloan JM. Association between inferior vena cava filter insertion in trauma patients and in-hospital and overall mortality. JAMA Surg. 2017;152(1):75–81.
93. Angel LF, Tapson V, Galgon RE, Restrepo MI, Kaufman J. Systematic review of the use of retrievable inferior vena cava filters. J Vasc Interv Radiol. 2011;22(11):1522–1530.e3.

Fluid Management and Hyperosmolar Therapy in Neurotrauma

20

Holly M. Stradecki-Cohan and Kristine H. O'Phelan

20.1 Introduction

Judicious fluid management after trauma is essential and, fluid management after brain trauma has some fundamental differences when compared with overall post traumatic resuscitation. First, the brain itself is enclosed by the skull and therefore swelling after injury will elevate intracranial pressure (ICP). Appropriate fluid management is essential in supporting brain perfusion during periods of elevated ICP and hyperosmolar fluids can be utilized to reduce elevated pressures. Second, the primary function of the brain is to allow for the generation of action potentials. This is governed by tightly regulated, energy-dependent ionic gradients between the intra- and extracellular spaces. To allow for generation and maintenance of these gradients, there is, by default, a need to prevent free flow of ions not only across cell membranes, but also from the intravascular space (initial area of entry of IV fluids) to the brain parenchyma. While ions, such as sodium, have nearly free permeability from the intravascular space to the parenchyma of other organs (e.g., liver, spleen, lung, intestine), an intact blood–brain barrier (BBB) prevents similar diffusion. When the brain is damaged, the BBB protection is impaired directly impacting the severity of traumatic brain injury (TBI).

In this chapter, we will examine fluid management in TBI in both acutely and after the patient has been stabilized. We will discuss how approaches have changed in targeting blood pressure goals and volume status. In addition, we will discuss hyperosmolar therapy and its indication in TBI as well as adverse effects of these solutions.

H. M. Stradecki-Cohan · K. H. O'Phelan (✉)
Department of Neurology, Miller School of Medicine, The University of Miami, Miami, FL, USA
e-mail: Hc3427@cumc.columbia.edu; kophelan@med.miami.edu

E. Brogi et al. (eds.), *Traumatic Brain Injury*, Hot Topics in Acute Care Surgery and Trauma, https://doi.org/10.1007/978-3-031-50117-3_20

20.2 Acute Resuscitation: Blood Pressure Targets

In the hyperacute setting, volume resuscitation after trauma has been generally targeted at closure of base deficit with blood pressure goals dependent on injury type: penetrating, blunt, or associated with TBI. Permissive arterial hypotension in penetrating (SBP 60–70 mmHg, [1]) and blunt (SBP goal 70–80 mmHg, [2]) trauma without TBI is beneficial over more aggressive blood pressure targets. In these patients, over resuscitation contributes to dilutional coagulopathy and higher blood pressures may promote clot disruption [1, 3]. However, after TBI, cerebral hypotension is associated with worse outcome. In a multicenter, observational study, the odds of 30-day mortality for TBI patients was tripled if the presenting SBP < 90 mmHg, doubled if SBP < 100 mmHg, and 1.5 times greater if SBP < 120 mmHg [4]. Currently, the Brain Trauma Foundation recommends maintaining SBP ≥100 mmHg in patients 50–69 years old or ≥ 110 mmHg in those 15–49 or > 70 years old after head injury [5]. These recommendations are taken directly from the work of Berry *et al.*, which examined the association of presenting SBP to mortality [6]. In this retrospective cohort of 15,733 patients with isolated moderate or severe TBI, the authors evaluated SBP as a dichotomous variable, "hypotensive or not hypotensive." Serial logistic regressions were performed with hypotensive SBP being defined at different targets. The optimal SBP for hypotension was determined from the model with best fit and highest discriminatory index in each age group [6]. More recent reports suggest that higher SBP targets are provide greater benefit in patients with isolated head injuries. A retrospective analysis of 154,725 patients with isolated, moderate to severe TBIs found that early and overall hospital mortality was reduced when initial blood pressures were > 110 mmHg regardless of age [7]. A subgroup analysis compared presenting systolic blood pressures between 90 and 109 mmHg vs. 110 and 129 mmHg matching patients on several characteristics. The higher presenting blood pressures resulted in reduced hospital mortality (4.9 vs. 3.2%) without statistically significant ventilated days (5.6 +/– 11.6 vs. 6.5 =/– 8.3, *p* 0.370) or 30-day ventilator free days (17.9 +/– 12.1 vs. 18.1 +/– 11.7 *p* = 0.851) suggesting SBP goals should be between 110 and 129 mmHg [7]. Another report of 94,411 patients with isolated, nonpenetrating TBI found that systolic blood pressures <110 or > 150 mmHg resulted in increased mortality for those with moderate or severe TBI regardless of age [8]. When analyzed by age, systolic blood pressure < 120 mmHg was associated with worse outcomes in patients >65 years old regardless of TBI severity suggesting this may be a more appropriate threshold [8]. Taken together, a SBP target of ≥110 mmHg is likely appropriate for patients with isolated TBI, but slightly higher goals may have more supporting evidence in the future.

In the case of polytrauma with concurrent head injury, the ability to limit hemorrhage with permissive hypotension is directly at odds with the goal of augmenting blood pressure to prevent secondary brain injury. To address this not uncommon situation, the 2019 World Society of Emergency Surgery (WSES), a group of intensivists, emergency surgeons, and neurosurgeons formed consensus recommendations. They suggest that after polytrauma with TBI, blood pressure goals should be

SBP > 100 mmHg or MAP >80 mmHg during acute resuscitation [9]. In the case of difficult to control intraoperative bleeding, lower pressures can be utilized but only for the minimal time necessary to achieve hemostasis [9]. These blood pressure targets are higher than the previously accepted 2013 European Task Force for Advanced Bleeding Care in Trauma which recommended SBP ≥ 80 mmHg [10]. Currently no randomized studies have been done to determine the effect of higher blood pressure targets on patient outcomes. In line with the higher BP recommendations, an observational study which included TBI patients with or without polytrauma, showed an 18.8% decrease in odds of death for each 10-point increase in lowest presenting SBP [11]. A more recent retrospective study of 1791 trauma patients with TBI noted a U-shaped relationship between blood pressure at triage and mortality [12]. While a presenting SBP between 130 and 149 mmHg was associated with the lowest risk of mortality, statistically significant differences were only found at SBP < 90 or > 190 mmHg supporting the 2019 WSES recommendations [12].

It is important to note that these studies are all retrospective and compare the blood pressures on presentation to outcomes of interest. While many adjust for severity of injury, patient age, and other potential confounders, the values above do not reflect the blood pressures targeted by the treating team. As such, prospective studies are needed to determine if blood pressure augmentation to specific targets do improve outcomes in patients after TBI (with or without other traumatic injuries).

20.3 Acute Resuscitation: Fluid Selection

The choice of resuscitation fluid in the hyperacute setting, including crystalloids, colloids, blood products, and hyperosmolar agents is still evolving for both general trauma patients as well as those with TBI as there are few interventional studies which have been performed at this early timepoint.

For non-TBI trauma patients, resuscitation with large volumes of crystalloid is generally avoided due to adverse effect on hemostasis (discussed above), diffuse tissue edema, and concern for abdominal compartment syndrome [10]. The use of colloids in this setting is also unclear as a Cochrane analysis of critically ill patients (including trauma, burns, and sepsis) found no effect on mortality or renal function with use of colloids vs. crystalloids, and suggested that crystalloids can be preferred due to lower costs [13]. For the non-TBI trauma patient, balanced crystalloids solutions (e.g., Lactated Ringers, Hartmann's solution) may be preferred as they are less likely to worsen acid-base disturbances. Some consideration is given to potential interaction of the bicarbonate in Lactated Ringer's with calcium in blood products if the same line is used for administration of blood. Infusion of blood products can be considered pending patient response to initial fluid challenges, mechanism or injury, and suspicion for hemorrhage (for further discussion elsewhere [14, 15]).

Common balanced crystalloids are more physiological in terms of pH and ion composition but can be hypotonic compared to 0.9% normal saline (Table 20.1). The Isotonic Solutions and Major Adverse Renal Events Trial (SMART) examined

Table 20.1 Composition of IVF and hyperosmolar therapies used in neurotrauma

	Sodium (mEq/L)	Chloride (mEq/L)	Buffer (mEq/L)	Osmolarity (mOsm/L)	Typical Bolus Dosing
Crystalloids					
Human plasma	135–145	96–108	22–30 HCO_3	285–295	–
0.9% sodium chloride	154	154	–	308	–
Lactated ringers	130	109	28 lactate	273	–
Hartmann's solution	131	112	28 lactate		–
Plasma-Lyte	140	98	27 acetate23 gluconate	295	–
Hypertonic					
3% sodium chloride	513	513	–	1026	150–250 mL
3% acetate buffered sodium chloride	513	273	240 acetate	1026	150–250 mL
7.45% sodium chloride	1274	1274	–	2548	100 mL
23.4% sodium chloride	4004	4004	–	8008	30 mL
20% mannitol	–	–	–	1098	0.5–1.5 g/kg
25% mannitol	–	–	–	1375	0.5–1.5 g/kg

the use of balanced crystalloids versus 0.9% normal saline for resuscitation in critically ill patients [16]. Block randomization and coordination of care allowed for randomization to occur at hospital presentation. A subgroup analysis of including those patients with TBI showed no difference in in-hospital mortality with either fluid type, however, fewer patients were discharged home in the balanced crystalloid group [17]. Of note, plasma-lyte was used more often than lactated ringers in that study (82.9% vs. 17.1%). These results are similar to the subgroup analysis of the Balanced Solutions in Intensive Care (BaSICs) study, which have showed post-resuscitation use of balanced solutions were associated with significantly higher 90-day mortality in patients with TBI than normal saline 34,375,394 [18]. Additionally, a retrospective analysis of prehospital administration of LR versus 0.9% NS to trauma patients found higher mortality in the LR treated group in patients with TBI but not trauma patients without head injury [19]. A caveat in this study was that baseline injury was more severe in the LR resuscitated group [19]. Taken together, 0.9% normal saline is preferred over balanced crystalloid solutions for acute resuscitation in patients with TBI.

Hypertonic saline solutions have not been associated with improvement in outcomes when used during resuscitation after TBI. In a double blind, randomized trial of 229 patients, prehospital administration of 250 mL 7.5% normal saline to comatose patients with severe TBI did not improve mortality or 6-month GOS-E score over Lactated Ringer's [20]. Initial serum sodium was elevated despite effectively raising serum sodium and there were nonsignificant trends in reduced ICP (10 vs. 15 mmHg, $p = 0.08$) and reduced duration of CPP < 70 mmHg (9.5 vs. 17 h, $p = 0.06$) in the HTS treated group [20]. Notably, these trends excluded patients who did not require ICP monitoring (i.e., rapid deterioration or improvement) and therefore possibly masked any treatment effect. Additionally, while prehospital treatment was randomized, subsequent hospital administration of hyperosmolar fluids was determined by the treating physician and were not different between groups [20]. There were no differences in adverse events (e.g., renal failure) reported due to hyperosmotic therapy [20]. A more recent metanalysis compared prehospital administration of either HTS (7.5% sodium chloride) or HTS with dextran (7.5% sodium chloride with 6% or 12% dextran) to normal crystalloids in patients with severe TBI [21]. There was no difference between in mortality (composite survival at 28 days or hospital discharge) or GOS-E scores between HTS or HTS with dextran compared to the normal crystalloid group. As the goal of this analysis was to examine hypertonic solutions in resuscitation, the "normal crystalloid group" was comprised of normal saline or Lactated Ringer's administration [21]. Currently, there is not adequate justification for use of hypertonic fluids for acute resuscitation in all TBI patients.

The use of albumin for fluid resuscitation after TBI is not recommended. The Saline versus Albumin Fluid Evaluation (SAFE) Study was a blinded, prospective, randomized trial comparing mortality outcomes with use of 4% albumin versus normal saline for resuscitation in patients admitted to ICU [22]. In this initial report, a preplanned subgroup analysis of patients with TBI found higher risk of mortality in the 28-day study period with albumin administration (RR = 1.62, $p = 0.009$). A subsequent study examined variables known to influence TBI (age > 60, GCS < 9, MAP <50 mmHg, and traumatic SAH on initial CTB) and followed patients for a total of 24 months after randomization [23]. Patients with severe TBI (GCS 3–8 on admission) had higher risk of mortality at 24 months if treated with albumin overall and when adjusted for covariates (RR 1.88, 95% CI 1.31–2.70, $p < 0.001$; adjusted risk 2.38, 95% CI 1.33–4.26, $p = 0.003$). This was not observed for patients with moderate TBI (GCS 9–12; RR 0.74, 95% CI 0.31–1.79, $p = 0.50$; adjusted risk 0.38, 95% CI 0.10–1.49, $p = 0.17$) [23]. Subsequent study of this data suggested that albumin administration was associated with worsening cerebral edema at 1 week as compared to saline control possibly due to albumin extravasation through injured BBB or that was slightly hypotonic compared to normal saline [24]. As such, albumin for fluid resuscitation should be avoided in severe TBI acutely and during hospital admission if no other indications exist.

20.4 Acute Resuscitation: Blood Product, Steroids, and Tranexamic Acid

Early transfusion of blood products in the setting of hemorrhagic shock is indicated after trauma as it maintains organ perfusion and avoids over resuscitation with IV solutions [15]. Anemia has been associated with worse outcome in TBI and traditional goal of HgB 7.0 g/dL is considered adequate after brain injury though currently without evidence. As such, the Transfusion strategies in Acute brain-injured patients (TRAIN) trial was preformed comparing transfusion at a HgB > 7 g/dL versus 9 g/dL for patients with brain injury including TBI; results from this work are pending [25]. Trauma and TBI lead to coagulopathy and platelet dysfunction through mechanisms not fully understood 35,071,780 [26]. In a retrospective analysis, plasma transfusion within 4 h of isolated TBI was not associated with improvement in overall mortality (OR 1.18, 0.71–1.96) but was associated with improved survival in a subset of patients with multifocal hemorrhages (OR 3.34 1.20–9.35, 27,776,795 [27]). In a small, retrospective analysis, viscoelastic guided platelet transfusion was associated with a decrease in mortality (OR 0.23, 0.06–0.92, $p = 0.038$) in patients with TBI and noted platelet dysfunction 30,124,626 [28]. Newer approaches to blood product administration after TBI will likely be developed as more information from future studies employing these mechanisms.

Corticosteroids were previously employed as empiric treatment after TBI. The rationale was that secondary brain injury may be regulated by inflammation and mitigation of inflammation by steroids would be beneficial. However, the Corticosteroids Randomization After Significant Head injury (CRASH) trial was a prospective randomized, blinded trial which was stopped early due to adverse effects of treatment [29]. Specifically, adults who presented within 8 h of TBI having a GCS $\leq$ 14 were randomized to receive methylprednisolone (2 g over 1 h then 0.4 g/h over next 48 h) or placebo. The group treated with methylprednisolone had higher 2-week mortality [RR 1.18, 1.09–1.27, $p = 0.0001$ [29]]. As such, steroids are not currently recommended for acute TBI treatment if there is no other prominent indication.

The use of tranexamic acid (TXA) after trauma with significant extracranial hemorrhage is beneficial. The Clinical Randomization of an Antifibrinolytic in Significant Hemorrhage-2 (CRASH-2) trial, a large ($n = 20{,}211$), double blinded, placebo control study, enrolled adult trauma patients with significant extracranial bleeding or at risk for significant bleeding 23,477,634. Patients were administered TXA (1 g over 10 min then 1 g over 8 h). Mortality within 4 weeks was significantly reduced in patients that received TXA within 3 h of injury 23,477,634 [30]. A subsequent study examined 270 of these patients who were noted to also have TBI and found that TXA administration trended to reduce hematoma expansion, number of new hemorrhages, and reduction in new ischemic lesions in the brain [31]. This prompted the subsequent CRASH-3 trial which enrolled adult patients who presented within 3 h of a TBI and having intracranial hemorrhage and/or GCS $\leq$ 12, and no significant extracranial hemorrhage requiring immediate transfusions [32]. While the TXA trended toward improved mortality (RR 0.94, 95% CI 0.86–1.02), this primary outcome was not significant. Prespecified subgroup analysis excluding patients presenting with GCS 3 and bilaterally nonreactive pupils was also not significant, but with a trend toward improvement in those treated with TXA (RR 0.89, 95% CI 0.80–1.00). However, TXA treatment did significantly reduce mortality in patient with mild to moderate but not severe TBI, the latter group making up 39% of the study patients and likely influencing the primary outcome. Moreover, there was no difference in the incidence of adverse effects including ischemic injury, increased disability, or seizures suggesting that TXA after head injury is safe [32]. Taken together, use of TXA may be appropriate for selected patients with mild to moderate TBI.

20.5 Blood Pressure Management

Outside the hyperacute resuscitation period, theories on optimal blood pressure targets have been shifting over the past 50 years. Currently, two general approaches exist for the management of blood pressure after TBI: the less employed Lund concept aimed at reducing hydrostatic pressure to prevent cerebral edema and the more widely used cerebral perfusion pressure (CPP) approach aimed at augmenting blood pressure to overcome elevated ICP.

First reported in 1994 and still utilized in some parts of Scandinavia today, the Lund approach attempts to prevent cerebral edema through volume neutral, low blood pressure states. Cerebral autoregulation and BBB permeability are disrupted in the damage brain. Proponents of this approach believe that cerebral edema is driven primarily by increased capillary hydrostatic pressure (promoting fluid leakage) and decreased intravascular oncotic pressure (reducing intravascular fluid sequestration) [33–35]. Therefore, this approach argues for aggressive control of hypertension with agents that will not cause dilation of the cerebral vasculature (B1 antagonist, metoprolol; alpha 2 antagonist, clonidine; ATII antagonism) and use of products that augment plasma oncotic pressure (albumin and blood transfusions). There is strict avoidance of vasopressors and a focus on reducing physiologic stressors which would elevate blood pressure [34, 35]. By maintaining normotension and plasma oncotic pressure, proponents argue that this prevents cerebral edema progression. By proactively preventing edema expansion and therefore ICP elevation, brain perfusion will remain adequate. The Lund approach has been shown to provide some improvement in mortality in centers in Sweden [33, 36, 37]. However, critics note that these were small studies including only 11 [33], 53 [36], and 38 patients [37]. Additionally, outcomes were evaluated in comparison to historical, rather than contemporaneous control groups.

Developed in parallel was the alternative movement aimed at overcoming the detrimental effects of cerebral edema by optimizing cerebral perfusion pressure [(CPP); CPP = mean arterial pressure (MAP)—ICP]. This approach was developed at a time when elevated ICPs were successfully lowered using ventriculostomy and mannitol infusions. Despite effectively achieving physiologic ICP targets, there was not an improvement in patient outcomes. When trying to understand why this was the case, one had to evaluate the detrimental effects of ICP elevations—namely a reduction of cerebral perfusion. If ICP targets were reached in the setting of lowering MAP, there would be no improvement in cerebral perfusion. By targeting CPP directly not only by reducing ICP, but also by augmenting MAP, proponents of this theory believed better patient outcomes could be achieved. In this sentiment and in contrast to what would be expected from the Lund theory, a small safety study showed that elevation of MAP after TBI did not worsen cerebral edema [38]. With this data, Rosner et al. published the first study examining the effect of targeting CPP > 70 mmHg in patients after TBI [39]. Using CSF drainage, mannitol boluses, vasopressors and volume expansion to augment CPP, the authors showed improvement in survival compared to historical controls [39]. While a CPP > 70 mmHg was the minimum CPP allowed, further augmentation of CPP was pursued if ICP values were spontaneously lower at higher CPP values, if ICP values were increasing, or if there was evidence of specific wave forms on the ICP monitoring [39].

Currently, the Brain Trauma Foundation recommends achieving CPP of 60–70 mmHg in all patients after severe TBI [5]. The reluctance to recommend higher CPPs comes from concern of development of acute respiratory distress syndrome (ARDS) found from the landmark study by Robertson et al. [40]. This randomized trial compared CPP-guided (CPP > 70 mmHg) versus ICP-guided (with CPP > 50 mmHg) treatment strategies of 189 patients who remained comatose after TBI. While the CPP strategy was associated with reduced secondary ischemia, it was also associated with a five-fold increase in the development of ARDS. As such, there was no mortality benefit between groups [40]. Development of ARDS was attributed to increase use of fluids and pressors needed to augment MAP for CPP goals. This association is likely to be called into question as new approaches are aimed at defining optimal CPP (CPPopt). CPPopt is a more dynamic and individualized target based on a patient's own cerebral autoregulatory abilities and localized oxygen demand and will likely more precisely guide therapy. Using CPPopt, a small, retrospective study of 38 patients with severe TBI noted that there was no association between optimal CPP and development of ARDS [41]. These results were echoed in a larger study of 113 patients after severe TBI where there were no differences in CPPopt values in patients that eventually did or did not develop ARDS [42].

A drawback to targeting CPP is the requirement for ICP monitoring. Direct measurements of ICP require invasive monitors (e.g., intraventricular monitors, subarachnoid screws/"bolts") and require trained personal for the insertion and device management. While noninvasive devices to measure cerebral autoregulation are being developed and their roles in TBI just beginning to be defined, intraventricular catheters do have the added benefit of draining CSF to temporize ICP elevations. Extensive discussion on invasive vs. noninvasive ICP monitoring can be found elsewhere [43].

20.6 Volume Status After TBI

As optimal blood pressures and perfusion targets have been evolving, ideal volume status for patients after TBI has had similar flux. Prior to the 1980s, a negative fluid balance was thought to prevent progression of cerebral edema likely from evidence of mannitol reducing ICP and causing diuresis [44]. However, later work examining ICP, cerebral perfusion pressure (CPP), and fluid balance after TBI overturned this assumption. In their retrospective analysis of 392 patients enrolled in the National Acute Brain Injury Study: Hypothermia (NABIS:H), Clifton et al. found that a fluid balance of −596 mL or more in the first 96 h after TBI was associated with poor outcome [44]. Hypovolemia was an independent predictor of poor outcome and not due to effects on ICP or CPP. Conversely, a large, multicenter, prospective observational study examined fluid management practices in patients with TBI in 55 hospitals in Europe and Australia with data collected in the CENTER-TBI and

OzENTER-TBI studies [45]. This study revealed the large variability in fluid management after TBI across the centers. Using these inherent differences, hypervolemia was associated with increased mortality and lower GOS-E score at 6 months [45]. Volume status did not correlate to CPP values [45]. Detrimental effects of hypervolemia, in efforts to augment CPP, has been associated with development of ARDS as discussed above [40]. However, when euvolemia is targeted and CPP goals individualized, CPP targets are not correlated to ARDS development [42]. Therefore, best practice would target euvolemia in patients after TBI and multiple means to assess volume status should be used including responsiveness to fluid administration, accurate input and output measures, daily weights, respiratory-dependent stroke volume variability, and utilization of bedside ultrasound (discussed in greater detail [15, 46]).

20.7 Hyperosmotic Therapies

Hyperosmolar therapy is used in TBI to help mitigate the effects of cerebral edema, namely ICP elevation, brain compression, and herniation. After TBI, areas of disrupted BBB allow for inappropriate diffusion of electrolytes and solutes from the intravascular space to the brain parenchyma. In addition, necrosed cells will release their intracellular contents to the extracellular space. Together, this will increase the osmotic drivers in the brain parenchyma encouraging the flow of water into the extravascular space exacerbating brain edema and ICP elevation.

With administration of hypertonic fluids, the intravascular osmolarity is increased creating an osmolar gradient. This gradient will drive brain parenchymal fluid from the extracellular space into the vasculature. To allow for the generation of a gradient, there cannot be a free flow of fluids from the intravascular to parenchymal space—i.e. there must be an intact blood–brain barrier (BBB). Therefore, when hyperosmolars are employed, they predominantly reduce brain water content (and therefore brain volume) of "healthy" brain tissue and not in areas of damaged brain with a dysfunctional BBB [47].

20.8 Overview of Hypertonic Fluids

Hypertonic fluids have been used to reduce ICPs after TBI for years and have a variety of compositions (summarized in Table 20.1). However, there is limited evidence on use of hyperosmotic therapies in improvement neurologic outcome after TBI despite good efficacy in reducing ICP [48–51]. Typically, the initial choice of hyperosmotic are between two crystalloid solutions, hypertonic saline and mannitol. The main difference in these solutions is the effect on volume status.

HTS will increase intravascular volume, increase preload thereby promoting cerebral perfusion if cardiac function is intact. Hypertonic saline can result in platelet aggregation dysfunction, hypokalemia, and hyperchloremic metabolic acidosis [52]. In the USA, hypertonic saline boluses are typically administered as 250 mL of

3% NaCl or 30 mL of 23.4% NaCl. In Europe, 100 mL of 7.45% NaCl is often used. Typically, HTS can reduce elevated ICP within 5 min with "effects" lasting 12 h [53]. Conversely, mannitol reduces volume status through osmotic diuresis. It can be considered a better choice in a patient with volume overload and may provide neuroprotection through ability to act as a free radical scavenger [54]. Mannitol is contraindicated in patients with anuresis as it will not achieve effective osmotic diuresis and may worsen acute kidney injury. To reduce ICP, mannitol can be given in 0.5–1.5 mg/kg bolus with onset time of 10 min and duration of 4 to 6 h [55]. Notably, mannitol may have a "rebound effect" in which ICP may rise above the baseline pressures prior to mannitol administration. This has been theorized to occur due to mannitol deposition in brain parenchyma in areas of disrupted BBB. While rebound has been shown in patients with brain tumors [56, 57], the degree this occurs after TBI is not well established.

Currently, the Neurocritical Care Society's Guidelines recommend employing HTS over mannitol for treatment of elevated ICP after TBI due to the benefits of enhancing intravascular volume and possibly promoting better cerebral perfusion [49]. The writing group acknowledges that this is based on low-quality evidence and was highlighted in recent commentary [58]. After this recommendation, a Cochran analysis found no difference in functional outcomes, early or 6-month mortality with use of mannitol versus HTS for treatment of ICP elevation [59]. Overall, agent selection should depend on patient volume status, cardiac function, kidney function, and local availability of hyperosmotic fluid. In the setting of refractory ICP, those parameters will change after administration of hypertonic fluids; as such a strategy of alternating agents may be employed.

20.9 Hypertonic Saline: Bolus Versus Continuous Therapy

Hypertonic saline may be administered in continuous infusions, in boluses in response to changes in symptoms/ICP, or a combination of the two strategies. Intuitively, using a symptom-based approach allows one to have more means to react to exam changes. Additionally, with continuous exposure to hyperosmolar solutions, it is possible that the cellular response would be to generate osmotic materials to restore cell size and acclimate to a hypertonic environment [47, 60]. In theory, this would make the dehydrating effect of a hyperosmotic therapy less effective. However, when bolus vs. continuous infusion of hypertonic saline was examined in a retrospective study of patients with severe TBI, there was no difference in neurologic outcome, effect ICP reduction, duration of hospitalization, or survival between treatment groups [61]. Patients treated with continuous infusion group did have higher rates of AKI and hyperchloremia than the bolus administered patients [61]. More recently, the Continuous hyperosmolar therapy (20% HTS) in Brain-Injured patient (COBI) trial compared early initiation of continuous HTS vs. standard of care. In the intervention group, patients were given an initial bolus of HTS and were kept on continuous infusion for a minimum of 48 h (with the duration extended until 12 h after ICP normalized). There was no statistical difference in functional outcome (GOS-E at 6 months) between groups. The authors noted more than expected variability in outcomes which may have limited the ability to detect improvements in the intervention group [62]. A posthoc analysis of this study data did not find an increase incidence of kidney injury with the dosing strategies either [63]. Currently, Neurocritical Care Guidelines do not recommend one strategy over the other due to lack of high-quality evidence [49]. Therefore, the choice should be individualized based on patient presentation, lab values (discussed below), and goal of therapy. Mannitol is only administered in bolus dosing.

20.10 Adverse Effects of Hypertonics: Kidney Injury

Regardless of frequency, laboratory values including sodium, chloride, and measured serum osmoles should be monitored when using hypertonic fluids. For the use of hypertonic saline, there are no studies comparing optimal serum sodium level for control of ICP. The neurocritical care guidelines only suggest avoiding hyponatremia and any ranges other than this in practice are typically arbitrarily set by patient care team [49]. Hypernatremia to an upper limit 155–160 mEq/L Na is generally tolerated as higher levels may cause platelet dysfunction [64]. Along with sodium, serum chloride will be elevated with repeated use of HTS and should be kept below 110–115 mEq/L to prevent AKI [49]. Hyperchloremia contributes to renal injury through tubular chloride mediated vasoconstriction of the afferent arteriole [65]. Additionally, elevated chloride can result in hyperchloremic metabolic acidosis. To overcome the effects of hyperchloremia and continue with a sodium based hyperosmotic, a hypertonic solution with 1:1 sodium chloride:sodium acetate may be used. A retrospective, single center study found that compared to HTS, HTS/sodium acetate can effectively increase serum osmolarity without causing prolonged elevation in serum chloride suggesting it is a useful alternative in cases of hyperchloremia [66]. As formulation is nonstandard and requires pharmacy preparation, its availability is highly institution dependent.

Unlike sodium, serum mannitol concentration is not routinely measured. Instead, serum osmolality and osmole gap are used as surrogate markers with osmole gap correlating more directly with serum mannitol concentration [67]. Doses of mannitol may be titrated to effect on ICP as needed, however, most clinicians will agree that a serum osmolality >320 mOsms/mL or an osmole gap >20 mOsm/kg will preclude use of additional dose due to concern for kidney function and lack of benefit [67].

In cases of refractory ICP, alternating strategies based on laboratory values, kidney function, and patient response to treatment can be utilized to achieve the desired reduction in ICP levels in addition to appropriate sedation, analgesia, and positioning.

20.11 Summary

Overall, the presence of head injury in the trauma patient should lead to considerations to promote brain perfusion and prevent secondary brain injury. The need for higher target blood pressures and avoidance of hypotonic solutions may provide better outcomes post-TBI. While there is no consensus on dosing strategy for hypertonic solutions, careful monitoring of laboratory values and clinical response can guide the treatment team to reduce elevated intracranial pressure and support essential cerebral perfusion. Individualized patient data will likely refine the definition of optimal cerebral perfusion pressures and strategies to achieve them.

References

1. Bickell WH, Wall MJ, Pepe PE, Martin RR, Ginger VF, Allen MK, Mattox KL. Immediate versus delayed fluid resuscitation for hypotensive patients with penetrating torso injuries. N Engl J Med. 1994;331(17):1105–9. https://doi.org/10.1056/NEJM199410273311701.
2. Dutton RP, Mackenzie CF, Scalea TM. Hypotensive resuscitation during active hemorrhage: impact on in-hospital mortality. J Trauma. 2002;52(6):1141–6. https://doi.org/10.1097/00005373-200206000-00020.
3. Cherkas D. Traumatic hemorrhagic shock: advances in fluid management. Emerg Med Pract. 2011;13(11):1–19; quiz 19-20.
4. Fuller G, Hasler RM, Mealing N, Lawrence T, Woodford M, Juni P, Lecky F. The association between admission systolic blood pressure and mortality in significant traumatic brain injury: a multi-centre cohort study. Injury. 2014;45(3):612–7. https://doi.org/10.1016/j.injury.2013.09.008.
5. Carney N, Totten AM, O'Reilly C, Ullman JS, Hawryluk GW, Bell MJ, Ghajar J. Guidelines for the management of severe traumatic brain injury, fourth edition. Neurosurgery. 2017;80(1):6–15. https://doi.org/10.1227/NEU.0000000000001432.
6. Berry C, Ley EJ, Bukur M, Malinoski D, Margulies DR, Mirocha J, Salim A. Redefining hypotension in traumatic brain injury. Injury. 2012;43(11):1833–7. https://doi.org/10.1016/j.injury.2011.08.014.
7. Gaitanidis A, Breen KA, Maurer LR, Saillant NN, Kaafarani HMA, Velmahos GC, Mendoza AE. Systolic blood pressure <110 mm hg as a threshold of hypotension in patients with isolated traumatic brain injuries. J Neurotrauma. 2021;38(7):879–85. https://doi.org/10.1089/neu.2020.7358.
8. Asmar S, Chehab M, Bible L, Khurrum M, Castanon L, Ditillo M, Joseph B. The emergency department systolic blood pressure relationship after traumatic brain injury. J Surg Res. 2021;257:493–500. https://doi.org/10.1016/j.jss.2020.07.062.
9. Picetti E, Rossi S, Abu-Zidan FM, Ansaloni L, Armonda R, Baiocchi GL, Catena F. WSES consensus conference guidelines: monitoring and management of severe adult traumatic brain injury patients with polytrauma in the first 24 hours. World J Emerg Surg. 2019;14:53. https://doi.org/10.1186/s13017-019-0270-1.
10. Spahn DR, Bouillon B, Cerny V, Coats TJ, Duranteau J, Fernández-Mondéjar E, Rossaint R. Management of bleeding and coagulopathy following major trauma: an updated European guideline. Crit Care. 2013;17(2):R76. https://doi.org/10.1186/cc12685.
11. Spaite DW, Hu C, Bobrow BJ, Chikani V, Sherrill D, Barnhart B, Adelson PD. Mortality and prehospital blood pressure in patients with major traumatic brain injury: implications for the hypotension threshold. JAMA Surg. 2017;152(4):360–8. https://doi.org/10.1001/jamasurg.2016.4686.
12. Huang HK, Liu CY, Tzeng IS, Hsieh TH, Chang CY, Hou YT, Wu MY. The association between blood pressure and in-hospital mortality in traumatic brain injury: evidence from a 10-year analysis in a single-center. Am J Emerg Med. 2022;58:265–74. https://doi.org/10.1016/j.ajem.2022.05.047.
13. Lewis SR, Pritchard MW, Evans DJ, Butler AR, Alderson P, Smith AF, Roberts I. Colloids versus crystalloids for fluid resuscitation in critically ill people. Cochrane Database Syst Rev. 2018;8(8):CD000567. https://doi.org/10.1002/14651858.CD000567.pub7.

14. Coppola S, Froio S, Chiumello D. Fluid resuscitation in trauma patients: what should we know? Curr Opin Crit Care. 2014;20(4):444–50. https://doi.org/10.1097/MCC.0000000000000115.
15. Wise R, Faurie M, Malbrain MLNG, Hodgson E. Strategies for intravenous fluid resuscitation in trauma patients. World J Surg. 2017;41(5):1170–83. https://doi.org/10.1007/s00268-016-3865-7.
16. Semler MW, Self WH, Wanderer JP, Ehrenfeld JM, Wang L, Byrne DW, Group, S. I. a. t. P. C. C. R. Balanced crystalloids versus saline in critically ill adults. N Engl J Med. 2018;378(9):829–39. https://doi.org/10.1056/NEJMoa1711584.
17. Lombardo S, Smith MC, Semler MW, Wang L, Dear ML, Lindsell CJ, Investigators, I. S. a. M. A. R. E. T. S. I. a. V. L. H. S. P. Balanced crystalloid versus saline in adults with traumatic brain injury: secondary analysis of a clinical trial. J Neurotrauma. 2022;39(17–18):1159–67. https://doi.org/10.1089/neu.2021.0465.
18. Zampieri FG, Machado FR, Biondi RS, Freitas FGR, Veiga VC, Figueiredo RC, members, B. i. a. t. B. Effect of intravenous fluid treatment with a balanced solution vs 0.9% saline solution on mortality in critically ill patients: the BaSICS randomized clinical trial. JAMA. 2021;326(9):1–12. https://doi.org/10.1001/jama.2021.11684.
19. Rowell SE, Fair KA, Barbosa RR, Watters JM, Bulger EM, Holcomb JB, Schreiber MA. The impact of pre-hospital administration of Lactated ringer's solution versus normal saline in patients with traumatic brain injury. J Neurotrauma. 2016;33(11):1054–9. https://doi.org/10.1089/neu.2014.3478.
20. Cooper DJ, Myles PS, McDermott FT, Murray LJ, Laidlaw J, Cooper G, Investigators HS. Prehospital hypertonic saline resuscitation of patients with hypotension and severe traumatic brain injury: a randomized controlled trial. JAMA. 2004;291(11):1350–7. https://doi.org/10.1001/jama.291.11.1350.
21. Bergmans SF, Schober P, Schwarte LA, Loer SA, Bossers SM. Prehospital fluid administration in patients with severe traumatic brain injury: a systematic review and meta-analysis. Injury. 2020;51(11):2356–67. https://doi.org/10.1016/j.injury.2020.08.030.
22. Finfer S, Bellomo R, Boyce N, French J, Myburgh J, Norton R, Investigators SS. A comparison of albumin and saline for fluid resuscitation in the intensive care unit. N Engl J Med. 2004;350(22):2247–56. https://doi.org/10.1056/NEJMoa040232.
23. Myburgh J, Cooper DJ, Finfer S, Bellomo R, Norton R, Bishop N, Health, G. I. f. I. Saline or albumin for fluid resuscitation in patients with traumatic brain injury. N Engl J Med. 2007;357(9):874–84. https://doi.org/10.1056/NEJMoa067514.
24. Cooper DJ, Myburgh J, Heritier S, Finfer S, Bellomo R, Billot L, Group, A. A. N. Z. I. C. S. C. T. Albumin resuscitation for traumatic brain injury: is intracranial hypertension the cause of increased mortality? J Neurotrauma. 2013;30(7):512–8. https://doi.org/10.1089/neu.2012.2573.
25. Taccone FS, Badenes R, Rynkowski CB, Bouzat P, Caricato A, Kurtz P, Vincent JL. TRansfusion strategies in acute brain INjured patients (TRAIN): a prospective multicenter randomized interventional trial protocol. Trials. 2023;24(1):20. https://doi.org/10.1186/s13063-022-07061-7.
26. El-Swaify ST, Refaat MA, Ali SH, Abdelrazek AEM, Beshay PW, Kamel M, Basha AK. Controversies and evidence gaps in the early management of severe traumatic brain injury: back to the ABCs. Trauma Surg Acute Care Open. 2022;7(1):e000859. https://doi.org/10.1136/tsaco-2021-000859.
27. Chang R, Folkerson LE, Sloan D, Tomasek JS, Kitagawa RS, Choi HA, Holcomb JB. Early plasma transfusion is associated with improved survival after isolated traumatic brain injury in patients with multifocal intracranial hemorrhage. Surgery. 2017;161(2):538–45. https://doi.org/10.1016/j.surg.2016.08.023.
28. Furay E, Daley M, Teixeira PG, Coopwood TB, Aydelotte JD, Malesa N, Brown CVR. Goal-directed platelet transfusions correct platelet dysfunction and may improve survival in patients with severe traumatic brain injury. J Trauma Acute Care Surg. 2018;85(5):881–7. https://doi.org/10.1097/TA.0000000000002047.
29. Roberts I, Yates D, Sandercock P, Farrell B, Wasserberg J, Lomas G, collaborators, C. t. Effect of intravenous corticosteroids on death within 14 days in 10008 adults with clinically

significant head injury (MRC CRASH trial): randomised placebo-controlled trial. Lancet. 2004;364(9442):1321–8. https://doi.org/10.1016/S0140-6736(04)17188-2.
30. Roberts I, Shakur H, Coats T, Hunt B, Balogun E, Barnetson L, Guerriero C. The CRASH-2 trial: a randomised controlled trial and economic evaluation of the effects of tranexamic acid on death, vascular occlusive events and transfusion requirement in bleeding trauma patients. Health Technol Assess. 2013;17(10):1–79. https://doi.org/10.3310/hta17100.
31. Perel P, Al-Shahi Salman R, Kawahara T, Morris Z, Prieto-Merino D, Roberts I, Wardlaw J. CRASH-2 (Clinical Randomisation of an Antifibrinolytic in Significant Haemorrhage) intracranial bleeding study: the effect of tranexamic acid in traumatic brain injury—a nested randomised, placebo-controlled trial. Health Technol Assess. 2012;16(13):iii–xii. https://doi.org/10.3310/hta16130; 1-54.
32. Roberts I, Shakur-Still H, Aeron-Thomas A, Beaumont D, Belli A, Brenner A, Williams J. Tranexamic acid to reduce head injury death in people with traumatic brain injury: the CRASH-3 international RCT. Health Technol Assess. 2021;25(26):1–76. https://doi.org/10.3310/hta25260.
33. Asgeirsson B, Grände PO, Nordström CH. A new therapy of post-trauma brain oedema based on haemodynamic principles for brain volume regulation. Intensive Care Med. 1994;20(4):260–7. https://doi.org/10.1007/BF01708961.
34. Grände PO. The "Lund Concept" for the treatment of severe head trauma—physiological principles and clinical application. Intensive Care Med. 2006;32(10):1475–84. https://doi.org/10.1007/s00134-006-0294-3.
35. Grände PO. Critical evaluation of the Lund concept for treatment of severe traumatic head injury, 25 years after its introduction. Front Neurol. 2017;8:315. https://doi.org/10.3389/fneur.2017.00315.
36. Eker C, Asgeirsson B, Grände PO, Schalén W, Nordström CH. Improved outcome after severe head injury with a new therapy based on principles for brain volume regulation and preserved microcirculation. Crit Care Med. 1998;26(11):1881–6. https://doi.org/10.1097/00003246-199811000-00033.
37. Naredi S, Edén E, Zäll S, Stephensen H, Rydenhag B. A standardized neurosurgical neurointensive therapy directed toward vasogenic edema after severe traumatic brain injury: clinical results. Intensive Care Med. 1998;24(5):446–51. https://doi.org/10.1007/s001340050594.
38. Rosner MJ, Daughton S. Cerebral perfusion pressure management in head injury. J Trauma. 1990;30(8):933–40. https://doi.org/10.1097/00005373-199008000-00001; discussion 940-931.
39. Rosner MJ, Rosner SD, Johnson AH. Cerebral perfusion pressure: management protocol and clinical results. J Neurosurg. 1995;83(6):949–62. https://doi.org/10.3171/jns.1995.83.6.0949.
40. Robertson CS, Valadka AB, Hannay HJ, Contant CF, Gopinath SP, Cormio M, Grossman RG. Prevention of secondary ischemic insults after severe head injury. Crit Care Med. 1999;27(10):2086–95. https://doi.org/10.1097/00003246-199910000-00002.
41. Moreira M, Fernandes D, Pereira E, Monteiro E, Pascoa R, Dias C. Is there a relationship between optimal cerebral perfusion pressure-guided management and PaO. Acta Neurochir Suppl. 2018;126:59–62. https://doi.org/10.1007/978-3-319-65798-1_13.
42. Thiara S, Griesdale DE, Henderson WR, Sekhon MS. Effect of cerebral perfusion pressure on acute respiratory distress syndrome. Can J Neurol Sci. 2018;45(3):313–9. https://doi.org/10.1017/cjn.2017.292.
43. Harary M, Dolmans RGF, Gormley WB. Intracranial pressure monitoring-review and avenues for development. Sensors (Basel). 2018;18(2):465. https://doi.org/10.3390/s18020465.
44. Clifton GL, Miller ER, Choi SC, Levin HS. Fluid thresholds and outcome from severe brain injury. Crit Care Med. 2002;30(4):739–45. https://doi.org/10.1097/00003246-200204000-00003.
45. Wiegers EJA, Lingsma HF, Huijben JA, Cooper DJ, Citerio G, Frisvold S, Groups, O.-T. C. Fluid balance and outcome in critically ill patients with traumatic brain injury (CENTER-TBI and OzENTER-TBI): a prospective, multicentre, comparative effectiveness study. Lancet Neurol. 2021;20(8):627–38. https://doi.org/10.1016/S1474-4422(21)00162-9.

46. Elhassan MG, Chao PW, Curiel A. The conundrum of volume status assessment: revisiting current and future tools available for physicians at the bedside. Cureus. 2021;13(5):e15253. https://doi.org/10.7759/cureus.15253.
47. Mohney N, Alkhatib O, Koch S, O'Phelan K, Merenda A. What is the role of hyperosmolar therapy in hemispheric stroke patients? Neurocrit Care. 2020;32(2):609–19. https://doi.org/10.1007/s12028-019-00782-9.
48. Burgess S, Abu-Laban RB, Slavik RS, Vu EN, Zed PJ. A systematic review of randomized controlled trials comparing hypertonic sodium solutions and mannitol for traumatic brain injury: implications for emergency department management. Ann Pharmacother. 2016;50(4):291–300. https://doi.org/10.1177/1060028016628893.
49. Cook AM, Morgan Jones G, Hawryluk GWJ, Mailloux P, McLaughlin D, Papangelou A, Shutter L. Guidelines for the acute treatment of cerebral edema in neurocritical care patients. Neurocrit Care. 2020;32(3):647–66. https://doi.org/10.1007/s12028-020-00959-7.
50. Miyoshi Y, Kondo Y, Suzuki H, Fukuda T, Yasuda H, Yokobori S, Committee, J. R. C. J. N. T. F. a. t. G. E. Effects of hypertonic saline versus mannitol in patients with traumatic brain injury in prehospital, emergency department, and intensive care unit settings: a systematic review and meta-analysis. J Intensive Care. 2020;8:61. https://doi.org/10.1186/s40560-020-00476-x.
51. Pigott A, Rudloff E. Traumatic brain injury-a review of intravenous fluid therapy. Front Vet Sci. 2021;8:643800. https://doi.org/10.3389/fvets.2021.643800.
52. Doyle JA, Davis DP, Hoyt DB. The use of hypertonic saline in the treatment of traumatic brain injury. J Trauma. 2001;50(2):367–83. https://doi.org/10.1097/00005373-200102000-00030.
53. Alnemari AM, Krafcik BM, Mansour TR, Gaudin D. A comparison of pharmacologic therapeutic agents used for the reduction of intracranial pressure after traumatic brain injury. World Neurosurg. 2017;106:509–28. https://doi.org/10.1016/j.wneu.2017.07.009.
54. Mizoi K, Suzuki J, Imaizumi S, Yoshimoto T. Development of new cerebral protective agents: the free radical scavengers. Neurol Res. 1986;8(2):75–80. https://doi.org/10.1080/01616412.1986.11739734.
55. Witherspoon B, Ashby NE. The use of mannitol and hypertonic saline therapies in patients with elevated intracranial pressure: a review of the evidence. Nurs Clin North Am. 2017;52(2):249–60. https://doi.org/10.1016/j.cnur.2017.01.002.
56. Palma L, Bruni G, Fiaschi AI, Mariottini A. Passage of mannitol into the brain around gliomas: a potential cause of rebound phenomenon. A study on 21 patients. J Neurosurg Sci. 2006;50(3):63–6.
57. Sankar T, Assina R, Karis JP, Theodore N, Preul MC. Neurosurgical implications of mannitol accumulation within a meningioma and its peritumoral region demonstrated by magnetic resonance spectroscopy: case report. J Neurosurg. 2008;108(5):1010–3. https://doi.org/10.3171/JNS/2008/108/5/1010.
58. Quintard H, Meyfroidt G, Citerio G. Hyperosmolar agents for TBI: all are equal, but some are more equal than others? Neurocrit Care. 2020;33(2):613–4. https://doi.org/10.1007/s12028-020-01063-6.
59. Chen H, Song Z, Dennis JA. Hypertonic saline versus other intracranial pressure-lowering agents for people with acute traumatic brain injury. Cochrane Database Syst Rev. 2020;1(1):CD010904. https://doi.org/10.1002/14651858.CD010904.pub3.
60. Diringer MN. New trends in hyperosmolar therapy? Curr Opin Crit Care. 2013;19(2):77–82. https://doi.org/10.1097/MCC.0b013e32835eba30.
61. Maguigan KL, Dennis BM, Hamblin SE, Guillamondegui OD. Method of hypertonic saline administration: effects on osmolality in traumatic brain injury patients. J Clin Neurosci. 2017;39:147–50. https://doi.org/10.1016/j.jocn.2017.01.025.
62. Roquilly A, Moyer JD, Huet O, Lasocki S, Cohen B, Dahyot-Fizelier C, Network, A. S. G. a. t. S. F. d. A. R. S. R. Effect of continuous infusion of hypertonic saline vs standard care on 6-month neurological outcomes in patients with traumatic brain injury: the COBI randomized clinical trial. JAMA. 2021;325(20):2056–66. https://doi.org/10.1001/jama.2021.5561.
63. Huet O, Chapalain X, Vermeersch V, Moyer JD, Lasocki S, Cohen B, Network, A. S. G. a. t. S. F. d. A. R. S. R. Impact of continuous hypertonic (NaCl 20%) saline solution on renal

outcomes after traumatic brain injury (TBI): a post hoc analysis of the COBI trial. Crit Care. 2023;27(1):42. https://doi.org/10.1186/s13054-023-04311-1.
64. Tan TS, Tan KH, Ng HP, Loh MW. The effects of hypertonic saline solution (7.5%) on coagulation and fibrinolysis: an in vitro assessment using thromboelastography. Anaesthesia. 2002;57(7):644–8. https://doi.org/10.1046/j.1365-2044.2002.02603.x.
65. Rein JL, Coca SG. "I don't get no respect": the role of chloride in acute kidney injury. Am J Physiol Renal Physiol. 2019;316(3):F587–605. https://doi.org/10.1152/ajprenal.00130.2018.
66. Holden DN, Yung FH, Entezami P. Hypertonic saline buffered with sodium acetate for intracranial pressure management. Clin Neurol Neurosurg. 2021;201:106435. https://doi.org/10.1016/j.clineuro.2020.106435.
67. García-Morales EJ, Cariappa R, Parvin CA, Scott MG, Diringer MN. Osmole gap in neurologic-neurosurgical intensive care unit: its normal value, calculation, and relationship with mannitol serum concentrations. Crit Care Med. 2004;32(4):986–91. https://doi.org/10.1097/01.ccm.0000120057.04528.60.

Neurosurgical Treatment of Traumatic Brain Injury and the Role of Decompressive Hemicraniectomy

21

M. Grutza, A. Unterberg, and A. Younsi

21.1 Introduction

Traumatic brain injury (TBI) remains one of the leading causes of morbidity and mortality worldwide [1]. Severe injuries, defined by a Glasgow Coma Scale (GCS) score between 3 and 8, are often associated with space-occupying lesions and secondary processes such as edema and hematoma expansion. Because of the rigid nature of the dura mater and the skull, these processes may lead to an elevation of the intracranial pressure (ICP), which in turn results in a vicious cycle of reduced cerebral blood flow, ischemia, and further ICP elevation, potentially culminating in herniation [2]. It is therefore no surprise that neurosurgical techniques to evacuate hematomas and reduce elevated ICP were established millennia ago, with signs of skull trepanation, the earliest forerunner of modern craniotomies, found in skeletons dating back to the neolithic period [3]. Despite our better understanding of the heterogeneity and complexity of TBI in the last decades, neurosurgical intervention has remained the mainstay of its treatment, and procedures such as decompressive craniectomies (DCs) to reduce refractory ICP, initially reported by Kocher and Cushing over a century ago [4], are still performed today. Moreover, in the era of broadly available imaging and modern monitoring techniques, the utilization of cranial computed tomography (CT) scans and ICP monitoring devices has led to a faster and more accurate diagnosis of cranial pathologies following TBI, permitting swift and precise surgeries. In this chapter, such cranial injuries and their state-of-the-art neurosurgical treatment will be described.

M. Grutza · A. Unterberg · A. Younsi (✉)
Department of Neurosurgery, University Hospital Heidelberg, Heidelberg, Germany
e-mail: martin.grutza@med.uni-heidelberg.de; andreas.unterberg@med.uni-heidelberg.de; alexander.younsi@med.uni-heidelberg.de

E. Brogi et al. (eds.), *Traumatic Brain Injury*, Hot Topics in Acute Care Surgery and Trauma, https://doi.org/10.1007/978-3-031-50117-3_21

21.2 Skull Fractures

21.2.1 Calvarial Fractures

Calvarial fractures can be divided into open or closed fractures, whereby open fractures are defined as a connection between the exterior of the skull and the subdural space. Calvarial fractures are also typically classified as linear, accounting for the majority of cases, or depressed, making up only 11% of cases. Potential mechanisms of skull fractures after TBI include blunt or focal force on the skull [5].

Linear fractures without intracranial injuries are treated primarily conservatively; a surgical approach is in most cases not necessary. Furthermore, isolated skull fractures without associated intracranial injuries are generally associated with a good prognosis. In contrast, depressed fractures causing neurological deterioration or compression of brain tissue may require surgical treatment. Open skull fractures may be accompanied by cerebrospinal fluid (CSF) leakage or prolapse of brain tissue. In these cases, neurosurgical treatment is mandatory. Especially in the presence of large intracranial hematoma, fracture displacement ≥1 cm, significant frontal sinus involvement, or pneumocephalus, neurosurgical treatment is often necessary [6].

Potential neurosurgical techniques for management of calvarial fractures are craniotomy or fracture elevation, with concomitant dural closure and wound debridement [7, 8]. Due to the risk for posttraumatic infection, such as meningitis, brain abscess or subdural empyema, treatment should ideally be performed within the first 6–8 h after injury [9]. Such complications might explain the higher mortality rate seen in severe TBI patients with isolated calvarial fractures [10].

21.2.2 Skull Base Fractures

Linear fractures resulting in fracture of the skull base are often caused by traffic accidents with a high-energy force frontal impact. Such fractures may occur in one or more parts of the temporal, occipital, sphenoid, frontal or ethmoid bone and can be classified into anterior fossa, middle fossa, and posterior fossa fractures. Skull base fractures can be found in 17% of all calvarial fractures; isolated skull base fractures occur in approximately 4% of patients with severe TBI [5].

Relevant skull base fracture types include frontobasal fractures and laterobasal fractures.

Signs of frontobasal fractures may include CSF leakage from the nose and/or ears and periorbital ecchymosis ("raccoon eyes"). Furthermore, retroauricular hemorrhage causing bruising over the mastoid process of the temporal bone ("Battle's sign") is frequently present in laterobasal fractures. Intracranial air collections or shadowing of air-filled bone compartments (paranasal sinuses, mastoid cells) might be indirect signs of skull base fractures even without the presence of a fracture gap as displayed on cranial CT scans. Thin-slice CT scans are recommended for further classification of such fractures. When uncertainty exists about whether leaking fluid is CSF, a sample of the fluid can collected and sent for testing to determine the presence of β2-transferrin. A positive result confirms the origin of the fluid as CSF.

Treatment of skull base fractures is mainly conservative. Some clinicians administer prophylactic antibiotics to prevent posttraumatic meningitis. However, no robust evidence concerning the clinical effects and benefits of antibiotics currently exists [11]. Neurosurgical intervention is recommended for severe dislocated bone fractures or persistent CSF fistulas. Surgery is normally performed after posttraumatic swelling has receded. Of note, complex frontobasal injuries often require a multidisciplinary approach that includes neurosurgery, oral and maxillofacial surgery, ear, nose, and throat surgery, and possibly other specialties. When concomitant large space-occupying intracranial hematomas are present, neurosurgical consultation should be sought immediately.

Complications of skull base fractures such as meningitis [12], empyema, brain abscess, carotid artery injuries with carotid-cavernous fistulas, or permanent cranial nerve lesions can occur and worsen the prognosis [13].

21.3 Epidural Hematomas

Epidural hematomas (EDH) are defined as blood collections between the dura mater and the skull. EDHs are typically seen as lens-shaped hyperdensities on cranial CT scans due to adhesions between dura and skull that restrict spread of the hematoma (Fig. 21.1). These adhesions increase with age; thus, older patients are less frequently affected by epidural hematomas.

Potential mechanisms for the occurrence of EDH are traumatic injuries of the middle meningeal artery or its branches. Injury of a dural venous sinus or a calvarial fracture are less common causes. Typical clinical signs are headache with nausea and vomiting. The disease progression may include rapid neurological deterioration such as progressive worsening of level of consciousness with ipsilateral pupillary dilation and contralateral hemiparesis. The so-called "lucid interval" encompassing initial brief posttraumatic unconsciousness, a subsequent period of regained alertness, and then renewed, secondary worsening of consciousness is present in only a small percentage of cases. A high degree of vigilance is needed because clinical deterioration may occur in a delayed manner, even several hours after injury.

Treatment of a large EDH consists of immediate surgical evacuation via craniotomy. Identification and obliteration of the bleeding source are necessary. In line with current guidelines, surgical treatment of EDH is indicated when the hematoma volume is greater than 30 cm^3 regardless of the patients' GCS score [14]. Conservative management might be considered in patients with [15] GCS score > 9 [16], no focal neurologic deficits [17], hematoma volume < 30 cm^3, and [7] midline shift <5 mm; however, close neurological and imaging monitoring are mandatory. It has been recommended that the first follow-up cranial CT scan should be performed 4–6 h after the initial trauma [18, 19]. In patients taking antithrombotic medication, surgery may be indicated even for small EDHs and may often be preceded by medical drug reversal [16].

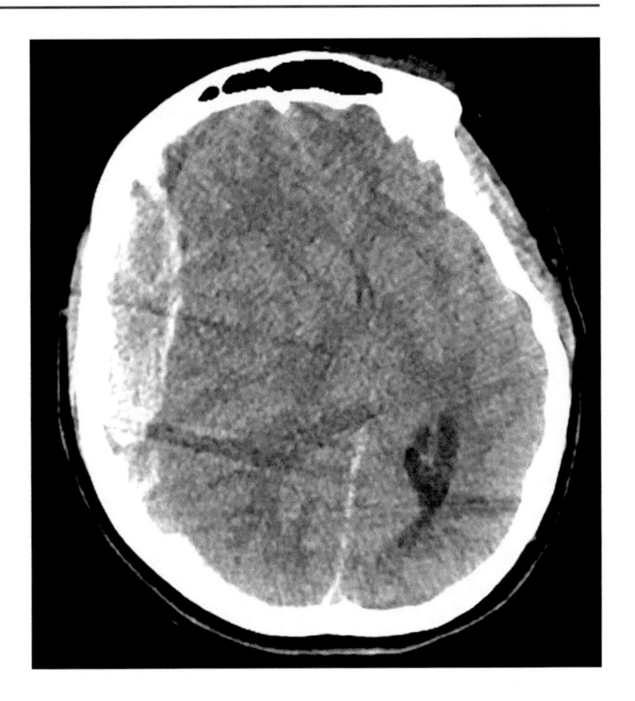

Fig. 21.1 Typical lens-shaped configuration of an EDH with midline shift

The prognosis of EDH depends on the patient's neurological status at the time of surgery. The absence of concomitant intracranial injuries as well as the promptness of emergency surgical intervention are predictors for good outcomes, and the mortality in such cases is relatively low [17, 20, 21].

21.4 Subdural Hematomas

Subdural hematomas (SDH) are defined as blood collections between the brain surface and the dura mater. The suspected underlying mechanisms are rupture of bridging veins in 25% or injuries of small vessels on the contused brain surface in 75% of cases. With respect to the injury severity and the temporal course of the bleeding, SDH can be divided into acute subdural hematoma (aSDH) and subacute and chronic subdural hematoma (sSDH and cSDH).

21.4.1 Acute Subdural Hematomas

The acute form of SDH is a frequent sequela of severe TBI. In young patients, aSDHs are mostly attributable to high-energy traumas such as traffic or sport accidents, while low-energy traumas such as falls from a standing or sitting position are the most common cause in older patients. Typical symptoms are headaches, nausea, and vomiting. In many cases, aSDH can lead to substantial impairment of consciousness or even to coma. These phenomena are caused by the space-occupying effect of the hematoma on the brain tissue, and patients might present with signs of cerebral herniation. A "lucid interval" is scarce, and contralateral hemiparesis with ipsilateral pupil dilation are classic clinical signs for large aSDHs.

On cranial CT scans, aSDHs present as crescent-shaped hyperdensities and often extend over large portions of a cerebral hemisphere (Fig. 21.2).

The indications for surgical evacuation of an aSDH via craniotomy are based on a patient's' neurological symptoms and imaging findings. Indications for surgery include impaired level of consciousness after trauma and/or focal neurological findings with an SDH width of >10 mm or midline shift >5 mm [22].

The typical surgical approach for aSDH evacuation consists of a craniotomy with opening of the dura mater, removal of the hematoma, and meticulous hemostasis. While a DC is usually only performed when the aSDH is accompanied by significant cerebral injury and corresponding brain swelling, its routine use for aSDH evacuation is currently under clinical investigation in the "RESCUE-ASDH" randomized clinical trial (RCT) [23]. Patients with concomitant parenchymal injuries or with continued poor level of alertness after surgery often receive an ICP monitor for neuromonitoring.

Conservative management remains an option for patients with mild neurological symptoms, a midline shift <5 mm, and an aSDH diameter < 10 mm. Close monitoring of such patients in an intermediate or intensive care unit is warranted. In case of secondary clinical deterioration, increasing ICP, or signs of cerebral herniation, immediate surgical therapy may be needed.

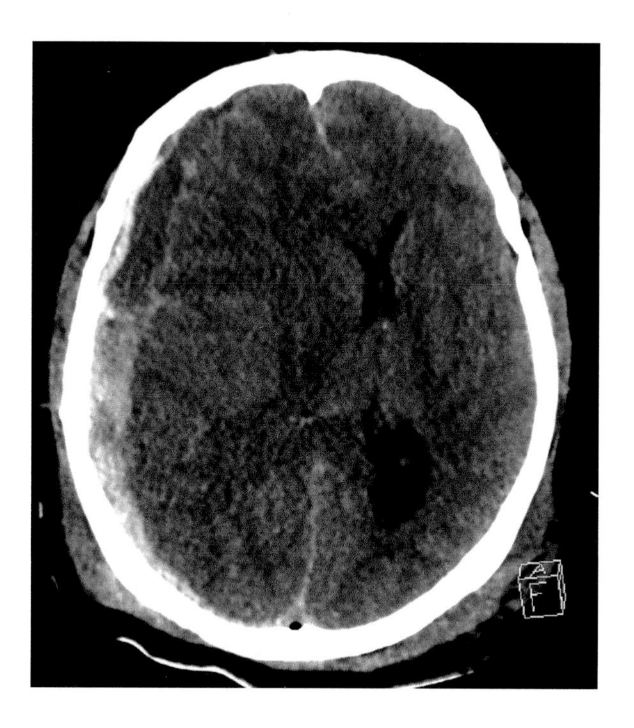

Fig. 21.2 Cranial CT scan of a large space-occupying aSDH with marked midline shift and subfalcine herniation in a patient with severe TBI

The prognosis of aSDH is often poor, with a mortality rate between 40 and 70%. Negative predictors include higher age, worse neurological condition at the time of presentation, and the presence of concomitant injuries [22].

21.4.2 Subacute and Chronic Subdural Hematoma

In contrast to acute SDH, subacute SDH (sSDH) might not become symptomatic until 3–20 days after TBI. Chronic SDH (cSDH) may lead to symptoms only months after an even mild head injury. In both entities, clinical signs are often nonspecific and can include dizziness, headaches or impaired concentration. Neurological deficits such as hemiparesis or sensory disturbances can also occur. The prevalence of sSDH and cSDH is higher in older patients since bridging veins are under greater tension due to physiological brain atrophy and are thus more susceptible to trauma-induced laceration or avulsion. Notably, the incidence of cSDH is increasing due to the global trend of increasing life expectancy [24].

Cranial CT scans demonstrate sSDH and cSDH as a concave subdural fluid collection with age-related hypodense (old), isodense (intermediate), and/or hyperdense (fresh) hematoma components (Fig. 21.3).

Hematoma evacuation via creation of one or more bur holes and insertion of a subdural or subgaleal drain is the mainstay of treatment for cSDH. In rare cases,

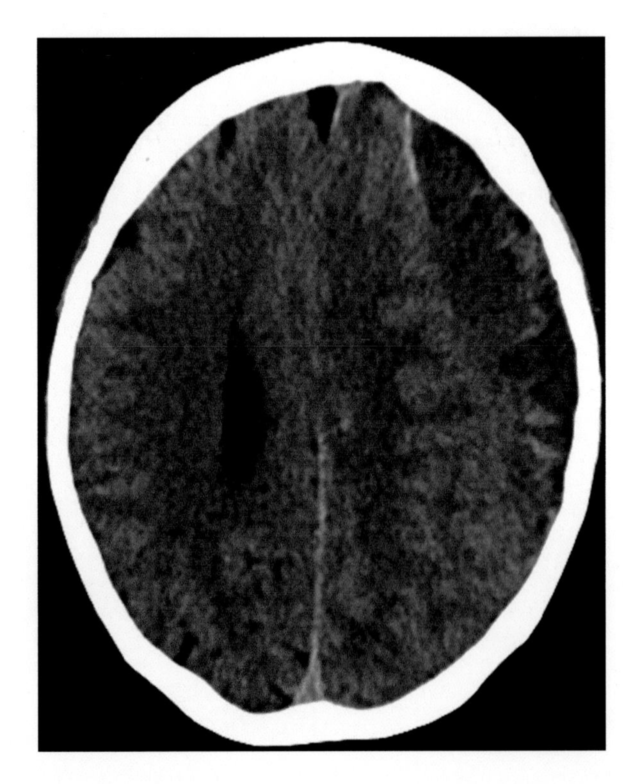

Fig. 21.3 Cranial CT of a space-occupying cSDH on the left side in a 75-year-old patient after mild TBI 6 weeks ago

when a sSDH or cSDH is complicated by the presence of organized hematomas, prominent membranes, or hematoma recurrence, craniotomy with evacuation of fresh hematoma components and resection of membranes might be necessary.

Indications for surgical evacuation of sSDH and cSDH include the presence of neurologic symptoms or deficits and hematoma diameter greater than the width of the skull or > 1 cm [25].

Emerging adjuncts to surgery such as the embolization of the meningeal artery or treatment with corticosteroids or statins are the subject of current research efforts [26–28].

The prognosis of cSDH is generally good. Successful drainage is achieved in almost 90% of cases. However, hematoma recurrence remains a challenge, with rates ranging between 5% and 30% [29, 30].

21.5 Traumatic Intracerebral Hematoma

Traumatic intracerebral hematomas (ICH) or contusions occur in the brain parenchyma after rupture of deep-seated, smaller brain vessels following TBI. On cranial CT, ICHs are initially hyperdense with the development of pronounced perifocal edema within days of the injury. Especially, in the presence of such risk factors as antithrombotic medication, polytrauma, old age, alcohol abuse, or mass transfusions, a repeat CT scan is advisable after 4–6 h (Fig. 21.4). ICHs often progress over several days, potentially increasing significantly in size and causing substantial mass effect ("delayed traumatic intracerebral hemorrhage").

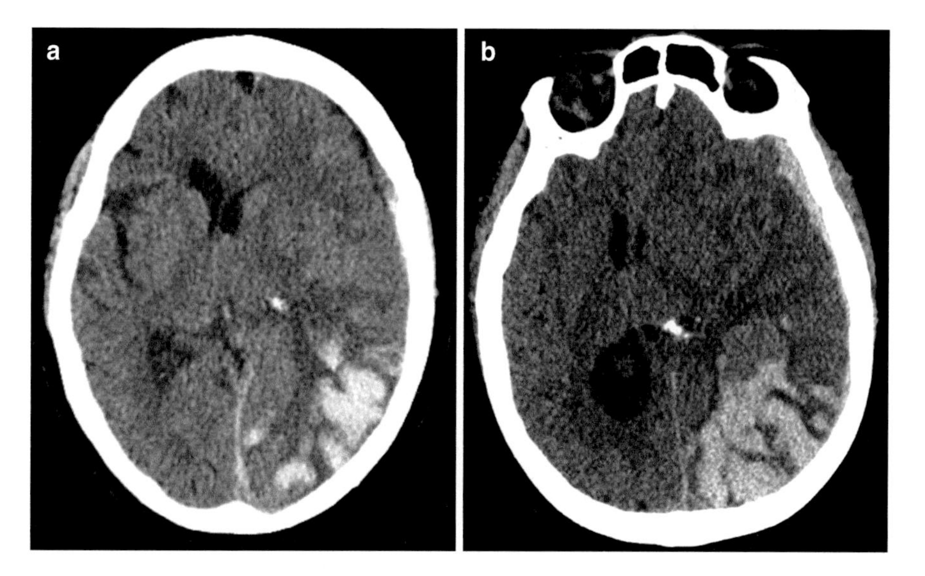

Fig. 21.4 Typical progression of a traumatic ICH over time. (**a**) Initial cranial CT of a comatose patient after severe TBI. (**b**) 6-h follow-up cranial CT after implantation of an ICP probe and increase of ICP values >20 mmHg

The neurologic symptoms of ICH depend on the severity of the initial brain injury as well as the size and location of the hemorrhage. If eloquent areas are affected, neurological deficits might occur. With larger hemorrhages, decrease in level of consciousness or even coma is common.

Indications for surgical ICH evacuation include mass effect on cranial CT imaging, refractory increase in ICP (if an ICP monitor is in place), or neurological deterioration. The primary goal of surgery is the evacuation or reduction of the intracranial lesion to reduce ICP and subsequently to prevent further secondary brain damage [31–34].

Extension of the ICH into the ventricular system is considered a prognostically unfavorable sign since it can lead to impaired CSF circulation, which might progress to hydrocephalus. In such cases, the placement of an external ventricular drainage (EVD) is often necessary and might need to be followed by the implantation of a ventriculoperitoneal shunt (VPS) for long-term management.

21.6 Posttraumatic Intracranial Hypertension

The posttraumatic elevation of ICP due to space-occupying lesions and brain edema, with its vicious cycle of reduced cerebral blood flow, ischemia and further intracranial hypertension, is a feared sequela of TBI because it can lead to brain herniation and death. Thus, invasive monitoring of ICP has become a mainstay in the treatment of TBI. Nevertheless, ICP-guided therapy is not without controversy among experts, and definitive evidence for the benefit of ICP monitoring with a clear relationship to improved outcome does not exist yet [35, 36].

21.6.1 Invasive ICP Monitoring

Although noninvasive ICP monitoring is currently under investigation, invasive ICP monitoring via the surgical placement of an intraparenchymal probe or an EVD so far remains the only way to reliably measure ICP. Intraparenchymal probes can be inserted at the bedside via a simple cannulated screw, whereas EVDs often require a bur hole trepanation and are associated with higher rates of infections and surgical complications. On the other hand, EVDs are less expensive and offer the capability of draining CSF and thus lowering the ICP. Nevertheless, no guideline for the use of parenchymal ICP probes vs. EVDs for ICP monitoring currently exists [15, 37].

The current Brain Trauma Foundation (BTF) guidelines suggest ICP monitoring for all TBI patients with a GCS score < 9 and pathological findings on cranial CT imaging. In unconscious patients with unremarkable cranial CT findings, ICP monitoring should still be considered if two of the following criteria are present [37]: age > 40 years, unilateral or bilateral motor deficits, or systolic blood pressure < 90 mmHg.

21.7 Decompressive Craniectomy

DC is a surgical procedure in which a large section of the skull is removed, and the underlying dura mater is opened. Primary DC refers to leaving a large bone flap out during surgery immediately after injury for evacuation of a large traumatic mass lesion.

Surgical decompression via a craniectomy and dural expansion with the goal to lower posttraumatic intracranial hypertension was performed as early as 1901 by Emil Theodor Kocher [4]. After the technique faded into the background for an extended period in the 1970s due to unsatisfactory results [38], it has experienced a renaissance in recent decades [39–41]. DC is usually performed when intracranial hypertension refractory to conservative treatment is present after TBI and no other means to control raised ICP and ensure adequate cerebral perfusion pressure are available.

Several surgical variants have been described, including bifrontal craniectomy, hemicraniectomy, and bilateral craniectomies.

The effect of DC on clinical outcomes in patients with refractory traumatic intracranial hypertension remains unclear. Following numerous single-center studies, the multicenter DECRA trial, published in 2011, analyzed the impact of DC on 155 adults under the age of 60 years with severe diffuse TBI and refractory intracranial hypertension versus standard care. The intervention significantly lowered ICP and prevented its refractory increase in the early postinjury phase. However, after surgical decompression, significantly worse neurologic outcomes after 6 and 12 months were observed in comparison to patients randomized to the non-DC group [42, 43]. In contrast, the multicenter RESCUE-ICP trial, published in 2016, which analyzed the clinical outcome of 405 patients aged between 18 and 65 years after DC vs. maximal conservative ICP therapy, demonstrated improvement of neurologic outcome 6 and 12 months postinjury [44]. Several differences between these RCTs must be noted. While bifrontal craniectomies were performed if ICP was elevated above 20 mmHg for 15 min within a 1-h period during the first 3 days after TBI in the DECRA trial, patients in the RESCUE-ICP trial were randomized to receive either a bifrontal craniectomy or a hemicraniectomy when ICP was above 25 mmHg for 1–12 h any time after TBI. RESCUE-ICP aimed to assess the effectiveness of DC as a last-tier treatment for late refractory ICP elevation, while DECRA focused on the effect of bifrontal DC for early moderate intracranial hypertension in patients without surgical mass lesions.

Even though the benefits of DC are still debated, a recent update to the BTF guidelines, incorporating the RESCUE-ICP trial results, now recommends the following [45]:

- To perform secondary DC for late (but not for early) refractory ICP elevation.
- To create a large frontotemporoparietal hemicraniectomy (> 15 cm in diameter).

More detailed indications to perform a DC that have been in place for a longer time are listed below [40]:

- Patient age < 50 years.
- GCS score > 3 at admission.
- Signs of brain swelling on cranial CT.
- ICP elevation refractory to conservative treatment.
- ICP elevation correlating with clinical deterioration.
- Irreversible brainstem damage likely without treatment.

Nevertheless, the decision to perform a DC for the treatment of posttraumatic intracranial hypertension must be taken individually and must be based on the presumed desires of the patient. Whether this surgical approach should be the first choice for the treatment of aSDH remains unclear until results of the "RESCUE-ASD" trial are available [23].

21.7.1 Cranioplasty After Decompressive Craniectomy

Cranial reconstruction using autologous bone (such as the surgically removed bone flap stored in the patient's abdominal wall or a freezer) or allografts (metal or plastic) should be performed as early as the patient's condition permits [46]. Cranioplasty may alleviate cognitive and functional deficits by reinstating regular CSF dynamics and improving brain perfusion. Recent analyses on the effects of cranioplasty timing on neurological recovery favor early cranioplasty [47].

21.7.2 Ventriculoperitoneal Shunt Placement for Posttraumatic Hydrocephalus

Posttraumatic hydrocephalus (PTH) is a well-known phenomenon occurring after moderate or severe TBI, with a prevalence ranging between 0.9% and 29% [48, 49]. It is defined by progressive accumulation of CSF and dilation of the ventricles from disorders of the CSF circulation and reabsorption after the traumatic event. PTH is frequently associated with patients' secondary neurological deterioration. Thus, prompt management is warranted [50, 51]. The diagnosis is usually based on both cranial CT imaging findings showing substantial enlargement of the ventricles and clinical manifestations of hydrocephalus.

Several factors have been previously described as potential risk factors for the development of PTH, such as severity of trauma, GCS score on admission, and DC. The rates of PTH after DC range from 11.9 to 36% [49, 50, 52]. Potential underlying mechanisms for the development of PTH after DC might be based on the conversion of the cranium from a closed system into an open "box." Thus, alterations of CSF hemodynamics might take place, including arachnoid adhesions in the basal cisterns, loss of pulsatile intracranial CSF dynamics, and impaired venous drainage into the sagittal sinus [49, 50, 52].

The mainstay of PTH treatment is the placement of a VPS since most patients have substantially reduced brain compliance related to impaired CSF absorption

[49, 50]. In a study on 140 patients suffering from PTH, the insertion of a VPS resulted in significant improvement of consciousness, behavior, memory, and gait, especially in those patients with an acute neurological deterioration before surgery [51]. Nevertheless, complications associated with VPS placement in the context of PTH can be high. In TBI patients who underwent DC, the appropriate timing of VPS vs. cranioplasty must be considered. While the individual patients' situation eventually dictates the order of those two surgical procedures, recent evidence suggests that cranioplasty should be performed before VPS placement and that a simultaneous approach should be avoided to drastically reduce the risk of complications [53, 54].

21.8 Outlook

Current research in the field of TBI is focusing on the identification and experimental treatment of pathophysiological mechanisms that contribute to the development of secondary brain damage. Such research might be helpful to develop new neuroprotective and regenerative therapeutic approaches. However, promising preclinical results have yet to be translated to successful clinical trials. Thus, research focusing on the optimization of existing treatments for TBI, including the above-mentioned neurosurgical approaches, is still warranted. Today, pragmatic RCTs and large repositories of prospectively collected data from observational studies or registries allowing for comparative effectiveness research might overcome the preexisting problems of disease heterogeneity and complexity in TBI research [55, 56].

References

1. James SL, Theadom A, Ellenbogen RG, Bannick MS, Montjoy-Venning W, Lucchesi LR, Abbasi N, Abdulkader R, Abraha HN, Adsuar JC, Afarideh M. Global, regional, and national burden of traumatic brain injury and spinal cord injury, 1990–2016: a systematic analysis for the Global Burden of Disease Study 2016. Lancet Neurol. 2019;18(1):56–87. https://doi.org/10.1016/S1474-4422(18)30415-0.
2. Stevens RD, Shoykhet M, Cadena R. Emergency neurological life support: intracranial hypertension and herniation. Neurocrit Care. 2015;23 Suppl 2(Suppl 2):S76–82. https://doi.org/10.1007/s12028-015-0168-z.
3. Campillo D. Neurosurgical pathology in prehistory. Acta Neurochir. 1984;70(3–4):275–90. https://doi.org/10.1007/BF01406656.
4. Kocher T. Hirnerschütterung, Hirndruck und chirurgische Eingriffe bei Hirnkrankheiten. A. Hölder. 1901; https://books.google.de/books?id=XzM_AAAAQAAJ.
5. Gennarelli D, Grahahm T. Pathology of brain damage after head injury. In: Cooper P, Golfinos G, editors. Head injury. 4th ed. New York, NY: Morgan Hill; 2000.
6. Heary RF, Hunt CD, Krieger AJ, Schulder M, Vaid C. Nonsurgical treatment of compound depressed skull fractures. J Trauma. 1993;35(3):441–7. https://doi.org/10.1097/00005373-199309000-00018.
7. Bullock MR, Chesnut R, Ghajar J, Gordon D, Hartl R, Newell DW, Servadei F, Walters BC, Wilberger J. Surgical management of depressed cranial fractures. Neurosurgery. 2006a;58(3 Suppl):S56–60. https://doi.org/10.1227/01.NEU.0000210367.14043.0E; discussion Si-iv.

8. Wan Y, Li X, Qian C, Xue Z, Yang S, Wang Y. The comparison between dissociate bone flap cranioplasty and traditional cranioplasty in the treatment of depressed skull fractures. J Craniofac Surg. 2013;24(2):589–91. https://doi.org/10.1097/SCS.0b013e3182801bae.
9. Rehman L, Ghani E, Hussain A, Shah A, Noman MA, Khaleeq-Uz-Zaman. Infection in compound depressed fracture of the skull. J Coll Physicians Surg Pak. 2007;17(3):140–3.
10. Tseng W-C, Shih H-M, Su Y-C, Chen H-W, Hsiao K-Y, Chen I-C. The association between skull bone fractures and outcomes in patients with severe traumatic brain injury. J Trauma. 2011;71(6):1611–4. https://doi.org/10.1097/TA.0b013e31823a8a60; discussion 1614.
11. Ratilal BO, Costa J, Sampaio C, Pappamikail L. Antibiotic prophylaxis for preventing meningitis in patients with basilar skull fractures. Cochrane Database Syst Rev. 2011;8:CD004884. https://doi.org/10.1002/14651858.CD004884.pub3.
12. Dagi TF, Meyer FB, Poletti CA. The incidence and prevention of meningitis after basilar skull fracture. Am J Emerg Med. 1983;1:295–8.
13. Resnick DK, Subach BR, Marion DW. The significance of carotid canal involvement in basilar cranial fracture. Neurosurgery. 1997;40(6):1177–81. https://doi.org/10.1097/00006123-199706000-00012.
14. Bullock MR, Chesnut R, Ghajar J, Gordon D, Hartl R, Newell DW, Servadei F, Walters BC, Wilberger JE. Surgical management of acute epidural hematomas. Neurosurgery. 2006c;58(3 Suppl):S7–15; discussion Si-iv.
15. Bales JW, Bonow RH, Buckley RT, Barber J, Temkin N, Chesnut RM. Primary external ventricular drainage catheter versus intraparenchymal ICP monitoring: outcome analysis. Neurocrit Care. 2019;31(1):11–21. https://doi.org/10.1007/s12028-019-00712-9.
16. Beynon C, Hertle DN, Unterberg AW, Sakowitz OW. Clinical review: traumatic brain injury in patients receiving antiplatelet medication. Crit Care. 2012;16(4):228. https://doi.org/10.1186/cc11292.
17. Bricolo AP, Pasut LM. Extradural hematoma: toward zero mortality. A prospective study. Neurosurgery. 1984;14(1):8–12. https://doi.org/10.1227/00006123-198401000-00003.
18. Cucciniello B, Martellotta N, Nigro D, Citro E. Conservative management of extradural haematomas. Acta Neurochir. 1993;120(1–2):47–52. https://doi.org/10.1007/BF02001469.
19. Hamilton M, Wallace C. Nonoperative management of acute epidural hematoma diagnosed by CT: the neuroradiologist's role. AJNR Am J Neuroradiol. 1992;13(3):852–3.
20. Khaled CN, Raihan MZ, Chowdhury FH, Ashadullah ATM, Sarkar MH, Hossain SS. Surgical management of traumatic extradural haematoma: experiences with 610 patients and prospective analysis. Indian J Neurotrauma. 2008;5(2):75–9. https://doi.org/10.1016/S0973-0508(08)80004-4.
21. Seelig JM, Becker DP, Miller JD, Greenberg RP, Ward JD, Choi SC. Traumatic acute subdural hematoma: major mortality reduction in comatose patients treated within four hours. N Engl J Med. 1981;304(25):1511–8. https://doi.org/10.1056/NEJM198106183042503.
22. Bullock MR, Chesnut RM, Ghajar J, Gordon DS, Hartl R, Newell DW, Servadei F, Walters BC, Wilberger JE. Surgical management of acute subdural hematomas. Neurosurgery. 2006d;58(3 Suppl):S16–24; discussion Si-iv, 58, S2-16.
23. Kolias AG, Li LM, Guilfoyle MR, Timofeev I, Corteen EA, Pickard JD, Kirkpatrick PJ, Menon DK, Hutchinson PJ. Decompressive craniectomy for acute subdural hematomas: time for a randomized trial. Acta Neurochir. 2013;155(1):187–8. https://doi.org/10.1007/s00701-012-1531-x.
24. Stubbs DJ, Vivian ME, Davies BM, Ercole A, Burnstein R, Joannides AJ. Incidence of chronic subdural haematoma: a single-centre exploration of the effects of an ageing population with a review of the literature. Acta Neurochir. 2021;163(9):2629–37. https://doi.org/10.1007/s00701-021-04879-z.
25. Kolias AG, Chari A, Santarius T, Hutchinson PJ. Chronic subdural haematoma: modern management and emerging therapies. Nat Rev Neurol. 2014;10(10):570–8. https://doi.org/10.1038/nrneurol.2014.163.
26. Hutchinson PJ, Edlmann E, Bulters D, Zolnourian A, Holton P, Suttner N, Agyemang K, Thomson S, Anderson IA, Al-Tamimi YZ, Henderson D, Whitfield PC, Gherle M, Brennan

PM, Allison A, Thelin EP, Tarantino S, Pantaleo B, Caldwell K, Kolias AG. Trial of dexamethasone for chronic subdural hematoma. N Engl J Med. 2020;383(27):2616–27. https://doi.org/10.1056/NEJMoa2020473.

27. Ironside N, Nguyen C, Do Q, Ugiliweneza B, Chen C-J, Sieg EP, James RF, Ding D. Middle meningeal artery embolization for chronic subdural hematoma: a systematic review and meta-analysis. J Neurointerv Surg. 2021;13(10):951–7. https://doi.org/10.1136/neurintsurg-2021-017352.
28. Jiang R, Zhao S, Wang R, Feng H, Zhang J, Li X, Mao Y, Yuan X, Fei Z, Zhao Y, Yu X, Poon WS, Zhu X, Liu N, Kang D, Sun T, Jiao B, Liu X, Yu R, Zhang J. Safety and efficacy of atorvastatin for chronic subdural hematoma in Chinese patients: a randomized ClinicalTrial. JAMA Neurol. 2018;75(11):1338–46. https://doi.org/10.1001/jamaneurol.2018.2030.
29. El-Kadi H, Miele VJ, Kaufman HH. Prognosis of chronic subdural hematomas. Neurosurg Clin N Am. 2000;11(3):553–67.
30. Machulda MM, Haut MW. Clinical features of chronic subdural hematoma: neuropsychiatric and neuropsychologic changes in patients with chronic subdural hematoma. Neurosurg Clin N Am. 2000;11(3):473–7.
31. Bullock MR, Chesnut R, Ghajar J, Gordon D, Hartl R, Newell DW, Servadei F, Walters BC, Wilberger JE. Guidelines for the surgical management of traumatic brain injury author group: acknowledgments. Neurosurgery. 2006b;58(3):S2–vi; https://journals.lww.com/neurosurgery/Fulltext/2006/03001/Guidelines_for_the_Surgical_Management_of.6.aspx.
32. Gudeman SK, Kishore PR, Miller JD, Girevendulis AK, Lipper MH, Becker DP. The genesis and significance of delayed traumatic intracerebral hematoma. Neurosurgery. 1979;5(3):309–13.
33. Kaufman HH, Moake JL, Olson JD, Miner ME, duCret RP, Pruessner JL, Gildenberg PL. Delayed and recurrent intracranial hematomas related to disseminated intravascular clotting and fibrinolysis in head injury. Neurosurgery. 1980;7(5):445–9. https://doi.org/10.1227/00006123-198011000-00003.
34. Young HA, Gleave JR, Schmidek HH, Gregory S. Delayed traumatic intracerebral hematoma: report of 15 cases operatively treated. Neurosurgery. 1984;14(1):22–5. https://doi.org/10.1227/00006123-198401000-00006.
35. Chesnut RM, Temkin N, Carney N, Dikmen S, Rondina C, Videtta W, Petroni G, Lujan S, Pridgeon J, Barber J, Machamer J, Chaddock K, Celix JM, Cherner M, Hendrix T. A trial of intracranial-pressure monitoring in traumatic brain injury. N Engl J Med. 2012;367(26):2471–81. https://doi.org/10.1056/NEJMoa1207363.
36. Robba C, Graziano F, Rebora P, Elli F, Giussani C, Oddo M, Meyfroidt G, Helbok R, Taccone FS, Prisco L, Vincent J-L, Suarez JI, Stocchetti N, Citerio G. Intracranial pressure monitoring in patients with acute brain injury in the intensive care unit (SYNAPSE-ICU): an international, prospective observational cohort study. Lancet Neurol. 2021;20(7):548–58. https://doi.org/10.1016/S1474-4422(21)00138-1.
37. Carney N, Totten AM, O'Reilly C, Ullman JS, Hawryluk GWJ, Bell MJ, Bratton SL, Chesnut R, Harris OA, Kissoon N, Rubiano AM, Shutter L, Tasker RC, Vavilala MS, Wilberger J, Wright DW, Ghajar J. Guidelines for the management of severe traumatic brain injury, fourth edition. Neurosurgery. 2017;80(1):6–15. https://doi.org/10.1227/NEU.0000000000001432.
38. Cooper PR, Rovit RL, Ransohoff J. Hemicraniectomy in the treatment of acute subdural hematoma: a re-appraisal. Surg Neurol. 1976;5(1):25–8.
39. Gaab MR, Rittierodt M, Lorenz M, Heissler HE. Traumatic brain swelling and operative decompression: a prospective investigation. Acta Neurochir Suppl. 1990;51:326–8. https://doi.org/10.1007/978-3-7091-9115-6_110.
40. Guerra WK, Gaab MR, Dietz H, Mueller JU, Piek J, Fritsch MJ. Surgical decompression for traumatic brain swelling: indications and results. J Neurosurg. 1999;90(2):187–96. https://doi.org/10.3171/jns.1999.90.2.0187.
41. Hutchinson PJ, Menon DK, Kirkpatrick PJ. Decompressive craniectomy in traumatic brain injury—time for randomised trials? In: Acta neurochirurgica, Vol 147, Issue 1; 2005. p. 1–3. https://doi.org/10.1007/s00701-004-0400-7.

42. Cooper DJ, Rosenfeld JV, Murray L, Arabi YM, Davies AR, D'Urso P, Kossmann T, Ponsford J, Seppelt I, Reilly P, Wolfe R. Decompressive craniectomy in diffuse traumatic brain injury. N Engl J Med. 2011;364(16):1493–502. https://doi.org/10.1056/NEJMoa1102077.
43. Cooper DJ, Rosenfeld JV, Murray L, Arabi YM, Davies AR, Ponsford J, Seppelt I, Reilly P, Wiegers E, Wolfe R. Patient outcomes at twelve months after early decompressive craniectomy for diffuse traumatic brain injury in the randomized DECRA clinical trial. J Neurotrauma. 2020;37(5):810–6. https://doi.org/10.1089/neu.2019.6869.
44. Hutchinson PJ, Kolias AG, Timofeev IS, Corteen EA, Czosnyka M, Timothy J, Anderson I, Bulters DO, Belli A, Eynon CA, Wadley J, Mendelow AD, Mitchell PM, Wilson MH, Critchley G, Sahuquillo J, Unterberg A, Servadei F, Teasdale GM, Kirkpatrick PJ. Trial of decompressive craniectomy for traumatic intracranial hypertension. N Engl J Med. 2016;375(12):1119–30. https://doi.org/10.1056/NEJMoa1605215.
45. Hawryluk GWJ, Rubiano AM, Totten AM, O'Reilly C, Ullman JS, Bratton SL, Chesnut R, Harris OA, Kissoon N, Shutter L, Tasker RC, Vavilala MS, Wilberger J, Wright DW, Lumba-Brown A, Ghajar J. Guidelines for the management of severe traumatic brain injury: 2020 update of the decompressive craniectomy recommendations. Neurosurgery. 2020;87(3):427–34. https://doi.org/10.1093/neuros/nyaa278.
46. Halani SH, Chu JK, Malcolm JG, Rindler RS, Allen JW, Grossberg JA, Pradilla G, Ahmad FU. Effects of cranioplasty on cerebral blood flow following decompressive craniectomy: a systematic review of the literature. Neurosurgery. 2017;81(2):204–16. https://doi.org/10.1093/neuros/nyx054.
47. Ozoner B. Cranioplasty following severe traumatic brain injury: role in neurorecovery. Curr Neurol Neurosci Rep. 2021;21(11):62. https://doi.org/10.1007/s11910-021-01147-6.
48. Nasi D, Gladi M, Di Rienzo A, di Somma L, Moriconi E, Iacoangeli M, Dobran M. Risk factors for post-traumatic hydrocephalus following decompressive craniectomy. Acta Neurochir. 2018;160(9):1691–8. https://doi.org/10.1007/s00701-018-3639-0.
49. Rufus P, Moorthy RK, Joseph M, Rajshekhar V. Post traumatic hydrocephalus: incidence, pathophysiology and outcomes. Neurol India. 2021;69(Supplement):S420–8. https://doi.org/10.4103/0028-3886.332264.
50. Chen H, Yuan F, Chen S-W, Guo Y, Wang G, Deng Z-F, Tian H-L. Predicting posttraumatic hydrocephalus: derivation and validation of a risk scoring system based on clinical characteristics. Metab Brain Dis. 2017;32(5):1427–35. https://doi.org/10.1007/s11011-017-0008-2.
51. Mazzini L, Campini R, Angelino E, Rognone F, Pastore I, Oliveri G. Posttraumatic hydrocephalus: a clinical, neuroradiologic, and neuropsychologic assessment of long-term outcome. Arch Phys Med Rehabil. 2003;84(11):1637–41. https://doi.org/10.1053/s0003-9993(03)00314-9.
52. Kaen A, Jimenez-Roldan L, Alday R, Gomez PA, Lagares A, Alén JF, Lobato RD. Interhemispheric hygroma after decompressive craniectomy: does it predict posttraumatic hydrocephalus?: clinical article. J Neurosurg. 2010;113(6):1287–93. https://doi.org/10.3171/2010.4.JNS10132.
53. Heo J, Park SQ, Cho SJ, Chang JC, Park HK. Evaluation of simultaneous cranioplasty and ventriculoperitoneal shunt procedures. J Neurosurg. 2014;121(2):313–8. https://doi.org/10.3171/2014.2.JNS131480; Epub 2014 Mar 21.
54. Mustroph CM, Malcolm JG, Rindler RS, Chu JK, Grossberg JA, Pradilla G, Ahmad FU. Cranioplasty infection and resorption are associated with the presence of a ventriculoperitoneal shunt: a systematic review and meta-analysis. World Neurosurg. 2017;103:686–93. https://doi.org/10.1016/j.wneu.2017.04.066; Epub 2017 Apr 19.
55. Rasmussen MS, Andelic N, Pripp AH, Nordenmark TH, Soberg HL. The effectiveness of a family-centred intervention after traumatic brain injury: a pragmatic randomised controlled trial. Clin Rehabil. 2021;35(10):1428–41. https://doi.org/10.1177/02692155211010369.

56. van Essen TA, Lingsma HF, Pisică D, Singh RD, Volovici V, den Boogert HF, Younsi A, Peppel LD, Heijenbrok-Kal MH, Ribbers GM, Walchenbach R, Menon DK, Hutchinson P, Depreitere B, Steyerberg EW, Maas AIR, de Ruiter GCW, Peul WC. Surgery versus conservative treatment for traumatic acute subdural haematoma: a prospective, multicentre, observational, comparative effectiveness study. Lancet Neurol. 2022;21(7):620–31. https://doi.org/10.1016/S1474-4422(22)00166-1.

22 Multiple Trauma Management: Treatment of Abdominal Injury in Combination with Trauma Brain Injury

Matthew Bartek, Kristin Sonderman, and Ali Salim

22.1 Statement of the Problem

Trauma care is characterized by the need to make impactful decisions under conditions of uncertainty with time limitations. Nowhere is this more apparent than with a patient that presents with polytrauma involving head and abdominal injuries where diagnosis, prioritization, and treatment must all occur concurrently. In the management of traumatic brain injuries, the goal is avoidance of secondary injury from ischemia caused either by hypotension, hemorrhage, or hypoxia.

Intra-abdominal bleeding is the most common cause of death in the trauma patient. For patients with traumatic brain injury, a combination of hemorrhage and intracranial hypertension most often leads to demise [1]. When both injuries are suspected, diagnosing and prioritizing the management of each problem are challenging and depend on a number of factors including: the hemodynamic stability of the patient, the appropriateness of cross sectional imaging, clinical presentation, availability of clinical resources, and prognostication. Reducing the time to laparotomy and craniotomy improves survival and so proper triage, diagnosis, and prioritization becoming even more important in this group of patients [2].

M. Bartek (✉)
Division of Trauma, Emergency Surgery, and Surgical Critical Care and Division of Palliative Care and Geriatrics, Massachusetts General Hospital, Boston, MA, USA
e-mail: mbartek@mgb.org

K. Sonderman
Surgery, Harvard Medical School, Division of Trauma, Burn, and Surgical Critical Care, Brigham and Women's Hospital, Boston, MA, USA
e-mail: ksonderman@bwh.harvard.edu

A. Salim
Surgery, Harvard Medical School, Division Chief, Trauma, Burn and Surgical Critical Care, Brigham and Women's Hospital, Boston, MA, USA
e-mail: asalim1@bwh.harvard.edu

E. Brogi et al. (eds.), *Traumatic Brain Injury*, Hot Topics in Acute Care Surgery and Trauma, https://doi.org/10.1007/978-3-031-50117-3_22

The clinical questions that face the trauma surgeon when presented with a patient suffering polytrauma to the head and abdomen include:

1. What is the correct diagnostic workup, based on the patient's clinical condition? Notably, is the patient hemodynamically stable enough for cross sectional imaging?
2. What is the right operative plan in order to appropriately address the suspicion of both abdominal and head injury?
3. How can secondary traumatic brain injury be avoided?

22.2 Epidemiology and Burden of Disease

In the USA, injury accounts for approximately 280,000 deaths, amounting to an incidence of 85 per 100,000 per year. The pattern of injury is changing with the aging population, with motor vehicle collisions giving way to falls as the causative factor [3].

Historically, traumatic brain injury (TBI) accounted for 60% of all trauma-related deaths, though more recent analyses place this proportion lower at 30% [4, 5]. In the USA, TBI accounts for approximately 280,000 hospitalizations and 53,000 deaths, though these estimates do not account for military injuries nor those who did not seek medical attention [6]. This amounts to an age-standardized incidence of 333 per 100,000 per year [7]. However, simple mortality and hospitalization statistics do not tell the whole story; morbidity including the need for rehabilitation, the burden on caregivers, and long-term changes to function all contribute to the burden of disease. Some estimates place a prevalence of those living with TBI-related disability at five million, approximately 1.5% of the US population [6, 7].

Few studies report on the impact of combined traumatic brain injury and polytrauma in particular. Jakob et al. recently queried the National Trauma Data Bank, noting that over a 10-year period, 25,585 patients were noted to have severe head and abdominal blunt trauma, representing approximately 10% of those patients with severe abdominal trauma [1].

22.3 Classification of Injury

The Glasgow coma scale is the most widely used classification scheme for traumatic brain injury. It has the benefit of relying only on clinical data that can quickly be calculated in the field or trauma bay. In addition to this, the abbreviated injury scale (AIS) score for the head is used once the full extent of injuries are known and ranges from "1" to "6" [6, 8]. Head injury can be classified as severe, moderate, and mild based on GCS: Severe TBI is defined as having a GCS ≤ 8, moderate is defined as having a GCS 9–11, and mild is defined as having a GCS ≥ 12. The limitations are in assessing patients that are intubated, sedated, or intoxicated.

Abdominal injuries can be classified based on the organ injured and the degree to which it is injured, with each organ system having its own rating scheme. Other anatomic injury classification schemes include the injury severity score (ISS) which summarizes multiple anatomic injuries in one patient across six anatomic regions, the revised trauma score (RTS) which incorporates the GCS with systolic blood pressure and respiratory rate, and the trauma-related injury severity score (TRISS) which combines anatomic and physiologic scores [9].

22.4 Pathophysiology and the Interaction Between Head and Abdominal Injury

Primary injury to the brain occurs from mechanical forces causing direct damage to brain tissue at the time of the injury [4]. This initial injury to the brain can lead to derangements in autoregulation of cerebral blood flow that can lead to further brain injury. With polytrauma, systemic hemodynamic changes can further lead to secondary injury.

Secondary brain injury is mediated by a variety of mechanisms that take place over the course of hours to days after the initial insult including: electrolyte imbalances, inflammatory responses, ischemia from vasospasm or vascular injury, and/or free-radical injury to cell membranes. The downstream effect is neuronal cell death and increased intracranial pressure. Mitigating secondary brain injury in the clinical setting means avoiding secondary brain insults including hypotension, hypoxemia, elevated intracranial pressure, maintaining cerebral perfusion pressure, and avoiding hyperglycemia [4, 10].

22.5 Management

The foundation of the management of complex trauma patients such as those with suspected combined head and abdominal injury is the same as that for any trauma patient: beginning with A, B, C—airway, breathing, and circulation, as spelled out by the Advanced Trauma and Life Support (ATLS) principles [11]. After obtaining a secure airway and evaluating for chest trauma requiring intervention, the trauma team must determine whether active hemorrhage is present and if so, how it should be managed. This is outlined below in the section titled "Is it safe to obtain cross sectional imaging." Once a decision is made to pursue operative intervention, the team must decide upon the resources and teams which must be available. This is further detailed below in the section titled "What is the right procedure?".

Few studies have directly investigated management strategies for patients who have suffered both head injury and polytrauma thus guidelines rely largely on expert opinion. In 2019, the World Society of Emergency Surgeons (WSES) assembled an international conference to establish guidelines for the management of severe adult TBI polytrauma patients in the first 24 h after injury [12]. Despite varying practice patterns, the group established 16 clinical recommendations which obtained a high-level of agreement among participants. These are included below in Table 22.1.

Table 22.1 Summary of consensus conference recommendations [2]

Number	Recommendation	Agreement (%)
1	All exsanguinating patients (life-threatening hemorrhage) require immediate intervention (surgery and/or interventional radiology) for bleeding control	100
2	Patients without life-threatening hemorrhage or following measures to obtain bleeding control (in case of life-threatening hemorrhage) require urgent neurological evaluation [pupils + Glasgow coma scale motor score (if feasible), and brain computed tomography (CT) scan] to determine the severity of brain damage (life-threatening or not)	100
3	After control of life-threatening hemorrhage is established, all salvageable patients with life-threatening brain lesions require urgent neurosurgical consultation and intervention	100
4	Patients (without or after control of life-threatening hemorrhage) at risk for intracranial hypertension (IH)[a] (without a life-threatening intracranial mass lesion or after emergency neurosurgery) require intracranial pressure (ICP) monitoring regardless of the need of emergency extra-cranial surgery (EES) [16, 17]	97.5
5	We recommend maintaining systolic blood pressure (SBP) > 100 mmHg or mean arterial pressure (MAP) > 80 mmHg during interventions for life-threatening hemorrhage or emergency neurosurgery. In cases of difficult intraoperative bleeding control, lower value may be tolerated for the shortest possible time	82.5
6	We recommend red blood cell (RBC) transfusion for hemoglobin (Hb) level < 7 g/dL during interventions for life-threatening hemorrhage or emergency neurosurgery. Higher threshold for RBC transfusions may be used in patients "at risk" (i.e., the elderly and/or patients with limited cardiovascular reserve due to pre-existing heart disease)	97.5
7	We recommend maintaining an arterial partial pressure of oxygen (PaO_2) level between 60 and 100 mmHg during interventions for life-threatening hemorrhage or emergency neurosurgery	95
8	We recommend maintaining an arterial partial pressure of carbon dioxide ($PaCO_2$) level between 35 and 40 mmHg during interventions for life-threatening hemorrhage or emergency neurosurgery	97.5
9	In cases of cerebral herniation, awaiting or during emergency neurosurgery, we recommend the use of osmotherapy and/or hypocapnia (temporarily)	90
10	In cases requiring intervention for life-threatening systemic hemorrhage, we recommend, at a minimum, the maintenance of a platelet (PLT) count >50.000/mm^3. In cases requiring emergency neurosurgery (including ICP probe insertion), a higher value is advisable	100
11	We recommend maintaining a prothrombin time (PT)/activated partial thromboplastin time (aPTT) value of <1.5 normal control during interventions for life-threatening hemorrhage or emergency neurosurgery (including ICP probe insertion)	92.5
12	We recommend, if available, that point-of-care (POC) tests [e.g., thromboelastography (TEG) and rotational thromboelastometry ROTEM] be utilized to assess and optimize coagulation function during interventions for life-threatening hemorrhage or emergency neurosurgery (including ICP probe insertion)	90

Table 22.1 (continued)

Number	Recommendation	Agreement (%)
13	During massive transfusion protocol initiation, we recommend the transfusion of RBCs/plasma/PLTs at a ratio of 1/1/1. Afterwards, this ratio may be modified according to laboratory values	92.5
14	We recommend maintaining a cerebral perfusion pressure (CPP) $\geq$ 60 mmHg when ICP monitoring becomes available. This value should be adjusted (individualized) based on neuromonitoring data and the cerebral autoregulation status of the individual patient	95
15	In the absence of possibilities to target the underlying pathophysiologic mechanism of IH, we recommend a stepwise approach [18], where the level of therapy, in patients with elevated ICP, is increased step by step, reserving more aggressive interventions, which are generally associated with greater risks/adverse effects, for situations when no response is observed	97.5
16	We recommend the development of protocols, in conjunction with local resources and practices, to encourage the implementation of a simultaneous multisystem surgery (SMS) [including radiologic interventional procedures] in patients requiring both intervention for life-threatening hemorrhage and emergency neurosurgery for life-threatening brain damage	100

[a]Patients in coma with radiological signs of intracranial hypertension

Of note, a key decision between Recommendation 1 and Recommendation 2 is the clinical determination of whether hemorrhage is "life-threatening" and if the patient can proceed without reasonable risk to obtain cross sectional imaging—the answer to this question relies largely on clinical judgment and is discussed further below. Many of their recommendations pertain to neurosurgical expertise and are beyond the scope of this discussion. Other specific recommendations from this paper are discussed in the corresponding subsections below.

22.6 Is It Safe to Obtain Cross Sectional Imaging?

After a patient arrives and undergoes a primary and secondary survey, the next question for the trauma team will be where the patients should proceed to next. Cross sectional imaging plays a particularly important role in the polytrauma patient: it helps identify sources of bleeding that may be best approached by interventional radiology, it can help with surgical planning, and it can diagnose the degree of head injury prior to an intervention for bleeding [13, 14]. Whether or not a patient can safely undergo CT scan, however, will largely be a clinical determination that incorporates a patient's injury pattern and physical exam, vital signs, and degree of fluid responsiveness.

Several have attempted to determine the safety of whole body CT scan in patients who present with hemodynamic abnormalities using retrospective trauma databases [14–17]. We advocate a conservative approach to scanning for two reasons: first, to avoid further deterioration in the scanner where a patient cannot receive ongoing resuscitation, and second, to mitigate the harmful effects of hypotension when head injury is suspected by addressing hemorrhage perhaps even more aggressively than if the injury was confined to the abdomen.

We categorize patients based on their initial vital signs and clinical assessment following the primary survey. Those patients who show signs of shock should be further classified based on their degree of fluid responsiveness into three groups after an initial bolus of fluid [11]:

1. Rapid responders.
2. Transient responders.
3. Non-responders.

We use this classification to assess the degree of potential hemorrhage and to plan further diagnostic studies and interventions. Transient- and non-response could signify class II shock or greater with blood loss exceeding 40% of blood volume. These patients should be evaluated in the trauma bay with careful monitoring while the surgical team plans an intervention based on the injury pattern.

22.7 What Is the Right Procedure?

Hemorrhage control remains the top priority in these polytrauma patients. In the case that there is still a diagnostic dilemma, we opt for a damage control laparotomy to assess the degree of injury, manage emergent sources of hemorrhage, and intentionally plan for a return to the operating room at a later date for definitive repair of the identified injuries. This involves, at times, leaving patients in intestinal discontinuity and placing a temporary abdominal closure so as to decrease operative time.

Among patients with combined blunt head and abdominal trauma, only a small fraction in retrospective analyses have required combined laparotomy/craniotomy procedures, ranging from 0.4–1.5% [1, 18]. Craniotomy alone is also rare in these patients, occurring 2.1–8% of the time. These data give credence to Advanced Trauma Life Support Guidelines recommending an urgent laparotomy for patients in shock with signs of intra-abdominal hemorrhage [11]. Three main clinical indicators have emerged as ways to inform the evaluation of these patients: lateralizing neurological symptoms, Glasgow coma scale, and response to fluid resuscitation.

In the 1990s, two studies examined hypotensive blunt trauma patients with suspected head injury. While in both studies the incidence of combined craniotomy and laparotomy were noted to be low, recommendations diverged: Thomason et al. examined hypotensive patients with blunt abdominal injury and, given that the rate of urgent laparotomy was 8.5 times higher than craniotomy, recommended proceeding to laparotomy with consideration to whether intracranial pressure monitoring is necessary [19]. Contrarily, Winchell et al. noted that, in hypotensive patients (defined as systolic blood pressure < 100 mmHg either in the field or in the resuscitation suite) who responded to fluid resuscitation, CT scan can be performed safely despite delaying the time to operation [20]. A more recent analysis of hypotensive patients presenting with combined blunt head and abdominal trauma noted that a GCS of 7–8 was most predictive for the need to undergo combined procedures. Moreover, they found that in hypotensive patients who require laparotomy and have a GCS score > 8, the likelihood of requiring craniotomy was very low, suggesting that laparotomy without CT evaluation is a good approach. Of note, their study was not able to evaluate whether fluid responsiveness can be used to triage patients [1].

As discussed above, a critical decision occurs often in the trauma bay of whether to obtain cross sectional imaging in the injured patient. For those patients who cannot undergo CT scan prior to operative or angiographic intervention, there are several options. Portable CT scanning products exist and allow patients to proceed directly to the operating room for hemorrhage control, while allowing for immediate subsequent neurosurgical evaluation and possible intervention [21]. Simultaneous surgery has been utilized as a damage control method in military centers and decreases the time to intervention for each injury in a polytraumatized patient [2, 22]. Single institution reports of hybrid rooms with angiography, trauma resuscitation, and operating capabilities have advocated for greater adoption across trauma centers, though the proportion of trauma patients who would truly benefit from these combined abilities is notably small [23, 24].

In summary, while large-scale data are lacking, when faced with the inability to perform a CT scan of the head due to hemodynamic instability, obtaining early neurosurgical involvement and joint decision-making on timing of imaging verses combined neurosurgical intervention without imaging requires a prompt multidisciplinary discussion. This is especially important when the GCS score is 7–8 and/or the patient has lateralizing symptoms indicative of a significant head injury that may necessitate neurosurgical intervention.

22.8 Resuscitative and Clinical Goals Post-Procedure

The resuscitative and hemodynamic goals post-procedure are driven by the presence of a traumatic brain injury and are addressed in detail elsewhere. Of note, these thresholds are far more stringent that would otherwise be the case given abdominal injury alone. Below is a summary of consensus guidelines:

- Red Blood Cell transfusion threshold: Hemoglobin (Hg) threshold of ≥7 g/dL with higher thresholds for patients who are "at risk" including elderly or those with pre-existing heart disease [2]. This recommendation maintains that bleeding itself has been adequately controlled and if not, blood should be transfused at a more liberal Hg level.
- Oxygenation: Maintain normoxia (PaO_2 60–100 mmHg) and normocapnia ($PaCO_2$ 35–45 mmHg) while avoiding hyperventilation and major hypoxia, especially in the first 24 h after injury [2, 26].
- Platelet transfusion threshold: Maintain platelet count >50,000/mm^3 and higher if emergency neurosurgical intervention was performed (including the placement of an intracranial pressure monitor device) [2].

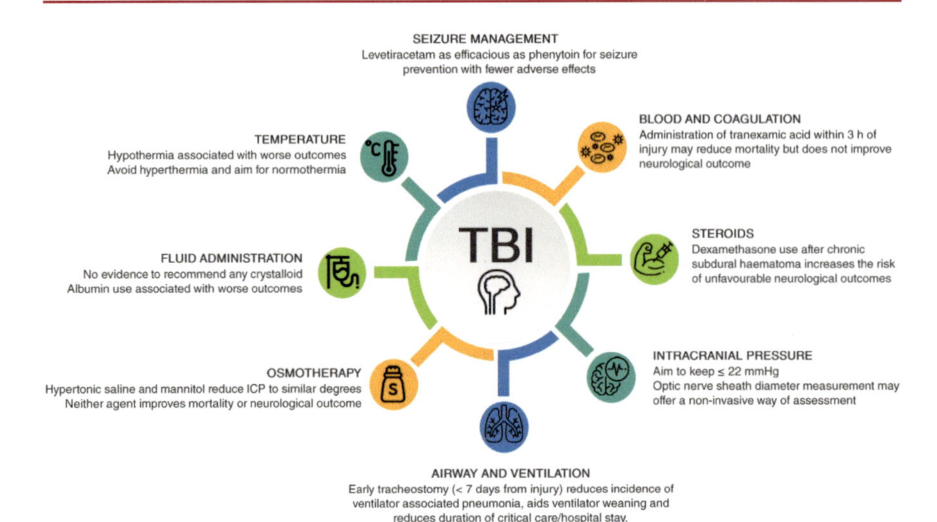

Image 22.1 Summary of recent evidence-based recommendations for the management of traumatic brain injury (TBI) [25]

- Blood Pressure: Systolic Blood Pressure (SBP) > 100 mmHg or mean arterial pressure (MAP) > 80 mmHg [2], though in the context of TBI alone, these thresholds are in fact higher with a target MAP >90 mmHg [25]. Importantly, permissive hypotension has been shown to improve survival and post-procedural cerebral oxygenation in animal models, prior to a definitive hemorrhage control operation in order to avoid further bleeding due to higher blood pressures [27] (Image 22.1).

22.9 Prognostication and Early Palliative Care

The presence of multiorgan injury should prompt other considerations outside of the immediate surgical and physiologic management of specific injuries. The American College of Surgeons Trauma Quality Improvement Program recommends that all trauma patients be screened for palliative care needs including identifying a healthcare proxy, performing a prognostication assessment, and assessing the emotional support needs of the patient and their family within the first 24 h of hospitalization and addressing Goals of Care and offering time-limited trials when appropriate during a family meeting within 72 h of hospitalization [28]. Moreover, Palliative Care—either by specialist teams or by multidisciplinary trauma teams—is indicated for patients who are at risk for functional disability and complex discharge needs, even when death is less likely [29]. There is evidence that Palliative Care consultation including the use of goals of care conversations and embracing a model of concurrent palliation and treatment in seriously-ill patients is lacking in surgical and trauma intensive care units [30–34].

It is our practice to perform primary palliative care early in the care for these polytrauma patients, giving families our "best guess" of subsequent need for intervention, prognosis, and discharge needs, while emphasizing the dynamic nature of trauma patients, especially early in their hospitalization. If the patient or family has particularly challenging social, emotional, or coping difficulties, we work closely with our trauma social worker and often consult the specialty palliative care team.

Early prognostication can aid in family discussions to assure that care plans honor what is most important to patients and their families, allowing them to gain a realistic understanding of the likely outcomes following their injury. In fact, the mortality rate from traumatic brain injury alone approaches 50% with survivors suffering debilitation from injury [35]. While many prognostic tools have been reported, none are widely accepted, perhaps owing to the difficulty to predicting functional outcomes in traumatic brain injury early in the disease course.

Several analyses and predictive tools are worth highlighting. Perel et al. developed a web-based prognostic calculator for all patients with head injury—from mild to moderate, using clinical data that are easily available to physicians [36]. Their model provides the risk of 14-day mortality and the risk of unfavorable outcome at 6 months, which they define as death, vegetative state, or severe disability and is available to use. For the prediction of mortality, especially early in the disease course, the Revised Injury Severity Classification II (RISC II) score has been shown to be best when compared to several other trauma scoring schemes [37]. The RISC II score includes several clinical factors including the AIS of the worst and second worst injuries, age, sex, pupil size, and several lab values [38].

22.10 What Are the Right Outcomes to Examine?

Traditionally, mortality has guided decision-making in polytrauma patients. However, family discussions may demand a more nuanced reflection of what patients can expect and how to proceed after initial stabilization. Understanding the right way to convey the concept of "quality of life"—from both research and clinical perspectives—is nuanced. There are no universally accepted outcome measures for patients with traumatic brain injury nor with abdominal trauma taken separately, let alone together, and so we have highlighted several that can guide decision-making [39].

The Glasgow outcome scale (GOS) attempts to capture global outcomes after TBI and consists of five categories: (1) "good recovery"; (2) "moderate disability"; (3) "severe disability"; (4) "persistent vegetative state"; (5) "dead" [40, 41]. Developed in 1975, the scoring system recognized the impact that traumatic brain injury has on mental, cognitive, and functional health. This outcome scale was expanded eight categories in 1998 as the Glasgow outcome scale extended (GOSE) and these two tools remain the cornerstone of outcome tracking for TBI. Values are obtained via interviews at various time points post-injury. Of note, many clinical trials which utilize the GOSE dichotomize the outcomes to being "favorable" and "unfavorable," the distinction of which is not standardized. This can simplify logistic modeling of the outcome, but reduces the nuances of the 8-point scale [41]. The Function Status Examination (FSE) is another measure which was developed in 2001 to evaluate changes to functional status as a result of TBI. It covers physical, social, and psychological domains, with data gathered through structured interviews. The coding for each domain is determined by these structured interviews and a branched-tree question and answer schema [42]. Dikmen et al. compared FSE and GOSE as outcome measures in TBI and found that FSE is more strongly correlated to TBI indices of severity than GOSE, concluding that the FSE may be more valuable as a functional outcome measure in TBI [43].

Other patient reported outcome measures are worth mentioning in the context of trauma [44]. In 2014, Hoffman et al. performed a systematic review of outcome measures used in studies which evaluate function and disability after major trauma to assess the degree to which the reported outcome measured captured the range of health outcomes that may be pertinent in trauma [39]. They evaluated 38 outcome measures identified in 34 studies noting that the Study Short Form Health Survey (SF-36) and European Quality of Life Questionnaire (EQ-5D) were the most used measures.

A multi-institutional project is underway to create validated patient reported outcomes (PROs) in trauma. The Functional Outcomes and Recovery after Trauma Emergencies (FORTE) project was born out of a recommendation from the National Academies of Sciences, Engineering, and Medicine (formerly the Institute of Medicine) for PRO inclusion in trauma registries with the purpose of improving trauma quality and initial work has already shown the feasibility of this approach [45]. The FORTE project collects data on employment status, residential status, quality of life, overall health status pre- and post-injury in order to track these outcomes against clinical data. Initial reporting has shown the burden of both physical pain and mental health after trauma [46].

References

1. Jakob DA, Benjamin ER, Cho J, Demetriades D. Combined head and abdominal blunt trauma in the hemodynamically unstable patient: what takes priority? J Trauma Acute Care Surg. 2021;90(1):170–6.
2. Picetti E, Rossi S, Abu-Zidan FM, Ansaloni L, Armonda R, Baiocchi GL, et al. WSES consensus conference guidelines: monitoring and management of severe adult traumatic brain injury patients with polytrauma in the first 24 hours. World J Emerg Surg. 2019;14(1):1–9.
3. Ferrah N, Cameron P, Gabbe B, Fitzgerald M, Martin K, Beck B. Trends in the nature and management of serious abdominal trauma. World J Surg. 2019;43(5):1216–25. https://doi.org/10.1007/s00268-018-04899-4.
4. El-Swaify ST, Refaat MA, Ali SH, Abdelrazek AEM, Beshay PW, Kamel M, et al. Controversies and evidence gaps in the early management of severe traumatic brain injury: back to the ABCs. Trauma Surg Acute Care Open. 2022;7(1):1–9.
5. Gennarelli TA, Champion HR, Sacco WJ, Copes WS, Alves WM. Mortality of patients with head injury and extracranial injury treated in trauma centers. J Trauma. 1989;29(9):1193–202; http://journals.lww.com/00005373-198909000-00002.
6. Centers for Disease Control and Prevention. Traumatic brain injury in the United States: epidemiology and rehabilitation. National Center for Injury Prevention and Control; Division of Unintentional Injury Prevention; 2015.

7. James SL, Bannick MS, Montjoy-Venning WC, Lucchesi LR, Dandona L, Dandona R, et al. Global, regional, and national burden of traumatic brain injury and spinal cord injury, 1990-2016: a systematic analysis for the global burden of disease study 2016. Lancet Neurol. 2019;18(1):56–87.
8. Gennarelli TA, Wodzin E. AIS 2005: a contemporary injury scale. Injury. 2006;37(12):1083–91.
9. Weiser TG. Trauma and multiple injury. In: Principles and practice of surgery. 8th ed; 2023. p. 111–25.
10. Wisler JR, Ii PRB. Multiply injured patient with brain trauma: management of competing priorities in the brain injured patient: dealing with the unexpected. 2011
11. American College of Surgeons. Committee on trauma. Advanced trauma life support, ATLS. Anaesthesia: Student Course Manual; 2018. p. 119–5.
12. Picetti E, Maier RV, Rossi S, Kirkpatrick AW, Biffl WL, Stahel PF, et al. Preserve encephalus in surgery of trauma: online survey. (P.E.S.T.O). World J Emerg Surg. 2019;14(1):1–8.
13. Salim A, Sangthong B, Martin M, Brown C, Plurad D, Demetriades D, et al. Whole body imaging in blunt multisystem trauma patients without obvious signs of injury: results of a prospective study. Arch Surg. 2006;141(5):468–75.
14. Ordoñez CA, Herrera-Escobar JP, Parra MW, Rodriguez-Ossa PA, Mejia DA, Sanchez AI, et al. Computed tomography in hemodynamically unstable severely injured blunt and penetrating trauma patients. J Trauma Acute Care Surg. 2016;80(4):597–603.
15. Ordoñez CA, Parra MW, Holguín A, García C, Guzmán-Rodríguez M, Padilla N, et al. Whole-body computed tomography is safe, effective and efficient in the severely injured hemodynamically unstable trauma patient. Colomb Med. 2020;51(4):1–8.
16. Tsutsumi Y, Fukuma S, Tsuchiya A, Ikenoue T, Yamamoto Y, Shimizu S, et al. Computed tomography during initial management and mortality among hemodynamically unstable blunt trauma patients: a nationwide retrospective cohort study. Scand J Trauma Resusc Emerg Med. 2017;25(1):1–8.
17. Huber-Wagner S, Biberthaler P, Häberle S, Wierer M, Dobritz M, Rummeny E, et al. Whole-body CT in haemodynamically unstable severely injured patients—a retrospective, multicentre study. PLoS One. 2013;8(7):e68880.
18. Wisner DH, Victor NS, Holcroft JW. Priorities in the management of multiple trauma: intracranial versus intra-abdominal injury. J Trauma. 1993;35:217–78.
19. Thomason M, Messick J, Rutledge R, Meredith W, Reeves LTR, Cunningham P, et al. Head CT scanning versus urgent exploration in the hypotensive blunt trauma patient. J Trauma. 1993;34:40–5.
20. Winchell RJ, Hoyt DB, Simons RK. Use of computed tomography of the head in the hypotensive blunt-trauma patient. Ann Emerg Med. 1995;25(6):737–42.
21. Rumboldt Z, Huda W, All JW. Review of portable CT with assessment of a dedicated head CT scanner. Am J Neuroradiol. 2009;30(9):1630–6.
22. Moore JM, Thomas PAW, Gruen RL, Chan P, Rosenfled JV. Simultaneous multisystem surgery: an important capability for the civilian trauma hospital. Clin Neurol Neurosurg. 2016;148:13–6. https://doi.org/10.1016/j.clineuro.2016.06.012.
23. Carver D, Kirkpatrick AW, D'Amours S, Hameed SM, Beveridge J, Ball CG. A prospective evaluation of the utility of a hybrid operating suite for severely injured patients: overstated or underutilized? Ann Surg. 2020;271(5):958–61.
24. Kinoshita T, Yamakawa K, Matsuda H, Yoshikawa Y, Wada D, Hamasaki T, et al. The survival benefit of a novel trauma workflow that includes immediate whole-body computed tomography, surgery, and interventional radiology, all in one trauma resuscitation room: a retrospective historical control study. Ann Surg. 2019;269(2):370–6.
25. Wiles MD. Management of traumatic brain injury: a narrative review of current evidence. Anaesthesia. 2022;77(S1):102–12.
26. Picetti E, Rosenstein I, Balogh ZJ, Catena F, Taccone FS, Fornaciari A, et al. Perioperative management of polytrauma patients with severe traumatic brain injury undergoing emergency extracranial surgery: a narrative review. J Clin Med. 2022;11(1):18.

27. Vrettos T, Poimenidi E, Athanasopoulos P, Balasis S, Karagiorgos N, Siklis T, et al. The effect of permissive hypotension in combined traumatic brain injury and blunt abdominal trauma: an experimental study in swines. Eur Rev Med Pharmacol Sci. 2016;20(4):620–30.
28. ACS TQIP palliative care best practices guidelines. 2017.
29. Fiorentino M, Hwang F, Pentakota SR, Livingston DH, Mosenthal AC. Palliative care in trauma: not just for the dying. J Trauma Acute Care Surg. 2019;87(5):1156–63.
30. O'Connell K, Maier R. Palliative care in the trauma ICU. Curr Opin Crit Care. 2016;22(6):584–90.
31. Schulz V, Novick RJ. The distinct role of palliative care in the surgical intensive care unit. Semin Cardiothorac Vasc Anesth. 2013;17(4):240–8.
32. Benjenk I, Prather C, Schockett E, Sarani B, Estroff JM. Variation in palliative care consultation among severely injured patients. J Palliat Med. 2019;22(5):474–5.
33. Lilley EJ, Lee KC, Scott JW, Krumrei NJ, Haider AH, Salim A, et al. The impact of inpatient palliative care on end-of-life care among older trauma patients who die after hospital discharge. J Trauma Acute Care Surg. 2018;85(5):992–8.
34. Ferre AC, Demario BS, Ho VP. Narrative review of palliative care in trauma and emergency general surgery. Ann Palliat Med. 2022;11(2):936–46.
35. Turgeon AF, Lauzier F, Zarychanski R, Fergusson DA, Léger C, McIntyre LA, et al. Prognostication in critically ill patients with severe traumatic brain injury: the TBI-prognosis multicentre feasibility study. BMJ Open. 2017;7(4):1–7.
36. Perel PA, Olldashi F, Muzha I, Filipi N, Lede R, Copertari P, et al. Predicting outcome after traumatic brain injury: practical prognostic models based on large cohort of international patients. BMJ. 2008;336(7641):425–9.
37. Girshausen R, Horst K, Herren C, Bläsius F, Hildebrand F, Andruszkow H. Polytrauma scoring revisited: prognostic validity and usability in daily clinical practice. Eur J Trauma Emerg Surg. 2022;0123456789:1. https://doi.org/10.1007/s00068-022-02035-5.
38. Lefering R, Huber-Wagner S, Nienaber U, Maegele M, Bouillon B. Update of the trauma risk adjustment model of the TraumaRegister DGU™: the revised injury severity classification, version II. Crit Care. 2014;18(5):1–12.
39. Hoffman K, Cole E, Playford ED, Grill E, Soberg HL, Brohi K. Health outcome after major trauma: what are we measuring? PLoS One. 2014;9(7):e103082.
40. Watanabe T, Kawai Y, Iwamura A, Maegawa N, Fukushima H, Okuchi K. Outcomes after traumatic brain injury with concomitant severe extracranial injuries. Neurol Med Chir (Tokyo). 2018;58(9):393–9.
41. Wilson L, Boase K, Nelson LD, Temkin NR, Giacino JT, Markowitz AJ, et al. A manual for the Glasgow outcome scale-extended interview. J Neurotrauma. 2021;38(17):2435–46.
42. Dikmen S, Machamer J, Miller B, Doctor J, Temkin N. Functional status examination: a new instrument for assessing outcome in traumatic brain injury. J Neurotrauma. 2001;18(2):127–40.
43. Dikmen S, Machamer J, Manley GT, Yuh EL, Nelson LD, Temkin NR. Functional status examination versus Glasgow outcome scale extended as outcome measures in traumatic brain injuries: how do they compare? J Neurotrauma. 2019;36(16):2423–9.
44. Ritschel M, Kuske S, Gnass I, Andrich S, Moschinski K, Borgmann SO, et al. Assessment of patient-reported outcomes after polytrauma—instruments and methods: a systematic review. BMJ Open. 2021;11(12):e050168.
45. Rios-Diaz AJ, Herrera-Escobar JP, Lilley EJ, Appelson JR, Gabbe B, Brasel K, et al. Routine inclusion of long-term functional and patient-reported outcomes into trauma registries: the FORTE project. J Trauma Acute Care Surg. 2017;83(1):97–104.
46. Castillo-Angeles M, Herrera-Escobar JP, Toppo A, Sanchez SE, Kaafarani HM, Salim A, et al. Patient reported outcomes 6 to 12 months after interpersonal violence: a multicenter cohort study. J Trauma Acute Care Surg. 2021;91(2):260–4.

The Brain-Abdominal Interaction

23

Wojciech Dabrowski, Chaira Robba, Neha S. Dangayach, and Manu L. N. G. Malbrain

Learning Objectives

- Understand the complex communication pathways involved in the brain–gut interaction.
- Recognize the impact of intra-abdominal pressure on brain function and neurological injuries.
- Explore the role of the nervous system in mediating brain–gut communication.
- Investigate the influence of the gut microbiome on brain function and neurological disorders.
- Examine the involvement of the immune system and hormonal communication in the brain–gut interaction.

W. Dabrowski (✉)
First Department of Anaesthesiology and Intensive Therapy Medical University of Lublin, Lublin, Poland

C. Robba
Department of Anaesthesia and Intensive Care, IRCCS Policlinico San Martino, Genoa, Italy

N. S. Dangayach
Departments of Neurosurgery and Neurology, Icahn School of Medicine at Mount Sinai, New York, NY, USA

Manu L. N. G. Malbrain
First Department of Anaesthesiology and Intensive Therapy Medical University of Lublin, Lublin, Poland

International Fluid Academy, Lovenjoel, Belgium

Medical Data Management, Medaman, Geel, Belgium

E. Brogi et al. (eds.), *Traumatic Brain Injury*, Hot Topics in Acute Care Surgery and Trauma, https://doi.org/10.1007/978-3-031-50117-3_23

23.1 Introduction

In critically ill patients with traumatic and non-traumatic systemic injuries, neuroinflammation and neurological complications frequent cause of morbidity and mortality. In fact, brain injury directly or via its association with other systemic complications, and extracerebral organ dysfunction commonly known as the brain–heart, lung or gut interactions can increase mortality [1–3]. These interactions are a complex communications mediated via neurohormonal, immunological pathways or cellular responses [4]. Interestingly, these interactions are bidirectional and brain-injury-related extracerebral organ dysfunction can worsen the primary brain injury and cause secondary brain injuries such as cerebral edema, seizures, ischemia, etc.

Traumatic brain injury (TBI) is associated with primary and secondary neurological injuries. Neurological injury in TBI occurs in two phases: an early phase, which results from a mechanical injury and a late phase which includes worsening cerebral edema, seizures, vasospasm, infarcts, etc. The initial traumatic event induces a cascade of biochemical, hormonal, and humoral activation leading to widespread organ dysfunction and secondary neurological injuries [5, 6]. Autonomic imbalance and hyperactivity seem to play a crucial role in the pathophysiology of multiorgan dysfunction after a traumatic event. Additionally, rapid increase in catecholamine release resulted from the hypothalamic-pituitary-adrenal axis activation increases vascular tone and may contribute to excessive systemic inflammation and subsequently vascular barrier dysfunction inducing or intensifying organ damage [7–10]. The intestines are particularly susceptible to such disorders, and brain–gut interactions have been well studied for more than 50 years. A decrease in splanchnic perfusion following a catecholamine surge and microbial dysbiosis are the two main mechanisms of impaired gut function after brain injury [4]. Additionally, the gastrointestinal tract has an extensive intrinsic nervous system that integrates control of intestine function with autonomic regulation separated from the central nervous system [11]. This system is termed the enteric nervous system (ENS) and it is responsible for transmitting the gut reflexes to the brain through sympathetic ganglia. Vascular barrier dysfunction leads to impaired intestinal motility and subsequently uncontrolled fluid shift to the interstitial space which further increases the risk of intra-abdominal pressure (IAP) elevation. This increase in IAP is detrimental to cerebral homeostasis and may worsen the primary and secondary neurological injuries by concomitantly increasing intracranial pressure (ICP) [12, 13].

23.1.1 The Brain–Gut Interaction: Role of IAP

IAP is the steady-state pressure within the abdominal cavity and determined by the elastic abdominal wall and viscera. A sustained or repeated elevation of IAP above 12 mmHg is defined as intra-abdominal hypertension (IAH) [14, 15].

An increase in IAP may causes organ dysfunction in the intra-abdominal and extra-abdominal compartments including the brain. Yet, the threshold at which IAP adversely affects brain function has not been determined. In an animal study, ischemic damage was observed in the CA1 hippocampal region of rats with sustained IAH at 25 mmHg [13]. The mechanisms of brain injury due to elevated IAP include a mechanical effect that impedes venous return due to elevated intra-thoracic pressure as well as impaired resorption of CSF. Increased IAP causes a cephalic displacement of the diaphragm, thereby decreasing the volume of the thoracic cavity and elevating intra-thoracic pressure. It has been found that 20–80% of IAP can be transmitted to the intra-thoracic cavity [16]. An increase in intra-thoracic pressure compresses intra-thoracic veins and then impairs cerebral venous outflow increasing intracranial pressure (ICP) and decreasing cerebral perfusion pressure (CPP) [15, 17–20]. According to the modified Monro-Kellie approach, intracranial compartments, which include brain parenchyma, cerebrospinal fluid (CSF), arterial and venous structures are interdependent and an increase in one of them can lead to a potential increase in ICP [21]. Additionally, elevated IAP compresses vertebral veins thereby impairs the absorption of cerebrospinal fluid in the sacral plexus leading to increase in ICP [20, 22]. Hence, IAH can play an important role in the brain–gut interaction, inducing or worsen brain injury (Fig. 23.1). Other organ-organ crosstalk phenomena are illustrated in Fig. 23.2.

23.1.2 The Brain–Gut Interaction: The Role of Nervous System

The brain–gut interaction consists in an information exchange between the brain and the intestine, which has been extensively studied over the last few years. Brain–gut interactions were first described in 1904 by Pavlov, who showed increased

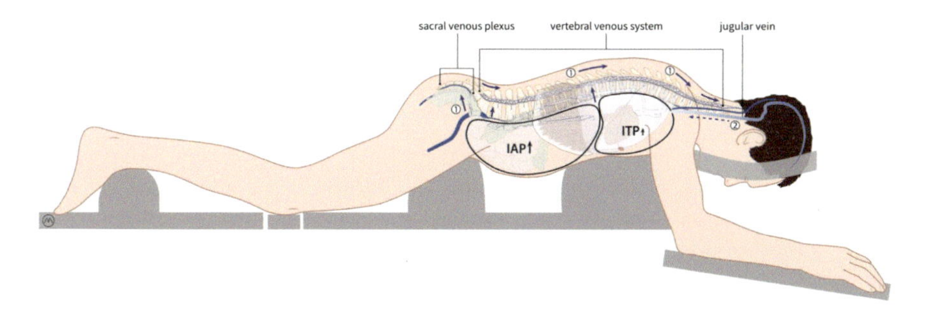

Fig. 23.1 Schematic drawing illustrating the concept of the two pathways. (Adapted with permission from Depauw et al. (Depauw PRAM, Groen RJM, Van Loon J, Peul WC, Malbrain MLNG, De Waele JJ. The significance of intra-abdominal pressure in neurosurgery and neurological diseases: a narrative review and a conceptual proposal. Acta Neurochir (Wien). 2019 May;161(5):855–864. doi: 10.1007/s00701-019-03868-7. Epub 2019 Mar 25. PMID: 30911831; PMCID: PMC6483957))In the first pathway, an increase in IAP can cause backflow through the sacral venous plexus and the vertebral venous into the spinal canal. This can cause congestion of venous blood in the spinal canal and can cause flow of venous blood into the brain. In the second pathway, an increase in IAP can cause an increase in ITP (intra-thoracic pressure) which in turn results in a back pressure on the jugular veins and decreases the drainage of the CSF and the venous blood. (Drawing made by Medical Visuals in collaboration with Dr. Paul Depauw)

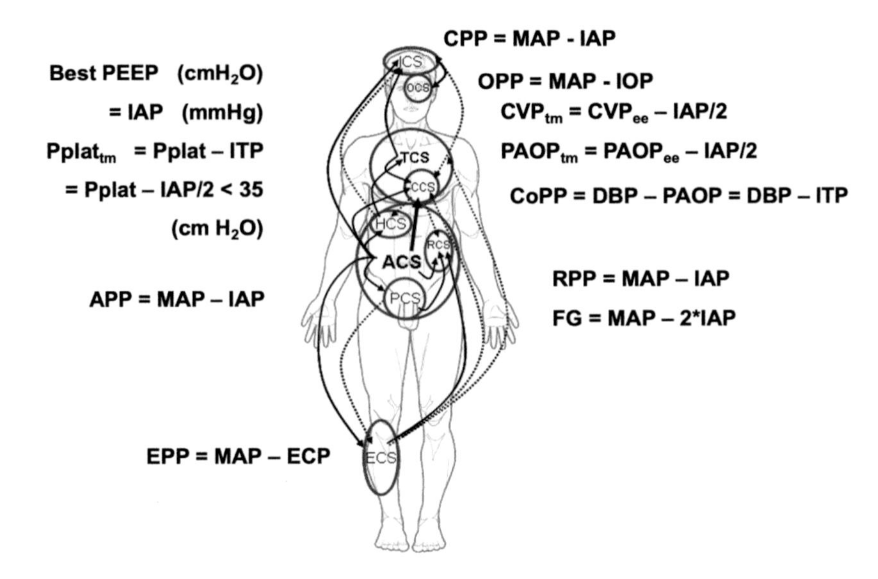

ACS: abdominal compartment syndrome
CCS: cardiac compartment syndrome
ECS: extremity compartment syndrome
HCS: hepatic compartment syndrome
ICS: intracranial compartment syndrome
RCS: renal compartment syndrome
OCS: orbital compartment syndrome
PCS: pelvic compartment syndrome
TCS: thoracic compartment syndrome

Fig. 23.2 Polycompartment syndrome and organ–organ crosstalk interactions between different compartments (adapted with permission from Malbrain ML, Roberts DJ, Sugrue M, De Keulenaer BL, Ivatury R, Pelosi P, Verbrugge F, Wise R, Mullens W. The polycompartment syndrome: a concise state-of-the-art review. Anaesthesiol Intensive Ther. 2014 Nov-Dec;46(5):433–50. doi: 10.5603/AIT.2014.0064. PMID: 25432560)The arrows indicate possible interactions between different compartmentsSolid lines show direct effects by mechanical pressure forcesDotted lines show indirect distant effects between compartments*ACS* abdominal compartment syndrome, *CCS* cardiac compartment syndrome, *ECS* extremity compartment syndrome, *HCS* hepatic compartment syndrome, *ICS* intracranial compartment syndrome, *RCS* renal compartment syndrome, *OCS* orbital compartment syndrome, *PCS* pelvic compartment syndrome, *TCS* thoracic compartment syndrome

secretion of gastric and pancreatic juices after experimental stimulation of different brain regions [23]. This interaction is bidirectional. Brain injury can have profound effects on intestinal function, and gut ENS and microflora can modulate the central nervous system, which has been was confirmed in several neurodegenerative diseases [24, 25]. The brain communicates with the gut through four main pathways: the vagus nerve, ENS, the immune system, and gut microbiome metabolism. The nervous system plays a dominant role in this communication because gastrointestinal tract is the most enervated extracranial organ in human body. The ENS is composed of enteric neurons, interneurons, and enteric glial cells distributed in the intestinal wall, which are distributed in small ganglia in all gastrointestinal tract from the upper esophagus to the anal sphincter. The ENS contains approximately 400–600 million neurons and functions independently from the central nervous system (CNS) regulating intestinal secretion and motility, and the integrity of the epithelial barrier between the gut lumen and cells, maintaining a healthy mucosal barrier [11, 26]. It also interacts with the gut endocrine and immune system influencing nutrient absorption. However, the autonomic nervous system also controls intestine function through parasympathetic innervation via the vagus nerve and sympathetic innervation via the splanchnic ganglion [27]. Interestingly, the gut microbiota can modulate the activity of the brainstem neurons, mainly in the nucleus tractus solitaries, by stimulation of intestinal vagal afferent nerves. In turn, the stimulated brainstem nerves transmit signals to the gut via efferent sympathetic nerves and celiac-superior mesenteric ganglion, which is responsible for the gut motility [28, 29]. This interaction can be responsible for functional disorders of the gastrointestinal tract in TBI patients. Clinical analysis showed important feeding intolerance in approximately 50% of patients treated for severe TBI during the first week after injury [30]. Experimental study confirmed TBI-related dysmotility showing impaired transit of intestinal contents and smooth muscle contractility between 1 and 7 days after injury [31]. Consistent with experimental findings, clinical observation showed that continuous feeding was better tolerated than bolus feeding.

Signals from the gut to the brain are also transmitted by sensory visceral afferents, which are responsible among others for modification of immune function, but can be stimulated by gut inflammation [32]. These neurons originating from the dorsal root ganglia play an important role in splanchnic circulation, intestinal secretion, and mucosal homeostasis and inflammation [33, 34]. A decrease in splanchnic circulation due to catecholamine surge following shock or TBI, further leads to sympathetic inhibition of gut motility via noradrenergic neurons in paravertebral ganglia [27, 35]. Hence, TBI-related gut dysfunction results directly from the brain injury and TBI-related ENS activation.

23.1.3 Role of Microbiome in the Brain–Gut or the Gut–Brain Interactions

The gut microbiome affects the brain function via multiple pathways, and the brain can modulate the composition of the gut microbiota [36]. This brain–gut axis is associated with the activation of autonomic nervous system, immunological system, and neuroendocrine responses to stress or injury. The gut microbiome can communicate with the ENS and the brain directly or indirectly. An activation of the autonomic nervous system and/or ENS can induce changes in the gut microbiome affecting mucus secretion and modulating gut motility [36, 37]. Additionally, both systems modulate the epithelial integrity [38]. The maintenance of epithelial permeability via ENS is multifactorial including altering the distribution of tight junction proteins, and modulation of mucin secretion, immune barrier, and electrolyte transport through intestinal epithelium [38]. It is worth highlighting that the intestinal epithelium is a semi-permeable and energy-dependent barrier restricting the movement of macromolecules, ions, and water. Therefore, every disorder that can affect adenosine triphosphate (ATP) and hypoxia increases paracellular and transcellular permeability, and commensal bacteria translocation across the epithelial layer [39]. These pathologies also favor bacterial toxins translocation, particularly *Clostridium difficile* toxin A and cholera toxins, which activate ENS to intensify intestinal motility [40]. However, direct effect of commensal bacteria on enteric neurons has not been well documented. Some probiotics such as *Lactobacillus rhamnosis*, *Lactobacillus rueteri*, or *Bacterioides fragilis* activate myenteric after-hyperpolarization neurons, which are part of ENS's afferent neurons [41, 42]. Experimental studies confirmed than ENS activity was strongly reduced in dysbiotic mice indicating that the commensal bacteria have ENS-modulating properties [43].

Some bacteria are able to produce neurotransmitters such as serotonin, noradrenaline, dopamine, acetylcholine, and histamine, that are released into the bloodstream and affect not only the ENS but also extra-abdominal organs including the brain [44]. Additionally, some of the bacterial fermentation products such as short-chain fatty acids, which may modulate the release of neuropeptides including serotonin and peptide YY. When these short-chain fatty acids are absorbed into the blood, they may also affect extra-abdominal organs and can modulate the blood–brain barrier (BBB) permeability [45, 46]. Several preclinical studies documented that a manipulation on the gut microbiome composition can improve or impair the brain plasticity affecting inter-neuronal signaling and receptor expressions [47, 48]. Experimental observation of functional properties in hippocampal microglia cells and synaptic transmission in mice receiving non-absorbable antibiotics, showed an increase in microglia density, without changes in their morphology, depression in hippocampal glutamatergic spontaneous, and evoked transmission [49]. Clinical studies also confirmed a strong relationships between the gut microbiota and neuropsychological condition. Use of antibiotics increases subcortical and frontoparietal brain connectivity improving cognitive function [50]. Importantly, disorders in the intestinal microbiota are associated with several neurological diseases such as bipolar diseases, depression, Parkinson's disease autism, and Alzheimer's disease [51–53]. Patients treated for Parkinson's disease have a significant reduction in *Prevotellaceae* and increase in *Enterobacteriaceae* species in the fecal samples [54, 55]. Experimental study confirmed that *Prevotellaceae* bacterial family affect spatial memory via hippocampal theta rhythmogenesis modulation [56]. The diversity of gut microbiome has been also been noted in patients treated for Alzheimer's disease [57]. In patients treated for major depression, an increase in *Bacterioidates* and *Proteobacteria* and decrease in *Firmicutes* in fecal samples has been described. *Firmicutes* bacteria are able to synthesize serotonin and perhaps a decrease in these bacteria may contribute to a serotonin deficiency in patients with depression [58, 59]. It was also documented that modulating the gut microbiota with probiotics containing large abundance of *Lactobacillus rhamnosus* could reduce stress- and anxiety-related behavior via afferent vagus nerve signals [60]. Taken together, it can be stated that the composition of gut microbiota plays a crucial role in the brain function, and any disorder that affects gut bacterial homeostasis may induce or intensify brain injury.

23.1.4 Immune System in the Brain–Gut Interaction

The gut is the largest immune organ in the humans and contains many immune cells including dendric cells, enterocytes, macrophages, and innate lymphoid cells. All of them can produce and release pro- and anti-inflammatory cytokines and chemokines. Additionally, commensal bacteria and their metabolites possess immunomodulatory properties [61]. The short-chain fatty acid, butyrate downregulates gut immune system and decrease abundance of bacteria producing short-chain fatty acids correspond to the severity of inflammation [62]. Experimental studies have shown that increase in bacteria producing high concentration of butyrate improve blood–brain barrier (BBB) integrity after destruction by upregulation of tight junction protein expression [63]. Inappropriate stimulation of the gut-associated immune system may intensify proinflammatory cytokine production, such as interleukin (IL) IL-1β, IL-6, tumor necrosis factor α (TNF-α) leading to BBB injury, and activation of microglia and astrocytes [64]. Additionally, the gut microbiota plays an important role in T-helper cell 17 (Th17) cell differentiation, an important class of CD4+ helper T-cells, which can infiltrate into the brain stimulating the microglial cells [65]. On the other hand, TBI-induced severe systemic inflammatory response with circulating cytokines can also impair function and act locally on cytokine receptors on vagal afferents altering the gut–brain signaling [66]. Alterations of the microbiota associated with immune depression in elderly patients can increase the risk of developing dementia and memory dysfunction [67, 68]. Numerous studies have also described an important role of toll-like receptors (TLR), which are highly present in the intestinal wall, and play a crucial role in initiating an immune response after stroke [69–71]. Interestingly, the intensity of immune activation and inflammatory response strongly correspond to severity of cognitive disorders after stroke [70–72]. Additionally, TLR2 and TLR5 are regulated by microbiota, and decrease in TLR expression can induce an inflammatory response to the microbiome [72, 73]. Disorders in microbiome are frequently correlated with progression of multiple sclerosis and correspond to severity of nerve demyelination [74]. An increase in abundance of *Faecalibacteria, Lachnospiraceae,* and *Anaerostipes, bacteria producing* butyrate can suppress central nervous system demyelination and enhance remyelination [75]. In the light of this interaction between the gut, the microbiota and the brain, and the role of gastrointestinal disorders in inflammation, there is a need to better understand how modulation of the gut microbiota may help in improving outcomes in patients with neurological disorders.

23.1.5 The Hormonal Communication Between the Brain and the Gut

Although the nervous and immunological communications between the brain and the gut are abundant, the hormonal pathway is also an important aspect of the brain–gut axis [76–78]. The intestine contains many endocrine cells that release different hormones that modulate brain–gut interaction. The hormonal response in the proximal part of intestine corresponds to feeding, whereas a response in the distal part depends on microbiota activity and composition [78]. The stomach can affect the brain function via release of stable gastric pentadecapeptide (BPC 157), which was found in the human gastric juice [79]. Several experimental studies documented a beneficial role of BPC 157 in reduction of brain edema, size of hemorrhagic post-traumatic lacerations, and intracerebral bleeding [80]. Additionally, BPC 157 can limit an experimental demyelination reducing the risk of severe encephalopathy [81]. Another endocrine cell localized in the ileum and colon can secrete peptide YY that binds to receptors expressed in the ENS, vagal afferent, and the brain [82]. The microbiome and mucosal enterochromaffin cells are the sources of serotonin. Serotonin is Dr. Jekyll and Mr. Hyde for the gut [83]. A positive property of serotonin is associated with the activation of intestinal reflexes and regulation the immune system. It also has a protective effect on neuronal and intestinal cells enhancing their regeneration. On the other hand, serotonin can induce severe gut inflammation. Serotonin plays a crucial role in the brain function. However, experimental studies have documented that the release of gut-produced serotonin to circulating blood is very low and it does not cross the BBB, which suggest this serotonin cannot modulate the brain function [84], but this should be confirmed in future studies.

The endocannabinoid system acting through cannabinoid receptors (CB1 and CB2) widely distributed in gastrointestinal tract that regulates gut motility and control intestinal inflammation [85]. In the brain, the endocannabinoid system is involved in the pathophysiology of stress and plays an important role in neurotransmission. The activation of CB1 inhibits pain perception in the gut [86]. Activation of this receptor alleviates the stress-induced brain damage including the activation of the hypothalamic-pituitary-adrenal response and anxiety [87]. Interestingly, an inhibition of CB1 increase gut motility reducing intestinal permeability, particularly for toxic metabolites and bacteria [88]. Hence, the modulation of cannabinoid receptors in the brain and gut can be promising option for therapy in patients treated for brain injury complicated by gut dysfunction. Figure 23.3 summarizes the gut–brain axis.

23.1.6 Conclusions

The brain–gut interaction is a multifaceted phenomenon with significant implications for critically ill patients. The interplay between the brain and gut involves various pathways, including intra-abdominal pressure, the nervous system, the gut microbiome, the immune system, and hormonal communication. The abdomen can

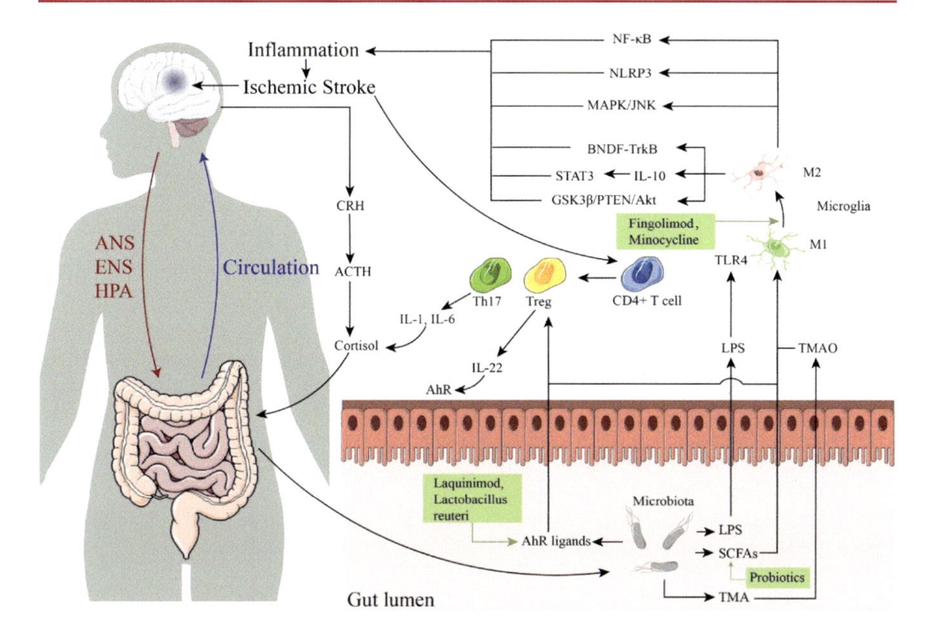

Fig. 23.3 The specific immune-related pathways in the post-ischemic stroke (IS) gut–brain axis and some drugs that targeting gut–brain axis of IS. *ANS* autonomic nervous system, *ENS* enteric nervous system, *HPA* hypothalamic-pituitary-adrenal, *CRH* corticotropin-releasing hormone, *ACTH* corticotropin-releasing hormone, *IL* interleukin, *TLR4* toll-like receptor 4, *LPS* lipopolysaccharide, *SCFAs* short-chain fatty acids, *TMA* trimethylamine, *TMAO* trimethylamine N-oxide, *NF-κB* nuclear factor kappa B, *NLRP3* NOD-like receptor thermal protein domain associated protein 3, *AhR* aryl hydrocarbon receptor. (Adapted from Zhou SY, Guo ZN, Yang Y, Qu Y, Jin H. Gut–brain axis: Mechanisms and potential therapeutic strategies for ischemic stroke through immune functions. Frontiers in Neuroscience. 2023 Jan 27;17:1081347)

impair brain function through reduction of venous outflow from cerebral circulation as an effect of increased IAP, afferent stimulation of the vagus nerve (neuronal connectivity), immune and hormonal pathways. In turn, the brain can affect the gut function through efferent stimulation, hormonal, and endocannabinoid pathways. Hence, the nervous system acts as a key mediator in transmitting signals between the brain and gut, while the gut microbiome participates in all of these pathophysiological mechanisms, playing an important role in many neurological diseases. The modulation of the gut microbiome maybe a promising therapeutical target for improving outcomes in patients with neurological injuries. Additionally, the microbiota is an integral part of the brain–gut interactions. Therefore, this axis should be termed as the brain–gut–microbiota crosstalk.

Take-Home Messages

- Intra-abdominal pressure can have detrimental effects on brain function and contribute to neurological injuries.
- The nervous system acts as a crucial communication pathway between the brain and gut.

- The gut microbiome plays a significant role in brain function and can contribute to neurological disorders.
- Dysregulation of the immune system in the gut–brain interaction leads to inflammation and cognitive impairments.
- Hormonal communication between the brain and gut influences their interaction and can be targeted for therapeutic interventions.

References

1. Battaglini D, De Rossa S, Godoy DA. Crosstalk between the nervous system and systemic organs in acute brain injury. Neurocrit Care. 2023;1:1. https://doi.org/10.1007/s12028-023-01725-1.
2. Zhao B, Li T, Fan Z, Yang Y, Shu J, Yang X, Wang X, Luo T, Tang J, Xiong D, Wu Z, Li B, Chen J, Shan Y, Tomlinson C, Zhu Z, Li Y, Stein JL, Zhu H. Heart-brain connections: phenotypic and genetic insights from magnetic resonance imagines. Science. 2023;380(6648):abn6598. https://doi.org/10.1126/science.abn6598.
3. Ziaka M, Exadaktylos A. ARDS associated acute brain injury: from the lung to the brain. Eur J Med Res. 2022;27(1):150. https://doi.org/10.1186/s40001-022-00780-2.
4. Husain-Syed F, McCullogh PA, Brik H-W, Renker M, Brocca A, Seeger W, Ronco C. Cardio-pulmonary-renal interactions. J Am Coll Cardiol. 2015;65:2433–48. https://doi.org/10.1016/j.j.
5. Lee S, Hwang H, Yamal JM, Goodman JC, Aisiku IP, Gopinath S, Robertson CS. IMPACT probability of poor outcome and plasma cytokine concentrations are associated with multiple organ dysfunction syndrome following traumatic brain injury. J Neurosurg. 2019;131(6):1931–7.
6. McDonald SJ, Sharkey JM, Sun M, Kaukas LM, Shultz SR, Turner RJ, Leonard AV, Brady RD, Corrigan F. Beyond the brain: peripheral interactions after traumatic brain injury. J Neurotrauma. 2020;37(5):770–81.
7. Kinoshita K. Traumatic brain injury: pathophysiology for neurocritical care. J Intensive Care. 2016;4:29.
8. Elder GA, Gama Sosa MA, De Gasperi R, Stone JR, Dickstein DL, Haghighi F, Hof PR, Ahlers ST. Vascular and inflammatory factors in the pathophysiology of blast-induced brain injury. Front Neurol. 2015;6:48. https://doi.org/10.3389/fneur.2015.00048.
9. Ajmo CT Jr, Collier LA, Leonardo CC, Hall AA, Green SM, Womble TA, Cuevas J, Willing AE, Pennypacker KR. Blockade of adrenoreceptors inhibits the splenic response to stroke. Exp Neurol. 2009;218(1):47–55. https://doi.org/10.1016/j.expneurol.2009.03.044.
10. Corps KN, Roth TL, McGavern DB. Inflammation and neuroprotection in tgraumatic brain injury. JAMA Neurol. 2015;72(3):355–62. https://doi.org/10.1001/jamaneurol.2014.3558.
11. Furness JB. Types of neurons in the enteric nervous system. J Auton Nerv Syst. 2000;81(1–3):87–96.
12. Depauw PRAM, Groen RJM, Van Loon J, Peul WC, Malbrain MLNG, De Waele JJ. The significance of intra-abdominal pressure in neurosurgery and neurological diseases: a narrative review and a conceptual proposal. Acta Neurochir. 2019;161(5):855–64.
13. Jarosz B, Dabrowski W, Marciniak A, Wacinski P, Rzecki Z, Kotlinska E, Pilat J. Increase in intra-abdominal pressure raises brain venous pressure, leads to brain ischaemia and decreases brain magnesium content. Magnes Res. 2012;25(2):89–98. https://doi.org/10.1684/mrh,2012.0310.
14. Kirkpatrick AW, Roberts DJ, De Waele J, Jaeschke R, Malbrain MLNG, De Keulenaer B, Duchesne J, Bjorck M, Leppaniemi A, Ejike JC, Sugrue M, Cheatham M, Ivatury R, Ball CG, Reintam Blaser A, Regli A, Balogh ZJ, D'Amours S, Debergh D, Kaplan M, Kimball E, Olvera C. Paediatric guidelines sub-committee for the world society of the abdominal compartment syndrome. Intra-abdominal hypertension and abdominal compartment syndrome: update consensus definitions and clinical practice guidelines from the world society of the abdominal compartment syndrome. Intensive Care Med. 2013;39:1190–206. https://doi.org/10.1007/s00134-013-2906-z.

15. Pereira BM. Abdominal compartment syndrome and intra-abdominal hypertension. Curr Opin Crit Care. 2019;25:688–96. https://doi.org/10.1097/MCC.0000000000000665.
16. Malbrain ML. Is it wise not to think about intraabdominal hypertension in the ICU? Curr Opin Crit Care. 2004;10:132–45.
17. Dabrowski W. Changes in intra-abdominal pressure and central venous and brain venous blood pressure in patients during extracorporeal circulation. Med Sci Monit. 2007;13(12):CR548–54.
18. Kotlinska-Hasiec E, Dabrowski W, Rzecki Z, Rybojad B, Pilat J, De Keulenaer B, Malbrain MLNG. Association between intra-abdominal pressure and jugular bulb saturation in critically ill patients. Minerva Anestesiol. 2014;80:785–95.
19. Depauw PRAM, van Eijsb F, Wensingc C, Geuzed R, van Santbrinke H, Malbrain M, De Waele JJ. The spine intra-abdominal pressure (SIAP) trial. A prospective, observational, single arm, monocentre study looking at the evolutions of the IAP prior, during and after spine surgery. J Clin Neurosci. 2023;113:93–8.
20. Deeren DH, Dits H, Malbrain MLNG. Correlation between intra-abdominal and intracranial pressure in nontraumatic brain injury. Intensive Care Med. 2005;31:1577–81. https://doi.org/10.1007/s00134-005-2802-2.
21. Josephs LG, Este-McDonald JR, Birkett DH, Hirsch EF. Diagnostic laparoscopy increases intracranial pressure. J Trauma. 1994;36:815–8.
22. De Laet I, Citerio G, Malbrain ML. The influence of intra-abdominal hypertension on the central nervous system: current insights and clinical recommendations, is it all in the head. Acta Clin Belg. 2007;62(suppl 1):89–97.
23. Wood JD. The first nobel prize for integrated system physiology: Ivan Petrovich Pavlov, 1904. Physiology (Bethesda). 2004;19:326–30. https://doi.org/10.1152/physiol.00034.2004.
24. Galgano M, Toshkezi G, Qiu X, Russell T, Chin L, Zhao LR. Traumatic brain injury current treatment strategies and future endeavors. Cell Transplant. 2017;26(7):1118–30. https://doi.org/10.1177/0963989717714102.
25. Li XJ, You XY, Wang CY, Li XL, Sheng YY, Zhuang PW, Zhang YJ. Bidirectional brain-gut-microbiota axis in increased intestinal permeability induced by central nervous system injury. CNS Neurosci Ther. 2020;26(8):783–90. https://doi.org/10.1111/cns.13401.
26. Hibberd T, Spencer NJ, Brookes S, Costa M, Yew WP. Enteric control of the sympathetic nervous system. Adv Exp Med Biol. 2022;1383:89–103. https://doi.org/10.1007/978-3-031-05843-1_9.
27. Browing KN, Travagli RA. Central nervous system control of gastrointestinal motility and secretion and modulation of gastrointestinal functions. Compr Physiol. 2014;4:1339–68.
28. Muller PA, Schneeberger M, Matheis F, Wang P, Kerner Z, Ilanges A, Pellegrino K, Del Marmol J, Castro TBR, Furuichi M, Perkins M, Han W, Rao A, Pickard AJ, Cross JR, Honda K, de Araujo I, Mucida D. Microbiota modulate sympathetic neurons via a gut-brain circuit. Nature. 2020;583:441–6.
29. Li L, Yang J, Liu T, Shi Y. Role of the gut-microbiotametabolite-brain axis in the pathogenesis of preterm brain injury. Biomed Pharmacother 2023;165:115243. https://doi.org/10.1016/j.biopha.2023.115243.
30. Rhoney DH, Parker D Jr, Formea CM, Yap C, Coplin WM. Tolerability of bolus versus continuous gastric feeding in brain-injured patients. Neurol Res. 2002;24:613–20.
31. Sun B, Hu C, Fang H, Zhu L, Gao N, Zhu J. The effects of lactobacillus acidophilus on the intestinal smooth muscle contraction through PKC/MLCK/MLC signalling pathway in TBI mouse model. PLoS One. 2015;10(6):e0128214. https://doi.org/10.1371/journal.pone.0128214.
32. Holzer P. Role of visceral afferent neurons in mucosal inflammation and defence. Curr Opin Pharmacol. 2007;7(6):563–9.
33. Evangelista S. Role of sensory neurons in restitution and healing of gastric ulcers. Curr Pharm Des. 2006;12:2977–84.
34. Agirman G, Yu KB, Hsiao EY. Signaling inflammation across the gut-brain axis. Science. 2021;374(6571):1087–92. https://doi.org/10.1126/science.abi6087.
35. Spencer NJ, Hongzhen H. Enteric nervous system: sensory transduction, neural circuits and gastrointestinal motility. Nat Rev Gastroenterol Hepatol. 2020;17(6):338–51.

36. Mayer EA, Tillisch K, Gupta A. Gut/brain axis and the microbiota. J Clin Invest. 2015;125:926–38.
37. Sharkey KA, Beck PL, McKay DM. Neuroimmunophysiology of the gut: advances and emerging concepts focusing on the epithelium. Nat Rev Gastroenterol Hepatol. 2018;15:765–83.
38. Sharkey KA, Savidge TC. Role of enteric neurotransmission in host defense and protection of gastrointestinal tract. Auton Neurosci. 2014;181:94–106.
39. Nazli A, Yang PC, Jury J, Howe K, Watson JL, Söderholm JD, Sherman PM, Perdue MH, McKay DM. Epithelia under metabolic stress perceive commensal bacteria as a threat. Am J Pathol. 2004;164:947–57.
40. Farthing MJ. Enterotoxins and the enteric nervous system—a fatal arrtaction. Int J Med Microbiol. 2000;290(4–5):491–6. https://doi.org/10.1016/S1438-4221(00)80073-9.
41. Al-Nedawi K, Mian MF, Hossain N, Karim K, Mao YK, Forsythe P, Min KK, Stanisz AM, Kunze WA, Bienenstock J. Gut commensal microvesicles reproduce parent bacterial signals to host immune and enteric nervous system. FASEB J. 2015;29:684–95.
42. Chanpong A, Borrelli O, Thapar N. The potential role of microorganisms on enteric nervous system development and disease. Biomol Ther. 2023;13(3):447. https://doi.org/10.3390/biom13030447.
43. McVey Neufeld KA, Mao YK, Bienenstock J, Foster JA, Knuze WA. The microbiome is essential for normal gut intrinsic primary afferent neuron excitability in the mouse. Neurogastroenterol Motil. 2013;25:183–e188. https://doi.org/10.1111/nno.12049.
44. Clarke SC, Stilling RM, Kennedy PJ, Stanton C, Cryan JF, Dinan TG. Minireview: gut microbiota: the neglected endocrine organ. Mol Endocrinol. 2014;28:1221–38.
45. Vijay Morris ME. Role of monocarboxylate transporters in drug delivery to the brain. Curr Pharm Das. 2014;20:1487–98.
46. Kekuda R, Manoharan P, Baseler W, Sundram U. Monocarboxylate 4 mediated butyrate transport in a rat intestinal epithelial cell line. Dig Dis Sci. 2013;58:660–7.
47. Diaz Heijtz R, Wang S, Anuar F, Qian Y, Björkholm B, Samuelsson A, Hibberd ML, Forssberg H, Pettersson S. Normal gut microbiota modulates brain development and behavior. Proc Natl Acad Sci U S A. 2011;108:3047–52.
48. Loughman A, Ponsonby AL, O'Hely M, Symeonides C, Collier F, MLK T, Carlin J, Ranganathan S, Allen K, Pezic A, Saffery R, Jacka F, Harrison LC, Sly PD, Vuillermin P, BIS Investigator Group. Gut microbiota composition during infancy and subsequent behavioural outcomes. EBioMedicine. 2020;52:102640. https://doi.org/10.1016/j.ebiom.2020.102640.
49. Cordella F, Sanchini C, Rosito M, Ferrucci L, Pediconi N, Cortese B, Guerrieri F, Pascucci GR, Antonangeli F, Peruzzi G, Giubettini M, Basilico B, Pagani F, Grimaldi A, D'Alessandro G, Limatola C, Ragozzino D, Di Angelantonio S. Antibiotisc treatment modulates microglia0synapses interaction. Cell. 2021;10(10):2648. https://doi.org/10.3390/cells10102648.
50. Ahluwalia V, Wade JB, Heuman DM, Hammeke TA, Sanyal AJ, Sterling RK, Stravitz RT, Luketic V, Siddiqui MS, Puri P, Fuchs M, Lennon MJ, Kraft KA, Gilles HC, White MB, Noble NA, Bajaj JS. Enhancement of functional connectivity, working memory and inhibitory control on multi-modal brain MR imaging with Rifaximin in cirrhosis: implications for the gut-liver-brain axis. Metab Brain Dis. 2014;29:1017–25.
51. Montagnani M, Bottalico L, Potenza MA, Charitos IA, Colella M, Santacroce L. The crosstalk between gut moscobiota and nervous system. A bidirectional interaction between miscroorganisms and metabolome. Int J Mol Sci. 2023;24(12):10322. https://doi.org/10.3390/ijms241210322.
52. Cryan JF, O'Riordan KJ, Sandhu K, Peterson V, Dinan TG. The gut microbiome in neurological disorders. Lancet Neurol. 2020;19(2):179–94. https://doi.org/10.1016/S1474-4422(19)30365-4.
53. Chen Y, Xu J, Chen Y. Regulation of neurotransmitters by gut microbiota and effects on cognition in neurological disorders. Nutrients. 2021;13(6):2099. https://doi.org/10.3390/nu13062099.
54. Scheperjans F, Aho V, Pereira PA, Koskinen K, Paulin I, Pokkonen E, Haapaniemi E, Kaakkola S, Eerola-Rautio J, Pohja M, Kinnunen E, Murros K, Auvinen P. Gut microbiota are related

to Parkinson's diseases and clinical phenotype. Mov Disord. 2015;30(3):350–8. https://doi.org/10.1002/mds.26069.
55. Unger MM, Spiegel J, Dillmann KU, Grundmann D, Philippeit H, Bürmann J, Faβbender K, Schwiertz A, Schäfer KH. Short chain fatty acids and gut microbiota differ between patients with Parkinson's disease and age-matched controls. Parkinsonism Relat Disord. 2016;32:66–72. https://doi.org/10.1016/parkreldis.2016.08.019.
56. Zhang S, Zeng L, Ma J, Xu W, Qu Y, Wang X, An X, Wang Q, Wu Y, Wang D, Chen H, Ai J. Gut *Prevotellaceae*-GABAergic septohippocampal pathway mediates spatial memory impairment in high-fat diet-fed ovariectomized mice. Neurobiol Dis. 2023;177:105993. https://doi.org/10.1016/j.nbd.2023.105993.
57. Jung JH, Kim G, Byun MS, Lee JH, Yi D, Park H, Lee DY. KBASE research group gut microbiome alterations in preclinical Alzheimer's disease. PLoS One. 2022;17(11):e0278276. https://doi.org/10.1371/journal.pone.0278276.
58. Jang H, Ling Z, Zhang Y, Mao H, Ma Z, Yin Y, Wang W, Tang W, Tan Z, Shi J, Li L, Ruan B. Altered fecal microbiota composition in patients with major depressive disorders. Brain Behav Immun. 2015;48:186–94. https://doi.org/10.1016/j.bbi.2015.03.016.
59. Sugiyama Y, Mori Y, Nara M, Kotani Y, Nagai E, Kawada H, Kitamura M, Hirano R, Shimokawa H, Nakagawa A, Minami H, Gotoh A, Sakanaka M, Iida N, Koyanagi T, Katayama T, Okamoto S, Kurihara S. Gut bacterial aromatic amine productionL aromatic acid decarboxylase and its effect on peripheral serotonine production. Gut Microbes. 2022;14(1):2128605. https://doi.org/10.1080/19490976.2022.2128605.
60. Bravo JA, Forsythe P, Chew MV, Escaravage E, Savignac HM, Dinan TG, Binenstock J, Cryan JF. Ingestion of lactobacillus strain regulates emontional behavior and central GABA receptor expression in a mouse via the vagus nerve. Proc Natl Acad Sci USA. 2011;108(38):16050–5. https://doi.org/10.1073/pnas.1102999108.
61. Gensollen T, Iyer SS, Kasper DL, Blumberg RS. How colonization by microbiota in elderly shapes the immune system. Science. 2016;352(6285):539–44. https://doi.org/10.1126/science.ssd9378.
62. Magnuson MK, Isaksson S, Ohman L. The anti-inflammatory immune regulation induced by butyrate is impaired in inflamed intestinal mucosa from patients with ulcerative colitis. Inflammation. 2020;43:507–17. https://doi.org/10.1007/s10753-019-01133-8.
63. Braniste V, Al-Asmakh M, Kowal C, Anuar F, Abbaspour A, Tóth M, Korecka A, Bakocevic N, Ng LG, Kundu P, Gulyás B, Halldin C, Hultenby K, Nilsson H, Hebert H, Volpe BT, Diamond B, Pettersson S. The gut microbiota influences blood-brain barrier permeability in mice. Sci Transl Med. 2014;6:263ra158. https://doi.org/10.1126/scitranslmed.3009759.
64. Logsdon AF, Erickson MA, Rhea EM, Salameh TS, Banks WA. Gut reactions: how the blood-brain barrier connects the microbiome and the brain. Exp Biol Med. 2018;243(2):159–65. https://doi.org/10.1177/1535370217743766.
65. Luo A, Leach ST, Barres R, Hesson LB, Grimm MC, Simar D. The microbiota and epigenetic regulation of T helper 17/regulatory T cells: in search of a balanced immune system. Front Immunol. 2017;8:417. https://doi.org/10.3389/fimmu.2017.00417.
66. Moughnyeh MM, Brawner KM, Kennedy BA, Yeramilli VA, Udayakumar N, Graham JA, Martin CA. Stress and the gut-brain axis: implications for cancer, inflammation and sepsis. J Surg Res. 2021;266:336–44. https://doi.org/10.1016/j.jss2021.02.055.
67. Sakurai K, Toshimitsu T, Okada E, Anzai S, Shiraishi I, Inamura N, Kobayashi S, Sashihara T, Hisatsune T. Effects of *Lactiplantibacillus plantarum* OLL2712 on memory function in older adults with declining memory. A randomized placebo-controlled trial. Nutrients. 2022;14(20):4300. https://doi.org/10.3390/nu14204300.
68. Saji N, Murotani K, Hisada T, Tsuduki T, Sugimoto T, Kimura A, Niida S, Toba K, Sakurai T. The relationship between the gut microbiome and mild cognitive impairment in patients without dementia: a cross-sectional study conducted in Japan. Sci Rep. 2019;9(1):19227. https://doi.org/10.1038/s41598-019-55851-y.
69. Chamorro Á, Meisel A, Planas AM, Urra X, van de Beek D, Veltkamp R. The immunology of acute stroke. Nat Rev Neurol. 2012;8:401–10. https://doi.org/10.1038/nrneurol.2012.98.

70. Bao Y, Wang L, Du C, Ji Y, Dai Y, Jiang W. Association between systemic immune inflammation index and cognitive impairment after acute ischemic stroke. Brain Sci. 2023;13(3):464. https://doi.org/10.3390/brainsci13030464.
71. Wei H, Yu C, Zhang C, Ren Y, Guo L, Wang T, Chen F, Li Y, Zhang X, Wang H, Liu J. Butyrate ameliorates chronic alcoholic central nervous damage by suppressing microglia-mediated neuroinflammation and modulating the microbiome-gut-brain axis. Biomed Pharmacother. 2023;160:114308. https://doi.org/10.1016/j.biopha.2023.114308.
72. Ye T, Youan S, Kong Y, Yang H, Wei H, Zhang Y, Jin H, Yu Q, Liu J, Chen S, Sun J. Effect of probiotic fungi against cognitive impairment in mice via regulation of the fungal microbiota-gut-brain axis. J Agric Food Chem. 2022;70(29):9026–38. https://doi.org/10.1021/acs.jafc.2c03142.
73. Sommer F, Backhed F. The gut microbiota—masters of host development and physiology. Nat Rev Microbiol. 2013;11:227–38. https://doi.org/10.1038/nrmicro2974.
74. Cantoni C, Lin Q, Dorsett Y, Ghezzi L, Liu Z, Pan Y, Chen K, Han Y, Li Z, Xiao H, Gormley M, Liu Y, Bokoliya S, Panier H, Suther C, Evans E, Deng L, Locca A, Mikesell R, Obert K, Newland P, Wu Y, Salter A, Cross AH, Tarr PI, Lovett-Racke A, Piccio L, Zhou Y. Alterations of host-gut microbiome interactions in multiple sclerosis. EBioMedicine. 2022;76:103798. https://doi.org/10.1016/j.ebiom.2021.103798.
75. Chen T, Noto D, Hoshino Y, Mizuno M, Miyake S. Butyrate suppresses demyelination and enhances remyelination. J Neuroinflammation. 2019;16:165. https://doi.org/10.1186/s12974-019-1552-y.
76. Ushiama S, Ishimaru Y, Narukawa M, Yoshioka M, Kozuka C, Watanabe N, Tsunoda M, Osakabe N, Asakura T, Masuzaki H, Abe K. Catecholamines facilitate fuel expenditure and protect against obesity via novel network of the gut-brain axis in transcriptional factor skn-1 deficient mice. EBioMedicine. 2016;8:60–71. https://doi.org/10.1016/jebiom.2016.04.031.
77. Makris AP, Karianaki M, Tsamis KI, Paschou SA. The role of the gut-brain axis in depression: endocrine, neural and immune pathways. Hormones (Athens). 2021;20(1):1–12. https://doi.org/10.1007/s42000-020-00236-4.
78. Regnier M, Van Hul M, Knauf C, Cani PD. Gut microbiome, endocrine control of gut barrier function and metabolic diseases. J Endocrinol. 2021;248(2):R67–82. https://doi.org/10.1530/JOE-20-0473.
79. Sikiric P, Seiwerth S, Brcic L, Blagaic AB, Zoricic I, Sever M, Klicek R, Radic B, Keller N, Sipos K, Jakir A, Udovicic M, Tonkic A, Turkovic B, Mise S, Anic T. Stable gastric pentadecapeptide BPC 157 in trials for inflammatory bowel disease (PL-10,PLD-116,PL 14736, Pliva, Croatia). Full and distended stomach, and vascular response. Inflammopharmacology. 2006;14:214–21. https://doi.org/10.1007/s10787-006-1531-7.
80. Tudor M, Jandric I, Marovic A, Gjurasin M, Perovic D, Radic B, Blagaic AB, Kolenc D, Brcic L, Zarkovic K, Seiwerth S, Sikiric P. Traumatic brain injury in mice and pentadecapeptide BPC 157 effect. Regul Pept. 2010;160(1–3):26–32. https://doi.org/10.1016/j.regpep.2009.11.012.
81. Sikiric P, Seiwerth S, Rucmsn R, Kolenc D, Vuletic BL, Drmic D, Grgic T, Strbe S, Zukanovic G, Crvenkovic D, Madzarac G, Rukavina I, Sucic M, Baric M, Starcevic N, Krstonijevic Z, Bencic ML, Filipcic I, Rokotov DS, Vlainic J. Brain-gut axis and pentadecapeptide BPC 157: theoretical and practical implications. Curr Neuropharmacol. 2016;14:857–65. https://doi.org/10.2174/1570159XI3666160502153022.
82. De Silva A, Salem V, Long CJ, Makwana A, Newbould RD, Rabiner EA, Ghatei ME, Bloom SR, Matthews PM, Beaver JD, Dhillo WS. The gut hormones PYY 3-36 n gut hormones and GLP-1 7-36 amide reduce food intake and modulate brain activity in appetite centers in humans. Cell Metab. 2011;14(5):700–6. https://doi.org/10.1016/j.cmet.2011.09.010.
83. Mawe G, Hoffman J. Serotonin signalling in the gut—functions, dysfunctions and therapeutic targets. Nat Rev Gastroenterol Hepatol. 2013;10(8):473–86. https://doi.org/10.1038/nrgastro.2013.105.
84. Yano JM, Yu K, Donaldson GP, Shastri GG, Ann P, Ma L, Magler CR, Ismagilov RF, Mazmanian SK, Hsiao EY. Indigenous bacteria from the gut microbiota regulate host serotonin biosynthesis. Cell. 2015;151:923.

85. Sharkey KA, Wiley JW. The role of endocannabinoid system in the brain-gut axis. Gastroenterology. 2016;151(2):252–66. https://doi.org/10.1053/j.gastro.2016.04.015.
86. Malik Z, Baik D, Schey R. The role of cannabinoids in regulation of nausea and vomiting, and visceral pain. Curr Gastroenterol Rep. 2015;17:429. https://doi.org/10.1007/s11894-015-0429-1.
87. Morena M, Patel S, Bains JS, Hill MN. Neurobiological interactions between stress and the endocannabinoid system. Neuropsychopharmacology. 2016;41:80–102. https://doi.org/10.1038/npp.2015.166.
88. Pacher P, Kunos G. Modulating the endocannabinoid system in human health and disease—successes and failures. FEBS J. 2013;280:1918–43. https://doi.org/10.1111/febs.12260.

Seizure: Prophylaxis and Treatment in Acute Brain Injury

24

Rembrandt R. VanDruff, Kyle J. Leneweaver, and Matthew J. Martin

Prophylaxis for post-traumatic seizures is a current practice to avoid the morbidity and potential secondary brain injury associated with post-traumatic seizure development. The benefits and efficacy of this strategy must be weighed against the potential harm, cost, and side effects of the anticonvulsants. In this chapter, we will review the historical background for prophylaxis, present the available randomized and non-randomized data, and suggest guidelines for therapy.

24.1 Background

24.1.1 Nomenclature, Incidence, and Risk Factors

Epilepsy may not immediately follow traumatic brain injury (TBI) [1]. Rather, neuronal remodeling lowers the seizure threshold, during a latent period of post-traumatic epileptogenesis. Sometimes this latent period may be as long as a several-week-long seizure-free interval [2]. Thus, the Brain Trauma Foundation categorizes post-traumatic seizures (PTS) into early (<7 days) and late (>7 days) after the initial insult. Post-traumatic epilepsy (PTE) is defined as recurrent seizures >7 days post-injury, and the incidence is higher after TBI than the incidence found in the general population [3]. Status epilepticus has historically held multiple definitions, initially regarded as continuous seizure activity over 30 minutes, or multiple seizures within a 30-minute period without fully regaining consciousness. In 2012,

R. R. VanDruff (✉) · M. J. Martin
LAC+USC Medical Center, Los Angeles, CA, USA
e-mail: rembrandt.vandruff@med.usc.edu; matthew.martin@med.usc.edu

K. J. Leneweaver
Ascension Medical Group, Pensacola, FL, USA
e-mail: kyle.leneweaver@ascension.org

E. Brogi et al. (eds.), *Traumatic Brain Injury*, Hot Topics in Acute Care Surgery and Trauma, https://doi.org/10.1007/978-3-031-50117-3_24

guidelines from the Neurocritical Care Society amended this definition to 5 min or more of continuous clinical and/or electrographic seizure activity or recurrent seizure activity without recovery (returning to baseline) between seizures. Evidence had emerged that merely 5 min of seizure activity could lead to permanent neuronal damage and pharmacoresistance, and generalized non-status seizures typically stop before this time [4]. It should be noted that PTS and PTE are separate entities from paroxysmal sympathetic hyperactivity (PSH) or "neuro-storming;" with continuous EEG data revealing no focal or generalized epileptiform activity during storming [5]. Of note, anticonvulsants do not treat or prevent PSH [6].

Historical data suggests that clinical seizures are observed in 2–16% of patients after brain injury [7]. Data from continuous electroencephalogram (EEG) suggests that subclinical incidence is higher, up to 30% [8]. In 1993, Stuart Yablon wrote an elegant and thorough review of the incidence and risk factors for PTS up to that point [9], reporting on data from military, civilian, pediatric, and rehabilitation settings. In military settings, reports from World War I [10], II [11], and up through the Vietnam War [12] were among the first data sets to indicate the incidence of PTS. Expectedly these reports showed penetrating head wounds to be a major risk factor. Yablon noted that "studies in civilian settings appeared later though probably are more relevant to most physicians," and identified late PTS incidence of 4–7% and early PTS incidence of around 5% in adults and 10% in children.

Annegers and colleagues at the University of Texas conducted multiple population-based studies of PTS based on a powerful data set from a single county in Minnesota that helped to define risk factors [13]. A retrospective evaluation of over 4500 patients spanned several decades with an overall incidence of 3%, and a 17% incidence in severe TBI. Multivariate analysis identified the significant risk factors for late seizures being age of 65 years or older, brain contusion with subdural hematoma (SDH), skull fracture, loss of consciousness, or amnesia for more than 1 day [14]. The study did not comment on early seizure risk factors. Yablon's review identified risk factors for seizure development including patient characteristics of chronic alcoholism, family history of epilepsy, and age (adults trended toward late PTS and children to immediate/early PTS). The injury characteristics include focal deficits, depressed skull fractures, cerebral contusions, retained bone/metal fragments, prolonged duration of post-traumatic amnesia, and intracranial hemorrhage particularly in the subdural space. Additional risk factors for early seizures from other data sets include the severity of the TBI (depressed GCS $\leq$10), epidural hematoma, immediate seizures, and linear skull fracture [15]. Early seizures are a risk factor for late seizures [16].

24.1.2 Pathophysiology

Neuronal trauma lowers seizure threshold through excitatory and inhibitory neuromessenger imbalances involving elevated cortical glutamate signaling and decreased GABA [17]. How do seizures worsen brain injury outcomes? The answer likely lies in the hallmark principle of prevention of secondary brain injury through avoidance factors that can result in inadequate oxygen delivery to the brain, such as hypotension and hypoxia. The significantly increased cerebral metabolic rate during seizure activity causes a secondary ischemic insult through increased oxygen demand and consumption [18]. The relationship of seizures, and subsequently seizure prophylaxis to neurological outcomes including mortality and meaningful neurologic recovery has been controversial, stemming from initial data that "early PTS have not been associated with worse outcomes." [19]

The notion that outcomes may not be worse even if seizure activity occurs probably stems from a 1997 single-institution prospective non-randomized study in China. Over 3300 adults with severe TBI were given anticonvulsants only if a seizure occurred. The overall incidence of early seizures was just over 3% which was consistent with the data from Annegers and associates. There was no statistical difference between brain parenchymal damage seen in patients who had early seizures and those who did not. Furthermore, patients with early seizures had a lower overall mortality rate that achieved statistical significance [20]. The authors of this paper suggested that early PTS may actually be an indication of preservation of brain function, representing relatively intact lateral corticospinal tracts, allowing the seizure activity to occur in the first place.

24.2 Randomized Studies

24.2.1 Refuting Prophylaxis

Early data did not support the use of routine seizure prophylaxis, showing no benefit of prophylactically administered phenytoin in the prevention of early PTS. In 1983, Young and colleagues randomized 244 patients with severe head injury into either a phenytoin or placebo group. They showed no significant difference in early seizures between the treated and placebo groups, as well as similar times from injury to first seizure [21]. Furthermore, the authors separately published a randomized trial following 179 patients for 18 months, with the same study design and similar results, concluding no benefit of prophylactically administered phenytoin in the prevention of late PTS. [22] In 1992, Manaka and colleagues examined delayed administration of seizure prophylaxis, and found no difference in late PTS in patients who were randomized to phenobarbital vs. placebo starting 1 month after the index TBI [23].

24.2.2 Supporting Prophylaxis

In 1990, Temkin and colleagues renewed enthusiasm for PTS prophylaxis as they conducted the earliest landmark study showing the benefit of phenytoin prophylaxis on PTS. Their group randomized 404 patients with TBI to a 1-year regimen of therapeutic phenytoin and followed patients for 2 years. Primary data analysis, according to intention-to-treat, revealed a significant change from Young's data in 1983: 3.6% of the patients assigned to phenytoin had early seizures, as compared with 14.2% of patients assigned to placebo ($p < 0.001$). Late seizures had no statistical difference [24].

Later that decade, Temkin's group aimed to find the optimal duration of therapy for seizure prophylaxis. 132 patients were assigned to a 1-week course of phenytoin, 120 were assigned to a 1-month course of valproate (VPA), and 127 were assigned to a 6-month course of valproate, with a 2-year follow-up. No benefit to valproate was shown over phenytoin in the prevention of early seizures, and neither drug prevented late seizures [25]. Furthermore, there was a statistically insignificant trend towards higher mortality in valproate arms. Thus, the standard of a 1-week duration of phenytoin supplanted the prior longer duration of therapy. Further use and study of valproate were discouraged after these findings were confirmed in 2000. In this study, 1 week of phenytoin was compared to 1-month and 6-month regimens of VPA. There was, again, a trend toward higher mortality in VPA group and no improvement in PTS prevention [26]. These studies supported the concept of a short course of seizure prophylaxis aimed at preventing early PTS and with no significant impact on the incidence or severity of late PTS.

The novel anticonvulsant levetiracetam (LEV) emerged on the market in the late 1990s and was granted FDA approval in oral form in 1999, followed by intravenous in 2006. Enthusiasm for the drug stems from its lower risk profile compared to phenytoin or fosphenytoin, especially in older patients and those with renal impairment, as well as its freedom from serum level monitoring requirements. In 2010, Szaflarski and colleagues conducted a prospective, randomized, single-blinded trial comparing intravenous LEV to intravenous phenytoin. This was a small study that enrolled 52 TBI patients with 18 in the phenytoin group. There were no differences in seizure occurrence, and the LEV arm trended towards better long-term neurologic outcomes. The authors concluded that LEV could represent a safe alternative to phenytoin for seizure prophylaxis [27]. Although this was a randomized trial, the Brain Trauma Foundation team noted issues with randomization and other parameters including sample size and allocation assignment and hence has considered it a Class 3 study [19]. More recently, a 2016 trial by Khan and colleagues randomized 154 patients with TBI to LEV versus phenytoin for 1 week. There was no difference in the overall incidence of PTS between LEV (9%) compared to phenytoin (5.2%) or in subgroup analyses based on the severity of TBI. It is important to note that there was no analysis of medication-related adverse effects or neurologic outcomes, and that the study population was relatively young (maximum age of 48 years) and included both children and adult patients [28].

24.3 Non-Randomized Studies and Additional Landmark Papers

In 1999, Haltiner and colleagues at the University of Washington studied, "side effects and mortality associated with use of phenytoin for early posttraumatic seizure prophylaxis" in their paper of the same name. The data from Temkin's 1990 trial was analyzed secondarily and found to support the safety of the phenytoin drug profile and risk/benefit ratio in a 1- or 2-week prophylactic protocol. Increased side effects occurred during the second week, and they concluded that the most favorable prophylactic protocol was 1 week of prophylaxis [29].

In 2001, Temkin performed a meta-analysis including an elegant summary of the landmark work on the subject of anti-epileptogenesis over the prior decades, looking at seizures from multiple causes including 13 clinical trials related to TBI-related seizures. The paper referenced several prospective and even randomized trials on PTE that did not come to pass due to "substantial problems with recruitment and retention" including several that "were stopped before reaching their planned sample sizes." These studies were conducted with several other well-established anticonvulsants but would not otherwise be at the forefront of knowledge as they have not been frequently referenced in the other common literature on this topic, for example, the BTF guidelines [30].

Controversy over the risk/benefit profile of PTS prophylaxis was revisited as recently as 2013 when Bhullar and colleagues completed a retrospective cohort study entitled, "More harm than good: Antiseizure prophylaxis after traumatic brain injury does not decrease seizure rates but may inhibit functional recovery." They examined 93 patients retrospectively who were divided into phenytoin prophylaxis and no prophylaxis groups and found no difference in disposition, mortality by head injury, or discharge to rehabilitation, but did find a significantly longer hospital stay and worse functional outcomes in the phenytoin prophylaxis group [31].

In 2008, Jones and colleagues at the University of Pittsburgh conducted a comparative study of 32 patients who prospectively received LEV for seizure prophylaxis and underwent spot EEG testing and then were compared to a historical cohort of 41 patients who received phenytoin. A few more subclinical seizures in the LEV group were noted but they had no difference in the outcome [32].

In 2013, Inaba and colleagues conducted a prospective, observational trial of 813 patients comparing levetiracetam to phenytoin in the prevention of early PTS. There was no difference in seizure rate, adverse drug reaction or mortality between the groups, further supporting the safe use of levetiracetam for early PTS prophylaxis with an equivalent efficacy profile compared to phenytoin [33].

A 2016 meta-analysis of the three prospective discussed here and four retrospective studies comparing LEV and phenytoin in PTS concluded patients treated with either drug have similar incidences of early seizures after TBI, with a Level III evidence grade [34]. A 2018 meta-analysis that included four randomized and 12 non-randomized studies of a mixed population of TBI and non-TBI craniotomy patients suggested a trend towards a decrease in early PTS in the LEV group and no difference in overall seizures, late seizures, or mortality [35].

24.4 Guidelines

Guidelines for prophylactic anticonvulsants tend to vary by institution and the authors will provide general suggestions here based on the practices of our institutions. Despite the presence of randomized data, the Brain Trauma Foundation (BTF)

Table 24.1 Suggested indications for seizure prophylaxis following TBI

Indications for traumatic brain injury (TBI) seizure prophylaxis
• Glasgow coma scale (GCS) score of 10 or less
• Immediate seizures
• Linear or depressed skull fracture
• Penetrating head injury
• Subdural, epidural, or intracerebral hematoma
• Cortical contusion
• Age ≥ 65 years
• Chronic alcoholism
• Acute on chronic subdural hematoma requiring neurosurgical intervention

makes no Level I recommendations on this particular topic. They provide two Level IIA recommendations, as follows: "Prophylactic use of phenytoin or valproate is not recommended for preventing late PTS. Phenytoin is recommended to decrease the incidence of early PTS (within 7 days of injury), when the overall benefit is felt to outweigh the complications associated with such treatment. However, early PTS have not been associated with worse outcomes."

The principal Trauma and Neurotrauma Professional Societies and their specific recommendations currently are as follows. The Eastern Association for the Surgery of Trauma (EAST), Western Trauma Association (WTA), the American Association of Neurological Surgeons (AANS), and the Neurocritical Care Society do not publish specific practice guidelines on the topic. The American Association for the Surgery of Trauma (AAST) makes no independent recommendations other than supporting the BTF guidelines.

At our institution, all patients with a TBI and any of the risk factors listed in Table 24.1 receive seizure prophylaxis for a seven-day duration.

24.4.1 Approaches to Prophylaxis, Small Subarachnoid and SDH in Mild TBI

Many institutions use a universal prophylaxis approach. The inclusion criteria in Table 24.1 are based on the risk factors previously mentioned and a broad definition encompassing all the criteria for starting anti-seizure prophylaxis from Temkin's 1990 data and onwards. If the patient was on an anticonvulsant prior to admission, we continue their home medication at the same dose, and levels are checked as needed.

Some institutions use a selective approach and withhold prophylaxis for mild TBIs with a positive head computed tomography (CT). Conspicuous by its absence in many institutional indications is the subarachnoid hemorrhage (SAH), which seems to derive either no benefit or the smallest benefit to PTS prophylaxis among all intracranial bleed patterns [36]. In the initial non-contrast CT head it is difficult to tell whether a trauma patient has a traumatic SAH or an aneurysmal SAH, and of course, an aneurysmal SAH may have led to the trauma and not vice versa. Most of these are followed by a CT angiogram of the head and neck. In 2007 Rosengart and colleagues at the University of Chicago compiled data from four prior randomized trials of anticonvulsant prophylaxis in aneurysmal SAH, concluding that it was associated with increased complications and worse outcomes [37]. Current guidelines from multiple neurologic and neurosurgical organizations recommend against routine administration of seizure prophylaxis in the setting of non-traumatic SAH.

Some institutions also use a selective approach that also omits prophylaxis in small SDH, i.e., <4 mm. The data supporting this are nascent. A recent prospective, multicenter study from groups at Pittsburgh and Cooper University supports this stance. A total of 490 patients with a positive head CT and GCS 13–15 were enrolled, without an observed improvement in PTS reduction in the prophylaxis group [38].

A future area of study is the investigation of which positive head scans have blood volume small enough to have a minor risk increase in seizure activity. The Marshall [39] and Rotterdam [40] classification of head CTs may help elucidate this for future researchers [41]. Joseph and colleagues have developed [42] and validated [43] the Brain Injury Guidelines (BIG) to standardize the management of traumatic brain injuries of varying severity, including the role of repeat head CT and the need for neurosurgical consultation. Unfortunately, seizure incidence and treatment were not included in the BIG schema and thus were not studied, but this categorization is promising to investigate which TBIs can safely go home without prophylaxis.

24.4.2 Treatment of Clinical Seizures and Duration of Therapy

With regard to the duration of therapy, 1 week is typical for a prophylactic strategy, as discovered in Temkin's 1999 data. There may be indications for a longer duration of therapy. If an early seizure occurs, the strategy changes from prophylactic to therapeutic. A benzodiazepine is the initial therapy of choice for convulsive status epilepticus (SE), which includes seizures lasting longer than 5 min, according to high-quality evidence supported by national guidelines from the American Epilepsy Society [44]. Current consensus guidelines recommend an initial dose of lorazepam 4 mg intravenously, although other benzodiazepines may be utilized per local protocols at individual centers.

After 20 min of SE, there is no evidence-based preferred therapy of choice. The decision is to either increase or change the existing anticonvulsant or add additional anticonvulsant agents with complementary mechanisms of action. In our institution, many scenarios exist, but we will start by checking drug levels (if applicable) and optimizing that anti-epileptic. Most patients who seize on therapeutic fosphenytoin/phenytoin will receive a bolus of levetiracetam (usually 20–60 mg/kg) and then start on scheduled levetiracetam. If already on levetiracetam but not at maximum doses, we will re-bolus and increase to 1500 mg every 12 hours. For patients with refractory or super-refractory SE, there has been an interesting and growing body of literature supporting the use of the NMDA-receptor antagonist ketamine as an effective salvage therapy. A 2014 systematic review of 23 articles found that ketamine was successful in stopping seizure activity in 56.5% of adults and 63.5% of pediatric patients with refractory or super-refractory SE [45]. The role of ketamine in preventing and treating seizures in the TBI population remains unknown but is an area of active interest given the increasing use of ketamine for pain control, procedural sedation, and anesthesia in the trauma population.

The therapeutic duration for patients who develop PTS or SE remains unclear. Our institutions continue treatment for at least three to 6 months, with Neurology colleagues following in both the inpatient and outpatient settings. There is significant heterogeneity from institution to institution with care dictated by expert opinion. Some use EEG in patients with a persistent GCS compromise despite appropriate care to evaluate for subclinical seizures, and if discovered, will increase the treatment dose of the antiepileptic or start a second antiepileptic until the EEG findings have resolved. Other duration increases may include high-risk surgical patients, i.e., those that require craniectomy, as there is retrospective data to suggest that these patients are at higher risk of seizures [46].

24.4.3 Miscellaneous: Drugs, Levels, Routes, Cost, Dosage, and Special Populations

Phenytoin, for the reasons above, has proven to be a measurable and reliable drug. It is the most studied anticonvulsant in trauma with a safety profile well-established over several decades. There are data to suggest worse cognitive effects in phenytoin subjects when compared to placebo. Dikmen and colleagues measured neurobehavioral assessments in 244 patients and found that phenytoin-receiving patients had worse scores at the 1-month mark, but no difference at 1 year [47]. This may be of particular concern in older patients who are more prone to adverse effects of anticonvulsants, hospital delirium, and drug–drug interactions. Although age is not mentioned in most guidelines on this topic, it is reasonable to have a higher threshold for the administration of seizure prophylaxis in the elderly population given the increased risk profile compared to the small potential benefit.

With regard to drug dosage, we give fosphenytoin 20 mg/kg IVPB for one dose, then start phenytoin 100 mg IV or PO q8h for a total of 7 days. The loading dose is based on the 1990s University of Washington data which used 20 mg/kg. Young's paper from 1983 observed that no seizures occurred in patients whose phenytoin plasma concentration reached 12 mcg/ml or higher [22]. All of the randomized data was conducted with intravenous loading doses of phenytoin, except for Young in 1983 which combined intravenous and intramuscular routes. At our institution, we do not obtain a steady-state level for a prophylactic strategy. We consider therapeutic ranges as 10–20mcg/ml of total phenytoin or 1–2mcg/ml free phenytoin level. An adjustment to the phenytoin level is required in patients with low albumin and thus we obtain a current albumin level. Free phenytoin levels may be useful in patients with low protein states or on hemodialysis for monitoring the treatment of TBI seizures. This is typically a send-out lab with a turnaround time of several days.

Valproate is likely no better than phenytoin, as shown in randomized data [25] as well as an underpowered retrospective study without statistical significance [48]. The BTF Guidelines of 2016 note that "at the present time there is insufficient evidence to recommend levetiracetam over phenytoin regarding efficacy in preventing early post-traumatic seizures and toxicity." In our institution, if a patient meets Table 24.1 criteria and is ≥80 years of age, is on renal replacement therapy (hemodialysis, peritoneal dialysis, or continuous renal replacement therapy), or is on medications that significantly interact with phenytoin, it is our practice to give levetiracetam 20 mg/kg IVPB for one loading dose and then initiate 7 days of maintenance levetiracetam at 500–750 mg IV or PO q12h. Other institutions use fixed-dose levetiracetam 1000 mg loading dose IVPB followed by 500 mg PO or IVPB twice daily for 7 days, and reduce doses for patients greater than 80 years of age to 500 mg IVPB load with dosing of 250 mg PO or IVPB twice daily for 7 days.

The course of phenytoin is generally less costly than the course of levetiracetam. A 2010 cost-utility analysis found that phenytoin is "more cost-effective than levetiracetam at all reasonable prices," including the cost of drawing levels [49]. However, levetiracetam has become cheaper over time since this data were published. Some institutions avoid phenytoin entirely and thus avoid the need for send-out levels and potential unknown home medication drug interactions [50].

More data is needed to draw significant conclusions among special populations with traumatic brain injury including the realms of pediatric, adolescent, pregnant, and geriatric patients.

24.5 Further Reading and Conclusion

We would like to highlight two additional resources for our readers. First, the Brain Trauma Foundation's Guidelines for the management of severe TBI (most recent publishing, fourth Edition, 2016) provides what we believe to be the most robust adjunct reference on the topic. See Chap. 11, "Seizure Prophylaxis." The authors provide excellent summaries of the available evidence: Tables 11–1, 2, and 3. Eleven relevant studies were available to review at the time of that writing, with the most recent one from the Inaba group in 2013. Since then, there have not been any additional landmark papers to change decision-making on this topic. The appendices of the BTF guidelines delineate how the authors graded their evidence and excluded some studies. Three studies were excluded from the seizure chapter (Appendix F, see pages 230–231) as they did not meet the inclusion criteria (Appendix E).

Second, a Cochrane review from 2015 provides an elegant breakdown of all the data up until the time of its publishing [51]. Kara Thompson and colleagues at Dalhousie University in Canada analyzed the literature to compare anticonvulsant and neuroprotective agents' efficacy with placebo, usual care, or other pharmacologic agents for the prevention of PTE in any severity of TBI. They concluded that there is "low-quality evidence that early treatment with an AED compared with placebo or standard care reduced the risk of early post-traumatic seizures. There was no evidence to support a reduction in the risk of late seizures or mortality. There was insufficient evidence to make any conclusions regarding the effectiveness or safety of other neuroprotective agents compared with placebo or for the comparison of phenytoin, a traditional AED, with another AED." Like many Cochrane reviews, it includes a "plain language" summary that may be helpful for sharing this treatment rationale with patients or their families.

References

1. Hameed MQ, Rotenberg A. Ceftriaxone treatment of TBI. In: Heidenreich K, editor. New therapeutics for traumatic brain injury: prevention of secondary brain damage and enhancement of repair and regeneration. 1st ed. San Diego: Elsevier Science; 2016. p. 235–49.
2. Pitkänen A, Kharatishvili I, Karhunen H, Lukasiuk K, Immonen R, Nairismägi J, et al. Epileptogenesis in experimental models. Epilepsia. 2007;48(Suppl 2):13–20.
3. Hirtz D, Thurman DJ, Gwinn-Hardy K, Mohamed M, Chaudhuri AR, Zalutsky R. How common are the "common" neurologic disorders? Neurology. 2007;68(5):326–37.
4. Brophy GM, Bell R, Claassen J, Alldredge B, Bleck TP, Glauser T, et al. Guidelines for the evaluation and management of status epilepticus. Neurocrit Care. 2012;17(1):3–23.
5. Wilson LD, Leath TC, Patel MB. Management of paroxysmal sympathetic hyperactivity after traumatic brain injury. In: Heidenreich K, editor. New therapeutics for traumatic brain injury: prevention of secondary brain damage and enhancement of repair and regeneration. 1st ed. San Diego: Elsevier Science; 2016. p. 145–58.
6. Perkes I, Baguley IJ, Nott MT, Menon DK. A review of paroxysmal sympathetic hyperactivity after acquired brain injury. Ann Neurol. 2010;68(2):126–35.
7. Frey LC. Epidemiology of posttraumatic epilepsy: a critical review. Epilepsia. 2003;44(Suppl 10):11–7.
8. Ronne-Engstrom E, Winkler T. Continuous EEG monitoring in patients with traumatic brain injury reveals a high incidence of epileptiform activity. Acta Neurol Scand. 2006;114(1):47–53.
9. Yablon SA. Posttraumatic seizures. Arch Phys Med Rehabil. 1993;74(9):983–1001.
10. Ascroft PB. Traumatic epilepsy after gunshot wounds of the head. Br Med J. 1941;1(4193):739–44.
11. Walker AE, Jablon S. A follow-up of head injured men of world war II. J Neurosurg. 1959;16:600–10.
12. Salazar AM, Jabbari B, Vance SC, Grafman J, Amin D, Dillon JD. Epilepsy after penetrating head injury. I. Clinical correlates: a report of the Vietnam head injury study. Neurology. 1985;35(10):1406–14.
13. Annegers JF, Grabow JD, Groover RV, Laws ER Jr, Elveback LR, Kurland LT. Seizures after head trauma: a population study. Neurology. 1980;30(7 Pt 1):683–9.
14. Annegers JF, Hauser WA, Coan SP, Rocca WA. A population-based study of seizures after traumatic brain injuries. N Engl J Med. 1998;338(1):20–4.
15. Temkin NR. Risk factors for posttraumatic seizures in adults. Epilepsia. 2003;44(Suppl 10):18–20.
16. Temkin NR, Dikmen SS, Winn HR. Management of head injury. Posttraumatic seizures. Neurosurg Clin N Am. 1991;2(2):425–35.
17. Hameed MQ, Rotenberg A. Ceftriaxone treatment of TBI. In: Heidenreich K, editor. New therapeutics for traumatic brain injury: prevention of secondary brain damage and enhancement of repair and regenertion. 1st ed. San Diego: Elsevier Science; 2016. p. 235–49.
18. Aisiku IP, Robertson C, Ngwenya LB. Critical care management of traumatic brain injury. In: Winn HR, editor. Youmans & Winn neurological surgery. 8th ed. Philadelphia: Elsevier; 2022. p. 3003–26.
19. Carney N, Totten AM, O'Reilly C, Ullman JS, Hawryluk GW, Bell MJ, et al. Guidelines for the management of severe traumatic brain injury, Fourth Edition. Neurosurgery. 2017;80(1):6–15.

20. Lee ST, Lui TN, Wong CW, Yeh YS, Tzuan WC, Chen TY, et al. Early seizures after severe closed head injury. Can J Neurol Sci. 1997;24(1):40–3.
21. Young B, Rapp RP, Norton JA, Haack D, Tibbs PA, Bean JR. Failure of prophylactically administered phenytoin to prevent early posttraumatic seizures. J Neurosurg. 1983;58(2):231–5.
22. Young B, Rapp RP, Norton JA, Haack D, Tibbs PA, Bean JR. Failure of prophylactically administered phenytoin to prevent late posttraumatic seizures. J Neurosurg. 1983;58(2):236–41.
23. Manaka S. Cooperative prospective study on posttraumatic epilepsy: risk factors and the effect of prophylactic anticonvulsant. Jpn J Psychiatry Neurol. 1992;46(2):311–5.
24. Temkin NR, Dikmen SS, Wilensky AJ, Keihm J, Chabal S, Winn HR. A randomized, double-blind study of phenytoin for the prevention of post-traumatic seizures. N Engl J Med. 1990;323(8):497–502.
25. Temkin NR, Dikmen SS, Anderson GD, Wilensky AJ, Holmes MD, Cohen W, et al. Valproate therapy for prevention of posttraumatic seizures: a randomized trial. J Neurosurg. 1999;91(4):593–600.
26. Dikmen SS, Machamer JE, Winn HR, Anderson GD, Temkin NR. Neuropsychological effects of valproate in traumatic brain injury: a randomized trial. Neurology. 2000;54(4):895–902.
27. Szaflarski JP, Sangha KS, Lindsell CJ, Shutter LA. Prospective, randomized, single-blinded comparative trial of intravenous levetiracetam versus phenytoin for seizure prophylaxis. Neurocrit Care. 2010;12(2):165–72.
28. Khan SA, Bhatti SN, Khan AA, Khan Afridi EA, Muhammad G, Gul N, et al. Comparison of efficacy of phenytoin and Levetiracetam for prevention of early post traumatic seizures. J Ayub Med Coll Abbottabad. 2016;28(3):455–60.
29. Haltiner AM, Newell DW, Temkin NR, Dikmen SS, Winn HR. Side effects and mortality associated with use of phenytoin for early posttraumatic seizure prophylaxis. J Neurosurg. 1999;91(4):588–92.
30. Temkin NR. Antiepileptogenesis and seizure prevention trials with antiepileptic drugs: meta-analysis of controlled trials. Epilepsia. 2001;42(4):515–24.
31. Bhullar IS, Johnson D, Paul JP, Kerwin AJ, Tepas JJ 3rd, Frykberg ER. More harm than good: antiseizure prophylaxis after traumatic brain injury does not decrease seizure rates but may inhibit functional recovery. J Trauma Acute Care Surg. 2014;76(1):54–61.
32. Jones KE, Puccio AM, Harshman KJ, Falcione B, Benedict N, Jankowitz BT, et al. Levetiracetam versus phenytoin for seizure prophylaxis in severe traumatic brain injury. Neurosurg Focus. 2008;25(4):E3.
33. Inaba K, Menaker J, Branco BC, Gooch J, Okoye OT, Herrold J, et al. A prospective multicenter comparison of levetiracetam versus phenytoin for early posttraumatic seizure prophylaxis. J Trauma Acute Care Surg. 2013;74(3):766–73.
34. Khan NR, VanLandingham MA, Fierst TM, Hymel C, Hoes K, Evans LT, et al. Should Levetiracetam or phenytoin be used for posttraumatic seizure prophylaxis? A systematic review of the literature and meta-analysis. Neurosurgery. 2016;79(6):775–82.
35. Zhao L, Wu YP, Qi JL, Liu YQ, Zhang K, Li WL. Efficacy of levetiracetam compared with phenytoin in prevention of seizures in brain injured patients: a meta-analysis. Medicine (Baltimore). 2018;97(48):e13247. https://doi.org/10.1097/MD.0000000000013247.
36. Yerram S, Katyal N, Premkumar K, Nattanmai P, Newey CR. Seizure prophylaxis in the neuroscience intensive care unit. J Intensive Care. 2018;6:17.
37. Rosengart AJ, Huo JD, Tolentino J, Novakovic RL, Frank JI, Goldenberg FD, et al. Outcome in patients with subarachnoid hemorrhage treated with antiepileptic drugs. J Neurosurg. 2007;107(2):253–60.
38. Pease M, Zaher M, Lopez AJ, Yu S, Egodage T, Semroc S, et al. Multicenter and prospective trial of anti-epileptics for early seizure prevention in mild traumatic brain injury with a positive computed tomography scan. Surg Neurol Int. 2022;13:241.
39. Marshall LF, Marshall SB, Klauber MR, Van Berkum CM, Eisenberg H, Jane JA, et al. The diagnosis of head injury requires a classification based on computed axial tomography. J Neurotrauma. 1992;9(Suppl 1):S287–92.

40. Maas AI, Hukkelhoven CW, Marshall LF, Steyerberg EW. Prediction of outcome in traumatic brain injury with computed tomographic characteristics: a comparison between the computed tomographic classification and combinations of computed tomographic predictors. Neurosurgery. 2005;57(6):1173–82.
41. Rojas K, Birrer K, Cheatham ML, Smith C. Seizure prophylaxis in patients with Traumatic Brain Injury (TBI). 2017. http://www.surgicalcriticalcare.net/Guidelines/Seizure%20prophylaxis%20in%20TBI%202017.pdf. Accessed 22 Nov 2022.
42. Joseph B, Friese RS, Sadoun M, Aziz H, Kulvatunyou N, Pandit V, et al. The BIG (brain injury guidelines) project: defining the management of traumatic brain injury by acute care surgeons. J Trauma Acute Care Surg. 2014;76(4):965–9.
43. Joseph B, Obaid O, Dultz L, Black G, Campbell M, Berndtson AE, et al. Validating the brain injury guidelines: results of an American Association for the Surgery of Trauma prospective multi-institutional trial. J Trauma Acute Care Surg. 2022;93(2):157–65.
44. Glauser T, Shinnar S, Gloss D, Alldredge B, Arya R, Bainbridge J, et al. Evidence-based guideline: treatment of convulsive status epilepticus in children and adults: report of the guideline Committee of the American Epilepsy Society. Epilepsy Curr. 2016;16(1):48–61.
45. Zeiler FA, Teitelbaum J, Gillman LM, West M. NMDA antagonists for refractory seizures. Neurocrit Care. 2014;20(3):502–13.
46. Huang YH, Liao CC, Chen WF, Ou CY. Characterization of acute post-craniectomy seizures in traumatically brain-injured patients. Seizure. 2015;25:150–4.
47. Dikmen SS, Temkin NR, Miller B, Machamer J, Winn HR. Neurobehavioral effects of phenytoin prophylaxis of posttraumatic seizures. J Am Med Assoc. 1991;265(10):1271–7.
48. Ma CY, Xue YJ, Li M, Zhang Y, Li GZ. Sodium valproate for prevention of early posttraumatic seizures. Chin J Traumatol. 2010;13(5):293–6.
49. Cotton BA, Kao LS, Kozar R, Holcomb JB. Cost-utility analysis of levetiracetam and phenytoin for posttraumatic seizure prophylaxis. J Trauma. 2011;71(2):375–9.
50. Dennis B, Guillamondegui O, Evans B, Atchison L, Beavers J. Practice management guidelines for seizure prophylaxis. Nashville, TN: Vanderbilt University Medical Center; 2021. https://www.vumc.org/trauma-and-scc/sites/default/files/public_files/Protocols/Seizure%20Prophylaxis%20PMG%202021.pdf. Accessed 22 Nov 2022.
51. Thompson K, Pohlmann-Eden B, Campbell LA, Abel H. Pharmacological treatments for preventing epilepsy following traumatic head injury. Cochrane Database Syst Rev. 2015;(8):CD009900.

Neuroendocrine Dysfunction After TBI

25

Yara Alfawares, George L. Yang, Rabindra Lamichhane, Abid Yaqub, and Laura B. Ngwenya

Neuroendocrine dysfunction is commonly observed after traumatic brain injury (TBI). In this setting, it is known as post-traumatic hypopituitarism (PTHP) and is defined as a failure of the neuroendocrine system after head trauma, manifesting as dysregulation of one or more of the pituitary hormones [1]. PTHP can take the form of growth hormone deficiency (GHD), hypogonadism, hypocortisolism, hypothyroidism, dysregulation of antidiuretic hormone (ADH), hyperprolactinemia, or combination of these. Here, we discuss epidemiology, clinical presentation, pathophysiology, diagnosis, and management of PTHP.

25.1 Epidemiology

The prevalence of PTHP, including both anterior and posterior pituitary dysfunction, ranges from 15 to 90% after injury. The breadth of this range is due to differences in criteria used for screening and diagnosis in different studies [2]. However, a general increase in prevalence is observed with increasing severity of TBI [3, 4].

Y. Alfawares · G. L. Yang
Department of Neurosurgery, University of Cincinnati College of Medicine, Cincinnati, OH, USA
e-mail: alfawaya@mail.uc.edu; yangege@ucmail.uc.edu

R. Lamichhane · A. Yaqub
Division of Endocrinology, Department of Medicine, University of Cincinnati College of Medicine Medical Sciences, Cincinnati, OH, USA
e-mail: lamichra@ucmail.uc.edu; yaqubad@ucmail.uc.edu

L. B. Ngwenya (✉)
Departments of Neurosurgery and Neurology & Rehabilitation Medicine University of Cincinnati College of Medicine, Cincinnati, OH, USA
e-mail: ngwenyla@ucmail.uc.edu

E. Brogi et al. (eds.), *Traumatic Brain Injury*, Hot Topics in Acute Care Surgery and Trauma, https://doi.org/10.1007/978-3-031-50117-3_25

In moderate to severe TBI, anterior pituitary dysfunction has a prevalence of 15–68% [5, 6]. GHD is the most common type, with a prevalence of 2–66% [2, 7]. It is followed in frequency by adrenal insufficiency, found in 0–60% of cases [2]. Other forms of PTHP include hypogonadism (0–29%), hypothyroidism (0–29%), and hyperprolactinemia (0–48%) [2].

Posterior pituitary dysfunction is characterized by disorders causing dysnatremia. Hyponatremia is the most common electrolyte abnormality observed acutely after TBI. It is seen in approximately 20% of patients, with about 60% of such cases caused by the syndrome of inappropriate antidiuretic hormone secretion (SIADH) [8, 9]. Alternatively, central diabetes insipidus (DI), associated with decreased ADH release and consequent hypernatremia, is identified in 15–28% of acute TBI cases [10].

25.2 Risk Factors

Risk factors for developing PTHP after TBI include age, fractures of the skull base, diffuse axonal injury, diffuse cerebral edema, intracranial hemorrhage, increased intracranial pressure (ICP), hypotension, hypoxia, and pre-existing endocrinopathy [1, 4, 11, 12]. Furthermore, blast TBI is associated with increased risk of PTHP compared to non-blast TBI [13]. Central DI in the acute phase after TBI may predict the development of anterior pituitary dysfunction in the chronic phase [11]. PTHP is less common in cases with cranial vault fractures [11].

25.3 Pathophysiology

The mechanisms underlying PTHP can be divided into primary and secondary types.

Primary injury involves direct damage to the hypothalamus, pituitary gland or the pituitary stalk via mechanical forces causing TBI or neighboring skull base fractures [14, 15]. Damage to the pituitary stalk could injure the pars tuberalis, in which gonadotropic, corticotropic, and thyrotropic neurons are located, resulting in the common forms of PTHP after TBI [16]. It could also lead to hyperprolactinemia after damage to the inhibitory neurons preventing the release of prolactin from the pituitary [17].

Secondary damage to the pituitary is caused by various mechanisms, including hypoxia, hemorrhage, hypotension, edema, raised ICP, and reduced cerebral perfusion [2, 18]. The pituitary gland's blood supply explains its relative susceptibility to ischemic injury [14]. The anterior pituitary derives its blood supply from the long portal veins branching from the superior hypophyseal artery and giving rise to the hypophyseal portal system [19]. These vessels course along the pituitary stalk and are at risk of primary injury with TBI or secondary injury from hypertension, hypotension, and edema [14]. Hence, the regions of the anterior pituitary gland peripheral to this blood supply and dependent upon it are particularly damaged by ischemic injury [14]. These regions include somatotropic and corticotropic neurons, the injury of which leads to the most common forms of PTHP: GHD and adrenal insufficiency [20].

This damage from ischemia is further compounded by the mitochondrial dysfunction seen after TBI, causing a reduction in oxidative metabolism [21]. The subsequent dependence on glycolysis reduces the efficiency of energy production from glucose metabolism. Thus, small fluctuations in glucose levels and perfusion can significantly affect energy production in regions such as the pituitary gland because of its already precarious blood supply [1].

Another proposed secondary injury mechanism is autoimmunity. Anti-pituitary antibodies (APAs) and anti-hypothalamus antibodies are present in TBI patients up to 5 years after injury [22]. This is thought to be a result of the disruption of the blood–brain barrier, exposing the brain to cells of the immune system that source such antibodies [2]. Indeed, there is a correlation between APA titers, the likelihood of PTHP, and GHD severity [23]. This is seen in patients with moderate to severe TBI and with repetitive mild TBI [24].

25.4 Acute Endocrinopathy

These pathophysiologic events contribute to both acute and chronic manifestations of PTHP. In the anterior pituitary, the physiological response to stress in the acute phase is an increase in sympathoadrenal function to maintain homeostasis by preserving energy and adjusting perfusion patterns to match need [25]. This is followed by a catabolic state in the subacute phase, generating substrates for repair [25]. This biphasic response, called the "ebb and flow," is associated with an overall increase in anterior pituitary function, especially in the release of ACTH, which aids in healing, preventing an excessive immune response, and recovery of hemodynamics after TBI [14, 25, 26]. Despite this, adrenal insufficiency is observed in some TBI patients within a week of injury and is considered a form of critical illness-related corticosteroid insufficiency, defined as cortisol levels lower than what would be expected in injured patients [27, 28]. This adrenal insufficiency typically presents with refractory hypotension, hypoglycemia, and hyponatremia [29]. Screening for adrenal insufficiency is discussed in the Screening section below.

The dysfunction of the posterior pituitary can appear as DI or SIADH, with corresponding hypernatremia and hyponatremia, respectively. Hypernatremia is associated with more extended hospital stays, worse prognosis, and increased mortality, while hyponatremia is mainly associated with longer hospital stays only [9, 30]. However, hyponatremia can also be fatal if it leads to cerebral edema, raised ICP, and subsequent herniation. Therefore, it is critical to identify and treat these conditions in the acute phase and continue until they resolve, which occurs in most cases [31].

The majority of SIADH cases are diagnosed within 48 h of injury [31]. Diagnosis is based on serum sodium, plasma osmolality, urine concentration, and the

Table 25.1 Diagnostic criteria for SIADH

Diagnostic criteria for SIADH
Decreased serum sodium concentration, < 135 mmol/L
Decreased effective plasma osmolality, < 275 mOsm/kg
Increased urine concentration, > 100 mOsm/kg
Clinical euvolemia
Increased urinary sodium, > 30 mmol/L
No recent use of diuretics
Exclusion of glucocorticoid and thyroid hormone deficiencies

Table 25.2 Diagnostic criteria for DI

Diagnostic criteria for DI
• Polyuria (increased urine volume), >2 mL/kg/h, OR > 300 mL/h for 2 consecutive hours
• Decreased urine osmolality, <300 mOsm/kg
• Increased plasma osmolality, >300 mOsm/kg
• Increased plasma sodium concentration, >145 mmol/L

exclusion of other conditions which can possibly cause hyponatremia after TBI, including reduced ACTH and subsequent cortisol deficiency and hypothyroidism [10]. Table 25.1 outlines the diagnostic criteria for SIADH [10].

It is important to note here that approximately 21% of cases of hyponatremia after TBI have iatrogenic causes, including but not limited to diuretics, inadequate fluid resuscitation, and the use of carbamazepine [31].

On the other hand, a decrease in the levels of ADH causes central DI, which typically manifests in the first 4–7 days after TBI and is initially indicated by polyuria [10]. Because most moderate and severe TBI patients are in a state of reduced level of consciousness or impaired cognitive status following injury, polydipsia is usually not a presenting or identifiable symptom. DI leads to hypernatremia if not treated, which is associated with increased mortality, as aforementioned. DI is diagnosed in the presence of hypotonic urine and polyuria, along with increased plasma osmolality [32]. Table 25.2 outlines the diagnostic criteria for DI. While most cases of DI resolve spontaneously within 2–5 days, management throughout the manifestation of the disease is crucial [10].

25.5 Chronic Endocrinopathy

Dysfunction of the anterior pituitary is more commonly observed in chronic PTHP. As outlined above in the Epidemiology section, the most common form is GHD, followed by secondary adrenal insufficiency. Cases of hypogonadism, secondary hypothyroidism, and hyperprolactinemia are also observed.

In contrast to the acute phase, clinical manifestations in the chronic phase after TBI are more apparent and are in line with symptoms expected to be observed in endocrinopathies not preceded by TBI [33]. Cognitive symptoms may include memory deficits, attention deficits, depression, anxiety, irritability, poor judgment, fatigue, lethargy, insomnia, poor sleep, diminished libido, and lack of emotional well-being [1, 34].

Of special note, Brain Injury Associated Fatigue and Altered Cognition (BIAFAC) is a recently defined syndrome that encompasses the constellation of symptoms experienced by patients with GHD, including fatigue, cognitive impairment, and depression [35]. Interestingly, patients with BIAFAC have been found to have reduced levels of circulating amino acids in serum, as well as changes in the gut microbiome, including decrease in *Prevotella* and *Bacteroides* spp. and an increase in Ruminococcaceae family bacteria [36, 37]. Both observations are implicated in the pathophysiology of the syndrome.

25.6 Special Populations

In addition to the above, some patient populations experience other manifestations of PTHP that deserve mention.

25.6.1 Pediatric

Studies examining PTHP in children are less abundant than those in adults. Nevertheless, it has been found that children with a history of TBI are 3.22 times more likely to have central endocrine diagnoses. This occurs more commonly in females than in males, with prevalence values of 64% and 36%, respectively [38].

In the acute phase, pediatric patients may experience DI or hypocortisolism, as seen in adults [39, 40]. GHD is the most prevalent chronic form of pituitary dysfunction after TBI [41]. This is followed by hypogonadism, in which children may exhibit a reduction in the progression of puberty [41]. Loss of menstrual regularity is another common observation in the first 6 months after TBI, seen in 22% of adolescent females [42]. However, some children exhibit contrasting presentations after TBI, where they have been observed to experience precocious puberty [42]. Most endocrine abnormalities resolve within 1 year after TBI [42].

25.6.2 Female Patients

Women with TBI are 21 times more likely to report amenorrhea than women without TBI, with a mean duration of 6.5 months (ranging from 1 to 60 months) [43]. Amenorrhea after TBI is correlated with lower GCS at admission, higher injury severity score and more extended hospital stay [43]. Those who continue to have periods are six times more likely to experience irregular periods [43].

Regarding pregnancy, there is no significant change in the ability to conceive or carry to term [43]. However, women with a history of TBI are less likely to have live births and are more likely to report difficulties after pregnancy, such as increased fatigue, depression, mobility problems, inability to concentrate, and lower extremity edema [43]. These observations are thought to be associated with PTHP [43].

25.6.3 Military

Studies have identified a high prevalence of PTHP in soldiers who experienced blast TBI, with GHD and deficiencies of follicle-stimulating hormone and luteinizing hormone being most common [44–46]. These deficiencies may be linked to mental health disorders such as anxiety [47]. Another study found that soldiers who experienced blast TBI were more likely to experience PTHP than soldiers who experienced non-blast TBI [48]. However, PTHP, specifically GHD, has also been observed in soldiers who experienced mild combat-related TBI [49].

25.6.4 Athletes

Athletes participating in aggressive or contact sports, such as soccer, boxing, and kickboxing, are at risk of developing PTHP due to a single TBI or chronic repetitive TBI [50–52].

25.7 Screening and Management

There are currently no official guidelines on screening TBI patients for PTHP, but neurosurgeons and endocrinologists have discussed recommendations [29, 53, 54].

During the acute hospital admission following TBI, they recommend no endocrine testing, including examination of serum cortisol levels, unless there is clinical suspicion for adrenal insufficiency due to symptoms such as refractory hypotension, hypoglycemia, or hyponatremia [29, 55]. Such adrenal insufficiency would warrant empiric treatment with hydrocortisone given as 50 mg IV or IM every 6–8 h or as 50–100 mg IV bolus followed by an infusion of 4–8 mg/h (Fig. 25.1) [29]. Endocrinology guidance should be sought for continued management of steroid supplementation.

After discharge, authors differ slightly on the specifics of screening, but most agree that it should be done. Ghigo et al. recommend that all patients with moderate to severe TBI, as well as those with mild TBI who were hospitalized for more than 24 hours or those presenting with symptoms, should be screened at 3 months and 12 months post-TBI (Fig. 25.1) [2, 55]. Meanwhile, Tan et al. recommend screening for any patient requiring admission for more than 48 h or less if they also exhibit some of the symptoms listed [29]. Screening for such patients is recommended at 3–6 months and 12 months after TBI [29].

Patients screened at 3–6 months and 12 months after injury should be tested as shown in Fig. 25.1 [29]. Any patients with abnormalities detected on screening should be referred to endocrinology. If adrenal insufficiency is detected, management should be initiated as shown in Fig. 25.1 [29].

Of note, routine screening for GHD at 3–6 months and 12 months after TBI is not recommended as most cases of GHD in PTHP resolve within 1 year of injury without intervention [29]. However, patients who exhibit symptoms of PTHP at 12 months post-TBI should be referred to endocrinology for evaluation and management of possible GHD [29].

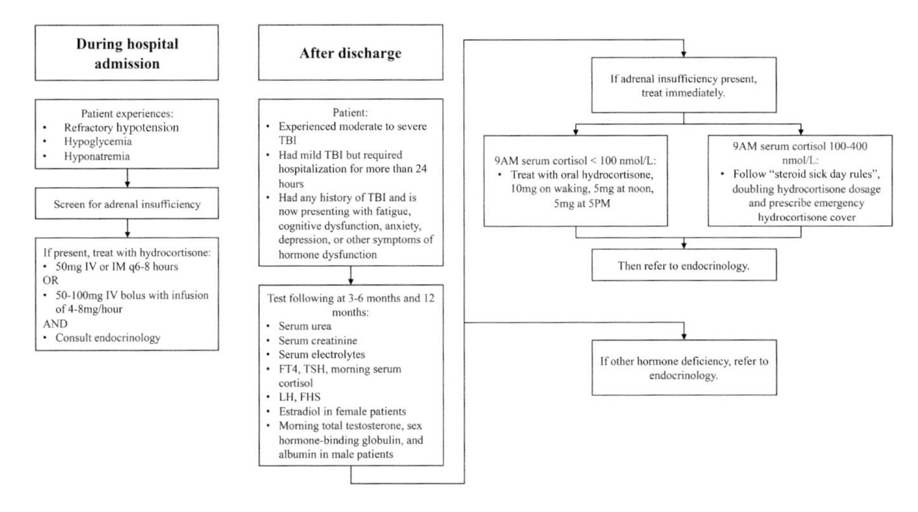

Fig. 25.1 Algorithm for management of endocrine abnormalities in TBI patients during initial hospitalization and after discharge

25.8 Conclusion

PTHP is common after TBI and can explain various sequelae experienced by patients in the chronic phase, such as cognitive and emotional impairment. The most common endocrine dysfunctions in the acute phase include secondary adrenal insufficiency, DI, and SIADH. In the chronic phase, GHD and secondary adrenal insufficiency are more common, and hypogonadism, secondary hypothyroidism, and hyperprolactinemia may also occur. Possible mechanisms underlying such dysfunction include direct injury during TBI or secondary injury via edema, ischemia, autoimmunity, and inflammation. Given the potential impact of PTHP on quality of life after TBI and the availability of treatment, at-risk patients should be screened for early identification and intervention.

References

1. Li M, Sirko S. Traumatic brain injury: at the crossroads of neuropathology and common metabolic endocrinopathies. J Clin Med. 2018;7:59.
2. Gray S, Bilski T, Dieudonne B, Saeed S. Hypopituitarism after traumatic brain injury. Cureus. 2019;11:e4163.
3. Schneider HJ, Schneider M, Saller B, et al. Prevalence of anterior pituitary insufficiency 3 and 12 months after traumatic brain injury. Eur J Endocrinol. 2006;154:259–65.
4. Klose M, Juul A, Poulsgaard L, Kosteljanetz M, Brennum J, Feldt-Rasmussen U. Prevalence of predictive factors of post-traumatic hypopituitarism. Clin Endocrinol. 2007;67:193–201.
5. Schneider HJ, Kreitschmann-Andermahr I, Ghigo E, Stalla GK, Agha A. Hypothalamopituitary dysfunction following traumatic brain injury and aneurysmal subarachnoid hemorrhage: a systematic review. JAMA. 2007;298:1429–38.
6. Emelifeonwu J, Flower H, Loan J, McGivern K, Andrews P. Prevalence of anterior pituitary dysfunction twelve months or more following traumatic brain injury in adults: a systematic review and meta-analysis. J Neurotrauma. 2020;37:217–26.

7. Gasco V, Cambria V, Bioletto F, Ghigo E, Grottoli S. Traumatic brain injury as frequent cause of hypopituitarism and growth hormone deficiency: epidemiology, diagnosis, and treatment. Front Endocrinol (Lausanne). 2021;12:634415.
8. Kleindienst A, Hannon MJ, Buchfelder M, Verbalis JG. Hyponatremia in neurotrauma: the role of vasopressin. J Neurotrauma. 2016;33:615–24.
9. Sherlock M, O'Sullivan E, Agha A, et al. Incidence and pathophysiology of severe hyponatraemia in neurosurgical patients. Postgrad Med J. 2009;85:171–5.
10. Tudor RM, Thompson CJ. Posterior pituitary dysfunction following traumatic brain injury: review. Pituitary. 2018;22:296–304.
11. Schneider M, Schneider HJ, Yassouridis A, Saller B, von Rosen F, Stalla GK. Predictors of anterior pituitary insufficiency after traumatic brain injury. Clin Endocrinol. 2008;68:206–12.
12. Kelly DF, Gonzalo IT, Cohan P, Berman N, Swerdloff R, Wang C. Hypopituitarism following traumatic brain injury and aneurysmal subarachnoid hemorrhage: a preliminary report. J Neurosurg. 2000;93:743–52.
13. Baxter D, Sharp D, Feeney C, et al. Pituitary dysfunction after blast traumatic brain injury. Ann Neurol. 2013;74:527–36.
14. Molaie AM, Maguire J. Neuroendocrine abnormalities following traumatic brain injury: an important contributor to neuropsychiatric sequelae. Front Endocrinol. 2018;9:176.
15. Bistritzer T, Theodor R, Inbar D, Cohen BE, Sack J. Anterior hypopituitarism due to fracture of the Sella turcica. Am J Dis Child. 1981;135:966–8.
16. Asa SL, Kovacs K, Bilbao JM. The pars tuberalis of the human pituitary. A histologic, immunohistochemical, ultrastructural and immunoelectron microscopic analysis. Virchows Arch A Pathol Anat Histopathol. 1983;399:49–59.
17. Simmons AN, Matthews SC. Neural circuitry of PTSD with or without mild traumatic brain injury: a meta-analysis. Neuropharmacology. 2012;62:598–606.
18. Dusick JR, Wang C, Cohan P, Swerdloff R, Kelly DF. Pathophysiology of hypopituitarism in the setting of brain injury. Pituitary. 2012;15:2–9.
19. Gorczyca W, Hardy J. Arterial supply of the human anterior pituitary gland. Neurosurgery. 1987;20:369–78.
20. Stieg MR. Advances in understanding hypopituitarism. F1000Res. 2017;6:178.
21. Verweij BH, Muizelaar JP, Vinas FC, Peterson PL, Xiong Y, Lee CP. Impaired cerebral mitochondrial function after traumatic brain injury in humans. J Neurosurg. 2000;93:815–20.
22. Guaraldi F, Grottoli S, Arvat E, Ghigo E. Hypothalamic-pituitary autoimmunity and traumatic brain injury. J Clin Med. 2015;4:1025–35.
23. Tanriverdi F, De Bellis A, Bizzarro A, et al. Antipituitary antibodies after traumatic brain injury: is head trauma-induced pituitary dysfunction associated with autoimmunity? Eur J Endocrinol. 2008;159:7–13.
24. Tanriverdi F, De Bellis A, Battaglia M, et al. Investigation of antihypothalamus and antipituitary antibodies in amateur boxers: is chronic repetitive head trauma-induced pituitary dysfunction associated with autoimmunity? Eur J Endocrinol. 2010;162:861–7.
25. Simsek T, Simsek HU, Cantürk NZ. Response to trauma and metabolic changes: posttraumatic metabolism. Ulus Cerrahi Derg. 2014;30:153–9.
26. Vanhorebeek I, Langouche L, Van den Berghe G. Endocrine aspects of acute and prolonged critical illness. Nat Clin Pract Endocrinol Metab. 2006;2:20–31.
27. Alavi SA, Tan CL, Menon DK, Simpson HL, Hutchinson PJ. Incidence of pituitary dysfunction following traumatic brain injury: a prospective study from a regional neurosurgical center. Br J Neurosug. 2016;30:302–6.
28. Olivecrona Z, Dahlqvist P, Koskinen LD. Acute neuro-endocrine profile and prediction of outcome after severe brain injury. Scand J Trauma Resusc Emerg Med. 2013;21:33.
29. Tan CL, Alavi SA, Baldeweg SE, et al. The screening and management of pituitary dysfunction following traumatic brain injury in adults: British neurotrauma group guidance. J Neurol Neurosurg Psychiatry. 2017;88:971–81.
30. Hoffman H, Jalal MS, Chin LS. Effect of hypernatremia on outcomes after severe traumatic brain injury: a nationwide inpatient sample analysis. World Neurosurg. 2018;118:e880–6.

31. Agha A, Thornton E, O'Kelly P, Tormey W, Phillips J, Thompson CJ. Posterior pituitary dysfunction after traumatic brain injury. J Clin Endocrinol Metab. 2004;89:5987–92.
32. Seckl J, Dunger D. Postoperative diabetes insipidus. BMJ. 1989;298:2–3.
33. Wijayatilake DS, Sherren PB, Jigajinni SV. Systemic complications of traumatic brain injury. Curr Opin Anaesthesiol. 2015;28:525–31.
34. Lorenzo M, Peino R, Castro AI, et al. Hypopituitarism and growth hormone deficiency in adult subjects after traumatic brain injury: who and when to test. Pituitary. 2005;8:233–7.
35. Urban RJ. A treatable syndrome in patients with traumatic brain injury. J Neurotrauma. 2020;37:1124–5.
36. Durham WJ, Foreman JP, Randolph KM, et al. Hypoaminoacidemia characterizes chronic traumatic brain injury. J Neurotrauma. 2017;34:385–90.
37. Urban RJ, Pyles RB, Stewart CJ, et al. Altered fecal microbiome years after traumatic brain injury. J Neurotrauma. 2020;37:1037–51.
38. Ortiz JB, Sukhina A, Balkan B, Harootunian G, et al. Epidemiology of pediatric traumatic brain injury and hypothalamic-pituitary disorders in Arizona. Front Neurol. 2020;10:1410.
39. Barzilay Z, Somekh E. Diabetes insipidus in severely brain damaged children. J Med. 1988;19:47–64.
40. Srinivas R, Brown SD, Chang Y, Garcia-Fillion P, Adelson PD. Endocrine function in children acutely following severe traumatic brain injury. Childs Nerv Syst. 2010;26:647–53.
41. Aimaretti G, Ambrosio MR, Somma CD, et al. Hypopituitarism induced by traumatic brain injury in the transition phase. J Endocrinol Investig. 2005;28:984–9.
42. Kaulfers AM, Backeljauw PF, Reifschneider K, et al. Endocrine dysfunction following traumatic brain injury in children. J Pediatr. 2010;157:894–9.
43. Colantonio A, Mar W, Escobar M, et al. Women's health outcomes after traumatic brain injury. J Womens Health (Larchmt). 2010;19:1109–16.
44. Undurti A, Colasurdo E, Sikkema C, et al. Chronic hypopituitarism associated with increased postconcussive symptoms is prevalent after blast-induced mild traumatic brain injury. Front Neurol. 2018;19:72.
45. Wilkinson C, Pagulayan K, Petrie E, et al. High prevalence of chronic pituitary and target-organ hormone abnormalities after blast-related mild traumatic brain injury. Front Neurol. 2012;3:11.
46. Lee J, Anderson L, Migula D, Yuen K, McPeak L, Garcia J. Experience of a pituitary clinic for US military veterans with traumatic brain injury. J Endocr Soc. 2021;5:bvab005.
47. Ciarlone SL, Statz J, Goodrich J, et al. Neuroendocrine function and associated mental health outcomes following mild traumatic brain injury in OEF-deployed service members. J Neurosci Res. 2020;98:1174–87.
48. Hannon MJ, Crowley RK, Behan LA, et al. Acute glucocorticoid deficiency and diabetes insipidus are common after acute traumatic brain injury and predict mortality. J Clin Endocrinol Metab. 2013;98:3229–37.
49. Ioachimescu A, Hampstead B, Moore A, Burgess E, Philips L. Growth hormone deficiency after mild combat-related traumatic brain injury. Pituitary. 2015;18:535–41.
50. Caglar AS, Tanriverdi F, Karaca Z, Unluhizarci K, Kelestimur F. Sports-related repetitive traumatic brain injury: a novel cause of pituitary dysfunction. J Neurotrauma. 2019;36:1195–202.
51. Gilis-Januszewska A, Kluczynski L, Hubalewska-Dydejczyk A. Traumatic brain injuries induced pituitary dysfunction: a call for algorithms. Endocr Connect. 2020;9:R112–23.
52. Hacioglu A, Kelestimur F, Taniverdi F. Pituitary dysfunction due to sports-related traumatic brain injury. Pituitary. 2019;22:322–31.
53. Wexler TL. Neuroendocrine disruptions following head injury. Curr Neurol Neurosci Rep. 2023;23(5):213–24. https://doi.org/10.1007/s11910-023-01263-5. Epub 2023 May 6. PMID: 37148402; PMCID: PMC10163581.
54. Mahajan C, Prabhakar H, Bilotta F. Endocrine Dysfunction after traumatic brain injury: an ignored clinical syndrome? Neurocrit Care. 2023;39(3):714–23. https://doi.org/10.1007/s12028-022-01672-3. Epub 2023 Feb 14. PMID: 36788181; PMCID: PMC10689524.
55. Ghigo E, Masel B, Aimaretti G, et al. Consensus guidelines on screening for hypopituitarism following traumatic brain injury. Brain Inj. 2005;19:711–24.

Infection Management in the Neurocritical Care Setting

26

Henry Chang and Paul Nyquist

26.1 Introduction

Central nervous system (CNS) infections are less commonly acquired in the community than other systemic infections [1]. Yet, CNS infections are significantly more frequent in patients with traumatic brain injury (TBI) and penetrating head trauma or neurosurgical procedures and instrumentation, all of which introduce pathogens into the protected CNS meningeal and parenchymal compartments and cerebrospinal fluid (CSF) [2]. We focus here on the diseases of meningitis, encephalitis, ventriculitis, brain abscess, and subdural empyema. These patients are usually treated in the intensive care unit (ICU) setting due to high risk for morbidity and mortality [3].

All CNS infections may present with a number of symptoms and findings, the most common of which are usually reported as fever, headache, and sometimes focal neurological symptoms. As with any infection, the cornerstones of treatment are appropriate antimicrobial therapy and source control. CNS infections are unique in that they require antimicrobials which are able to effectively cross the blood-brain barrier [4]. Additionally, patients with neurological injury frequently have prolonged ICU stays which increases the chance for multidrug resistant bacterial strains necessitating more potent antibiotics [5].

Supportive care is key, as these patients frequently exhibit complications including decreased consciousness, impaired respiratory drive, immobility, and seizures [6]. Physicians must be vigilant for evidence of elevated intracranial pressure (ICP) due to inflammation and cerebral edema or obstructive mass effect, as increasing ICPs and cerebral herniation can rapidly become life threatening.

H. Chang (✉) · P. Nyquist
Neuroscience Critical Care Division, Departments of Neurology, Neurosurgery, and Anesthesiology and Critical Care Medicine, Johns Hopkins University School of Medicine, Baltimore, MD, USA
e-mail: hchang26@jhu.edu; pnyquis1@jhmi.edu

E. Brogi et al. (eds.), *Traumatic Brain Injury*, Hot Topics in Acute Care Surgery and Trauma, https://doi.org/10.1007/978-3-031-50117-3_26

While this chapter focuses on primary CNS infections, it is worthwhile to note that TBI and neurocritical care patients are also at high risk to develop non-CNS infections [7]. Treatment of neurological injuries and disease often requires hyperosmolar solutions, vasoactive medications, and other therapies which commonly involve arterial and central lines and urinary catheters, thus increasing the risk of nosocomial bloodstream and urinary infections [2]. Pneumonias—both in patients with invasive ventilation and without—are also very common due to decreased consciousness, dysphagia (seen in up to 93% of TBI patients [8]), and impaired protective airway reflexes [9], accounting for up to 40% of neurosurgical ICU infections [10]. Urinary dysfunction is frequently seen (50–62% of cases) [11], and urinary retention increases the risk for cystitis. Additionally, TBI is believed to cause peripheral immune system dysfunction through decreased neuronal activation of inflammatory pathways [12], which likely increases the susceptibility of these patients to all of the above CNS and systemic infections.

26.2 Encephalitis and Meningitis

Encephalitis and meningitis are infections of the brain parenchyma and the meningeal layers surrounding the brain, respectively. Though they define separate pathologies, they often occur concurrently (termed meningoencephalitis) due to the physical continuity of these spaces, and they can present with a similar constellation of symptoms including fever, headache, and neurological findings [13].

Patients with bacterial meningitis are at risk for acute cerebral edema, hydrocephalus, elevated intracranial pressure, and ischemic stroke [14]. In community-acquired meningitis, the most common pathogens are Streptococcus pneumoniae and Neisseria meningitidis [15], while meningitis after neurosurgery or penetrating skull injury are more likely to be caused by Staphylococcus or a number of different colonizing or nosocomial organisms [16]. Viral encephalitis is typically a more indolent process but can also present similarly to bacterial meningitis, and it has also been implicated as a trigger for autoimmune encephalitis [3]. Herpes simplex virus is the most common pathogen and commonly affects the temporal lobes causing seizures, psychosis, hemiparesis, and aphasia [1]. Also frequently seen are West Nile virus infections which can cause obtundation and a poliomyelitis-like flaccid paralysis [1].

26.2.1 Diagnosis

Cerebrospinal fluid analysis is required for definitive diagnosis of meningitis [4]. A lumbar puncture should be performed with measurement of opening and closing pressures [15]. Adequate CSF should be collected to send for cell counts with differentials (analyzed twice in two separate tubes), protein, glucose, gram stain, cultures, and viral PCRs. Serum glucose should be obtained at the same time as the lumbar puncture for comparison [4].

Classic CSF findings suggestive of acute bacterial meningitis include elevated opening pressure, elevated protein, pleocytosis with polymorphonuclear predominance, and hypoglycorrhachia [17]. A positive gram stain and culture provides a definitive diagnosis of bacterial meningitis and identifies the causative organism. The CSF profile in viral meningitis usually features a milder degree of pleocytosis, elevated protein, and hypoglycorrhachia. Gram stain and cultures will be negative, but PCR studies are available for many common viruses and often are able to identify the infectious organism. Lactate may be useful in differentiating a bacterial from viral etiology if sampled prior to antimicrobial therapy, especially in neurosurgical or trauma patients [18]. Note that caution must be taken when interpreting the CSF values in non-infectious conditions such as intracranial bleeding, seizures, malignancies, and neuroinflammatory disorders, as the CSF profile in these other conditions may mimic that of an infection.

Blood cultures should be collected when working up meningitis, as they will be positive for the causative organism in 50–90% of cases, even when CSF cultures are negative [19].

Imaging is usually performed prior to the lumbar puncture to rule out an obstructive cause of elevated intracranial pressure, which would increase the risk of herniation. In most cases a computed tomography (CT) scan of the head without contrast is sufficient for this purpose. Magnetic resonance imaging (MRI) with and without contrast offers additional diagnostic utility when certain characteristic findings such as meningeal enhancement and lesions of the temporal lobe and/or basal ganglia are present (Table 26.1).

26.2.2 Management

Meningoencephalitis is considered an emergency and, when suspected, empiric treatment should be initiated without waiting for confirmatory testing results [4]. The most common bacterial pathogens are Neisseria meningitidis and Streptococcus pneumoniae. Treatment consists of a third generation cephalosporin as well as vancomycin (due to varying susceptibilities of N. meningitidis to cephalosporins). Aztreonam or meropenem may be used in place of the third generation

Table 26.1 CSF interpretation

	Gross appearance	Opening pressure (mmH2O	Glucose (mmol/L)	CSF:serum glucose ratio	Protein (mg/dL)	Lactate (mmol/L)	WBC (cells/uL)
Normal	Clear	<20	50–80	>0.4	15–45	<3.5	<5
Bacterial meningitis	Purulent	Elevated	Very low	Very low	High	Elevated	>1000
Viral meningitis	Clear/cloudy	Normal/elevated	Low	Low	High	Normal	5–200, lymphocytic predominance
Fungal meningitis	Clear/cloudy	Normal/elevated	Low	Low	High	Normal	

cephalosporin in patients with beta-lactam allergies. Additionally, adults who are immunocompromised or are over the age of 50 are at increased risk of Listeria monocytogenes infections so ampicillin (or sulfamethoxazole-trimethoprim in patients with beta-lactam allergies) should be started empirically as well.

When a pneumococcal meningitis is suspected, dexamethasone (0.15 mg/kg every 6 h) should be given up to 10–20 min prior to the first dose of antibiotics and continued for 2–4 days. Though steroids have not been shown to improve mortality, studies have shown decreased risk of neurological sequelae—particularly hearing loss—perhaps due to an attenuated inflammatory response [20].

If a viral encephalitis is expected, patients should be immediately started on empiric acyclovir (10 mg/kg ideal body weight every 8 h) until HSV encephalitis is ruled out with negative CSF PCR tests [1]. Acyclovir is associated with nephrotoxicity in patients with poor hydration status or preexisting renal disease, so it should be administered slowly over a period of 1 h and adequate hydration should be maintained during therapy [21].

26.3 Ventriculitis

Ventriculitis is an infection of the CSF and ventricular system of the brain [22]. Symptomatically, it may present similar to a meningoencephalitis, with fever and neurological findings. Most commonly it is related to the presence of a CSF shunt or external ventricular device (EVD), and the risk of ventriculitis varies depending on the type of device, insertion technique, management, frequency of CSF sampling, and length of time the device is in place. CSF shunt- and EVD-related infection is reported in 8–40% of patients, with most infections occurring 1–2 weeks after placement [23–26], and associated mortality rates are reported to be between 10% and 75% [25–27].

The most common pathogens involved in EVD and CSF shunt infections are Staphylococcus, Streptococcus, Propionibacterium, Candida, Aspergillus, and various Gram-negative organisms [17, 23]. In patients with traumatic brain injury or following neurosurgical procedures, aerobic Gram-negative bacilli (e.g., Pseudomonas) and Staphylococcus are the most common ventriculitis pathogens [17].

26.3.1 Diagnosis

Ventriculitis is diagnosed by a suggestive clinical picture of fever and neurological deficits in an at-risk patient and CSF studies consistent with a bacterial infection (e.g., elevated protein, pleocytosis with polymorphonuclear predominance, hypoglycorrhachia, and positive gram stain and cultures). The CSF may be sampled via lumbar puncture or directly from shunt or drain output. However, interpretation of these studies is often not straightforward in a patient with hardware or who has already suffered neurologic injury, as the CSF may falsely appear infectious due to inflammation and breakdown of the blood–brain barrier [25]. Gram stain and culture might also be positive from device colonization or contamination rather than a true infection [28]. A CSF lactate >4.0 mmol/L may be a helpful indicator of a true infection warranting treatment in the postoperative neurosurgical patient [17, 29], but thus far no single test has demonstrated the ability to reliably predict or exclude infectious ventriculitis [25].

26.3.2 Management

Ventriculitis should initially be treated empirically with vancomycin and either a cephalosporin (such as cefepime or ceftazidime) or meropenem. Treatment duration varies between 5 and 21 days depending on the organism and whether source control is successfully achieved [17, 25]. A fungal infection with Candida or Aspergillus species should be managed with voriconazole and amphotericin B for 2 weeks after the last negative CSF culture [25]. In some cases, intraventricular or intrathecal administration of microbial agents may be considered when standard intravenous therapy is not effective, though this practice remains controversial [3].

In addition to antimicrobial therapy, infected hardware should be removed, replaced, or externalized when appropriate [30]. Early device removal and re-implantation avoidance is associated with shorter illness duration [31]. Failure to achieve source control often limits success of the initial treatment and may result in infection recrudescence weeks to months after treatment. It is important to highlight that, in the case of EVDs, careful insertion and meticulous device care can prolong EVD use and minimize infection rates [27, 32]. On the other hand, neither antibiotic-impregnated catheters nor prophylactic systemic antibiotics appear to have any benefit, nor does the practice of routine EVD exchange [24, 33].

26.4 Brain Abscess

A brain abscess is a focal pus-filled infection in the brain parenchyma. It may occur as a complication after neurosurgical procedures, after head trauma with penetrating injury, and via contiguous spread from chronic oto-rhinological infections (particularly in immunocompromised patients) [34–36]. Patients may have a unilateral headache which progresses to fevers and neurological symptoms related to local mass effect from the abscess, such as lateralized sensorimotor weakness or focal seizures [37, 38]. Further complications include cerebral edema, ischemia, elevated ICP, and herniation [39].

In many cases, particularly in post-neurosurgical abscesses, polymicrobial infections are found. The most common pathogens are skin-colonizing bacteria, such as Staphylococcus, Streptococcus, and Gram-negative bacilli, among others [40, 41].

26.4.1 Diagnosis

The primary diagnostic test for a brain abscess is neuroimaging. On CT scan, a brain abscess appears as a well-demarcated hypodense lesion with a thin contrast-enhancing rim; however, the specificity of this finding is relatively poor due to the similar appearance of other lesions such as brain metastasis, hematoma, and radiation necrosis. A brain MRI is preferred for diagnosis and shows a diffusion restricting lesion with a contrast-enhancing rim [36, 37].

Identification of the infectious organism may be possible through surgical aspiration of the abscess. A lumbar puncture may also reveal positive CSF cultures if the abscess has ruptured into the ventricular system; however, this must be done with caution as lumbar puncture has been estimated to cause cerebral herniation in 15–20% of in patients with cerebral abscess [38].

26.4.2 Management

Upon diagnosis of a brain abscess, empiric antibiotic therapy should be initiated immediately [39]. Patients who have undergone neurosurgical procedures or have sustained head trauma with skull fractures should be started on vancomycin, cefepime, and metronidazole for 4–8 weeks, depending on clinical and radiological response and success with source control [36].

For abscesses larger than 2.5 cm in diameter, medical therapy alone may be ineffective and surgical drainage may be necessary [42]. However, surgery can also increase the risk for other complications when the abscess is located near eloquent brain, when the patient also has meningitis or ventriculitis, or in the setting of hydrocephalus which requires CSF diversion and instrumentation. The risks of benefits of surgery and its timing should be considered on an individualized basis.

26.5 Subdural Empyema

Subdural empyema is a bacterial infection of the space between the dura mater and the arachnoid meningeal layer. Due to the lack of anatomic barriers, infections in this contiguous space can spread along the entire convexity of the brain and even layer into the opposite hemisphere and/or the posterior fossa, potentially causing compression with elevated ICP and herniation [43, 44]. Subdural empyemas can be seen in patients with penetrating head trauma, chronic oto-rhinologic infections, and up to 4% of all neurosurgical cases [37]. The most common pathogens are Staphylococcus, Streptococcus, and Gram-negative bacilli, among others.

Patients usually develop headache, fever, and neurological symptoms within several weeks after the neurosurgical procedure. Neurological findings may include meningismus, somnolence, hemiplegia, and papilledema. Seizures occur in up to half of patients [44].

26.5.1 Diagnosis

Intracranial imaging should be performed in all patients with suspected subdural empyemas. On CT imaging, subdural empyemas appear as hypodense collections with contrast enhancement in the subdural space. MRI may be more sensitive than CT for visualizing subdural empyemas; they appear as diffusion restricting areas with decreased signal on T1-weighted imaging and increased signal on T2-weighted imaging [44].

Serological laboratory abnormalities may include leukocytosis and elevated C-reactive protein and erythrocyte sedimentation rate [45]. Blood cultures are usually collected but rarely isolate an organism if the infection is confined to the subdural space [46]. Lumbar puncture is not recommended in subdural empyemas as it is associated with increased risk for cerebral herniation.

26.5.2 Management

Empiric antibiotic therapy for subdural empyemas consists of vancomycin and cefepime for 3–6 weeks, depending on clinical response. In some cases where the patient appears well clinically and the subdural empyema is small, antibiotic therapy alone may be sufficient. However, the majority of patients should also undergo surgical drainage for source control. Surgical drainage may done via burr holes or craniotomy [43], and samples can be collected in the operating room for Gram stains and cultures, though unfortunately up to 53% of these patients may have negative surgery cultures [47], Table 26.2.

Table 26.2 Standard antibiotic treatments or common microorganisms in the neurocritical care unit

Microorganism	Standard therapy
Streptococcus pneumoniae	Vancomycin 15–30 mg/kg q8h or q12h, maintain serum trough concentrations of 15–20 ug/mL, plus ceftriaxone 2 g q12h
Neisseria meningitidis	Cetftriaxone 2 g q12h
Herpes simplex virus	Acyclovir 10 mg/kg IBW q8h
Listeria monocytogenes	Ampicillin 2 g q4h
Staphylococcus, methicillin sensitive	Nafcillin 2 g q4h or oxacillin 2 g q4h
Staphylococcus, methicillin resistant	Vancomycin 15–30 mg/kg q8h or q12h, maintain serum trough concentrations of 15–20 ug/mL
Pseudomonas aeruginosa	Cefepime 2 g q8h or ceftazidime 2 g q8h or meropenem 2 g q8h
ESBL gram-negative bacilli	Meropenem 2 g q8h
Candida	Lipid amphotericin B 3–5 mg/kg q24h
Aspergillus	Voriconazole 4 mg/kg q12h

ESBL extended spectrum beta-lactamase-producing, *mg/kg* milligrams per kilogram, *IBW* ideal body weight, *q4h* every 4 hours, *q8h* every 12 hours, *q12h* every 12 hours, *q24h* every 24 hours
Standard therapy per IDSA (Infectious Diseases Society of America) 2017 guidelines [48]

26.6 Conclusion

CNS infections—which include meningitis, encephalitis, ventriculitis, brain abscess, and subdural empyema—carry high risk for morbidity and mortality (about 30% for meningitis) [30], and increase in likelihood with penetrating trauma or neurosurgical procedures or instrumentation. Patients with TBI and neurological pathologies frequently have a constellation of findings including dysphagia, urinary dysfunction, and neuronal-mediated immune dysfunction, which additionally places them at greater risk for non-CNS infections such as pneumonia, urinary tract infections, and bloodstream infections. Prolonged ICU stays also predispose these patients to greater rates of infections with multidrug resistant bacteria. Clinicians must be aware of the high incidence of these infections and maintain a vigilant attitude toward identifying and treating them properly in the neurological intensive care setting.

References

1. Martin-Loeches I, Blake A, Collins D. Severe infections in neurocritical care. Curr Opin Crit Care. 2021;27(2):131–8.
2. Busl KM. Healthcare-associated infections in the Neurocritical care unit. Curr Neurol Neurosci Rep. 2019;19(10):76.
3. Robinson CP, Busl KM. Meningitis and encephalitis management in the ICU. Curr Opin Crit Care. 2019;25(5):423–9.
4. O'Horo JC, Sampathkumar P. Infections in Neurocritical care. Neurocrit Care. 2017;27(3):458–67.
5. Munari M, Franzoi F, Sergi M, de Cassai A, Geraldini F, Grandis M, et al. Extensively drug-resistant and multidrug-resistant gram-negative pathogens in the neurocritical intensive care unit. Acta Neurochir. 2022;164(3):859–65.
6. van de Beek D, de Gans J, Spanjaard L, Weisfelt M, Reitsma JB, Vermeulen M. Clinical features and prognostic factors in adults with bacterial meningitis. N Engl J Med. 2004;351(18):1849–59.
7. Rosenthal VD, Al-Abdely HM, El-Kholy AA, AlKhawaja SAA, Leblebicioglu H, Mehta Y, et al. International nosocomial infection control consortium report, data summary of 50 countries for 2010-2015: device-associated module. Am J Infect Control. 2016;44(12):1495–504.
8. Hansen TS, Engberg AW, Larsen K. Functional oral intake and time to reach unrestricted dieting for patients with traumatic brain injury. Arch Phys Med Rehabil. 2008;89(8):1556–62.
9. Berrouane Y, Daudenthun I, Riegel B, Emery MN, Martin G, Krivosic R, et al. Early onset pneumonia in neurosurgical intensive care unit patients. J Hosp Infect. 1998;40(4):275–80.
10. Laborde G, Grosskopf U, Schmieder K, Harders A, Klimek L, Hardenack M, et al. Nosocomial infections in a neurosurgical intensive care unit. Anaesthesist. 1993;42(10):724–31.
11. Giannantoni A, Silvestro D, Siracusano S, Azicnuda E, D'Ippolito M, Rigon J, et al. Urologic dysfunction and neurologic outcome in coma survivors after severe traumatic brain injury in the postacute and chronic phase. Arch Phys Med Rehabil. 2011;92(7):1134–8.
12. Hazeldine J, Lord JM, Belli A. Traumatic brain injury and peripheral immune suppression: primer and prospectus. Front Neurol. 2015;6:235.
13. Tunkel AR, Glaser CA, Bloch KC, Sejvar JJ, Marra CM, Roos KL, et al. The management of encephalitis: clinical practice guidelines by the Infectious Diseases Society of America. Clin Infect Dis. 2008;47(3):303–27.
14. Roos KL. Acute bacterial meningitis. Semin Neurol. 2000;20(3):293–306.

15. Kramer AH, Bleck TP. Neurocritical care of patients with central nervous system infections. Curr Infect Dis Rep. 2007;9(4):308–14.
16. van de Beek D, Drake JM, Tunkel AR. Nosocomial bacterial meningitis. N Engl J Med. 2010;362(2):146–54.
17. Tunkel AR, Hartman BJ, Kaplan SL, Kaufman BA, Roos KL, Scheld WM, et al. Practice guidelines for the management of bacterial meningitis. Clin Infect Dis. 2004;39(9):1267–84.
18. Dorsett M, Liang SY. Diagnosis and treatment of central nervous system infections in the emergency department. Emerg Med Clin North Am. 2016;34(4):917–42.
19. Heckenberg SGB, Brouwer MC, van de Beek D. Bacterial meningitis. Handb Clin Neurol. 2014;121:1361–75.
20. Shao M, Xu P, Liu J, Liu W, Wu X. The role of adjunctive dexamethasone in the treatment of bacterial meningitis: an updated systematic meta-analysis. Patient Prefer Adherence. 2016;10:1243–9.
21. Izzedine H, Launay-Vacher V, Deray G. Antiviral drug-induced nephrotoxicity. Am J Kidney Dis. 2005;45(5):804–17.
22. Lewis A, Wahlster S, Karinja S, Czeisler BM, Kimberly WT, Lord AS. Ventriculostomy-related infections: the performance of different definitions for diagnosing infection. Br J Neurosurg. 2016;30(1):49–56.
23. Armstrong W, Boulis N, McGillicuddy I. Infections of the central nervous system. In: Crockard H, Hoff J, editors. Neurosurgery: the scientific basis of clinical practice. 3rd ed; 2000. p. 757–83.
24. Ortiz R, Lee K. Nosocomial infections in neurocritical care. Curr Neurol Neurosci Rep. 2006;6(6):525–30.
25. Beer R, Lackner P, Pfausler B, Schmutzhard E. Nosocomial ventriculitis and meningitis in neurocritical care patients. J Neurol. 2008;255(11):1617–24.
26. Lozier AP, Sciacca RR, Romagnoli MF, Connolly ES. Ventriculostomy-related infections: a critical review of the literature. Neurosurgery. 2002;51(1):170–81; discussion 181–2.
27. Korinek AM, Reina M, Boch AL, Rivera AO, de Bels D, Puybasset L. Prevention of external ventricular drain—related ventriculitis. Acta Neurochir. 2005;147(1):39–45; discussion 45–6.
28. van Ek B, Bakker FP, van Dulken H, Dijkmans BA. Infections after craniotomy: a retrospective study. J Infect. 1986;12(2):105–9.
29. Leib SL, Boscacci R, Gratzl O, Zimmerli W. Predictive value of cerebrospinal fluid (CSF) lactate level versus CSF/blood glucose ratio for the diagnosis of bacterial meningitis following neurosurgery. Clin Infect Dis. 1999;29(1):69–74.
30. Ziai WC, Lewin JJ. Update in the diagnosis and management of central nervous system infections. Neurol Clin. 2008;26(2):427–68. viii.
31. Soavi L, Rosina M, Stefini R, Fratianni A, Cadeo B, Magri S, et al. Post-neurosurgical meningitis: management of cerebrospinal fluid drainage catheters influences the evolution of infection. Surg Neurol Int. 2016;7(Suppl 39):S927–34.
32. Lo CH, Spelman D, Bailey M, Cooper DJ, Rosenfeld J, v, Brecknell JE. External ventricular drain infections are independent of drain duration: an argument against elective revision. J Neurosurg. 2007;106(3):378–83.
33. Murphy RKJ, Liu B, Srinath A, Reynolds MR, Liu J, Craighead MC, et al. No additional protection against ventriculitis with prolonged systemic antibiotic prophylaxis for patients treated with antibiotic-coated external ventricular drains. J Neurosurg. 2015;122(5):1120–6.
34. Tenney JH. Bacterial infections of the central nervous system in neurosurgery. Neurol Clin. 1986;4(1):91–114.
35. Calfee DP, Wispelwey B. Brain abscess. In: Seminars in neurology, vol. 20. New York, NY: Thieme Medical Publishers, Inc; 2000. p. 353–60.
36. Vibha D, Garg D. Infections of the central nervous system (CNS) in the ICU. In: Infectious diseases in the intensive care unit. Singapore: Springer; 2020. p. 117–37.
37. Hall WA, Truwit CL. The surgical management of infections involving the cerebrum. Neurosurgery. 2008;62(Suppl 2):519–30. discussion 530-1.

38. Brouwer MC, Coutinho JM, van de Beek D. Clinical characteristics and outcome of brain abscess: systematic review and meta-analysis. Neurology. 2014;82(9):806–13.
39. Brouwer MC, Tunkel AR, McKhann GM, van de Beek D. Brain abscess. N Engl J Med. 2014;371(5):447–56.
40. Yang KY, Chang WN, Ho JT, Wang HC, Lu CH. Postneurosurgical nosocomial bacterial brain abscess in adults. Infection. 2006;34(5):247–51.
41. Honda H, Warren DK. Central nervous system infections: meningitis and brain abscess. Infect Dis Clin N Am. 2009;23(3):609–23.
42. Mamelak AN, Mampalam TJ, Obana WG, Rosenblum ML. Improved management of multiple brain abscesses: a combined surgical and medical approach. Neurosurgery. 1995;36(1):76–85; discussion 85–6.
43. Nathoo N, Nadvi SS, van Dellen JR, Gouws E. Intracranial subdural empyemas in the era of computed tomography: a review of 699 cases. Neurosurgery. 1999;44(3):529–35; discussion 535–6.
44. Fernández-de Thomas RJ, de Jesus O. Subdural empyema. Treasure Island, FL: StatPearls Publishing; 2022.
45. Wong AM, Zimmerman RA, Simon EM, Pollock AN, Bilaniuk LT. Diffusion-weighted MR imaging of subdural empyemas in children. AJNR Am J Neuroradiol. 2004;25(6):1016–21.
46. Madhugiri VS, Sastri BVS, Bhagavatula ID, Sampath S, Chandramouli BA, Pandey P. Posterior fossa subdural empyema in children—management and outcome. Childs Nerv Syst. 2011;27(1):137–44.
47. Osborn MK, Steinberg JP. Subdural empyema and other suppurative complications of paranasal sinusitis. Lancet Infect Dis. 2007;7(1):62–7.
48. Tunkel AR, Hasbun R, Bhimraj A, Byers K, Kaplan SL, Scheld WM, et al. 2017 Infectious Diseases Society of America's clinical practice guidelines for healthcare-associated Ventriculitis and meningitis. Clin Infect Dis. 2017;64(6):e34–65.

Traumatic Brain Injury in Pregnancy

27

Joshua Dilday and Kenji Inaba

27.1 TBI Epidemiology

Traumatic brain injury (TBI) is a significant health care issue, with over two million occurrences and 56,000 deaths per year [1, 2]. TBI also leads to significant morbidity, as over one million patients will experience some sort of short-term disability and 90,000 patients will progress to permanent disability [1]. Older adults are at an increased risk for TBI due to cerebral atrophy, stretching of the bridging veins, increased use of antiplatelet and anticoagulation medications. As the aging population increases, the health costs associated with TBI have seen a similar increase. One current estimate of the TBI healthcare burden is around 56 billion dollars [1]. Despite TBI often being seen in older adults, it does not discriminate and can often be a major factor related to overall traumatic morbidity and mortality in younger patients. In fact, TBI is the leading cause of death and disability in the trauma population [3].

Trauma is also the leading cause of non-obstetric maternal death, affecting up to 8% of all pregnancies [4, 5]. Guidelines exist regarding the initial management of the pregnant trauma patient and should be followed [6]. However, these guidelines lack specific TBI management recommendations. Making matters worse, pregnant patients with TBI have higher rates of both morbidity and mortality compared to non-pregnant patients [7, 8]. Although there have been significant advances in the understanding and treatment of TBI recently [9], Level 1 evidence is lacking and there remains a paucity of guidelines related to this patient group. Thus, with certain

J. Dilday
Division of Trauma and Acute Care Surgery, Medical College of Wisconsin, Milwaukee, WI, USA

K. Inaba (✉)
Trauma and Surgical Critical Care, LA General Medical Center/Keck Medicine of USC, Los Angeles, CA, USA
e-mail: Kenji.Inaba@med.usc.edu

E. Brogi et al. (eds.), *Traumatic Brain Injury*, Hot Topics in Acute Care Surgery and Trauma, https://doi.org/10.1007/978-3-031-50117-3_27

exceptions addressed here, the general TBI guidelines can be followed in the pregnancy population [9]. The concepts discussed here, while not exhaustive, are designed to provide a framework for the initial management of TBI in the pregnant patient.

27.1.1 Initial Management

As with any trauma scenario, the key to initial treatment of the pregnant TBI patient should be the basic principles of trauma resuscitation, focusing on a rapid assessment of airway, breathing, and circulation [10]. Maintaining a clear airway is of the utmost importance, as hypoxia should be avoided at all costs. Weight gain, reduced functional reserve capacity, and increased airway resistance in pregnancy warrant treating every pregnant patient as a "difficult airway." Pregnant patients have an increased risk of failed intubation and aspiration of gastric contents. If intubation is required, it should be followed by prompt gastric decompression via either a nasogastric or orogastric tube. Early development of hypoxia has been shown to increase mortality in TBI patients [11]. Ventilation should be monitored with a goal of normocarbia ($PaCO_2$ of 35–40 mmHg). This is of increased importance in the pregnant patient, as mild hyperventilation and hypocapnia are already present during pregnancy. This, combined with a decreased functional reserve capacity, increases the potential for respiratory compromise in a trauma scenario. While transient hyperventilation may be an early strategy that can be employed in impending brain herniation, deviations of $PaCO_2$ in either direction are associated with increased mortality [12].

The circulation assessment should be aimed at promoting adequate perfusion. Although permissive hypotension may be employed in other trauma scenarios, the goal blood pressure in TBI may be higher. Some have advocated for a goal SBP over 100 mmHg during the initial resuscitation period [13, 14]. The fetus is especially sensitive to any changes in circulatory flow and even minor changes can lead to significant reductions in uteroplacental perfusion and gas exchange. Additionally, vasopressors should be avoided as the uteroplacental vasculature is extremely sensitive to these agents.

If blood transfusions are required for resuscitation, fully cross matched or O-negative red blood cells should be used to prevent Rh alloimmunization. Minimal amount of fetal-maternal blood mixing can lead to sensitization in the Rh-negative mother, and anti-D IgG should be given to all Rh-negative pregnant patients within 72 h [6].

27.1.2 Secondary Injury

A major tenet of TBI management is prevention of secondary injury. The pathophysiology of secondary brain injury in TBI is complex, but proinflammatory cytokines, cerebral edema, and disruption of the blood–brain barrier are likely contributing factors [15]. While the initial insult may not be reversable, controlling certain factors can dimmish the chance of worsening or expanding injury and sequelae. Recent strategies shown to decrease the effects of secondary injury are aimed at providing blood flow and nutrition to the injured brain tissue. Thus, hypotension, hypoxia, and malnutrition should be avoided to simultaneously prevent secondary injury and promote neuronal recovery [3, 16].

27.1.3 Imaging

Although the unnecessary ionizing radiation should be avoided in pregnant patients, current guidelines state that radiographic studies needed for maternal evaluation and diagnosis should not be delayed [6]. For TBI, the imaging of choice is non-contrast enhanced computed tomography (CT) [9]. The risks of ionizing radiation are dose-dependent. However, the radiation burden of a head CT scan falls within the threshold deemed safe in pregnancy [6]. The risk of radiation exposure obviously increases with each additional CT scan. In order to categorize who needs additional imaging, the Brain Injury Guidelines (BIG) have classified TBI patients into tiered categories [17, 18]. The lowest category, deemed BIG 1, includes patients with small brain injuries who are not intoxicated or on anticoagulants/antiplatelets. Joseph et al. found that BIG 1 category patients can be safely observed without the need for repeat imaging [17, 18]. This has major implications in the pregnant population, as unnecessary radiation can be safely avoided in minor TBI.

27.1.4 Intracranial Hypertension

Elevations in intracranial pressure (ICP) are a feared complication which can lead to secondary brain injury. The initial prevention and treatment strategies are relatively benign, but more drastic measures may be indicated depending on the severity and duration. The Brain Trauma Foundation has separated these strategies into a tiered approach to help guide clinical decision-making [9]. Elevating the head, treating pain, and preventing hyperthermia are important early maneuvers that can safely be performed in the pregnant patient. The antipyretic of choice, acetaminophen, can also treat pain and is considered safe in pregnancy.

As previously mentioned, hyperventilation for early treatment of elevated ICP is controversial in the pregnant patient [19]. The physiological changes of pregnancy already promote a degree of baseline hypocarbia and fetal perfusion is sensitive to any changes in $PaCO_2$. Although some have advised aiming for a lower $PaCO_2$, others recommend maintaining levels on the lower end of normal maternal obstetric levels [20]. The use of prophylactic hyperventilation in TBI has been abandoned [9]. Because any significant alteration in $PaCO_2$ can increase mortality [12], we recommend maintaining levels as close to baseline as possible.

If additional measures are needed to treat intracranial hypertension, diuretic and osmotic therapies are used in the general population. Loop diuretics, mannitol, and hypertonic saline are common therapies used to acutely lower ICP. However, these agents remain controversial in pregnancy. Mannitol has a theoretical risk of fetal tissue accumulation affecting serum osmolality and dehydration has been observed in animal studies [21, 22]. However, reports of its use in pregnant patients have not demonstrated any adverse effects [7, 8, 23]. Hypertonic saline should be avoided in the pregnant population, as literature has not yet supported its fetal safety.

27.1.5 Specific Factors in Pregnancy

The impact of pregnancy on TBI may have a unique hormonal component. Progesterone, an endogenous steroid and sex hormone produced by the ovary and placenta, is significantly elevated during pregnancy. Besides promoting fetal development, progesterone may also promote remyelination and neural repair [24]. Progesterone levels are also elevated following TBI and some have found a potential neuroprotective effect in animal models [25–29]. The mechanism is not completely understood, but regulation of neural excitability, inflammation, antioxidants, and the blood–brain barrier have been proposed as reasons for the benefit seen in murine models [30].

However, the benefits of the progesterone in TBI have not been as robust in human studies. The SyNAPSe and the ProTECT III randomized controlled trials did not show any significant benefit of exogenous progesterone on TBI outcomes [31, 32]. Although the data is not exhaustive, there does not seem to be any current evidence to support the use of progesterone as a treatment for TBI [33–35]. In fact, despite the theoretical benefit of increased progesterone, pregnancy may actually lead to worse outcomes in TBI. Berry et al. found a trend toward increased mortality in pregnant patient with isolated TBI [2]. Davis et al. found that only postmenopausal women have better TBI outcomes than men and Farace et al. found that pregnant patients do worse [36–38]. The reasons for these discrepancies are unknown, but the combined hypercoagulability from pregnancy and TBI may be a contributing factor [2, 39].

27.2 Pregnancy-Specific Management

27.2.1 Treat the Mother

While treating the pregnant trauma patient may seem daunting at first, the initial strategies remain the same. The primary focus in any pregnant trauma scenario is to treat the mother. Any effort designed to optimize the mother's outcomes will only increase the chance of fetal survival. While there are certain caveats that should not be overlooked (e.g., placing a bump under the left flank to avoid uterine compression of the IVC, recognizing the relative anemia during pregnancy, and providing Rh antigen protection as indicated), the tenants of TBI management do not differ for the pregnant patient [6]. On the contrary, the strategy of avoiding secondary injury is even more important in this population as hypotension and hypoxia are less tolerated in both the pregnant mother and the fetus [8]. Prompt delivery of oxygen and avoidance of hypotension during resuscitation should be employed to treat both the TBI and the fetus.

The fetal response to any traumatic injury can be variable and obstetric expertise is warranted for any fetus of viable gestational age. Obstetric consultation and fetal monitoring are even more important of the variability in hemodynamic response in TBI. Severe TBI can present with prompt changes to both heart rate and blood pressure and the fetus should be monitored for any signs of downstream distress.

27.2.2 Fetal Monitoring

Obstetric consultations, fetal ultrasound, and biophysical profile should be considered in all pregnant TBI patients [5, 8]. Initial fetal monitoring should be considered in all pregnant patients presenting after a traumatic scenario and continuous monitoring should be performed for all fetuses of viable age (i.e., ≥ 23 weeks gestation). Monitoring should be continued for at least 4 h, as that duration of monitoring is sensitive for detecting immediate adverse fetal issues [40, 41]. In cases of significant respiratory, cardiac, or hemodynamic abnormalities, a longer period of monitoring is warranted based on the patient's individual characteristics [5].

Among other things, fetal monitoring may identify occasional uterine contractions, which are the most common finding after trauma [41]. These contractions are important to monitor, as their intensity and frequency may be the first predictive sign of uterine compromise. Maternal tachycardia and hypotension are late signs of shock, as the physiologic increase in maternal blood volume during pregnancy can mask hemodynamically significant distress. Alterations in uterine blood flow can occur despite normal maternal vital signs. Thus, uterine contractions should raise suspicion for the presence of possible fetal hypoperfusion [8, 42].

27.2.3 Delivery Considerations

As stated previously, pregnant patients carrying a viable fetus should be given special attention and ideally should be treated at a large volume trauma center [5]. After resuscitation and stabilization, a thorough assessment of the fetus should be performed. This should focus on identifying any placental abruption, placental hypoperfusion, and spontaneous rupture of membranes [6]. If preterm delivery is eminent, corticosteroids are recommended for pregnant women between 24 and 36 weeks of gestation [43].

In severe cases, delivery of the fetus may be necessary to improve the chance of maternal and fetal survival. While preterm delivery may be necessary in rare cases, all efforts should be made to allow for in utero fetal maturation. This may require ICU admission, steroids for pulmonary maturation, and tocolytic therapy [8]. There are little data regarding the safety of tocolytic therapy in TBI, but some reports have used oxytocin without significant adverse effects [44, 45]. However, oxytocin does have potential for significant vasodilation and care should be used to measure the lowest possible dose [8]. Some have recommended that intrauterine pregnancy only needs to be prolonged until 32 weeks, although this remains controversial [46].

Persistent distress in a viable fetus warrants emergent cesarean section as soon as the maternal condition has stabilized. Emergent cesarean section has the potential to be life-saving to the mother and the baby and should be considered early in devastating trauma scenarios [5, 8, 23]. In the case of maternal death despite cardiopulmonary resuscitation, perimortem cesarian sections can be performed with the hope of saving a viable fetus. However, it should be done within 5 min of unsuccessful maternal resuscitation in order to provide the best fetal outcomes [5, 8, 46].

Sometimes fetal maturation and health comes to the forefront of decision-making in the pregnant trauma scenario. No case is more severe than that of maternal brain death or poor maternal neurologic prognosis. These cases demand the utmost sensitivity and discussions with the family and obstetric team should be pursued in order to identify the next steps of management [8, 47–49]. Published recommendations, despite being limited, focus on the ethical consideration for the mother, but the principles of non-maleficence and justice should be followed when expressed wishes are unknown [50, 51]. The benefits of additional fetal maturation must be balanced against the risk and feasibility of continued medical support for the brain dead mother [8].

27.2.4 Long-Term Outcomes

There is not much difference in the long-term outcomes experienced between pregnant and not pregnant TBI patients. Two exceptions, however, include increased risk for postpartum depression and continued hormonal irregularities [8]. The combination of TBI with hormonal fluctuations pre-and post-delivery may lead to a higher risk of postpartum depression compared to those patients without TBI [52]. Additionally, women may experience irregular menses or amenorrhea after TBI, but these symptoms may not be permanent [8, 53]. The longevity and severity of post-injury symptoms seem to correlate with the severity of the initial TBI [53]. TBI may also affect future pregnancies. One study found previous TBI was associated with increased preterm delivery and cesarean sections [54].

27.3 Conclusion

Traumatic brain injury is a significant cause of morbidity and mortality in the pregnant trauma patient. Although there are minor differences, the treatment principles should be similar to those of the non-pregnant patient. Initial resuscitation should focus on maternal stability, as efforts to save the mother will simultaneously help save the baby. Avoiding secondary injury is crucial, hypoxia and hypotension should be avoided at all costs. The uteroplacental circulation is extremely sensitive and monitoring should be routinely performed with prompt obstetric consultation. As a rule, a multidisciplinary approach to both the initial management and the ethical considerations regarding end-of-life care should be pursued.

References

1. Wang KK, Larner SF, Robinson G, Hayes RL. Neuroprotection targets after traumatic brain injury. Curr Opin Neurol. 2006;19(6):514–9.
2. Berry C, Ley EJ, Mirocha J, Margulies DR, Tillou A, Salim A. Do pregnant women have improved outcomes after traumatic brain injury? Am J Surg. 2011;201(4):429–32.
3. Vella MA, Crandall ML, Patel MB. Acute management of traumatic brain injury. Surg Clin North Am. 2017;97(5):1015–30.
4. Muench MV, Canterino JC. Trauma in pregnancy. Obstet Gynecol Clin N Am. 2007;34(3):555–83. xiii
5. Mendez-Figueroa H, Dahlke JD, Vrees RA, Rouse DJ. Trauma in pregnancy: an updated systematic review. Am J Obstet Gynecol. 2013;209(1):1–10.
6. Jain V, Chari R, Maslovitz S, Farine D, Bujold E, Gagnon R, Basso M, Bos H, Brown R, Cooper S, et al. Guidelines for the management of a pregnant trauma patient. J Obstet Gynaecol Can. 2015;37(6):553–74.
7. Kazemi P, Villar G, Flexman AM. Anesthetic management of neurosurgical procedures during pregnancy: a case series. J Neurosurg Anesthesiol. 2014;26(3):234–40.
8. Leach MR, Zammit CG. Traumatic brain injury in pregnancy. Handb Clin Neurol. 2020;172:51–61.
9. Carney N, Totten AM, O'Reilly C, Ullman JS, Hawryluk GW, Bell MJ, Bratton SL, Chesnut R, Harris OA, Kissoon N, et al. Guidelines for the management of severe traumatic brain injury, fourth edition. Neurosurgery. 2017;80(1):6–15.
10. Gentleman D, Dearden M, Midgley S, Maclean D. Guidelines for resuscitation and transfer of patients with serious head injury. BMJ. 1993;307(6903):547–52.
11. Haddad SH, Arabi YM. Critical care management of severe traumatic brain injury in adults. Scand J Trauma Resusc Emerg Med. 2012;20:12.
12. Davis DP, Peay J, Sise MJ, Kennedy F, Simon F, Tominaga G, Steele J, Coimbra R. Prehospital airway and ventilation management: a trauma score and injury severity score-based analysis. J Trauma. 2010;69(2):294–301.
13. Manley G, Knudson MM, Morabito D, Damron S, Erickson V, Pitts L. Hypotension, hypoxia, and head injury: frequency, duration, and consequences. Arch Surg. 2001;136(10):1118–23.
14. Vos PE, Battistin L, Birbamer G, Gerstenbrand F, Potapov A, Prevec T, Stepan CA, Traubner P, Twijnstra A, Vecsei L, et al. EFNS guideline on mild traumatic brain injury: report of an EFNS task force. Eur J Neurol. 2002;9(3):207–19.
15. Bourgeois-Tardif S, De Beaumont L, Rivera JC, Chemtob S, Weil AG. Role of innate inflammation in traumatic brain injury. Neurol Sci. 2021;42(4):1287–99.
16. Robertson CS, Valadka AB, Hannay HJ, Contant CF, Gopinath SP, Cormio M, Uzura M, Grossman RG. Prevention of secondary ischemic insults after severe head injury. Crit Care Med. 1999;27(10):2086–95.
17. Joseph B, Friese RS, Sadoun M, Aziz H, Kulvatunyou N, Pandit V, Wynne J, Tang A, O'Keeffe T, Rhee P. The BIG (brain injury guidelines) project: defining the management of traumatic brain injury by acute care surgeons. J Trauma Acute Care Surg. 2014;76(4):965–9.
18. Joseph B, Obaid O, Dultz L, Black G, Campbell M, Berndtson AE, Costantini T, Kerwin A, Skarupa D, Burruss S, et al. Validating the brain injury guidelines: results of an American Association for the Surgery of Trauma prospective multi-institutional trial. J Trauma Acute Care Surg. 2022;93(2):157–65.

19. Curley G, Kavanagh BP, Laffey JG. Hypocapnia and the injured brain: more harm than benefit. Crit Care Med. 2010;38(5):1348–59.
20. Wang LP, Paech MJ. Neuroanesthesia for the pregnant woman. Anesth Analg. 2008;107(1):193–200.
21. Ross MG, Leake RD, Ervin MG, Fisher DA. Fetal lung fluid response to maternal hyperosmolality. Pediatr Pulmonol. 1986;2(1):40–3.
22. Burns PD, Linder RO, Drose VE, Battaglia F. The placental transfer of water from fetus to mother following the intravenous infusion of hypertonic mannitol to the maternal rabbit. Am J Obstet Gynecol. 1963;86:160–7.
23. Kho GS, Abdullah JM. Management of severe traumatic brain injury in pregnancy: a body with two lives. Malays J Med Sci. 2018;25(5):151–7.
24. Schumacher M, Hussain R, Gago N, Oudinet JP, Mattern C, Ghoumari AM. Progesterone synthesis in the nervous system: implications for myelination and myelin repair. Front Neurosci. 2012;6:10.
25. Schumacher M, Guennoun R, Stein DG, De Nicola AF. Progesterone: therapeutic opportunities for neuroprotection and myelin repair. Pharmacol Ther. 2007;116(1):77–106.
26. Wagner AK, McCullough EH, Niyonkuru C, Ozawa H, Loucks TL, Dobos JA, Brett CA, Santarsieri M, Dixon CE, Berga SL, et al. Acute serum hormone levels: characterization and prognosis after severe traumatic brain injury. J Neurotrauma. 2011;28(6):871–88.
27. Roof RL, Duvdevani R, Stein DG. Gender influences outcome of brain injury: progesterone plays a protective role. Brain Res. 1993;607(1–2):333–6.
28. Stein DG. Brain damage, sex hormones and recovery: a new role for progesterone and estrogen? Trends Neurosci. 2001;24(7):386–91.
29. Stein DG. The case for progesterone. Ann N Y Acad Sci. 2005;1052:152–69.
30. Schumacher M, Mattern C, Ghoumari A, Oudinet JP, Liere P, Labombarda F, Sitruk-Ware R, De Nicola AF, Guennoun R. Revisiting the roles of progesterone and allopregnanolone in the nervous system: resurgence of the progesterone receptors. Prog Neurobiol. 2014;113:6–39.
31. Skolnick BE, Maas AI, Narayan RK, van der Hoop RG, MacAllister T, Ward JD, Nelson NR, Stocchetti N. A clinical trial of progesterone for severe traumatic brain injury. N Engl J Med. 2014;371(26):2467–76.
32. Wright DW, Yeatts SD, Silbergleit R, Palesch YY, Hertzberg VS, Frankel M, Goldstein FC, Caveney AF, Howlett-Smith H, Bengelink EM, et al. Very early administration of progesterone for acute traumatic brain injury. N Engl J Med. 2014;371(26):2457–66.
33. Junpeng M, Huang S, Qin S. Progesterone for acute traumatic brain injury. Cochrane Database Syst Rev. 2011;(1):Cd008409.
34. Wang Z, Shi L, Ding W, Shao F, Yu J, Zhang J. Efficacy of progesterone for acute traumatic brain injury: a meta-analysis of randomized controlled trials. Mol Neurobiol. 2016;53(10):7070–7.
35. Korley F, Pauls Q, Yeatts SD, Jones CMC, Corbett-Valade E, Silbergleit R, Frankel M, Barsan W, Cahill ND, Bazarian JJ, et al. Progesterone treatment does not decrease serum levels of biomarkers of glial and neuronal cell injury in moderate and severe traumatic brain injury subjects: a secondary analysis of the progesterone for traumatic brain injury, experimental clinical treatment (ProTECT) III trial. J Neurotrauma. 2021;38(14):1953–60.
36. Davis DP, Douglas DJ, Smith W, Sise MJ, Vilke GM, Holbrook TL, Kennedy F, Eastman AB, Velky T, Hoyt DB. Traumatic brain injury outcomes in pre-and post-menopausal females versus age-matched males. J Neurotrauma. 2006;23(2):140–8.
37. Farace E, Alves WM. Do women fare worse: a metaanalysis of gender differences in traumatic brain injury outcome. J Neurosurg. 2000;93(4):539–45.
38. Berry C, Ley EJ, Tillou A, Cryer G, Margulies DR, Salim A. The effect of gender on patients with moderate to severe head injuries. J Trauma. 2009;67(5):950–3.
39. Wafaisade A, Lefering R, Tjardes T, Wutzler S, Simanski C, Paffrath T, Fischer P, Bouillon B, Maegele M. Acute coagulopathy in isolated blunt traumatic brain injury. Neurocrit Care. 2010;12(2):211–9.

40. ACOG educational bulletin, Obstetric Aspects of Trauma Management. Number 251, September 1998 (replaces Number 151, January 1991, and Number 161, November 1991). American College of obstetricians and gynecologists. Int J Gynaecol Obstet. 1999;64(1):87–94.
41. Pearlman MD, Tintinallli JE, Lorenz RP. A prospective controlled study of outcome after trauma during pregnancy. Am J Obstet Gynecol. 1990;162(6):1502–7; discussion 7–10.
42. Scorpio RJ, Esposito TJ, Smith LG, Gens DR. Blunt trauma during pregnancy: factors affecting fetal outcome. J Trauma. 1992;32(2):213–6.
43. ACOG Committee Opinion No. 475. Antenatal corticosteroid therapy for fetal maturation. Obstet Gynecol. 2011;117(2 Pt 1):422–4.
44. Kasper EM, Hess PE, Silasi M, Lim KH, Gray J, Reddy H, Gilmore L, Kasper B. A pregnant female with a large intracranial mass: reviewing the evidence to obtain management guidelines for intracranial meningiomas during pregnancy. Surg Neurol Int. 2010;1:95.
45. Goldschlager T, Steyn M, Loh V, Selvanathan S, Vonau M, Campbell S. Simultaneous craniotomy and caesarean section for trauma. J Trauma. 2009;66(4):E50–1.
46. Di Filippo S, Godoy DA, Manca M, Paolessi C, Bilotta F, Meseguer A, Severgnini P, Pelosi P, Badenes R, Robba C. Ten rules for the management of moderate and severe traumatic brain injury during pregnancy: an expert viewpoint. Front Neurol. 2022;13:911460.
47. Burkle CM, Tessmer-Tuck J, Wijdicks EF. Medical, legal, and ethical challenges associated with pregnancy and catastrophic brain injury. Int J Gynaecol Obstet. 2015;129(3):276–80.
48. Farragher RA, Laffey JG. Maternal brain death and somatic support. Neurocrit Care. 2005;3(2):99–106.
49. Whitney N, Raslan AM, Ragel BT. Decompressive craniectomy in a neurologically devastated pregnant woman to maintain fetal viability. J Neurosurg. 2012;116(3):487–90.
50. Siwatch S, Rohilla M, Singh A, Ahuja C, Jain K, Jain V. Pregnancy in a persistent vegetative State: a management dilemma. Case report, literature review and ethical concerns. J Obstet Gynaecol. 2020;70:310–3.
51. Anon. Brain death and pregnancy. Int J Gynaecol Obstet. 2011;115(1):84–5.
52. Uysal S, Hibbard MR, Robillard D, Pappadopulos E, Jaffe M. The effect of parental traumatic brain injury on parenting and child behavior. J Head Trauma Rehabil. 1998;13(6):57–71.
53. Colantonio A, Mar W, Escobar M, Yoshida K, Velikonja D, Rizoli S, Cusimano M, Cullen N. Women's health outcomes after traumatic brain injury. J Womens Health (Larchmt). 2010;19(6):1109–16.
54. Vaajala M, Kuitunen I, Nyrhi L, Ponkilainen V, Kekki M, Luoto T, Mattila VM. Pregnancy and delivery after traumatic brain injury: a nationwide population-based cohort study in Finland. J Matern Fetal Neonatal Med. 2022;25:1–8.

Traumatic Brain Injury in Pediatric Patients

28

Alfred Pokmeng See and Mark Proctor

28.1 Introduction

28.1.1 Epidemiology

Trauma is a significant driver of morbidity and mortality in children across the globe. The incidence ranges from 200 to 300 per 100,000 children, with a particular peak during infancy, and a rising trend with male predominance during the school-aged years through early adulthood [1]. It remains the leading cause of morbidity and mortality in children in the USA despite overall decreases in head trauma from motor vehicles [2].

Within the USA, there is significant disparity in the incidence and outcomes of traumatic brain injury (TBI). There are higher incidence and worse outcomes for children in rural areas, as care for children with TBI in more remote areas may result in delayed initial care and less access to therapy and mental health services [2].

28.1.2 Morbidity

The severity of injury is a significant driver of morbidity and mortality. The Glasgow Coma Scale (GCS) is adapted for pediatric applications and correlates with prognosis, and although it may be reported either as a composite or as component scores, there may be value in each separate component [3, 4]. Mortality rates may be as high as 74% in the most severely injured [5]. However, even in the subset with a low composite GCS score of 3 or 4, there may be good long-term outcome in as many as one in seven [6].

A. P. See · M. Proctor (✉)
Department of Neurosurgery, Boston Children's Hospital, Boston, MA, USA
e-mail: Mark.Proctor@childrens.harvard.edu

E. Brogi et al. (eds.), *Traumatic Brain Injury*, Hot Topics in Acute Care Surgery and Trauma, https://doi.org/10.1007/978-3-031-50117-3_28

28.1.3 Changes over Time

Despite legislative and public health measures to prevent and reduce trauma, pediatric TBI continues to increase, particularly driven by an increase in mild TBI [7]. However, there are some signs that certain mechanisms of injury are decreasing in frequency, coinciding with interventions for bicycling safety and sports programs [8, 9].

28.1.4 Features Unique to Children and Scenarios with Pediatric-Specific Data

Understanding of pediatric TBI is confounded by variability across the pediatric age range, including not only brain development but also changes in cerebrovascular regulation, systemic thrombosis regulation, bone development, and immune responses [10–12].

Findings and standards of care for TBI in adults may not be directly generalizable to pediatric TBI. However, some aspects of care are not amenable to study, or may not have been studied in children yet, and are therefore extrapolated from data derived from adult TBI.

28.1.5 Pathologic Processes

The primary injury may intuitively be a key component of severe TBI. The direct disruption of brain tissue may occur from a foreign body, large mechanical forces, or the rapid development of mass effect from blood products. That said, secondary processes may also have a significant impact on outcome and are discussed further below.

Imaging after brain injury may show blood product in many different compartments ranging from the scalp to epidural, subdural, subarachnoid, subpial, intraparenchymal, or intraventricular (Figs. 28.1 and 28.2).

Severe brain injury may also be associated with other pathophysiology that may cause neurologic compromise. This may include cardiac arrest or other systemic mechanisms of anoxic brain injury, or focal cerebrovascular processes, such as blunt cerebrovascular injury to the carotid or vertebral arteries. Although those are critical components of the management of a trauma patient, they are beyond the scope of this chapter.

28.1.6 Secondary Processes

Primary brain injury can be further worsened by secondary injury such as from intracranial hypertension as well as venous or arterial injury with associated stroke.

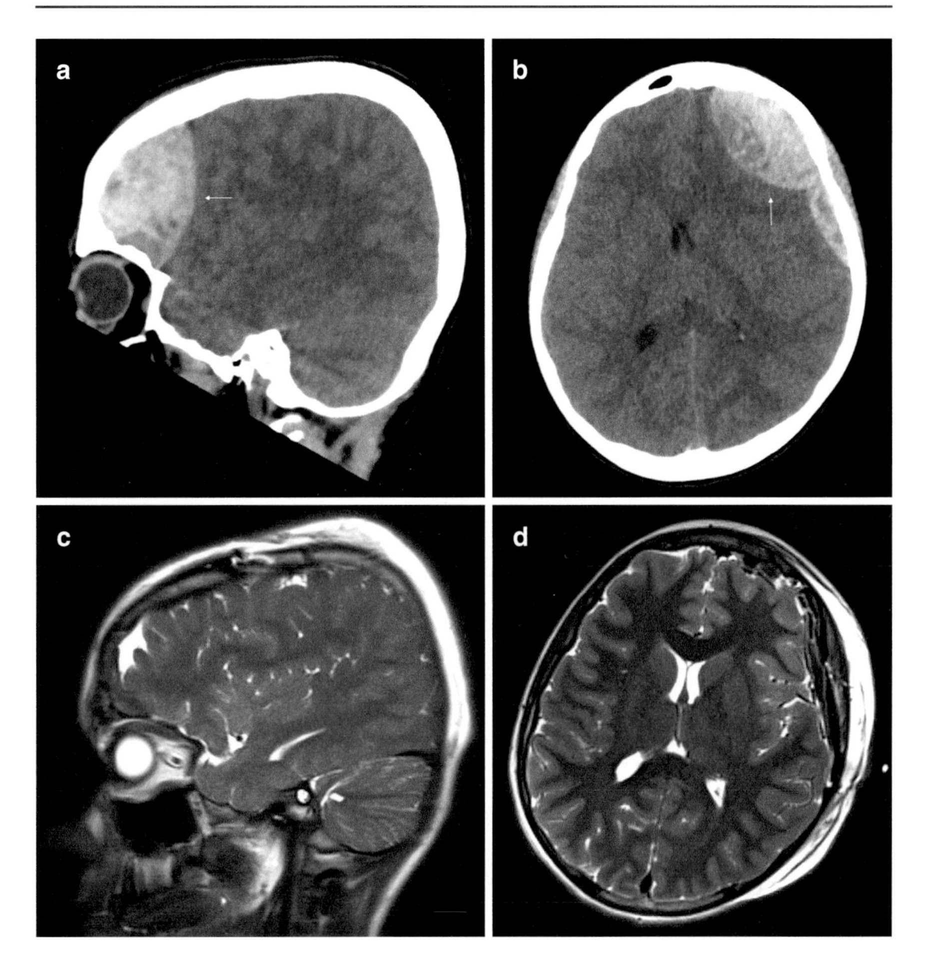

Fig. 28.1 A teenage child suffered a head strike while sledding and lost consciousness. He was brought to medical evaluation after regaining consciousness but having several episodes of emesis and was transferred for emergent surgical management after initial cranial imaging. (**a**) Sagittal non-contrast CT head demonstrates a frontal epidural hematoma (white arrow). (**b**) Axial plane of the same CT demonstrates the epidural hematoma (white arrow) and mass effect with displacement of the midline. (**c**) Sagittal T2 MRI after craniotomy for evacuation demonstrates resolution of the hematoma with trace fluid at the surgical site. (**d**) Axial plane of the same postoperative T2 MRI demonstrates the absence of epidural hematoma and the improvement of ventricular symmetry and midline course of the septum pellucidum. There is surgical site fluid visible as T2 prolongation in the extra-cranial soft tissue

Delayed hemorrhage or secondary obstructive hydrocephalus are common causes of intracranial hypertension which may indicate a need for emergent surgical intervention. In addition, edema typically progresses over several days after trauma and can cause delayed intracranial hypertension.

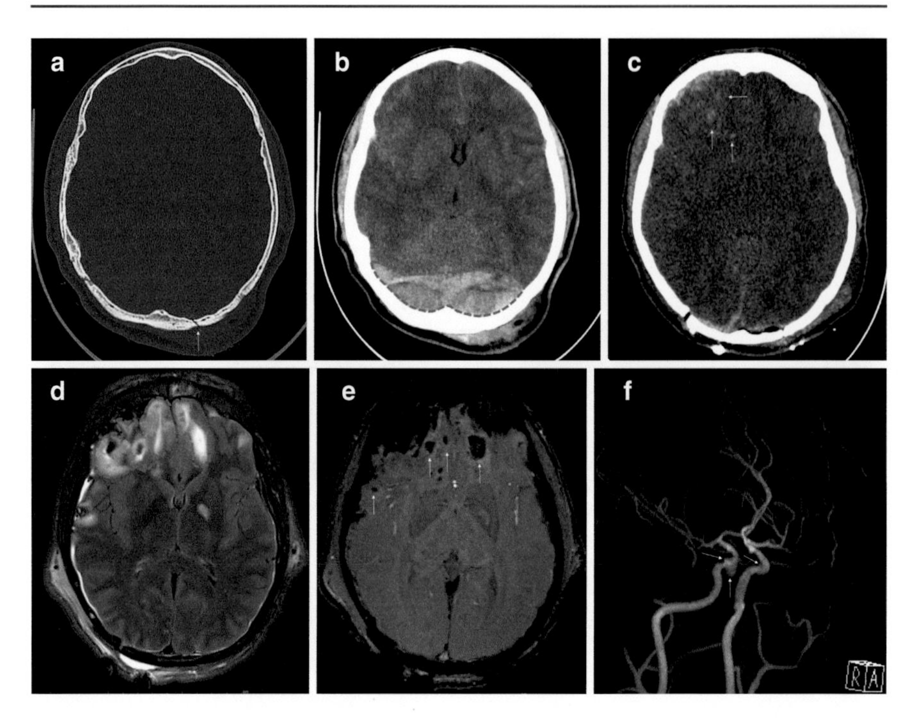

Fig. 28.2 A teenager fell from a moving vehicle with an occipital head strike, presenting with a severe TBI. Imaging reveals different components of TBI for which management involves different surgical and medical therapies. (**a**) Bone-windowing of a non-contrast CT head demonstrates a non-displaced occipital fracture (arrow). (**b**) Brain-windowing of the same CT head demonstrates an occipital epidural hematoma (blue dashed outline) requiring urgent surgical decompression and an overlying subgaleal hematoma in the soft tissue of the skin. (**c**) Postoperative non-contrast CT head demonstrates evacuation of the occipital hematoma with bilateral bone defects from the craniotomy and a small area of hypodensity from surgical site air. There is new evidence of evolving hyperdensities in the frontal lobe that are more prominent than before, consistent with parenchymal injury (white arrows). (**d**) T2 FLAIR sequence MRI brain demonstrates bifrontal right-more-than-left edema (blue dashed outline). The occipital surgical site is again visible with the right-sided extent of the craniotomy visible. (**e**) Susceptibility sequence MRI brain demonstrates areas of hemorrhage that are better defined due to the blooming effect of this sequence that amplifies signal inhomogeneity and increases sensitivity. (**f**) Three-dimensional reconstruction of a time-of-flight MR angiographic sequence. This slightly rotated view demonstrates both internal carotid arteries. The white arrows indicate areas of irregularity within the cavernous carotid. On one ICA, there is circumferential irregularity of the lumen both ventrally and dorsally, a dissection and pseudoaneurysm of the carotid. The other carotid has a small (submillimeter) dorsal irregularity which may be also a sequela of the trauma. He suffered post-traumatic seizures and multifocal infarcts from a traumatic cerebrovascular dissection. At 1 year, he had recovered his motor deficits and was able to resume work

28.1.7 Overall Management

Systemic derangements after severe TBI can alter the in-hospital trajectory as well as longer-term functional outcomes and therefore require careful management [13]. Many of these treatment decisions are implemented in the acute and early stages of management, often in the context of a multidisciplinary team with a protocolized pathway [14–16].

An expert panel with participants from critical care medicine, pediatric medicine, neurology, neurological surgery, epidemiology, and medical informatics, convened by the Brain Trauma Foundation, American Association of Neurological Surgeons, Congress of Neurological Surgeons, and Department of Defense, developed updated guidelines in 2019 based on evidence available at the time [16, 17]. Since that guideline statement, the Approaches and Decisions in Acute Pediatric TBI Trial (ADAPT) has reported new data in a cohort of about 1000 children with TBI.

While there are excellent resources and protocols in existence, the realities of patient care may often be very different. Often there remains significant variability in the management of TBI between institutions, particularly in pediatric TBI [18].

28.2 TBI Management

28.2.1 Areas of Consensus

Despite the paucity of prospective or controlled trials in severe TBI in children, there is expert consensus in areas based on both extrapolation from adult data and support from retrospective data. In certain circumstances, the management in children is adapted from adult severe TBI data based on pediatric-specific physiology.

Based on this, there is relative consensus on a number of management techniques:

- Initial assessment and communication of extent of injury should include component analysis of the GCS, which aids in both prognosis and team communication [3].
- Intracranial pressure (ICP) monitoring can guide medical and surgical management in aiming for a goal of less than 20 mmHg.
- Outcomes of ICP monitoring with a parenchymal monitor or an external ventricular drain are comparable. An EVD may provide an additional mechanism for managing ICP via drainage of cerebrospinal fluid [19].
- Cerebral perfusion pressure (CPP), as a calculated estimate based on ICP monitoring and systemic blood pressure monitoring, should have a goal of greater than 40 mm Hg, and potentially 50 mm Hg in adolescents.
- Hyperosmolar therapy can be an effective means of reducing elevated ICP to improve outcomes. There is increasing evidence that hypertonic saline, such as bolus or infusion dosing of 3% or boluses of 23.4%, may be more effective than mannitol [20].
- Sedation may be used in conjunction with other modes of ICP management, although studies have not been adequately controlled to identify medications such as fentanyl and midazolam as effective in altering ICP beyond achieving appropriate analgesia and sedation for a patient receiving medical interventions [21, 22]. There is also ongoing debate about whether certain agents may alter brain perfusion in an unfavorable fashion even while lowering ICP [23].

- Seizure prophylaxis is appropriate during the first 7 days after injury. There is no specific evidence to support a particular regimen of anti-seizure medication.
- Normothermia is an appropriate target for initial management after severe TBI in children. Hypothermia in a prophylactic fashion, or initiated within 8 h after injury, may increase mortality without evidence for improving neurologic outcomes.
- Surgical decompression, such as by craniectomy sometimes requiring excision of injured tissue, is a viable method of addressing elevated ICP, although the impact on mortality and outcomes is less certain [24–26].

28.3 Areas of Growing Evidence

28.3.1 Biomarkers

Molecular biomarkers in TBI have been studied for decades [27–29]. Radiologic findings do not capture the full extent of pathology or pathophysiology in TBI [30]. Furthermore, symptoms and patient report may not capture the ongoing physiological impact of TBI during recovery and may underrepresent the extent of injury [31]. Potential applications for molecular biomarkers range from assessment of mild brain injury that may otherwise involve a heterogeneous clinical presentation, to prognostication of severe brain injury, to more precise participant selection in research studies of neuroprotection [27]. Beyond the obvious attributes of sensitivity and specificity, several key attributes determine the practical application of a biomarker [32]:

- Volume of distribution: This can determine how accessible the biomarker is, such as for salivary, serum, urine, or cerebrospinal fluid sampling.
- Temporal distribution: This can determine if it is useful for early diagnostic characterization, delayed prognostication, etc. Most commonly used within 3–24 hours after injury.
- Temporal trend: This is a further nuance of how a biomarker changes after a specific insult and how it correlates with recovery.
- Mechanistic association: This is particularly important as it may determine the role of a biomarker in measuring treatment or recovery, or as a determinant of severity of injury.
- Multiple test availability: This is important for validation and reliability.

Logistical aspects such as availability of the test can also limit appropriate inclusion of biomarkers into guideline recommendations by professional societies, scientific organizations, and patient advocacy groups. Single manufacturer or limited supply chain pathways can limit reliable access to tests, and entry to the North American healthcare market involves significant regulatory barriers [33]. Biomarker development in other clinical areas has required significant coordinated investment by industry, academia, patient advocates, and regulatory agencies.

Particular concerns for pediatric TBI biomarkers include validation across different stages of brain and neurologic development, which is impacted by age and biologic sex [34, 35].

Biomarker development in children has a slight bias toward mild TBI and sports injuries. Only about 1 in 5 studies specifically evaluated a biomarker for severe TBI in children [36]. Many studies combine children with different injuries, but the mixture of different severities in a study may actually complicate mechanistic understanding, since different injuries have been found to have different effects on some circulating biomarkers [37]. Although S100B, neuron-specific enolase (NSE), ubiquitin C-terminal hydrolase (UCH-L1), and glial fibrillary acid protein (GFAP) are the most commonly studied serum biomarkers, many of these studies included mild TBI cohorts. Furthermore, S100B may be non-specific to brain injury and may have a lower signal-to-noise ratio in children due to age-related variability in normal levels [38–40]. NSE is susceptible to overestimation due to high circulating levels in red blood cells from the serological sample [41]. UCH-L1 and αII-spectrin breakdown product 145 kDa (SBDP1445) are neuron-specific and are released from the intracellular compartment after neuronal injury. UCH-L1 may also require disruption of the blood–brain barrier for systemic distribution [42]. UCH-L1, SBDP1445, and osteopontin (OPN) are altered in severe TBI [43–45]. One ongoing clinical trial for biomarkers in pediatric severe TBI is reported in ClinicalTrials.gov [46].

There is currently one serological biomarker (Brain Trauma Indicator, Banyan Biomarkers, Inc., approved February 13, 2018) for use in adults to assess the utility of CT scan after mild TBI. This enzyme-linked immunosorbent assay semiquantitatively measures ubiquitin C-terminal hydrolase-L1 (UCH-L1) and glial fibrillary acidic protein (GFAP) that are detected serologically within 12 h of injury and predicts CT results, with results in 3–4 h. If the level of either protein is greater than threshold (327 pg/mL UCH-L1, or 22 pg/mL GFAP), then the test is considered positive and is associated with acute lesions on head CT. The clinical utility of this biomarker is to reduce the use of cranial CT imaging in trauma patients. There is no approved biomarker for TBI in children or for severe TBI.

28.3.2 Thrombosis

In children who suffer TBI, venous thromboembolism (VTE) occurs in approximately 4.6 per 1000 hospitalizations, which is more than four-fold higher than in general pediatric hospitalizations, although still less than half the rate of adult inpatients [47]. About 44% of these may be associated with central venous catheterization. VTE tends to be associated with children 15 years and older, and with orthopedic or cranial surgeries, and accrue at a marginal risk of approximately 2% increase per day of hospitalization.

In North American practice, providers are implementing VTE prophylaxis in about 30% of children 12 and older within 48 h, and compared to those with other types of trauma, TBI patients may be less likely to receive pharmacoprophylaxis

[48]. There may be potential to improve outcomes through standardization by evaluating VTE risk and applying VTE prophylaxis accordingly [49].

One example of a pediatric TBI VTI risk-assessment tool (risk of clots in kids with trauma score, Yen 2016 [49])			
Factor	Score	Total score	Risk
Age		Ranges 0–23	Ranges 0–9%
0–12	0	>14	>1%
13–15	2	>16	>2%
16–21	4	>20	>5%
ISS			
0–8	0		
9–24	5		
25–75	7		
GCS			
9–15	0		
3–8	1		
Blood transfusion	2		
Intubation	4		
Major surgery	5		

In the absence of a widely adopted and easily applied risk-assessment tool, there remains variability in identifying age thresholds for routine post-TBI pharmacoprophylaxis, although the variations all fall in the early teenage years [50–52]. However, there have been fewer studies on the adverse effects of enoxaparin in children than in adults, and this may merit further follow-up monitoring as its application increases.

28.3.3 Response to Cerebral Perfusion Pressure

Although there is an age-dependent target for CPP, aside from control of ICP there is less clear evidence of the means by which to achieve the goal CPP. Calculated CPP does not account for cerebrovascular autoregulation, but is rather a surrogate measure to achieve adequate cerebral flow to match cerebral metabolic demand. Autoregulation is thought to function over a more limited range in children than in adults. Further alteration of autoregulation may occur in the setting of TBI and may be prognostic and may also increase the difficulty of matching blood flow to metabolic demand [11, 53–55].

In addition to the overall approach, nuances in management may have implications for cerebral blood flow and brain tissue oxygenation, potentially in either a congruent or incongruent fashion [56]. Aside from lowering the ICP, there remain several different options to improve CPP, with limited evidence on the comparative long-term benefit of each.

28.4 Areas of Uncertainty

28.4.1 Assessment

The GCS is a well-established and widely understood clinical scale for consciousness, having been applied to adult Advanced Trauma Life Support in 1980 and further adapted and validated in the care of children [3, 57–59]. In the research context, there are ongoing evolutions in the documentation of nuanced scores in settings where some components are not evaluable, such as verbal function in an intubated patient, or medically inappropriate due to neuromuscular blockade. Aside from considerations of appropriately grouping patients for better treatment and study design, GCS inadequately predicts prognosis; patients with the same score may have very different outcomes [6]. The evaluation and communication of neurological status following severe brain injury may be augmented by new clinical scales accounting for early clinical features. For example, the prognosis for higher and lower likelihood of poor outcomes may be improved with adjunctive metrics such as pupil reactivity [5, 6, 60, 61]. It remains unclear whether these will be broadly applied or implemented in standard protocols.

28.4.2 Invasive Brain Neuromonitoring

Advanced neuromonitoring has been studied in small series at single sites. In the research context there may be a number of markers that can be evaluated through neuromonitoring. However, in studying the clinical application of advanced neuromonitoring, most studies have used brain tissue oxygen ($PbrO_2$). However, there are a number of potential approaches to application. Some analyze absolute levels of $PbrO_2$, while others evaluate responsiveness of $PbrO_2$ to PaO_2. Mixed results in these studies in children demonstrate that there is not a good understanding of how to optimally use $PbrO_2$ in the care of severe pediatric TBI.

28.4.3 Hypothermia

There have been several prospective, multinational, randomized research studies into the neuroprotective effect of hypothermia after severe TBI. Unfortunately, despite optimism regarding its effect on ICP, the complications associated with this intervention have been significant [62–64]. The negative results of these studies were met with a number of editorial responses citing the preclinical scientific mechanisms, as well as meta-analyses of studies in adults. In summary, the current evidence does not support the application of prophylactic hypothermia for children with severe TBI. The difference in response to hypothermia seen in hypoxic or ischemic injury, such as in cardiac arrest, may derive from underlying pathophysiologic differences, such as the temporal course of neuronal injury and death.

28.4.4 Recovery

Long-term prognostication of outcome remains challenging, and this is a key limitation in counseling families after injury. Although it is known that there are significant rates of morbidity and dependency, there are subsets of children who recover to independence. Neurological rehabilitation programs often admit children with disordered consciousness, such as vegetative or minimally conscious states. Recovery of consciousness within the first months of rehabilitation tends to suggest potential for further improvement, potentially to the level of independence [65, 66]. In the absence of recovery by a year, significant impairment may be expected [67]. Different groups have found variable results when testing characteristics that may be observed earlier in the course of severe TBI, such as time to follow commands or post-traumatic amnesia [68, 69]. However, findings from mild TBI may not extrapolate to severe TBI. Furthermore, newer characterization of trajectories of recovery may begin to explain some of the divergent outcomes observed in small cohorts who have been previously reported [70].

28.5 Conclusion

Although the acute management of severe TBI in children is based on a strong consensus of expert opinion, there is limited information on the longer-term impact of management decisions. This includes limited prognostic ability beyond the apparent severity of the initial injury, as evaluated by a decade-old bedside metric, the GCS. We continue to have limited understanding of the biological mechanisms unique to each patient that determine clinical management responses, and we continue to rely primarily on ICP and CPP, although monitoring of regional blood flow and tissue oxygenation might be equally relevant. Although there have been advances in the care of adults with severe TBI, not all of these have been further validated in children, where neurodevelopmental changes create a variable physiologic environment. Over time, with advances in critical care monitoring that can more easily monitor and integrate all the physiological variables with appropriate treatment algorithms, we expect to see advances in the management of pediatric severe TBI.

References

1. GBD 2016 Traumatic Brain Injury and Spinal Cord Injury Collaborators. Global, regional, and national burden of traumatic brain injury and spinal cord injury, 1990-2016: a systematic analysis for the global burden of disease study 2016. Lancet Neurol. 2019;18(1):56–87.
2. Yue JK, Upadhyayula PS, Avalos LN, Cage TA. Pediatric traumatic brain injury in the United States: rural-urban disparities and considerations. Brain Sci. 2020;10(3):135.
3. Murphy S, Thomas NJ, Gertz SJ, Beca J, Luther JF, Bell MJ, et al. Tripartite stratification of the Glasgow coma scale in children with severe traumatic brain injury and mortality: an analysis from a multi-center comparative effectiveness study. J Neurotrauma. 2017;34(14):2220–9.

4. Van de Voorde P, Sabbe M, Rizopoulos D, Tsonaka R, De Jaeger A, Lesaffre E, et al. Assessing the level of consciousness in children: a plea for the Glasgow coma motor subscore. Resuscitation. 2008;76(2):175–9.
5. Brennan PM, Murray GD, Teasdale GM. Simplifying the use of prognostic information in traumatic brain injury. Part 1: the GCS-pupils score: an extended index of clinical severity. J Neurosurg. 2018;128(6):1612–20.
6. Fulkerson DH, White IK, Rees JM, Baumanis MM, Smith JL, Ackerman LL, et al. Analysis of long-term (median 10.5 years) outcomes in children presenting with traumatic brain injury and an initial Glasgow coma scale score of 3 or 4. J Neurosurg Pediatr. 2015;16(4):410–9.
7. Chen C, Peng J, Sribnick EA, Zhu M, Xiang H. Trend of age-adjusted rates of pediatric traumatic brain injury in U.S. emergency departments from 2006 to 2013. Int J Environ Res Public Health. 2018;15(6):1171.
8. Waltzman D, Womack LS, Thomas KE, Sarmiento K. Trends in emergency department visits for contact sports-related traumatic brain injuries among children—United States, 2001-2018. MMWR Morb Mortal Wkly Rep. 2020;69(27):870–4.
9. Sarmiento K, Haileyesus T, Waltzman D, Daugherty J. Emergency department visits for bicycle-related traumatic brain injuries among children and adults—United States, 2009-2018. MMWR Morb Mortal Wkly Rep. 2021;70(19):693–7.
10. Baller EB, Valcarcel AM, Adebimpe A, Alexander-Bloch A, Cui Z, Gur RC, et al. Developmental coupling of cerebral blood flow and fMRI fluctuations in youth. Cell Rep. 2022;38(13):110576.
11. Freeman SS, Udomphorn Y, Armstead WM, Fisk DM, Vavilala MS. Young age as a risk factor for impaired cerebral autoregulation after moderate to severe pediatric traumatic brain injury. Anesthesiology. 2008;108(4):588–95.
12. Fraunberger E, Esser MJ. Neuro-inflammation in pediatric traumatic brain injury-from mechanisms to inflammatory networks. Brain Sci. 2019;9(11):319.
13. McCredie VA, Alali AS, Scales DC, Rubenfeld GD, Cuthbertson BH, Nathens AB. Impact of ICU structure and processes of care on outcomes after severe traumatic brain injury: a multicenter cohort study. Crit Care Med. 2018;46(7):1139–49.
14. Alali AS, McCredie VA, Mainprize TG, Gomez D, Nathens AB. Structure, process, and culture of intensive care units treating patients with severe traumatic brain injury: survey of centers participating in the American College of Surgeons trauma quality improvement program. J Neurotrauma. 2017;34(19):2760–7.
15. Lujan S, Petroni G, Castellani P, Bollada S, Bell MJ, Velonjara J, et al. The status of quality improvement programs for pediatric traumatic brain injury care in Argentina. J Surg Res. 2021;265:71–8.
16. Kochanek PM, Tasker RC, Bell MJ, Adelson PD, Carney N, Vavilala MS, et al. Management of pediatric severe traumatic brain injury: 2019 consensus and guidelines-based algorithm for first and second tier therapies. Pediatr Crit care Med. 2019;20(3):269–79.
17. Kochanek PM, Tasker RC, Carney N, Totten AM, Adelson PD, Selden NR, et al. Guidelines for the management of pediatric severe traumatic brain injury, third edition: update of the brain trauma foundation guidelines, executive summary. Neurosurgery. 2019;84(6):1169–78.
18. Larsen GY, Schober M, Fabio A, Wisniewski SR, Grant MJC, Shafi N, et al. Structure, process, and culture differences of pediatric trauma centers participating in an international comparative effectiveness study of children with severe traumatic brain injury. Neurocrit Care. 2016;24(3):353–60.
19. Bell MJ, Rosario BL, Kochanek PM, Adelson PD, Morris KP, Au AK, et al. Comparative effectiveness of diversion of cerebrospinal fluid for children with severe traumatic brain injury. JAMA Netw Open. 2022;5(7):e2220969.
20. Kochanek PM, Adelson PD, Rosario BL, Hutchison J, Miller Ferguson N, Ferrazzano P, et al. Comparison of intracranial pressure measurements before and after hypertonic saline or mannitol treatment in children with severe traumatic brain injury. JAMA Netw Open. 2022;5(3):e220891.

21. Welch TP, Wallendorf MJ, Kharasch ED, Leonard JR, Doctor A, Pineda JA. Fentanyl and midazolam are ineffective in reducing episodic intracranial hypertension in severe pediatric traumatic brain injury. Crit Care Med. 2016;44(4):809–18.
22. Shein SL, Ferguson NM, Kochanek PM, Bayir H, Clark RSB, Fink EL, et al. Effectiveness of pharmacological therapies for intracranial hypertension in children with severe traumatic brain injury—results from an automated data collection system time-synched to drug administration. Pediatr Crit Care Med. 2016;17(3):236–45.
23. Bar-Joseph G, Guilburd Y, Tamir A, Guilburd JN. Effectiveness of ketamine in decreasing intracranial pressure in children with intracranial hypertension. J Neurosurg Pediatr. 2009;4(1):40–6.
24. Josan VA, Sgouros S. Early decompressive craniectomy may be effective in the treatment of refractory intracranial hypertension after traumatic brain injury. Childs Nerv Syst. 2006;22(10):1268–74.
25. Taylor A, Butt W, Rosenfeld J, Shann F, Ditchfield M, Lewis E, et al. A randomized trial of very early decompressive craniectomy in children with traumatic brain injury and sustained intracranial hypertension. Childs Nerv Syst. 2001;17(3):154–62.
26. Thomale UW, Graetz D, Vajkoczy P, Sarrafzadeh AS. Severe traumatic brain injury in children--a single center experience regarding therapy and long-term outcome. Childs Nerv Syst. 2010;26(11):1563–73.
27. Shore PM, Berger RP, Varma S, Janesko KL, Wisniewski SR, Clark RSB, et al. Cerebrospinal fluid biomarkers versus Glasgow coma scale and Glasgow outcome scale in pediatric traumatic brain injury: the role of young age and inflicted injury. J Neurotrauma. 2007;24(1):75–86.
28. Berger RP, Pierce MC, Wisniewski SR, Adelson PD, Clark RSB, Ruppel RA, et al. Neuron-specific enolase and S100B in cerebrospinal fluid after severe traumatic brain injury in infants and children. Pediatrics. 2002;109(2):E31.
29. Lo TYM, Jones PA, Minns RA. Pediatric brain trauma outcome prediction using paired serum levels of inflammatory mediators and brain-specific proteins. J Neurotrauma. 2009;26(9):1479–87.
30. Keightley ML, Sinopoli KJ, Davis KD, Mikulis DJ, Wennberg R, Tartaglia MC, et al. Is there evidence for neurodegenerative change following traumatic brain injury in children and youth? A scoping review. Front Hum Neurosci. 2014;8:139.
31. Kamins J, Bigler E, Covassin T, Henry L, Kemp S, Leddy JJ, et al. What is the physiological time to recovery after concussion? A systematic review. Br J Sports Med. 2017;51(12):935–40.
32. Wang KK, Yang Z, Zhu T, Shi Y, Rubenstein R, Tyndall JA, et al. An update on diagnostic and prognostic biomarkers for traumatic brain injury. Expert Rev Mol Diagn. 2018;18(2):165–80.
33. Khleif SN, Doroshow JH, Hait WN. AACR-FDA-NCI cancer biomarkers collaborative consensus report: advancing the use of biomarkers in cancer drug development. Clin cancer Res. 2010;16(13):3299–318.
34. Miskovic V, Ma X, Chou CA, Fan M, Owens M, Sayama H, et al. Developmental changes in spontaneous electrocortical activity and network organization from early to late childhood. NeuroImage. 2015;118:237–47.
35. Gozdas E, Holland SK, Altaye M. Developmental changes in functional brain networks from birth through adolescence. Hum Brain Mapp. 2019;40(5):1434–44.
36. Marzano LAS, Batista JPT, de Abreu AM, de Freitas Cardoso MG, de Barros JLVM, Moreira JM, et al. Traumatic brain injury biomarkers in pediatric patients: a systematic review. Neurosurg Rev. 2022;45(1):167–97.
37. Sorokina EG, Semenova ZB, Reutov VP, Arsenieva EN, Karaseva OV, Fisenko AP, et al. Brain biomarkers in children after mild and severe traumatic brain injury. Acta Neurochir Suppl. 2021;131:103–7.
38. Undén J, Bellner J, Eneroth M, Alling C, Ingebrigtsen T, Romner B. Raised serum S100B levels after acute bone fractures without cerebral injury. J Trauma. 2005;58(1):59–61.
39. Anderson RE, Hansson LO, Nilsson O, Dijlai-Merzoug R, Settergren G. High serum S100B levels for trauma patients without head injuries. Neurosurgery. 2001;48(6):1255–60.

40. Gazzolo D, Michetti F, Bruschettini M, Marchese N, Lituania M, Mangraviti S, et al. Pediatric concentrations of S100B protein in blood: age- and sex-related changes. Clin Chem. 2003;49(6 Pt 1):967–70.
41. Tolan NV, Vidal-Folch N, Algeciras-Schimnich A, Singh RJ, Grebe SKG. Individualized correction of neuron-specific enolase (NSE) measurement in hemolyzed serum samples. Clin Chim Acta. 2013;424:216–21.
42. Blyth BJ, Farahvar A, He H, Nayak A, Yang C, Shaw G, et al. Elevated serum ubiquitin carboxy-terminal hydrolase L1 is associated with abnormal blood-brain barrier function after traumatic brain injury. J Neurotrauma. 2011;28(12):2453–62.
43. Berger RP, Hayes RL, Richichi R, Beers SR, Wang KKW. Serum concentrations of ubiquitin C-terminal hydrolase-L1 and αII-spectrin breakdown product 145 kDa correlate with outcome after pediatric TBI. J Neurotrauma. 2012;29(1):162–7.
44. Metzger RR, Sheng X, Niedzwecki CM, Bennett KS, Morita DC, Zielinski B, et al. Temporal response profiles of serum ubiquitin C-terminal hydrolase-L1 and the 145-kDa alpha II-spectrin breakdown product after severe traumatic brain injury in children. J Neurosurg Pediatr. 2018;22(4):369–74.
45. Gao N, Zhang-Brotzge X, Wali B, Sayeed I, Chern JJ, Blackwell LS, et al. Plasma osteopontin may predict neuroinflammation and the severity of pediatric traumatic brain injury. J Cereb blood flow Metab. 2020;40(1):35–43.
46. Ducharme-Crevier L. Prediction of neurological outcome of children after a traumatic brain injury based on an integrated predictive model. ClinicalTrials.gov identifier: NCT04157634. [Internet]. https://clinicaltrials.gov/. 2019. https://clinicaltrials.gov/ct2/show/NCT04157634
47. Harris DA, Lam S. Venous thromboembolism in the setting of pediatric traumatic brain injury. J Neurosurg Pediatr. 2014;13(4):448–55.
48. Bigelow AM, Flynn-O'Brien KT, Simpson PM, Dasgupta M, Hanson SJ. Multicenter review of current practices associated with venous thromboembolism prophylaxis in pediatric patients after trauma. Pediatr Crit Care. 2018;19(9):e448–54.
49. Yen J, Van Arendonk KJ, Streiff MB, McNamara L, Stewart FD, Conner KG, et al. Risk factors for venous thromboembolism in pediatric trauma patients and validation of a novel scoring system: the risk of clots in kids with trauma score. Pediatr Crit Care. 2016;17(5):391–9.
50. Landisch RM, Hanson SJ, Cassidy LD, Braun K, Punzalan RC, Gourlay DM. Evaluation of guidelines for injured children at high risk for venous thromboembolism: a prospective observational study. J Trauma Acute Care Surg. 2017;82(5):836–44.
51. Thompson AJ, McSwain SD, Webb SA, Stroud MA, Streck CJ. Venous thromboembolism prophylaxis in the pediatric trauma population. J Pediatr Surg. 2013;48(6):1413–21.
52. Mahajerin A, Petty JK, Hanson SJ, Thompson AJ, O'Brien SH, Streck CJ, et al. Prophylaxis against venous thromboembolism in pediatric trauma: a practice management guideline from the eastern Association for the Surgery of trauma and the pediatric trauma society. J Trauma Acute Care Surg. 2017;82(3):627–36.
53. Lewis PM, Czosnyka M, Carter BG, Rosenfeld JV, Paul E, Singhal N, et al. Cerebrovascular pressure reactivity in children with traumatic brain injury. Pediatr Crit Care Med. 2015;16(8):739–49.
54. Figaji AA, Zwane E, Fieggen AG, Argent AC, Le Roux PD, Siesjo P, et al. Pressure autoregulation, intracranial pressure, and brain tissue oxygenation in children with severe traumatic brain injury. J Neurosurg Pediatr. 2009;4(5):420–8.
55. Udomphorn Y, Armstead WM, Vavilala MS. Cerebral blood flow and autoregulation after pediatric traumatic brain injury. Pediatr Neurol. 2008;38(4):225–34.
56. Friess SH, Bruins B, Kilbaugh TJ, Smith C, Margulies SS. Differing effects when using phenylephrine and norepinephrine to augment cerebral blood flow after traumatic brain injury in the immature brain. J Neurotrauma. 2015;32(4):237–43.
57. Collicott PE, Hughes I. Training in advanced trauma life support. JAMA. 1980;243(11):1156–9.
58. Raimondi AJ, Hirschauer J. Head injury in the infant and toddler. Coma scoring and outcome scale. Childs Brain. 1984;11(1):12–35.

59. Borgialli DA, Mahajan P, Hoyle JDJ, Powell EC, Nadel FM, Tunik MG, et al. Performance of the pediatric Glasgow coma scale score in the evaluation of children with blunt head trauma. Acad Emerg Med Off J Soc Acad Emerg Med. 2016;23(8):878–84.
60. Emami P, Czorlich P, Fritzsche FS, Westphal M, Rueger JM, Lefering R, et al. Impact of Glasgow coma scale score and pupil parameters on mortality rate and outcome in pediatric and adult severe traumatic brain injury: a retrospective, multicenter cohort study. J Neurosurg. 2017;126(3):760–7.
61. Balakrishnan B, VanDongen-Trimmer H, Kim I, Hanson SJ, Zhang L, Simpson PM, et al. GCS-pupil score has a stronger association with mortality and poor functional outcome than GCS alone in pediatric severe traumatic brain injury. Pediatr Neurosurg. 2021;56(5):432–9.
62. Hutchison JS, Ward RE, Lacroix J, Hébert PC, Barnes MA, Bohn DJ, et al. Hypothermia therapy after traumatic brain injury in children. N Engl J Med. 2008;358(23):2447–56.
63. Beca J, McSharry B, Erickson S, Yung M, Schibler A, Slater A, et al. Hypothermia for traumatic brain injury in children-a phase II randomized controlled trial. Crit Care Med. 2015;43(7):1458–66.
64. Adelson PD, Wisniewski SR, Beca J, Brown SD, Bell M, Muizelaar JP, et al. Comparison of hypothermia and normothermia after severe traumatic brain injury in children (cool kids): a phase 3, randomised controlled trial. Lancet Neurol. 2013;12(6):546–53.
65. Eilander HJ, Wijnen VJM, Schouten EJ, Lavrijsen JCM. Ten-to-twelve years after specialized neurorehabilitation of young patients with severe disorders of consciousness: a follow-up study. Brain Inj. 2016;30(11):1302–10.
66. Kramer ME, Suskauer SJ, Christensen JR, DeMatt EJ, Trovato MK, Salorio CF, et al. Examining acute rehabilitation outcomes for children with total functional dependence after traumatic brain injury: a pilot study. J Head Trauma Rehabil. 2013;28(5):361–70.
67. Rodgin S, Suskauer SJ, Chen J, Katz E, Davis KC, Slomine BS. Very long-term outcomes in children admitted in a disorder of consciousness after severe traumatic brain injury. Arch Phys Med Rehabil. 2021;102(8):1507–13.
68. Austin CA, Slomine BS, Dematt EJ, Salorio CF, Suskauer SJ. Time to follow commands remains the most useful injury severity variable for predicting WeeFIM® scores 1 year after paediatric TBI. Brain Inj. 2013;27(9):1056–62.
69. Suskauer SJ, Slomine BS, Inscore AB, Lewelt AJ, Kirk JW, Salorio CF. Injury severity variables as predictors of WeeFIM scores in pediatric TBI: time to follow commands is best. J Pediatr Rehabil Med. 2009;2(4):297–307.
70. Molteni E, Ranzini MBM, Beretta E, Modat M, Strazzer S. Individualized prognostic prediction of the long-term functional trajectory in pediatric acquired brain injury. J Pers Med. 2021;11(7):675.

Traumatic Brain Injury in Older Adults

29

Navpreet K. Dhillon and Mira H. Ghneim

29.1 Epidemiology

Adults 65 years and older represent the fastest growing population in the United States (U.S) [1]. In fact, by 2050, the population of older adults is expected to more than double to 80 million [2]. Currently older adults have more active lifestyles then prior generations, so are at increased risk of injury. The Centers for Disease Control and Prevention lists unintentional injuries as the seventh most common cause of death in older adults, with TBI accounting for over 150,000 cases [3, 4]. Outcomes after brain trauma can be devastating with high mortality rates and worse cognitive and functional outcomes in those who survive [5–7]. While many may be independent with activities of daily living (ADLs) prior to injury, the majority are dependent for one or more ADL after injury [8]. TBI clearly has several implications not only in this population, but for overall healthcare and related expenditures.

29.2 The Role of Aging and TBI

The unique properties and morphological changes of the aging brain makes it more susceptible to traumatic injury and worse outcomes. Parenchymal volume decreases by decade as the brain atrophies, leading to an increase in the size of the subdural space and increased mobility of the cerebral hemispheres [9]. Additionally, the dura becomes more adherent to the skull. These changes are coupled with fragile

N. K. Dhillon (✉)
Program in Trauma, University of Maryland School of Medicine, R Adams Cowley Shock Trauma Center, Baltimore, MD, USA
e-mail: navpreet.dhillon@som.umaryland.edu

M. H. Ghneim
University of Maryland School of Medicine, R Adams Cowley Shock Trauma Center, Baltimore, MD, USA
e-mail: mira.ghneim@som.umaryland.edu

E. Brogi et al. (eds.), *Traumatic Brain Injury*, Hot Topics in Acute Care Surgery and Trauma, https://doi.org/10.1007/978-3-031-50117-3_29

vascularity, which explains why certain injury types, such as subdural hematomas (SDH) and contrecoup injuries, are commonly seen, while others such as epidural hematomas (EDH) occur less frequently.

A well described central and systemic inflammatory process occurs following TBI, and a robust inflammatory response is correlated with worse outcomes. Animal models demonstrate an increased number of peripherally-derived monocytes in older animals compared to their younger counterparts in addition to an impaired anti-inflammatory response. Interestingly, knock-out mice which do not express certain inflammatory markers develop fewer deficits, implicating the role of the inflammatory response in outcomes [10]. Plasticity is imperative to recovery; alterations in signaling pathways related to plasticity can result in downstream changes that can lead to continued deficits in older patients [11]. Many older adults, not surprisingly, often have multiple baseline comorbidities including cerebrovascular disease, diabetes, hypertension, and depression [12]. In conjunction with the physiologic changes of the aging brain, these comorbidities have additional implications on survivability and overall recovery after injury.

29.3 Assessment and Considerations

Initial neurologic examinations and assessments differ in older patients when compared to their younger counterparts. While determining the Glasgow Coma Scale (GCS) score is important in TBI classification and for the assessment of injury severity, baseline dementia, cognitive function, and any visual or hearing impairments limit its use in older adults [13]. Abnormal pupillary response, which is indicative of increased intracranial pressure (ICP) and need for urgent surgical intervention [14], is often not useful in older adults. Preexisting conditions such as glaucoma and cataracts can alter the pupillary response. Additionally, with an atrophied brain, a larger volume of hemorrhage may need to be present before pupillary changes develop. Given the decreased reliability of the standard neurologic examination in this patient population, a computed tomography scan of the brain should be obtained in all older adults with suspicion for head injury [1].

29.4 Anticoagulant and Antiplatelet Agents

As the population continues to age, the number of older adults on antiplatelet and anticoagulant therapy for the treatment of atrial fibrillation, peripheral vascular disease, venous thromboembolism, and cerebrovascular disease continues to increase [15]. Commonly used antiplatelet and anticoagulant therapy include aspirin, clopidogrel, warfarin, and direct oral anticoagulants (DOACs). Prothrombin time, the international normalized ratio (INR), and thromboelastography are used to assess the effects of warfarin and antiplatelet therapy. Currently, there are no readily available laboratory tests to assess the effect of DOACs.

A primary concern in older adults with a history of antiplatelet and anticoagulant use who experience a traumatic injury is the increased risk of intracranial hemorrhage (ICH) and ICH progression. It has been reported that approximately 30% of trauma patients on preadmission anticoagulation present with ICH [16, 17]. A large prospective, multicenter study comparing outcomes after warfarin, clopidogrel, dabigatran, rivaroxaban, and apixaban by Kobayashi et al. showed that patients on aspirin had the highest rate and risk of ICH [18]. Surprisingly those on a DOAC were not at an increased risk for an ICH, progression of an ICH, or death. The rate of progression of an ICH occurred in one of five patients, irrespective of the agent involved. This study not only emphasized the high prevalence of ICH among those on antiplatelet agents and anticoagulants but also highlighted the clinical significance of aspirin, a medication commonly prescribed to older adults [19].

Recently, the Western Trauma Association developed guidelines for antiplatelet and anticoagulant reversal in trauma patients presenting with intracranial, spinal, cavitary, or extremity injury requiring surgical intervention [20]. However, practice management guidelines regarding the use of reversal agents in older adults presenting with a TBI and history of antiplatelet or anticoagulant use are lacking. The decision to administer reversal agents should be considered carefully within the given clinical context, indication for prior to admission anticoagulation, and the severity and consequences of ongoing bleeding. For example, in the setting of non-life-threatening ICH, providers may be more reluctant to reverse a patient with a mechanical valve if the perceived risk of ongoing bleeding is small. Reversal can be deferred in patients on warfarin if they have small hematomas on imaging, are neurologically intact, and with a mild elevation in their INR. However, based on the current available evidence and risk of expansion and neurological deterioration, patients with an ICH on a direct factor Xa inhibitor should be reversed [21]. On the other hand, when life-threatening ICH is identified, patients are candidates for reversal therapy.

Vitamin K or plasma can be administered to patients on warfarin, while different forms of prothrombin complex concentrate (PCC) can be used when reversing patients on warfarin, dabigatran (a direct thrombin inhibitor), or factor Xa inhibitors (apixaban and rivaroxaban). Additionally, providers should be aware of the available yet costly drug specific-reversal agents: idarucizumab (Praxbind), for dabigatran reversal and Andexanet Alfa, for factor Xa inhibitors. Platelet transfusion and desmopressin, or DDAVP, potentially can be used to mitigate the effects of antiplatelet therapy.

The literature regarding platelet transfusion is conflicting, with the PATCH trial showing worse outcomes in patients with nontraumatic ICH who received platelet transfusions [22]. The current Neurocritical Care Society and the Society of Critical Care Medicine guidelines recommend administering DDAVP to any patient with an ICH on antiplatelet therapy, and DDVAP plus platelet transfusion in patients requiring neurosurgical intervention [21].

29.5 Management Strategies in Older Adults

The principal tenant in the management of TBI in all patients, including older adults, is to prevent secondary brain injury by minimizing the incidence of post-injury hypotension and hypoxia. As mentioned previously, there are a number of changes in the aged brain that lead to lower ICPs, higher baseline cerebral perfusion pressures (CPP), and altered cerebral autoregulation. While these changes influence how prevention of the "second hit" is managed in older adults when compared to their younger counterparts, current guidelines do not specifically address the management of older adults with a TBI.

Conventionally, a systolic blood pressure (SBP) less than 90 mmHg is considered hypotensive and is associated with an increased risk of morbidity and mortality in TBI. However, this threshold does not apply to older adults who often, due to comorbidities and the physiologic changes in the cardiovascular system with aging, require higher baseline perfusion pressures. Therefore, a SBP greater than 90 mmHg may result in relative hypotension [23]. The Brain Trauma Foundation (BTF) guidelines recommend maintaining a SBP of at least 100 mmHg in patients aged 50–69 years and at least 110 mmHg in those older [24].

The role of ICP monitoring is not well defined in older adults due to the conflicting currently available data regarding improved outcomes [25–27]. As a result, the BTF guidelines do not have specific recommendations for ICP monitor use in this patient population. In fact, the only recommendation taking age into consideration is to initiate ICP monitoring with severe TBI with normal imaging in patients greater than 40 years if motor posturing is present or if the SBP is less than 90 mmHg. A recent study by Ghneim et al. of 3081 older adults presenting with an isolated TBI showed that less than 3% of patients who met BTF criteria for ICP monitoring underwent ICP monitor placement. As the utility and benefit of ICP monitoring in this patient population remains unclear, future studies that focus on clinical, patient-specific, and provider specific factors that influence the decision for ICP monitor placement is warranted [28].

If an ICP monitor is placed, the question arises about how to manage CPP, which is often used as a surrogate for cerebral blood flow (CBF) and tissue oxygenation. The current recommended CPP target for survival and favorable outcomes is between 60 and 70 mmHg [27] as higher CPPs have been associated with increased cardiopulmonary complications. The applicability of these guidelines to older adults is unknown due to the lack of studies that directly address CPP and outcomes in this population [1]. Additionally, as CBF and vascular reactivity decrease with aging, the changes seen in cerebral autoregulation with aging are not well understood. Recommendations regarding CPP management are not age-specific; identifying optimal CPP goals in older adults with TBI requires further investigation.

The BTF guidelines make recommendations regarding surgical intervention for the management of SDH and EDH based on size and clinical examination. These current guidelines are based on studies that fail to address age or any frailty markers as factors in selecting patients for operative intervention and often exclude older adults from the analysis. In older adults, due to cerebral atrophy, intracranial lesion size is not a valid indication for operative intervention. Additionally, these patients often harbor large mass lesions with relatively little mass effect because of the increased intracranial space rendering the clinical exam unreliable [1]. There is sparse literature addressing when surgical intervention is most beneficial in geriatric patients. Based on a single-center retrospective study, Petridis et al. conclude that older patients with a GCS score below 8 and bilateral pupillary abnormalities should not be surgically intervened given their poor prognosis [29]. Although we cannot make such recommendations, the study lends some insight into this matter. Recommendations for neurosurgical intervention should be based on a patient's baseline comorbidities, functional status, clinical and injury characteristics, neurosurgery evaluation, and goals of care.

29.6 Outcomes and Prognostication

Mortality, cognitive, and functional outcomes following TBI are worse in older adults compared to their younger counterparts. Factors such as age, admission GCS, Charlson Comorbidity Index, head Abbreviated Injury Scale score, and Injury Severity Score may predict mortality in this patient population [1]. Older adults are more likely to value function, independence, and freedom from symptoms over longevity, therefore the topic of prognostication becomes vitally important in this population after brain injury.

When compared to a younger patient with mild TBI, older patients have worse functional and cognitive outcomes with the same degree of injury [30]. However, the differences in outcomes may be minimized with rehabilitation. A prospective study involving four Level I trauma centers by Mosenthal et al. investigated patients with mild TBI and showed negligible differences in Functional Independence Measures scores with rehabilitation, suggesting that rehabilitation is instrumental in improving functional outcomes [7]. In contrast, severe TBI is associated with double the mortality rate in older patients compared to their younger counterparts [6]. As expected, outcomes in older adults with severe injury are worse but difficult to predict. Providers may be tempted to use neurologic status during the early hospital course as a surrogate for long-term prognosis, but this notion was invalidated by a retrospective, single-center study conducted by Lilley et al. where no difference in 12-month survival was observed based on change in neurologic status at 72 h from admission [8].

In addition to severity of the intracranial injury, age, baseline health status and physical function, and frailty should be considered during prognostication. It has been reported that between 44% and 78% of older adults are frail at the time of injury with a 15%–50% associated increased risk of mortality. Poor preinjury physical function is associated with 30% higher mortality and 50% worse physical function 1 year after injury [1].

Tools and scoring systems are often used to aid with prognostication. The applicability of these tools in older populations are variable. Presenting GCS does not reflect degree of injury in older adults [31], and thus tools that incorporate presenting GCS should be questioned. Other models, often validated in younger patients, should be used with caution in this subgroup [32]. The Palliative Performance Scale, which assesses functional performance and palliative care needs in seriously ill patients, shows promise as a prognostic tool in older trauma patients. This scale provides a score between 0 and 100. In a single-center study of geriatric trauma patients admitted to an ICU, those with a palliative performance scale score less than 80 had almost three times higher in-hospital mortality and eight times higher risk of discharge to dependent care [1].

29.7 Goals of Care Discussions and Palliative Care

In settings where dismal prognosis is certain or ongoing care would be inconsistent with the patient's wishes, it is reasonable to consider a thorough goals of care discussion with the individuals who are close to the patient. As mentioned previously in this chapter, prognostication after brain trauma is not a simple matter and initial clinical status does not necessarily reflect long-term prognosis. Furthermore, there is little consensus among providers regarding what constitutes a poor neurologic status [33].

Older adults with TBI have special palliative care needs, given the acute onset of injury and the devastating toll that the brain trauma has on the patient and family. Helping patients and families navigate the prognostic uncertainty with either recovery or end-of-life care involves challenges that make palliative care an essential component of the treatment plan. The majority of older patients make medical decisions based on benefits or burdens of treatment, and quality of life rather than quantity. Many will forego life-sustaining interventions if these will not result in improved functional or cognitive outcomes. Therefore, early structured palliative care consultation, identifying a healthcare proxy, determining the presence of advance directives within 24 h, and setting up a family meeting to discuss goals of care discussion within 72 h have resulted in earlier goals of care consensus and lower use of nonbeneficial life support [1].

In the event that de-escalation of care is deemed appropriate, it is imperative to involve individuals who are close to the patient and review any advanced directives, if they exist. Discussions regarding appropriateness of undergoing potentially invasive and life-sustaining measures including tracheostomy and/or feeding tube placement are imperative. Additional discussions should be held about what to do in the event the patient requires prolonged mechanical ventilation and is unable to be liberated from the ventilator.

29.8 Rehabilitation and Recovery

Rehabilitation plays a vital role in long-term outcomes in select older patients with brain injury. In a retrospective review of 52 individuals aged 55 years and older who were admitted to a rehabilitation unit, a substantial portion had significant functional gains and returned to home despite the severity of initial injury [34]. In another series, approximately 70% of patients admitted with mild brain injury regained functional independence after rehabilitation [7]. That being said, older patients may not fare as well as their younger counterparts after rehabilitation [35]. However, age alone does not impact functional improvement after rehabilitation

[36], suggesting that there are other factors, such as sex, that may influence outcomes after rehabilitation [37]. The benefits of rehabilitation are evident, but the optimal course of rehabilitation and specifically the role of neuro-rehabilitation are perhaps less defined in this subgroup.

29.9 Conclusion

TBI is a leading cause of trauma in older adults and is associated with an increased risk of mortality and worse cognitive and functional outcomes. Currently practice management guidelines for this patient population are lacking. Therefore, to address this important knowledge gap regarding management strategies and prognostication tools, future geriatric-centered research endeavors are warranted.

References

1. Stein DM, Kozar RA, Livingston DH, et al. Geriatric traumatic brain injury-what we know and what we don't. J Trauma Acute Care Surg. 2018;85(4):788–98. https://doi.org/10.1097/TA.0000000000001910.
2. Profile of older Americans|ACL administration for community living. https://acl.gov/aging-and-disability-in-america/data-and-research/profile-older-americans. Accessed 13 Nov 2022.
3. Fakhry SM, Shen Y, Biswas S, et al. The public health burden of geriatric trauma: analysis of 2,688,008 hospitalizations from centers for medicare and medicaid services inpatient claims. J Trauma Acute Care Surg. 2022;92(6):984–9. https://doi.org/10.1097/TA.0000000000003572.
4. Richmond R, Aldaghlas TA, Burke C, Rizzo AG, Griffen M, Pullarkat R. Age: is it all in the head? Factors influencing mortality in elderly patients with head injuries. J Trauma. 2011;71(1):E8–E11. https://doi.org/10.1097/TA.0b013e3181fbaa46.
5. Livingston DH, Lavery RF, Mosenthal AC, et al. Recovery at one year following isolated traumatic brain injury: a Western trauma association prospective multicenter trial. J Trauma. 2005;59(6):1298–304. https://doi.org/10.1097/01.ta.0000196002.03681.18; discussion 1304.
6. Mosenthal AC, Lavery RF, Addis M, et al. Isolated traumatic brain injury: age is an independent predictor of mortality and early outcome. J Trauma. 2002;52(5):907–11. https://doi.org/10.1097/00005373-200205000-00015.
7. Mosenthal AC, Livingston DH, Lavery RF, et al. The effect of age on functional outcome in mild traumatic brain injury: 6-month report of a prospective multicenter trial. J Trauma. 2004;56(5):1042–8. https://doi.org/10.1097/01.ta.0000127767.83267.33.
8. Lilley EJ, Williams KJ, Schneider EB, et al. Intensity of treatment, end-of-life care, and mortality for older patients with severe traumatic brain injury. J Trauma Acute Care Surg. 2016;80(6):998–1004. https://doi.org/10.1097/TA.0000000000001028.
9. Karibe H, Hayashi T, Narisawa A, Kameyama M, Nakagawa A, Tominaga T. Clinical characteristics and outcome in elderly patients with traumatic brain injury: for establishment of management strategy. Neurol Med Chir (Tokyo). 2017;57(8):418–25. https://doi.org/10.2176/nmc.st.2017-0058.
10. Chou A, Krukowski K, Morganti JM, Riparip LK, Rosi S. Persistent infiltration and impaired response of peripherally-derived monocytes after traumatic brain injury in the aged brain. Int J Mol Sci. 2018;19(6):E1616. https://doi.org/10.3390/ijms19061616.
11. Dj T, Furones C, Kang Y, Atkins CM. Age-dependent alterations in cAMP signaling contribute to synaptic plasticity deficits following traumatic brain injury. Neuroscience. 2013;231:231. https://doi.org/10.1016/j.neuroscience.2012.12.002.

12. Gardner RC, Dams-O'Connor K, Morrissey MR, Manley GT. Geriatric traumatic brain injury: epidemiology, outcomes, knowledge gaps, and future directions. J Neurotrauma. 2018;35(7):889–906. https://doi.org/10.1089/neu.2017.5371.
13. Rau CS, Wu SC, Chen YC, et al. Effect of age on Glasgow coma scale in patients with moderate and severe traumatic brain injury: an approach with propensity score-matched population. Int J Environ Res Public Health. 2017;14(11):1378. https://doi.org/10.3390/ijerph14111378.
14. Bullock MR, Chesnut R, Ghajar J, et al. Surgical management of traumatic parenchymal lesions. Neurosurgery. 2006;58(3 Suppl):S25–46. https://doi.org/10.1227/01.NEU.0000210365.36914.E3; discussion Si-iv.
15. Dossett LA, Riesel JN, Griffin MR, Cotton BA. Prevalence and implications of preinjury warfarin use: an analysis of the National Trauma Databank. Arch Surg. 2011;146(5):565–70. https://doi.org/10.1001/archsurg.2010.313.
16. Brewer ES, Reznikov B, Liberman RF, et al. Incidence and predictors of intracranial hemorrhage after minor head trauma in patients taking anticoagulant and antiplatelet medication. J Trauma. 2011;70(1):E1–5. https://doi.org/10.1097/TA.0b013e3181e5e286.
17. Reddy S, Sharma R, Grotts J, Ferrigno L, Kaminski S. Incidence of intracranial hemorrhage and outcomes after ground-level falls in geriatric trauma patients taking preinjury anticoagulants and antiplatelet agents. Am Surg. 2014;80(10):975–8.
18. Kobayashi L, Barmparas G, Bosarge P, et al. Novel oral anticoagulants and trauma: the results of a prospective American Association for the Surgery of Trauma multi-institutional trial. J Trauma Acute Care Surg. 2017;82(5):827–35. https://doi.org/10.1097/TA.0000000000001414.
19. O'Sullivan JW. Aspirin for the primary prevention of cardiovascular disease in the elderly. BMJ Evid Based Med. 2019;24(4):143–4. https://doi.org/10.1136/bmjebm-2018-111138.
20. Peck KA, Ley EJ, Brown CV, et al. Early anticoagulant reversal after trauma: a Western trauma association critical decisions algorithm. J Trauma Acute Care Surg. 2021;90(2):331–6. https://doi.org/10.1097/TA.0000000000002979.
21. Frontera JA, Lewin JJ, Rabinstein AA, et al. Guideline for reversal of antithrombotics in intracranial hemorrhage: a statement for healthcare professionals from the Neurocritical Care Society and Society of Critical Care Medicine. Neurocrit Care. 2016;24(1):6–46. https://doi.org/10.1007/s12028-015-0222-x.
22. Baharoglu MI, Cordonnier C, Al-Shahi Salman R, et al. Platelet transfusion versus standard care after acute stroke due to spontaneous cerebral haemorrhage associated with antiplatelet therapy (PATCH): a randomised, open-label, phase 3 trial. Lancet. 2016;387(10038):2605–13. https://doi.org/10.1016/S0140-6736(16)30392-0.
23. Brenner M, Stein DM, Hu PF, Aarabi B, Sheth K, Scalea TM. Traditional systolic blood pressure targets underestimate hypotension-induced secondary brain injury. J Trauma Acute Care Surg. 2012;72(5):1135–9. https://doi.org/10.1097/TA.0b013e31824af90b.
24. Carney N, Totten AM, O'Reilly C, et al. Guidelines for the management of severe traumatic brain injury, fourth edition. Neurosurgery. 2017;80(1):6–15. https://doi.org/10.1227/NEU.0000000000001432.
25. Shen L, Wang Z, Su Z, et al. Effects of intracranial pressure monitoring on mortality in patients with severe traumatic brain injury: a meta-analysis. PLoS One. 2016;11(12):e0168901. https://doi.org/10.1371/journal.pone.0168901.
26. Yuan Q, Wu X, Sun Y, et al. Impact of intracranial pressure monitoring on mortality in patients with traumatic brain injury: a systematic review and meta-analysis. J Neurosurg. 2015;122(3):574–87. https://doi.org/10.3171/2014.10.JNS1460.
27. Chesnut RM, Temkin N, Carney N, et al. A trial of intracranial-pressure monitoring in traumatic brain injury. N Engl J Med. 2012;367(26):2471–81. https://doi.org/10.1056/NEJMoa1207363.
28. Ghneim M, Albrecht J, Brasel K, et al. Factors associated with receipt of intracranial pressure monitoring in older adults with traumatic brain injury. Trauma Surg Acute Care Open. 2021;6(1):e000733. https://doi.org/10.1136/tsaco-2021-000733.

29. Petridis AK, Dörner L, Doukas A, Eifrig S, Barth H, Mehdorn M. Acute subdural hematoma in the elderly; clinical and CT factors influencing the surgical treatment decision. Cent Eur Neurosurg. 2009;70(2):73–8. https://doi.org/10.1055/s-0029-1224096.
30. Demetriades D, Kuncir E, Murray J, Velmahos GC, Rhee P, Chan L. Mortality prediction of head abbreviated injury score and Glasgow coma scale: analysis of 7,764 head injuries. J Am Coll Surg. 2004;199(2):216–22. https://doi.org/10.1016/j.jamcollsurg.2004.02.030.
31. Kehoe A, Rennie S, Smith JE. Glasgow coma scale is unreliable for the prediction of severe head injury in elderly trauma patients. Emerg Med J. 2015;32(8):613–5. https://doi.org/10.1136/emermed-2013-203488.
32. Staples JA, Wang J, Zaros MC, Jurkovich GJ, Rivara FP. The application of IMPACT prognostic models to elderly adults with traumatic brain injury: a population-based observational cohort study. Brain Inj. 2016;30(7):899–907. https://doi.org/10.3109/02699052.2016.1146964.
33. Turgeon AF, Lauzier F, Burns KEA, et al. Determination of neurologic prognosis and clinical decision making in adult patients with severe traumatic brain injury: a survey of Canadian intensivists, neurosurgeons, and neurologists. Crit Care Med. 2013;41(4):1086–93. https://doi.org/10.1097/CCM.0b013e318275d046.
34. Yap SGM, Chua KSG. Rehabilitation outcomes in elderly patients with traumatic brain injury in Singapore. J Head Trauma Rehabil. 2008;23(3):158–63. https://doi.org/10.1097/01.HTR.0000319932.15085.fe.
35. Flanagan SR, Hibbard MR, Riordan B, Gordon WA. Traumatic brain injury in the elderly: diagnostic and treatment challenges. Clin Geriatr Med. 2006;22(2):449–68. https://doi.org/10.1016/j.cger.2005.12.011; x.
36. Reeder KP, Rosenthal M, Lichtenberg P, Wood D. Impact of age on functional outcome following traumatic brain injury. J Head Trauma Rehabil. 1996;11:22–31. https://doi.org/10.1097/00001199-199606000-00006.
37. Graham JE, Radice-Neumann DM, Reistetter TA, Hammond FM, Dijkers M, Granger CV. Influence of sex and age on inpatient rehabilitation outcomes among older adults with traumatic brain injury. Arch Phys Med Rehabil. 2010;91(1):43–50. https://doi.org/10.1016/j.apmr.2009.09.017.

Part III

Final Considerations

Prognostication and Treatment-Limiting Decisions After Severe Traumatic Brain Injury

30

Jordan C. Petitt, Ahmed Kashkoush, and Michael L. Kelly

30.1 Introduction

Traumatic brain injury (TBI) is a major public health issue, affecting 50–60 million people per year with a global cost of approximately $400 billion annually [1]. TBI is a heterogenous disease and early measures of TBI severity have traditionally focused on levels of consciousness and neurological function. The Glasgow Coma Scale (GCS) was first developed in 1974 as a tool to assess coma and impaired consciousness in patients with brain damage. The GCS was one of the first measures of neurological function and remains an important marker of prognosis in these patients. Traditionally, patients with severe TBI are defined as having a GCS score of less than nine. They typically have worse outcomes, including prolonged unconscious or vegetative state, than patients with moderate (GCS score 9–12) or mild (GCS score 13–15) TBI.

Historically, early indicators of prognosis in severe TBI have included GCS, age, pupillary diameter and light reflex, hypotension, and CT scan features [2]. However, other parameters such as prothrombin time, hemoglobin, glucose, and various biomarkers may also have a role in determining outcomes in this patient population [3].

J. C. Petitt
Department of Neurological Surgery, Case Western Reserve University School of Medicine, MetroHealth Medical Center, Cleveland, OH, USA

A. Kashkoush
Department of Neurological Surgery, Cleveland Clinic Foundation, Cleveland, OH, USA

M. L. Kelly (✉)
Department of Neurological Surgery, Case Western Reserve University School of Medicine, MetroHealth Medical Center, Cleveland, OH, USA

Department of Neurosurgery, Case Western Reserve University School of Medicine, MetroHealth Medical Center, Cleveland, OH, USA
e-mail: mkelly4@metrohealth.org

E. Brogi et al. (eds.), *Traumatic Brain Injury*, Hot Topics in Acute Care Surgery and Trauma, https://doi.org/10.1007/978-3-031-50117-3_30

These variables have been used to create a multitude of prediction models over the past few decades to determine prognosis for a given individual and aid in clinical decision-making. The 2022 Lancet Commission on TBI concluded that despite the broad acceptance of prognostic models in TBI research, the use of these models in clinical practice is limited, which may be due to the low precision of these models in individual patients [1]. Additionally, robust prognostic models exist for moderate-to-severe TBI, but account for only 35% of the variance in outcomes [1]. Although prognostic research in TBI has come a long way, there is far more to explore. In this chapter, we describe the development of modern prognostication models in TBI and how prognostication science informs treatment-limiting decisions in patients with severe TBI.

30.2 TBI Prognostication

30.2.1 Early Models of Prognosis in Severe TBI

Early clinical prediction models in TBI began to emerge in the latter half of the 20th century. These prediction models typically revolved around age, pupillary diameter and light reflex, and eventually the GCS. With the advent of computed tomography (CT) in the 1970s, CT scan findings became another strong predictor of outcome in severe TBI. Later studies also showed that physiological variables such as hypotension were also associated with poor outcome. These five characteristics remain to this day the strongest predictors of outcome in patients with severe TBI [2].

30.2.1.1 Glasgow Coma Scale

The GCS is based on motor responsiveness, verbal performance, and eye opening. The GCS is scored from 3 to 15, with a higher score indicating less severe injury. The scale was first described in 1974 by Teasdale and Jennet as an objective measure of level of consciousness [4]. The GCS has become the most widely utilized clinical measure of severity in patients with severe TBI and is associated with long-term outcomes after severe TBI. Although it has a high degree of inter- and intra-rater reliability across various levels of experience, the GCS can be limited by acute injury factors in some patients. Prior to hospital arrival, patients with TBI might be sedated, paralyzed, and/or endotracheally intubated. These circumstances complicate instruction-based portions of the GCS and may be problematic in half of patients admitted to trauma centers. Studies have shown that patients with a GCS score of 3 have better overall outcomes than those with a score of 4 [5] because the exam in patients with a GCS score of 3 T ("T" denoting endotracheal intubation) is often confounded by other factors. Furthermore, the GCS has been shown to have poor predictive accuracy for Glasgow Outcome Scale (GOS) categories after hospital discharge [6]. Lack of reliability in initial GCS measurement is a major limitation in predicting outcome when the initial GCS score is low [2].

30.2.1.2 Age

Increased age is associated with a higher likelihood of a poor outcome in patients with severe TBI, especially when age is above 60 years. The effect of age on functional outcomes is multifactorial. Older individuals are at increased risk of medical comorbidities, polypharmacy, and frailty, which have all been associated with worse outcomes in TBI [7]. The Brain Trauma Foundation (BTF) concluded that age should be recorded as a continuous variable in prognostication study designs, and confounders such as pre-existing medical conditions should be further recorded and analyzed in patients to better understand their association with age and these comorbid conditions [2].

30.2.1.3 Pupils

Bilateral pupillary dilation and absence of pupillary light reflex are associated with poor outcome, including death, vegetative state, and/or severe disability after severe TBI. Uncal herniation from elevated intracranial pressure results in oculomotor nerve compression, causing reduced parasympathetic input to pupillary constrictor fibers, resulting in a dilated pupil. Of note, direct orbital trauma can sometimes cause a pupil to be dilated when no intracranial pathology is present. BTF guidelines specify that pupillary size greater than 4 mm can be considered dilated and that pupillary assessment should occur after reversal of hypotension and hypoxia [2].

30.2.1.4 Hypotension

Hypotension, defined as systolic blood pressure less than 90 mmHg, is known to have an association with poor outcome in TBI. Studies show hypotension to have a positive predictive value (PPV) of 67% for poor outcome and that the PPV for poor outcome increases to 79% when combined with hypoxia. Hypotensive episodes from the time of injury through intensive care unit stay are associated with poor outcome after severe TBI. In fact, a single recording of hypotension in the setting of TBI was associated with double the likelihood of mortality and marked increase in morbidity [8].

30.2.1.5 CT Scan

CT scan features are a strong early prognostic indicator for outcomes in severe TBI. The conventional classification of CT findings in severely head-injured patients was described by Gennarelli and colleagues in 1982 [9]. They described a difference between focal (extradural and subdural hematomas, intracerebral hematomas, and space-occupying contusions) and diffuse (absence of mass lesions, although small contusions without mass effect may be present) head injuries. In 1983, Lobato et al. described eight categories of head injury, subdividing patients with focal lesions [10]. In this study, it was determined that patients with pure extracerebral hematoma, single brain contusion, generalized brain swelling, and normal CT scan had significantly better outcomes compared to patients who had multiple brain contusions (either unilateral or bilateral) and patients with diffuse axonal injury (DAI). This new categorization by Lobato et al. was found to have a higher predictive value than Gennarelli's conventional categorization.

In 1991, Marshall et al. used the Traumatic Coma Data Bank (TCDB) to expand the categorization of diffuse injury to Diffuse Injury Types I–IV, taking into account signs of elevated ICP with compressed or absent basal cisterns, midline shift, and presence or absence of evacuated mass lesions [11]. The Marshall Classification was shown to have reasonable discrimination (AUC = 0.67). The BTF prognostic guidelines determined that abnormalities on initial CT examination, CT classification, compressed or absent basal cisterns, and traumatic subarachnoid hemorrhage (tSAH) are greatly associated with poor outcomes in severe TBI, with abnormalities in approximately 90% of patients who present with severe head injury. The BTF guidelines conclude that imaging provides the added benefit of identifying the need for operative intervention or ICP monitoring. However, new lesions may develop in 40% of patients with a normal CT scan on admission, which may be associated with delayed ICP elevations [2].

In 2005, using the tirilazad trials, Maas et al. developed the Rotterdam CT score [12]. Using logistic regression analysis, recursive partitioning, and internal validation with bootstrapping techniques, Maas et al. improved upon the performance of the Marshall Classification by adding intraventricular hemorrhage (IVH), tSAH, and a more detailed differentiation of mass lesions and basal cisterns to determine 6-month mortality in TBI patients (AUC = 0.77).

30.2.2 Developments in Prognostication Modeling

In the early 2000s, three systematic reviews collected and described known existing prognostic models for TBI. All three studies generally determined that prognostic models for TBI were largely lacking in quality and were not clinically practical.

In 2006, Hukkelhoven et al. examined validity of six models using four series of patients from the tirilazad trial [13], the International Selfotel Trial [14], the European Brain Injury Consortium (EBIC) survey [15], and the Traumatic Coma Data Bank (TCDB) [16]. All six models included age, pupillary reactivity, and either the GCS score or the GCS motor score, and some models included cause of injury, hypotension, hypoxia, injury severity score (ISS), and various CT scan characteristics. Discrimination in these models varied widely (AUC: 0.61–0.89) and calibration was poor in four of the six models, indicating that mortality prediction was overestimated. They concluded that models developed on baseline characteristics available on admission may provide satisfactory discrimination but poor calibration. In other words, TBI prognostication models prior to 2006 were able to separate patients with different outcomes, but the models were unable to produce unbiased estimates of the probability of outcomes. Therefore, these models could best be used for discriminative purposes such as ranking or classifying patients, but caution was needed when applying them to clinical decision-making and resource allocation [17].

In 2006, Perel et al. identified studies between 1990 and 2006 that examined at least two variables to predict any outcome in any type or severity of TBI. One hundred and two models were identified and only 7% of the models were from low- or middle-income countries (LMICs). Eighty-nine variables were included, with the most common being GCS score, age, and pupillary reactivity. Only 66% of models reported a measure of discrimination, 20% reported calibration, and only 11% were externally validated. They concluded that TBI prognostic models prior to 2006 suffered from small sample size, high variability in methodology, and limited external validity, and they lacked clinically practical application. Additionally, the authors highlighted that most trauma occurs in LMICs and that very few models were developed from these populations, thereby limiting global generalizability [18].

In 2008, Mushkudiani et al. identified all prognostic models for GOS from 1970 to 2005 for all TBI patients based on admission data. This approach differed from that of Perel et al. in that models for clinical course characteristics were excluded. This systematic review identified 31 studies, of which 24 were single-center and 22 had fewer than 500 patients. Age, GCS score, GCS motor, ISS, pupillary reactivity, and radiological characteristics were the most common prognostic variables in this study. Model validity was completed in 15 of the 31 studies, and only four studies were externally validated. Furthermore, although GOS was the primary endpoint in all studies, GOS outcomes were dichotomized inconsistently across studies. Discrimination was reported in 20 studies, while calibration was reported in five studies. The authors concluded that sample sizes of prognostic modeling studies in TBI prior to 2005 were too small to create valid prognostic models, and the generalizability of these models was limited by predominance of a single-center design and the absence of external validation [19].

The common theme described by these systematic reviews is the low methodological quality of TBI prognostication studies prior to 2006. Small sample sizes, single-center studies, varying statistical approaches, lack of performance assessment, little external validation, and lack of generalizability plagued these investigations and made these earlier models clinically problematic. Prognostic modeling on small samples provides limited power to identify predictive variables needed to create a precise model. Hukkelhoven et al. observed increased model performance once single-center models were refitted to the large multicenter tirilazad patient population [17]. Proposed future avenues for TBI prognostication included larger sample sizes that reflect the inherent heterogeneity of TBI, more powerful and precisely defined predictor variables, calibration and discrimination assessment, internal validation with bootstrapping, external validation on patients different in time and/or place, increased LMIC representation, statistical imputation for missing data, precisely defined outcomes, and an improved presentation format.

30.3 Current Status of Prognostication Models in TBI

Because of the state of prognostication studies in TBI in the early 2000s, large methodological changes were required to create more clinically relevant research that could aid in clinical decision-making. The Medical Research Council (MRC) Corticosteroid Randomization After Significant Head Injury (CRASH) Trial in 2008 and the International Mission for Prognosis and Analysis of Clinical Trials in

TBI (IMPACT) project created TBI prognostication models with larger sample sizes, improved validation, and extended modeling.

The CRASH trial was the largest clinical trial conducted in patients with TBI. Within 8 h of injury, 10,008 TBI patients with GCS score ≤ 14 were prospectively enrolled. Outcomes were based on GOS and included death, unfavorable outcome (death, vegetative state, severe disability), and favorable outcome (moderate disability or good recovery) at 6 months. Prognostic variables had standardized definitions and included age, sex, cause of injury, time from injury to randomization, GCS score at randomization, pupillary reactivity, CT results, presence of major extracranial injury, and level of income in the subject's country. A basic model and CT model were created, internal validity was assessed with bootstrap resampling, and external validity was assessed in an external cohort of 8,509 patients with moderate and severe TBI from 11 studies from the IMPACT project.

In the basic model, predictors included age, GCS score, pupillary reactivity, and major extracranial injury. GCS was found to be the strongest predictor of outcome in LMICs, age was the strongest predictor in high-income countries, and absence of pupillary reactivity was third strongest predictor in both regions. The CT model used predictors in the basic model in addition to petechial hemorrhages, third ventricle/basal cistern obliteration, SAH, midline shift (MLS), and non-evacuated hematoma. Obliteration of the third ventricle and MLS were the strongest predictors of mortality at 14 days, while non-evacuated hematoma was the strongest predictor of unfavorable outcome at 6 months. Model discrimination was excellent, and calibration was adequate, as six of the eight models had good calibration when evaluated with the Hosmer-Lemeshow goodness-of-fit test. External validation was in a cohort of patients from high-income countries only, excluded major extracranial injury and petechial hemorrhage, and showed good discrimination for both basic and CT models as well as excellent calibration for the CT model, but poorer calibration for the basic model. A clinical score using country, age, GCS score, pupillary reactivity, extracranial injury, and CT characteristics was created and showed expected risk of death at 14 days and death or severe disability at 6 months [5].

The IMPACT database was designed in 2007 and created a complete dataset from most clinical trials and organized epidemiologic studies conducted over the previous 20 years, accumulating 9,205 patients with severe and moderate brain injuries from eight randomized placebo-controlled trials and three observational studies [20]. Data included prehospital admission factors, postresuscitation assessments, acute management, and short- and long-term outcome. Multivariable prognostic analysis in TBI from the IMPACT Study found that age, GCS motor, pupillary response, and CT characteristics including Marshall CT classification and tSAH were strong predictors of outcome. A new finding was that prothrombin time (PT) was also a powerful independent prognostic factor but was only available for a limited number of patients. Hypotension, hypoxia, eye and verbal components of the GCS, glucose, platelets, and hemoglobin were also highlighted as important prognostic variables [21].

In 2008, Steyerberg et al. described the development and validation of prognostic scores based on admission characteristics [22]. In this study, predictors available at admission determined from the 8,509 IMPACT patients were externally validated in the 6,681 patients from the MRC CRASH Trial. Strongest predictors were found to be age, motor score, pupillary reactivity, and CT characteristics (tSAH). Prognostic models that included age, GCS motor score, and pupillary reactivity had an AUC between 0.66 and 0.84 at cross validation and improved by approximately 0.05 when considering CT characteristics (Marshall CT classification, tSAH, and EDH), secondary insults (hypotension and hypoxia), and lab parameters (glucose and hemoglobin). External validation showed adequate discriminative ability of the model (AUC = 0.80) and worse calibration; however, outcome prediction was better in patients from high-income countries in the CRASH trial. A web-based calculator was created for the various prediction models (http://www.tbi-impact.org/).

The CRASH trial and IMPACT project provided larger, more robust datasets, with improved statistical approaches for TBI prognostication. Previously known variables including age, GCS score, pupillary reactivity, CT characteristics, and presence of major extracranial injury were further confirmed as important variables in predicting TBI outcome. Additionally, new parameters including PT, hemoglobin, and glucose were now described as well [21].

A 2020 systematic review by Dijkland et al. provided an update on TBI prognostication models for moderate-to-severe TBI [3]. A total of 67 models were included that were mainly developed with logistic regression (94%) and internally validated with apparent or split-sample validation. Common predictors were GCS motor, age, pupillary reactivity, tSAH, IVH, hematoma, compression of cisterns and third ventricle, Marshall or RCT classifications, hypotension, glucose, hemoglobin, and coagulopathy. Newly included but less frequently used predictors included sex, mechanism of injury, ethnic group, cerebral perfusion pressure, and blood-based biomarkers. Mortality and unfavorable outcome (defined as either GOS 1–3 or GOS-Extended [GOS-E] 1–4) were the outcome measures assessed. The CRASH and IMPACT cohorts were used most often for external validation with large AUC variability. Extension models also arose during this time period. Biomarkers, extracranial injury, coagulation parameters, and dynamic predictors were added on to the IMPACT and CRASH models. These extended models showed mildly improved performance compared to the original versions, indicating that model improvements with other strong predictors may be used in the future. However, these model improvements have not been proven or externally validated yet [23–25]. Similar to previous conclusions, discrimination and calibration varied across studies; however, the IMPACT and CRASH prognostic models had adequate discriminative ability across various settings. Although calibration has not greatly improved, models are recommended for implementation into clinical practice, as long as they have been validated or updated for the specific clinical setting [3].

Future enhancement of TBI prognostication may exist through new avenues of data sharing, advanced modeling, and incorporation of new measurable data points. The Transforming Research and Clinical Knowledge in TBI (TRACK-TBI) multicenter study [26], Collaborative European Neurotrauma Effectiveness Research in TBI (CENTER-TBI) observational study [27], and Collaborative Research on Acute TBI in intensiVe Care Medicine in Europe (CREACTIVE) studies offer big data and improvements to the heterogeneity and inconsistency that surround TBI research [28]. Increased use of machine learning and dynamic modeling offer more variables to be considered during a patient's stay, which may lead to more accurate prognostication. Lastly, new data points may have potential use in the future. Biomarkers associated with TBI have demonstrated correlation with intracranial disease burden and may be an avenue for future exploration [29, 30].

30.4 Treatment-Limiting Decisions in Severe TBI

The increasing sophistication of TBI prognostication models has not necessarily been associated with major changes in decision-making for patients with severe TBI. Decision-making in severe TBI remains challenging and understudied. The time-dependent and unexpected nature of severe TBI limits patient participation in TBI decision-making and places enormous decisional burdens on family and friends. These decisions are further subject to geographic, institutional, and cognitive biases that limit generalizability in decision-making models and patterns.

Severe TBI poses a unique challenge to treatment decision-making in that patients often cannot communicate or lack insight due to neurological injury. TBI clinical decisions, such as the decision to offer surgery or to place a tracheostomy or PEG tube, must often be made acutely, without the patient's ability to participate in the treatment decision and without much family support. While impressive in their growing predictive abilities, prognostic models often rely on assumptions about "favorable" outcomes, which are culturally, geographically, and oftentimes institutionally or individually conditioned. These models assume a clinician's perspective and rarely account for patient perspectives or backgrounds. Moreover, the aging population in many Western nations is a growing challenge to standards for aggressiveness of care and notions of how to define desirable outcomes in severe TBI [31].

Prognostication variables such as GCS, age, pupillary reactivity, and CT characteristics (tSAH, IVH, compression of cisterns and third ventricle) have been consistently shown to be associated with worse outcomes in TBI [3]. However, how these known associations should impact clinical decision-making is unknown. Clinical trials in TBI have relied heavily on the GOS-E to assess long-term outcome in TBI. However, the GOS-E has known limitations and likely does not account for the spectrum of injury recovery and functional ability after TBI [32].

Several clinician-reported health status measures in addition to the GOS-E have been used to describe function after neurological injury, including the functional independence measure (FIM), modified Rankin scale (mRS), and Barthel Index (BI), to name just a few. The recent DECRA and RESCUEicp trials used GOS-E to examine the benefit of decompressive craniectomy in the setting of severe TBI [33, 34]. Both studies found that surgery was associated with more "unfavorable outcomes," but these two trials defined different cutoffs for "unfavorable" GOS-E outcomes in each study. The DECRA trial defined favorable outcome as GOS-E ≥ 5 (low moderate disability or better), while RESCUEicp defined favorable outcome as GOS-E ≥ 4 (upper severe disability or better). The lack of consensus around the concept of a "favorable" outcome limits the interpretation and the bedside application of these study findings in a real-world setting. More recent statistical methods have moved away from dichotomizing outcomes into "favorable" and "unfavorable" and now focus on the overall distribution of outcomes across an outcomes scale.

In addition to clinician-reported outcomes, patient-reported outcome measures are an expanding field of research in patients with neurological injury. Examples of these measures include the Stroke Impact Scale (SIS-16), the Patient Health Questionnaire (PHQ-9) for depression, and the EuroQol EQ-5D to assess global quality-of-life metrics. The NIH PROMISE outcome measures offer domain-specific patient self-reported outcomes scales and include the Quality of Life in Neurological Disorders (NeuroQoL) patient-reported health measures. While patient-reported outcomes measures offer great promise, their utility requires patient participation for meaningful results, which is a major limitation in severe TBI [35, 36]. The relationship between clinician-reported outcomes and patient-reported outcomes is poorly understood and limits the application of the largely clinician-reported prognostication research in TBI, which may not be generalizable across cultural, geographic, institutional, and even personal boundaries [35]. This limitation becomes even more important because patients rely on physicians to make best-interest determinations when they lose decision-making capacity, which is not reflected in TBI prognostication modeling to date [37].

Treatment resources and attitudes toward treatment vary across different geographic regions, cultural groups, and institutional boundaries, which heavily influences practice patterns associated with treatment-limiting decisions. Regional differences in causes of injury, patient characteristics, referral policy, time intervals, and outcomes in TBI have been described between Europe and North America [38]. Decisions and treatment in one location may not be reproducible in another. This may help explain the difference in calibration seen amongst prediction modeling studies. Factors such as regional trauma organization, triage protocols, and institutional treatment practice patterns limit the application of generalized prognostication models to support clinical decision-making [17]. This effect is heightened in LMICs. The CRASH trial was the first to highlight differences in TBI outcomes between high-income countries and LMICs [5]. Low GCS score was associated with even worse prognosis in patients from LMICs. The IMPACT project also noticed that prognostication improved when only considering high-income countries, showing that models from high-income countries are likely inappropriate to use in LMIC settings [5, 22].

Similarly, practice patterns in emergency neurosurgery procedures can vary widely. The 2005 International Surgical Trial in Intracerebral Haemorrhage (STICH) found significant variations in operative rates for intracerebral hemorrhage (ICH) amongst different countries [39]. The variation was not explained by population differences and was thought to be secondary to habits of physician training or institutional culture [35, 40]. Culture and training bias adds to the heterogeneity of clinical decision-making that complicates prognostication modeling and applicability worldwide. In fact, survey data show substantial variation in the rates and types of neurosurgical monitoring for intracranial hypertension among European neurotrauma centers participating in the CENTER-TBI study [41, 42]. Similarly, decisions regarding treatment-limiting decisions show significant variation across centers and physicians [31, 43, 44].

Treatment-limiting decisions are applied in approximately 50% of fatal cases of severe TBI, and decisions are typically based on predictions of poor prognosis [45]. Increased patient age, GCS, pupillary response, presence of comorbidities, vegetative state, and impaired neurological function are known factors associated with treatment-limiting decisions [46]. However, specific factors that are associated with variation in treatment-limiting decisions for severe TBI are poorly described and are likely influenced by regional, cultural, institutional, and even personal biases [45]. These factors are so influential that one study showed a 15-fold difference among intensivists in the same ICU in the decisions to limit life support [47].

The clinical characteristics of severe TBI combined with limitations in prognostic modeling and variable attitudes and approaches to medical treatment all create significant challenges to the standardization of TBI care worldwide. These challenges also demonstrate the vital importance of neurotrauma specialists who can interpret and apply complex clinical information for the benefit of a unique patient in a particular time and place. The neurotrauma specialist is the necessary bridge that connects the power of TBI prognostic modeling with treatment decisions for a particular patient with unique preferences and treatment goals. In the end, a truly shared decision-making process is the best model for promoting treatment decisions that reflect patient values in the setting of severe TBI [37].

30.5 Conclusion

Prognostication in patients with severe TBI has grown in sophistication and accuracy over the last several decades. Standard prognostic clinical factors such as age, GCS score, pupillary reactivity, and CT scan findings have been combined with more sophisticated grading scales, laboratory data, and advanced imaging modalities. These improvements have made prognostication more accurate but not necessarily more clinically useful or generalizable. The interaction between prognostication and treatment-limiting decision is poorly understood and strongly influenced by cultural, institutional, geographic, and even personal factors. Future research is needed to determine how these non-injury factors impact treatment-limiting decisions, particularly in LMICs worldwide. The application of prognostic modeling to individual patients in severe TBI is the noble obligation of the neurotrauma specialist, and one that allows medical science to best serve each unique patient in a relationship of shared decision-making.

Funding Statement No authors received funding from any funding agency in the public, commercial or not-for-profit sectors.

Competing Interests Statement The authors have no personal or institutional interest with regards to the authorship and/or publication of this manuscript.

Contributorship Statement MLK, JP, and AK were involved in the design, writing, and revisions of this manuscript. All authors have approved the manuscript as it is written.

References

1. Maas AIR, Menon DK, Manley GT, Abrams M, Åkerlund C, Andelic N, et al. Traumatic brain injury: progress and challenges in prevention, clinical care, and research. Lancet Neurol. 2022;21(11):1004–60. https://doi.org/10.1016/S1474-4422(22)00309-X.
2. Chestnut RM, Ghajar J, Maas AIR, Marion DW, Servadei F, Teasdale G, et al. Part 2: early indicators of prognosis in severe traumatic brain injury. J Neurotrauma. 2000;17:555–627.
3. Dijkland SA, Foks KA, Polinder S, Dippel DWJ, Maas AIR, Lingsma HF, et al. Prognosis in moderate and severe traumatic brain injury: a systematic review of contemporary models and validation studies. J Neurotrauma. 2020;37(1):1–13. https://doi.org/10.1089/neu.2019.6401.
4. Teasdale G, Jennett B. Assessment of coma and impaired consciousness. A practical scale. Lancet. 1974;2(7872):81–4. https://doi.org/10.1016/s0140-6736(74)91639-0.
5. Perel P, Arango M, Clayton T, Edwards P, Komolafe E, Poccock S, et al. Predicting outcome after traumatic brain injury: practical prognostic models based on large cohort of international patients. BMJ. 2008;336(7641):425–9. https://doi.org/10.1136/bmj.39461.643438.25.
6. Jennett B, Teasdale G, Braakman R, Minderhoud J, Knill-Jones R. Predicting outcome in individual patients after severe head injury. Lancet. 1976;1(7968):1031–4. https://doi.org/10.1016/s0140-6736(76)92215-7.
7. Tang OY, Shao B, Kimata AR, Sastry RA, Wu J, Asaad WF. The impact of frailty on traumatic brain injury outcomes: an analysis of 691 821 nationwide cases. Neurosurgery. 2022;91(5):808–20. https://doi.org/10.1227/neu.0000000000002116.
8. Chesnut RM, Marshall LF, Klauber MR, Blunt BA, Baldwin N, Eisenberg HM, et al. The role of secondary brain injury in determining outcome from severe head injury. J Trauma. 1993;34(2):216–22. https://doi.org/10.1097/00005373-199302000-00006.
9. Gennarelli TA, Spielman GM, Langfitt TW, Gildenberg PL, Harrington T, Jane JA, et al. Influence of the type of intracranial lesion on outcome from severe head injury. J Neurosurg. 1982;56(1):26–32. https://doi.org/10.3171/jns.1982.56.1.0026.
10. Lobato RD, Cordobes F, Rivas JJ, de la Fuente M, Montero A, Barcena A, et al. Outcome from severe head injury related to the type of intracranial lesion. A computerized tomography study. J Neurosurg. 1983;59(5):762–74. https://doi.org/10.3171/jns.1983.59.5.0762.
11. Marshall L, Gautille T, Klauber M, Eisenberg H, Jane J, Luerssen T, et al. The outcome of severe closed head injury. J Neurosurg. 1991;75:S28–36.
12. Maas AI, Hukkelhoven CW, Marshall LF, Steyerberg EW. Prediction of outcome in traumatic brain injury with computed tomographic characteristics: a comparison between the computed tomographic classification and combinations of computed tomographic predictors. Neurosurgery. 2005;57(6):1173–82. https://doi.org/10.1227/01.neu.0000186013.63046.6b; discussion -82.
13. Marshall LF, Maas AI, Marshall SB, Bricolo A, Fearnside M, Iannotti F, et al. A multicenter trial on the efficacy of using tirilazad mesylate in cases of head injury. J Neurosurg. 1998;89(4):519–25. https://doi.org/10.3171/jns.1998.89.4.0519.
14. Morris GF, Bullock R, Marshall SB, Marmarou A, Maas A, Marshall LF. Failure of the competitive N-methyl-D-aspartate antagonist Selfotel (CGS 19755) in the treatment of severe head injury: results of two phase III clinical trials. The Selfotel Investigators. J Neurosurg. 1999;91(5):737–43. https://doi.org/10.3171/jns.1999.91.5.0737.

15. Murray GD, Teasdale GM, Braakman R, Cohadon F, Dearden M, Iannotti F, et al. The European brain injury consortium survey of head injuries. Acta Neurochir. 1999;141(3):223–36. https://doi.org/10.1007/s007010050292.
16. Marshall LF, Becker DP, Bowers SA, Cayard C, Eisenberg H, Gross CR, et al. The National Traumatic Coma Data Bank. Part 1: design, purpose, goals, and results. J Neurosurg. 1983;59(2):276–84. https://doi.org/10.3171/jns.1983.59.2.0276.
17. Hukkelhoven CW, Rampen AJ, Maas AI, Farace E, Habbema JD, Marmarou A, et al. Some prognostic models for traumatic brain injury were not valid. J Clin Epidemiol. 2006;59(2):132–43. https://doi.org/10.1016/j.jclinepi.2005.06.009.
18. Perel P, Edwards P, Wentz R, Roberts I. Systematic review of prognostic models in traumatic brain injury. BMC Med Inform Decis Mak. 2006;6:38. https://doi.org/10.1186/1472-6947-6-38.
19. Mushkudiani NA, Hukkelhoven CW, Hernández AV, Murray GD, Choi SC, Maas AI, et al. A systematic review finds methodological improvements necessary for prognostic models in determining traumatic brain injury outcomes. J Clin Epidemiol. 2008;61(4):331–43. https://doi.org/10.1016/j.jclinepi.2007.06.011.
20. Marmarou A, Lu J, Butcher I, McHugh GS, Mushkudiani NA, Murray GD, et al. IMPACT database of traumatic brain injury: design and description. J Neurotrauma. 2007;24(2):239–50. https://doi.org/10.1089/neu.2006.0036.
21. Murray GD, Butcher I, McHugh GS, Lu J, Mushkudiani NA, Maas AI, et al. Multivariable prognostic analysis in traumatic brain injury: results from the IMPACT study. J Neurotrauma. 2007;24(2):329–37. https://doi.org/10.1089/neu.2006.0035.
22. Steyerberg EW, Mushkudiani N, Perel P, Butcher I, Lu J, McHugh GS, et al. Predicting outcome after traumatic brain injury: development and international validation of prognostic scores based on admission characteristics. PLoS Med. 2008;5(8):e165. https://doi.org/10.1371/journal.pmed.0050165; discussion e.
23. Czeiter E, Mondello S, Kovacs N, Sandor J, Gabrielli A, Schmid K, et al. Brain injury biomarkers may improve the predictive power of the IMPACT outcome calculator. J Neurotrauma. 2012;29(9):1770–8. https://doi.org/10.1089/neu.2011.2127.
24. Güiza F, Depreitere B, Piper I, Van den Berghe G, Meyfroidt G. Novel methods to predict increased intracranial pressure during intensive care and long-term neurologic outcome after traumatic brain injury: development and validation in a multicenter dataset. Crit Care Med. 2013;41(2):554–64. https://doi.org/10.1097/CCM.0b013e3182742d0a.
25. Raj R, Siironen J, Kivisaari R, Hernesniemi J, Skrifvars MB. Predicting outcome after traumatic brain injury: development of prognostic scores based on the IMPACT and the APACHE II. J Neurotrauma. 2014;31(20):1721–32. https://doi.org/10.1089/neu.2014.3361.
26. Yue JK, Vassar MJ, Lingsma HF, Cooper SR, Okonkwo DO, Valadka AB, et al. Transforming research and clinical knowledge in traumatic brain injury pilot: multicenter implementation of the common data elements for traumatic brain injury. J Neurotrauma. 2013;30(22):1831–44. https://doi.org/10.1089/neu.2013.2970.
27. Maas AI, Menon DK, Steyerberg EW, Citerio G, Lecky F, Manley GT, et al. Collaborative European NeuroTrauma effectiveness research in traumatic brain injury (CENTER-TBI): a prospective longitudinal observational study. Neurosurgery. 2015;76(1):67–80. https://doi.org/10.1227/NEU.0000000000000575.
28. Kelly ML. Big data and clinical research in traumatic brain injury. World Neurosurg. 2018;109:465–6. https://doi.org/10.1016/j.wneu.2017.09.155.
29. Whitehouse DP, Vile AR, Adatia K, Herlekar R, Roy AS, Mondello S, et al. Blood biomarkers and structural imaging correlations post-traumatic brain injury: a systematic review. Neurosurgery. 2022;90(2):170–9. https://doi.org/10.1227/NEU.0000000000001776.
30. Krausz AD, Korley FK, Burns MA. The current state of traumatic brain injury biomarker measurement methods. Biosensors (Basel). 2021;11(9):319. https://doi.org/10.3390/bios11090319.
31. Kashkoush A, Petitt JC, Ladhani H, Ho VP, Kelly ML, Group AAftSoTG-TS. Predictors of mortality, withdrawal of life-sustaining measures, and discharge disposition in octogenarians

with subdural hematomas. World Neurosurg. 2022;157:e179–e87. https://doi.org/10.1016/j.wneu.2021.09.121.
32. Manley GT, Maas AI. Traumatic brain injury: an international knowledge-based approach. JAMA. 2013;310(5):473–4. https://doi.org/10.1001/jama.2013.169158.
33. Cooper DJ, Rosenfeld JV, Murray L, Arabi YM, Davies AR, D'Urso P, et al. Decompressive craniectomy in diffuse traumatic brain injury. N Engl J Med. 2011;364(16):1493–502. https://doi.org/10.1056/NEJMoa1102077.
34. Hutchinson PJ, Kolias AG, Timofeev IS, Corteen EA, Czosnyka M, Timothy J, et al. Trial of decompressive craniectomy for traumatic intracranial hypertension. N Engl J Med. 2016;375(12):1119–30. https://doi.org/10.1056/NEJMoa1605215.
35. Kelly ML, Sulmasy DP, Weil RJ. Spontaneous intracerebral hemorrhage and the challenge of surgical decision making: a review. Neurosurg Focus. 2013;34(5):E1. https://doi.org/10.3171/2013.2.FOCUS1319.
36. Kelly ML, Rosenbaum BP, Kshettry VR, Weil RJ. Comparing clinician- and patient-reported outcome measures after hemicraniectomy for ischemic stroke. Clin Neurol Neurosurg. 2014;126:24–9. https://doi.org/10.1016/j.clineuro.2014.08.007.
37. Sulmasy DP, Hughes MT, Thompson RE, Astrow AB, Terry PB, Kub J, et al. How would terminally ill patients have others make decisions for them in the event of decisional incapacity? A longitudinal study. J Am Geriatr Soc. 2007;55(12):1981–8. https://doi.org/10.1111/j.1532-5415.2007.01473.x.
38. Hukkelhoven CW, Steyerberg EW, Farace E, Habbema JD, Marshall LF, Maas AI. Regional differences in patient characteristics, case management, and outcomes in traumatic brain injury: experience from the tirilazad trials. J Neurosurg. 2002;97(3):549–57. https://doi.org/10.3171/jns.2002.97.3.0549.
39. Mendelow AD, Gregson BA, Fernandes HM, Murray GD, Teasdale GM, Hope DT, et al. Early surgery versus initial conservative treatment in patients with spontaneous supratentorial intracerebral haematomas in the international surgical trial in intracerebral Haemorrhage (STICH): a randomised trial. Lancet. 2005;365(9457):387–97. https://doi.org/10.1016/S0140-6736(05)17826-X.
40. Hoff JT. Editorial comment—International variations in surgical practice for spontaneous intracerebral hemorrhage. Stroke. 2003;34(11):2597–8. https://doi.org/10.1161/01.STR.0000101663.71972.49.
41. Cnossen MC, Huijben JA, van der Jagt M, Volovici V, van Essen T, Polinder S, et al. Variation in monitoring and treatment policies for intracranial hypertension in traumatic brain injury: a survey in 66 neurotrauma centers participating in the CENTER-TBI study. Crit Care. 2017;21(1):233. https://doi.org/10.1186/s13054-017-1816-9.
42. van Essen TA, den Boogert HF, Cnossen MC, de Ruiter GCW, Haitsma I, Polinder S, et al. Variation in neurosurgical management of traumatic brain injury: a survey in 68 centers participating in the CENTER-TBI study. Acta Neurochir. 2019;161(3):435–49. https://doi.org/10.1007/s00701-018-3761-z.
43. DeMario BS, Stanley SP, Truong EI, Ladhani HA, Brown LR, Ho VP, et al. Predictors for withdrawal of life-sustaining therapies in patients with traumatic brain injury: a retrospective trauma quality improvement program database study. Neurosurgery. 2022;91(2):e45–50. https://doi.org/10.1227/neu.0000000000002020.
44. Truong EI, Stanley SP, DeMario BS, Tseng ES, Como JJ, Ho VP, et al. Variation in neurosurgical intervention for severe traumatic brain injury: the challenge of measuring quality in trauma center verification. J Trauma Acute Care Surg. 2021;91(1):114–20. https://doi.org/10.1097/TA.0000000000003114.
45. Turgeon AF, Lauzier F, Simard JF, Scales DC, Burns KE, Moore L, et al. Mortality associated with withdrawal of life-sustaining therapy for patients with severe traumatic brain injury: a Canadian multicentre cohort study. CMAJ. 2011;183(14):1581–8. https://doi.org/10.1503/cmaj.101786.

46. Bozkurt I, Umana GE, Deora H, Wellington J, Karakoc E, Chaurasia B. Factors affecting neurosurgeons' decisions to forgo life-sustaining treatments after traumatic brain injury. World Neurosurg. 2022;159:e311–e23. https://doi.org/10.1016/j.wneu.2021.12.056.
47. Garland A, Connors AF. Physicians' influence over decisions to forego life support. J Palliat Med. 2007;10(6):1298–305. https://doi.org/10.1089/jpm.2007.0061.

31 Clinical and Bioethical Perspective on Brain Death, Organ Donation, and Family Communication

Vincent Y. Wang

Brain death describes the ultimate demise of patients with a severe brain injury from either a traumatic or nontraumatic cause. While brain death has been accepted as a legal definition of death throughout the USA for over 40 years, clinical, legal and ethical issues related to brain death still exist. While brain death is accepted by most in the community, there remains a significant part of the population who view brain death with significant reservation. Therefore, it is important for providers of brain-injured patients to have a basic understanding of brain death and related issues.

31.1 History of Brain Death

Up until the 1950s, death was defined by irreversible loss of circulatory and respiratory function. After the development of ventilators, patients with devastating brain injury could be kept alive for prolonged periods. Keeping such patients alive, with no hope of recovery, created a significant burden to society [1]. It also created a legal dilemma because discontinuing these patients' life support would be considered criminal homicide [2]. At the same time, the field of organ transplantation believed that "live donors" would offer better success than cadaver donors [3]. This prompted Henry Beecher to establish the Ad hoc Committee of Harvard Medical School to examine the concept of brain death, which published its report in 1968 [4]. Commonly known as Beecher's report, the publication defined a state of "irreversible coma" as a new criterion of death [4]. The committee put forth the diagnostic criteria for irreversible coma, which describes a permanently nonfunctioning brain as follows [4]:

V. Y. Wang (✉)
Ascension Medical Group Seton Neurosurgery, Austin, TX, USA

Department of Neurosurgery, Dell Medical School, University of Texas Austin, Austin, TX, USA
e-mail: vywang@ascension.org

E. Brogi et al. (eds.), *Traumatic Brain Injury*, Hot Topics in Acute Care Surgery and Trauma, https://doi.org/10.1007/978-3-031-50117-3_31

1. Unreceptivity and unresponsivity—total unawareness and unresponsiveness to external stimuli and inner needs;
2. No movements or breathing—no spontaneous movement or breathing noted by a qualified physician over the period of 1 h. If the patient was on a respirator, no effort to breath spontaneously within 3 min after the respirator was turned off;
3. No reflexes, including pupillary reflex, ocular movements in response to cold caloric testing, blinking to threat, swallowing, cough, and gag;
4. Flat or isoelectric electroencephalogram (EEG), which provided confirmatory data and should be used whenever it is available.

These tests were to be repeated in 24 h to ensure that no changes had occurred [4].

In 1971, the state of Kansas adopted the first statute regarding brain death [2]. During the second half of the 1970s, the American Medical Association, American Bar Association, National Conference of Commissioners on Uniform State Laws, and the Hastings Center developed different model statues for brain death [2]. The President's Commission for the Study of Ethical Problems in Medicine and Biomedical and Behavioral Research was organized to clarify the legal and ethical issues surrounding brain death [3]. The President's Commission eventually developed the Uniform Determination of Death Act (UDDA), which stated the following:

> An individual who has sustained either (1) irreversible cessation of circulatory and respiratory function or (2) irreversible cessation of all functions of the entire brain, including the brainstem, is dead.
>
> A determination of death must be made in accordance with acceptable medical standards [5].

The UDDA language was eventually adopted by 48 states into their respective state statutes or case law in one form or another, thus codifying brain death as a legal definition of death [6]. Two states, Arizona and North Carolina, recognize brain death but have language different than UDDA.

31.2 Determination of Brain Death: American Academy of Neurology (AAN) Guideline

In 1995, the American Academy of Neurology (AAN) developed its own guideline used for determination of brain death. The guideline was updated in 2010 and reaffirmed in 2017 [7]. In 2023, the AAN published a new guideline for determination of brain death or death by neurological criteria. The 2023 AAN guideline contains a number of new updates. It combines the adult and pediatric guidelines, which had previously been separate [8]. The 2023 guideline also uses the terminology of "brain death/death by neurologic criteria" (BD/DNC) rather than the commonly used term brain death to clarify that BD/DNC refers to death of the entire person, not just the brain. There are recommendations in the guideline about which clinicians should perform the brain death exam, which should be someone who does not have any conflict of interest (including any clinicians who will be involved in the surgical recovery of organs) and who is appropriately trained and credentialed [8]. Importantly, both attending physicians and advanced practice providers (APP) may perform the brain death exam unsupervised as long as they are appropriately trained and credentialled. The 2023 guideline also has recommendations regarding consent for brain death testing, pregnant patients, determination of time of death, neuroendocrine function, and patients with a primary posterior fossa injury [8].

Much of the 2023 guideline is similar to the 2010 guideline, which established the prerequisites of the clinical evaluation, the clinical assessment (including a protocol for the apnea test), and the use of ancillary tests. The essential elements of the brain death exam include identification of an injury that results in loss of brain function, exclusion of confounding conditions, and a clinical examination that demonstrates unarousable lack of responsiveness, lack of brain reflexes, and apnea (see Checklist). Compared to the 2010 guideline, the 2023 guideline provides more specific criteria for the minimal period of time to determine permanency and also provides quantitative criteria for blood concentrations of drugs that may affect the central nervous system [8]. Special attention is emphasized for patients with primary posterior fossa injuries to ensure that their supratentorial compartment is also severely injured as demonstrated by imaging. There is also a recommendation that clinicians should make a reasonable attempt to inform family that a BD/DNC exam is to be done, but importantly, family consent is not needed for the BD/DNC exam [8].

For the clinical exam, the 2023 guideline is essentially the same as the 2010 guideline (see Checklist). The only additions are criteria from the pediatric guideline, since the new guideline is a combined adult and pediatric guideline. Essentially, BD/DNC could be declared if a patient shows no evidence of consciousness, motor function, and brainstem function, and confirmation is obtained with an apnea test. These neurological exam criteria are long-established for the use of brain death exam, going back to the 1968 Beecher report. Importantly, the current AAN guideline does not test the function of the neuroendocrine axis, which is an area of debate since the UDDA defines brain death as the death of the entire brain. The current guideline recommends that clinicians may perform BD/DNC test despite evidence of neuroendocrine function. Patients with catastrophic permanent brain injury may still have intact neuroendocrine function despite meeting brain death criteria based on previously published guideline [8].

While clinical exam (including the apnea test) is sufficient to determine brain death, sometimes the BD/DNC clinical exam cannot be completed due to factors like inability to correct metabolic derangements, inability to perform part of the exam due to other injuries such as spinal cord injuries and facial fractures, or uncertainty as to whether reflexes are cerebral or spinal in origin (Checklist). In such situations, ancillary testing in addition to the clinical exam can confirm the presence of brain death. Currently, the AAN approves three ancillary tests: four-vessel conventional digital subtraction angiography, radionuclide cerebral scintigraphy, and transcranial Doppler ultrasonography.

Conventional cerebral angiography has a long history as an ancillary test in brain death, and many consider it as the "gold standard" ancillary test [9–11]. However, conventional cerebral angiography is not widely available, and different techniques may lead to difference in interpretation [9]. Moreover, clinically brain-dead patients sometimes can still have some opacification intracranially, leading to potentially confounding interpretation [12, 13].

Radionuclide scanning to determine the presence of intracranial blood flow often uses 99mTC-HMPAO, which is a brain-specific radionuclide agent [14]. In the past, radionuclide scans consisted of planar images obtained after injection of the radiopharmaceutical agent, resulting in a radionuclide angiogram [14]. This can be used to evaluate anterior and posterior circulation. Recently, both the AAN and American College of Radiology recommended the use of SPECT along with planar projections for evaluation of brain death with radiopharmaceutical agents [14]. In a meta-analysis, SPECT has 88% sensitivity and 100% specificity for brain death evaluation [14].

Transcranial doppler (TCD) is a non-invasive test. TCD confirms brain death by looking for a distinctive cerebral blood flow pattern associated with cerebral circulatory arrest, like reversal of diastolic flow and systolic spike [15]. In a systematic review, Chang et al. showed that TCD is both highly sensitive (90%) and specific (98%) for determination of brain death. However, case reports of both false positives and false negatives exist [9, 15]. Similar to EEG, TCD does not evaluate the brainstem area well. TCD is operator-dependent, and procedures such as decompressive craniectomy also affect the result [15].

One important change in the 2023 guideline is that EEG is no longer considered as an approved ancillary test. EEG has a very long history as part of brain death determination. EEG is noninvasive and often readily available. However, it is prone to artifact, especially in the ICU, due to electrical noise [9]. Medications like sedatives and metabolic disorders will also affect EEG signals [16]. One of the criticisms of EEG as an ancillary test is that it only measures cortical electrical activity and cannot capture activity from the brainstem region well. Even if EEG can be supplemented with additional testing like auditory evoked potentials or somatosensory evoked potentials, electrodiagnostic tests will not be sufficient to test hemispheric and brainstem function [8].

Recently, a number of new ancillary tests have been studied for brain death determination, including MR angiography, bispectral index, somatosensory evoked potentials, and CT angiography [17]. In the 2023 guideline, it was felt that there was insufficient evidence to recommend these as ancillary tests [8]. But with continual advances in technology and increasing popularity in their clinical use, it is possible that technologies like CTA or MRA will eventually gain acceptance as ancillary tests.

Use of ancillary testing has been controversial. All current ancillary tests assess brain blood flow/perfusion. It is implied that if there is no blood flow to/in the brain, there cannot be any functional activity in the brain. Therefore, these tests are indirect assessments of brain function. Ancillary tests are indicated if there are conditions or situations that make it impossible to perform a clinical BD/DNC exam (including apnea test), but the guideline currently does not provide sufficient guidance when discrepancies arise between the BD/DNC clinical exam result and the ancillary test result. Theoretically, ancillary tests should be used to assist the clinical exam in determination of brain death, and therefore ancillary testing is not needed if the clinical exam confirms brain death. The current guideline also does not address the issue of institutional or state requirement for ancillary testing. There is significant state or institutional variation in terms of ancillary test use [18], and in fact one of the potential reasons for use of ancillary testing on the 2023 checklist is state or institutional requirement. That begs the potential scenario of a patient who meets clinical BD/DNC criteria by clinical exam, but the ancillary test (s) that was/were performed due to institutional requirement is/are inconclusive of brain death. Is this patient brain dead? This is potentially be addressed at the institutional policy level, but it is a potential area for future legal challenges as well.

It is generally felt that the AAN guideline can be considered as the standard for brain death determination. There has not been a known case in which a patient who was diagnosed with brain death using the AAN guideline has regained any brain function [19]. However, adoption of the AAN guideline is currently not mandatory in most states. Currently, only Nevada mandates the use of the AAN guideline for brain death determination [20]. This results in significant variability of the practice of brain death determination. Greer et al. evaluated 492 hospital policies and found that while 94% of policies described prerequisites for brain death assessment, many of the policies did not contain all the components as prescribed by the AAN published guideline [18]. Similarly, 98% of policies described the apnea test, but for individual components, compliance was around 60% [18]. At the individual provider level, deviations were even more pronounced. Shappell et al. reviewed the medical records of 226 brain death exams and found that only 45% strictly adhered to the AAN guidelines [21]. Compliance in academic medical centers was not any better. Braksick et al. surveyed physicians from three academic medical centers and found that only 25% completed all the brain death exam components without doing an unnecessary exam of the peripheral reflexes, which is not part of the AAN guideline exam [22]. Use of simulation training has been shown to improve residents' and fellows' competence in brain death determination and communication [23]. Such programs may help to reduce practice variability in the future.

The variability in brain death policy may reflect unsettled issues in brain death determination. For example, many different modifications have been published on apnea testing, and some have been endorsed by other countries' guidelines [24]. More recently, new technologies such as extracorporeal membrane oxygenation (ECMO) introduce a different set of challenges in apnea testing, and several studies have developed accommodations for apnea testing in patients on ECMO [25]. It is therefore not a surprise that compared to examination of brainstem reflexes, more variations exist in institutional policies for apnea testing.

31.3 Public Perception of Brain Death

Despite the fact that brain death has been legally accepted as a definition of death in the USA for over 40 years, studies have shown that few members of the public have a correct understanding of brain death [26]. In a survey of families of patients who are eligible organ donors, Siminoff et al. found that only 28% of participants were able to give a correct description of brain death [27]. Common misunderstandings included confusing brain death with coma or persistent vegetative state, believing that patients are alive on a machine, or believing a brain-dead patient will recover [27]. In another study involving the general public, participants showed significant confusion over the concepts of brain death, coma, or persistent vegetative state [28].

Such poor understanding of brain death is at least partly due to a lack of availability of correct information. Brain death is uncommon compared to cardiopulmonary death, with a recent study suggesting that there is one brain death for every 50 cardiopulmonary deaths [29]. In public media, misinformation about brain death is common. For example, in a 2018 study, 4 out of the top 10 Google websites and 6 out of the 10 most popular YouTube videos on "brain death" or "brain dead" contained inaccurate information [30]. Similarly, Lewis et al. evaluated 215 online articles on two highly publicized brain death cases (Jahi McMath and Marlise Muñoz) and found that 74% of the articles contain misinformation, and fewer than 30% had a teaching point [31]. In more traditional media like television and movies, Lewis et al. also found that only a small fraction of the productions provided an accurate portrayal of brain death [32]. In addition, there is also significant diversity in acceptance and understanding of brain death among those of different cultural backgrounds. While brain death is commonly accepted in Western culture, it is not as well accepted in many Eastern cultures such as Chinese or Japanese [33, 34]. In fact, some countries like China still do not have legislation or statues regarding brain death. Similarly, there is significant variation among different religious beliefs. A significant minority of Orthodox Jews and Muslims do not accept brain death as a determination of death [35–37]. Such principled objections to the concept of brain death, whether based on cultural or religious beliefs, are often more difficult to manage than objections based on lack of information [38].

31.4 Brain Death-Some Legal Perspectives

Brain death is recognized in all 50 states either through statutes or case laws. Thirty-eight states adopted the UDDA effectively word for word, while nine states adopt UDDA with the express qualification that brain death may only be used when an individual's respiratory and circulatory functions are maintained by artificial means [6]. The two states that vary from UDDA are Arizona and North Carolina. Arizona statute states "that determination of death must be made in accordance with accepted medical standards" without explicit reference to any organ system (s) (AZ Rev. Stat § 14–1107 (2015)) [39]. Brain death is accepted for the determination of death through common law, based on the Arizona Supreme Court decision in *State v.*

Fierro [40]. In North Carolina, recognition of brain death is permissive but not conclusive, as recognition of brain death "shall not preclude the use of other medically recognized criteria for determining whether and when a person has died" [41]. Interestingly, Georgia law also allows "the use of other medically recognized criteria for determining death" in addition to the standard UDDA criteria (O.C.G.A. 31–10-16 (2010)) [42].

Throughout the years, there have been a number of legal challenges to the concept of brain death. These legal cases become case laws and lead to modifications of statues. One of the most contentious issues surrounding death by neurological criteria is religious exemption. Currently New Jersey is the only state that recognizes religious exemption. The religious objection and exemption issue was brought into the spotlight in recent years by several high-profile cases. Perhaps the one that garnered the most attention was the case of Jahi McMath, who was a 13 year-old-girl who underwent a tonsil surgery in 2013 in California and suffered a significant complication, leading to cardiac arrest [43]. She was determined to be brain dead by 3 physicians and was then declared dead by Alameda County [43]. Family refused to withdraw organ support, and this led to several lawsuits. In an unusual turn of events, the hospital and family settled, and JM was transferred to New Jersey and maintained on life support, including mechanical ventilation and artificial feeding. She had a cardiopulmonary arrest in 2018.

Jahi McMath's case raised numerous issues. She was declared dead by California state law in 2013, and yet again in New Jersey in 2018 by cardiopulmonary criteria. This led to the realization that whether someone is alive or dead depends not just on their medical condition, but also what state they live in. The McMath case was followed in 2016 by the case of Israel Stinson, a 2-year-old California boy who suffered cardiac arrest and subsequent brain death after an asthma attack. Citing religious objection, the mother objected to discontinuation of life support, and a lengthy legal battle ensued. Israel remained on organ support in California for 1 month and was then transferred to a facility in Guatemala [43]. In a strange twist of events, Israel was transferred back to California several months later [43]. Upon arrival in California, the accepting facility did not want to continue organ support. After the court ruled in favor of the hospital, Israel Stinson's organ support was discontinued [43].

These two cases highlight the difficulties of handling religious objections. In both of these cases, although the court did not overturn the legal status that the patient was dead, the court in both situations allowed for prolonged organ support and eventual transfer of the patients to another facility. Neither of these cases resulted in any significant change in the legal status of brain death law in California. Perhaps one can consider both of these as religious accommodations, which are explicitly permitted under the California law [44]. However, these two cases highlight that we are not yet able to come up with an optimal solution when religious exemption is recognized in one state (or other part of the world), but not in most states in the USA.

Another controversial area is the process of determining brain death. The UDDA established cessation of all brain function as a legal criterion for death, as determined by acceptable medical standards. It was silent in terms of specific exam elements and tests. The intention was to allow the medical community to revise and update the criteria with advances in medical knowledge and technologies [45]. Most states do not have a defined set of criteria, relying primarily on the principle of "acceptable medical standards." Idaho has the additional qualification of being limited to the "usual and customary procedures of the community in which the determination of death is made" (ID Code § 54–1819, (2011)) [6]. The courts have accepted a number of different criteria for the determination of brain death [46]. The only state that specifies the protocol for brain death determination is Nevada [20]. The Nevada legislation was developed in response to the case of Arden Hailu (In re Guardianship of Hailu, 131 Nev. Adv. Op. 89 (Nov. 16, 2015)). In 2015, the Supreme Court of Nevada ruled that it was unclear whether the AAN guideline satisfied the "acceptable medical standard" by the medical communities [47]. The led to legislation in 2017 to codify the AAN guideline as the protocol to determine brain death in Nevada. As discussed above, there continues to be significant variation in hospital policies in terms of brain death determination. Such variation is potential ground for legal challenges of what constitutes brain death.

Lastly, the need for consent for brain death testing—especially the apnea test—is another contentious issue. Although this does not challenge the legitimacy of death by neurological criteria, it has the practical consequence of allowing family to opt out of brain death determination. Currently, states are split in terms of whether consent is required for the apnea test. Montana, for example, requires consent to be obtained prior to an apnea test, while Nevada, New York, and Virginia do not [45].

31.5 Management of the Brain-Dead Patient

31.5.1 Communication of Brain Death

Care of the brain dead does not end with the brain death examination. Communicating to the family about brain death and optimizing the condition of the brain dead for potential organ donation are two challenges faced by many providers. Delivering the news of brain death is a difficult task due to the general public's poor understanding of brain death. As many brain deaths are associated with a sudden event such as trauma, stroke, or subarachnoid hemorrhage, families often do not have time to prepare for the tragic death, and many will struggle with accepting the idea of brain death. Family may object to brain deaths due to informational, emotional or principled objections [38]. Understanding the source of objections will help practitioners respond to the refusal of acceptance of brain death [38]. Clear communication to family is the key. Avoidance of medical jargon, detailed explanation of the brain death exam, and potentially allowing some family members to be present during the brain death exam will help to improve the family's acceptance [48]. Such transparent communication is important as it helps to limit the amount of ambiguity of brain death, which is common among family members [49]. It is important to note that family members receiving a clear and consistent explanation of brain death are more likely to agree to organ donation [50].

31.5.2 Post-Brain Death Organ Support

In general, the court has been supportive of hospitals and providers withdrawing organ support once brain death has been determined, even if that is against a family's wishes [46, 49]. Despite the legal protection, many providers would continue organ support treatment such as intravenous fluid, nutrition or in some case antibiotics and vasopressors if the family requested [43]. Fear of litigation was the primary reason why such treatments were continued [43]. California, Illinois and New York have specific provisions that require hospitals to develop policies regarding "religious accommodations" [6]. In practice, these accommodations usually involve waiting for a few days after brain death before organ support is withdrawn.

If a brain-dead patient progresses to organ donation, ongoing support is needed to maintain the organs' viability from the time of brain death to the time of organ procurement. A detailed discussion of specific therapies for managing a brain-dead donor is beyond the scope of this chapter. In general, there is often significant hemodynamic instability around the time of brain herniation, starting with a sympathetic storm just prior to herniation and followed by hypotension after herniation [51]. Intravascular hypovolemia can occur due to peripheral vasodilatation and to diabetes insipidus, which occur frequently in brain-dead subjects [51, 52]. Therefore, close vital sign monitoring (including invasive monitoring), adequate fluid resuscitation and use of pressors when necessary are important to maintain organ perfusion [51, 52]. Other organ-protective therapies include lung protective ventilation, thyroid hormone and corticosteroid replacement, body temperature management, and close monitoring of coagulopathy [51].

31.6 Conclusion and Future Development

Despite having been accepted as a legal standard for determination of death, neurological criteria for determination of death continue to have many skeptics. Cases like that of Jahi McMath have forced the world to re-evaluate brain death and the process of determining it. In 2020, the Executive Committee of the Uniform Law Commission authorized a new study committee to update the Uniform Determination of Death Act [53]. Some of the issues for the committee to consider include the lack of uniformity of the standards for determining brain death, the neuroendocrine axis, and whether notice or consent is needed prior to the brain death exam [53]. The current AAN guideline has made recommendations regarding these issues, but they are unlikely to resolve these controversies. The issue of the neuroendocrine axis is especially interesting. Although the current UDDA defines death as "irreversible cessation of ALL functions of the entire brain," the hormonal function of the hypothalamus is not tested in most brain death protocols. This has led to the development of two camps of experts, with one camp advocating for formal recognition of the neuroendocrine axis as a brain function that needs to be tested as part of the brain death exam, and the other camp advocating for neurorespiratory criteria for brain death, which will not test neuroendocrine function [54, 55]. Fundamentally, this may require a revision to the definition of the phrase “ALL functions of the brain.” What are *all* functions of the brain? Even if we refine the definition to all known functions or functional networks of the brain, it will not be possible to test all of these functions/functional networks. Other areas that the AAN considers as priority of research include observation period, number of examinations, qualifications of examiner, and new ancillary tests like CT angiography [8].

As controversial as it may be, the concept of brain death is not going away. Some authors, in fact, consider that all human deaths are brain deaths to some extent [56]. If technologies like ECMO advance to the point at which we can one day maintain a patient without cardiac or respiratory function on machines for a prolonged period of time, brain death may become the main or even sole determinant of death in the future.

Brain Death/Death by Neurologic Criteria Checklist

Last Name	First name	DOB	MRN

PREREQUISITES FOR CLINICAL EXAMINATION	
1. Ascertainment that the patient has sustained a catastrophic, permanent brain injury caused by an identified mechanism that is known to lead to brain death/death by neurologic criteria (BD/DNC) (7a and 13a)	☐ Yes ☐ No Etiology:
2. Neuroimaging consistent with mechanism and severity of brain injury (in patients with primary posterior fossa injury, neuroimaging should demonstrate catastrophic supratentorial injury) (7c and 40)	☐ Yes ☐ No
3. Observation for permanency a) ≥48 hours after acute brain injury (particularly hypoxic ischemic brain injury) for patients ≤2-years-old (8) b) ≥24 hours after hypoxic ischemic brain injury for patients ≥2-years-old (9b) c) A sufficient amount of time after brain injury to ensure there is no potential for recovery of brain function as determined by the evaluator based on the pathophysiology of the brain injury (9a)	☐ Yes ☐ No Observation period (hours):
4. Core body temperature ≥ 36°C (for ≥24 hours for patients whose core body temperature has been ≤35.5°C [10a and b])	☐ Yes ☐ No Value:
5. Systolic blood pressure (SBP) ≥ 100 mm Hg and mean arterial pressure (MAP) ≥ 75 mm Hg for adults/SBP and MAP ≥ 5th percentile for age in children (for patients on venoarterial ECMO: MAP ≥ 75 mm Hg for adults/MAP ≥ 5th percentile for age in children) (11b and 11c)	☐ Yes ☐ No Value:
6. Exclusion of pharmacologic paralysis (if administered or suspected) through use of train-of-four stimulator or demonstration of deep tendon reflexes (12a)	☐ Yes ☐ No ☐ Not indicated
7. Drug levels for medications that may suppress central nervous system function are therapeutic/subtherapeutic (if available), pentobarbital level is <5 mcg/mL (if the patient received pentobarbital) and at least five half-lives for all other such drugs have passed (longer if there is renal/hepatic dysfunction or if the patient is obese or was hypothermic); (12a)	☐ Yes ☐ No
8. Alcohol blood level ≤ 80 mg/dL (if clinically indicated) (12a)	☐ Yes ☐ No ☐ Not indicated
9. Toxicology screen (urine and blood) is negative (if clinically indicated) (12a)	☐ Yes ☐ No ☐ Not indicated
10. Exclusion of severe metabolic, acid-base, and endocrine derangements; (12a)	☐ Yes ☐ No
11. A reasonable attempt has been made to inform the patient's family of the plan to perform a BD/DNC examination (35a)	☐ Yes ☐ No
Prerequisite Summary (check one):	
☐ All prerequisites were met	
☐ Unable to adequately correct metabolic derangements, but all other prerequisites were met, so will complete the neurologic examinations and apnea test(s) and if they are consistent with BD/DNC, will perform ancillary testing (12b)	
☐ One or more prerequisites were not met, so the evaluation was not completed	

CLINICAL EXAM *(must be completed to fullest extent possible)*	Yes	No	Not tested
12. Coma with unresponsiveness to visual, auditory, and tactile stimulation (15)	☐	☐	
13. Absent motor responses, other than spinally mediated reflexes, of the head/face, neck, and extremities after application of noxious stimuli to the head/face, trunk, and limbs (16a and 16b)	☐	☐	
14. Absent pupillary responses to bright light bilaterally (17)	☐	☐	☐
15. Absent oculocephalic reflex (unless there is concern for cervical spine or skull base integrity) (18a)	☐	☐	☐
16. Absent oculovestibular reflexes bilaterally (18b)	☐	☐	☐
17. Absent corneal reflexes bilaterally (19)	☐	☐	☐
18. Absent gag reflex (20)	☐	☐	☐
19. Absent cough reflex (20)	☐	☐	☐
20. Absence of sucking and rooting reflexes (patients <6-months only) (21)	☑	☐	☐
Clinical examination results (check one):			
☐ All elements of the ☐ First ☐ Second clinical exam were completed and findings were consistent with BD/DNC or all elements of the clinical exam except the oculocephalic reflex (18c) were completed and findings were consistent with BD/DNC			

☐	A portion of the clinical exam other than the oculocephalic reflex could not be assessed safely or it was unclear whether observed limb movements were spinally mediated (note that even if a person does not have all limbs, painful stimulation can still be provided to the torso as close to the termination of the limb as possible, so this does not necessitate ancillary testing); however, the remainder of the test was performed to the fullest extent possible and responses were consistent with BD/DNC. *(Ancillary testing is required.)* (14a) Reason(s) for incomplete testing (check all that apply): ☐ Anophthalmia; ☐ Corneal trauma or transplantation; ☐ Fracture of the base of the skull or petrous temporal bone; ☐ High cervical cord injury ☐ Ophthalmic surgery that influences pupillary reactivity; ☐ Severe facial trauma; ☐ Severe pre-existing neuromuscular disorder ☐ Severe orbital or scleral edema or chemosis; ☐ Limb movements that may be spinally mediated; ☐ Other (specify):
☐	One or more elements of the clinical exam were inconsistent with BD/DNC, so the patient does NOT meet criteria for BD/DNC (14b)
Attending name, signature, date, time.	

APNEA TEST	Yes	No
APNEA TESTING PREREQUISITES		
21. No hypoxemia, hypotension, hypovolemia (23)	☐	☐
22. pH is normal (7.35-7.45) and $Pa{CO_2}$ is normal (35-45 mm Hg) or if the patient is known to have chronic hypercarbia, $Pa{CO_2}$ is at baseline if baseline is known or at estimated baseline if baseline is not known (arterial blood gases [ABGs] should be taken from both the distal arterial line and the ECMO postcircuit oxygenator for patients on venoarterial ECMO) (24a-b and 26)	☐ Value:	☐
23. $Pa{O_2}$ > 200 mm Hg (25a)	☐ Value:	☐
APNEA TESTING PERFORMED	☐	☐
24. Apnea duration (minutes)		
25. Post-$Pa{CO_2}$ value (mm Hg)		
26. Post-pH value		
Final apnea testing results (check one):		
☐ Apnea confirmed – no respirations and targets reached (pH < 7.30 and final $Pa{CO_2}$ ≥ 60 mm Hg (8.0 kPa) and ≥ 20 mm Hg (2.7 kPa) above pre-apnea test baseline (≥ 20 mm Hg (2.7 kPa) above chronic baseline for patients known to have chronic hypercarbia whose baseline is known) *(Ancillary testing is required if patient is known/suspected to have chronic hypercarbia but baseline $Pa{CO_2}$ is not known.)* (25f)		
☐ Apnea testing is inconclusive (could not be completed and no respirations and targets not reached) due to: ☐ SBP < 100 mm Hg or MAP < 75 mm Hg or SBP/MAP < 5th percentile for age in children ☐ Progressive oxygen desaturation < 85% ☐ Cardiac arrhythmia with hemodynamic instability (25h)		
☐ Apnea testing is negative – one or more spontaneous respirations were seen; findings are not consistent with BD/DNC (25g)		
Attending name, signature, date, time.		

ANCILLARY TESTING	
27. Reason(s) for ancillary testing (27b):	☐ Inability to correct metabolic derangements ☐ Inability to complete all clinical tests (e.g., fracture of the cervical spine, skull base, orbits, face) ☐ Inability to complete apnea test due to risk of cardiopulmonary decompensation or inability to interpret $Pa{CO_2}$ level in a patient with chronic hypoxemia for whom chronic baseline is unknown ☐ Uncertainty regarding interpretation of spinally vs. cerebrally mediated motor responses ☐ Required by hospital/state guidelines
28. Type of ancillary testing performed (29-31)	☐ Conventional 4-vessel catheter angiography (digital subtraction angiography) ☐ SPECT radionuclide perfusion scintigraphy or planar radionucleotide angiography ☐ Transcranial doppler ultrasonography (adults only)
Final ancillary testing results (check one):	
☐ Ancillary testing results are consistent with BD/DNC	
☐ Ancillary testing results are <u>not</u> consistent with BD/DNC	
☐ Ancillary testing results are inconclusive	
Date/Time of testing	Date of interpretation of results
Attending name, signature, date, time.	

SUMMARY OF FINDINGS	
☐	**BRAIN DEATH/DEATH BY NEUROLOGIC CRITERIA DETERMINED CLINICALLY** • Prerequisites for clinical testing have been fulfilled, (Section II), and • Results of clinical exams, including apnea testing, have been fully completed and are consistent with BD/DNC (Section III, IV) Date *(YYYY-MM-DD)* and time of death (*HR:MM AM/PM)*: *(Time of death is the time during the final apnea test [if more than one performed] that the ABG results are reported and demonstrate that the* $Pa{CO_2}$ *and pH levels are consistent with BD/DNC criteria [36a].)*
☐	**BRAIN DEATH/DEATH BY NEUROLOGIC CRITERIA DETERMINED WITH CLINICAL ASSESSMENT AND ANCILLARY TESTING** • Results of clinical exams, including apnea testing, where tested are consistent with BD/DNC (Section III, IV), and • Ancillary testing has been performed and results are consistent with BD/DNC (Section V) Date *(YYYY-MM-DD)* and time of death (*HR:MM AM/PM)*: *(Time of death is the time an attending clinician (e.g., nuclear medicine physician or angiographer) documents in the medical record that the ancillary test results are consistent with BD/DNC [36b].)*
☐	**PATIENT DOES NOT MEET CRITERIA FOR BRAIN DEATH/DEATH BY NEUROLOGIC CRITERIA** Provide reasons:
Attending name, signature, date, time.	

References

1. Truog RD, Berlinger N, Zacharias RL, Solomon MZ. Brain death at fifty: exploring consensus, controversy, and contexts. Hast Cent Rep. 2018;48(Suppl 4):S2–5.
2. Capron AM. Beecher Dépassé: fifty years of determining death, legally. Hastings Cent Rep. 2018;48(Suppl 4):S14–S8.
3. De Georgia MA. History of brain death as death: 1968 to the present. J Crit Care. 2014;29(4):673–8.
4. A definition of irreversible coma. Report of the Ad Hoc Committee of the Harvard Medical School to examine the definition of brain death. JAMA. 1968;205(6):337–40.
5. https://www.uniformlaws.org/committees/community-home/librarydocuments?communitykey=155faf5d-03c2-4027-99ba-ee4c99019d6c&tab=librarydocuments&LibraryFolderKey=&DefaultView=. Accessed 21 Jun 2020.
6. Nikas NT, Bordlee DC, Moreira M. Determination of death and the dead donor rule: a survey of the current law on brain death. J Med Philos. 2016;41(3):237–56.
7. https://www.aan.com/Guidelines/home/GuidelineDetail/431.
8. Greer DM, Kirschen MP, Lewis A, Gronseth GS, Rae-Grant A, Ashwal S, et al. Pediatric and adult brain death/death by neurologic criteria consensus guideline: report of the AAN guidelines subcommittee, AAP, CNS, and SCCM. Neurology. 2023;1:1. https://doi.org/10.1212/WNL.0000000000207740.
9. Wijdicks EF. The case against confirmatory tests for determining brain death in adults. Neurology. 2010;75(1):77–83.
10. Robbins NM, Bernat JL. Practice current: when do you order ancillary tests to determine brain death? Neurol Clin Pract. 2018;8(3):266–74.
11. Bradac GB, Simon RS. Angiography in brain death. Neuroradiology. 1974;7(1):25–8.
12. Braum M, Ducrocq X, Huot JC, Audibert G, Anxionnat R, Picard L. Intravenous angiography in brain death: report of 140 patients. Neuroradiology. 1997;39(6):400–5.
13. Savard M, Turgeon AF, Gariépy JL, Trottier F, Langevin S. Selective 4 vessels angiography in brain death: a retrospective study. Can J Neurol Sci. 2010;37(4):492–7.
14. Sinha P, Conrad GR. Scintigraphic confirmation of brain death. Semin Nucl Med. 2012;42(1):27–32.
15. Chang JJ, Tsivgoulis G, Katsanos AH, Malkoff MD, Alexandrov AV. Diagnostic accuracy of transcranial Doppler for brain death confirmation: systematic review and meta-analysis. AJNR Am J Neuroradiol. 2016;37(3):408–14.
16. Szurhaj W, Lamblin MD, Kaminska A, Sediri H, Société de Neurophysiologie Clinique de Langue Française. EEG guidelines in the diagnosis of brain death. Neurophysiol Clin. 2015;45(1):97–104.
17. Wijdicks EF, Varelas PN, Gronseth GS, Greer DM, American Academy of Neurology. Evidence-based guideline update: determining brain death in adults: report of the quality standards subcommittee of the American Academy of Neurology. Neurology. 2010;74(23):1911–8.
18. Greer DM, Wang HH, Robinson JD, Varelas PN, Henderson GV, Wijdicks EF. Variability of brain death policies in the United States. JAMA Neurol. 2016;73(2):213–8.
19. Russell JA, Epstein LG, Greer DM, Kirschen M, Rubin MA, Lewis A, et al. Brain death, the determination of brain death, and member guidance for brain death accommodation requests: AAN position statement. Neurology. 2019;92:228.
20. https://www.leg.state.nv.us/Session/79th2017/Bills/AB/AB424_R1.pdf.
21. Shappell CN, Frank JI, Husari K, Sanchez M, Goldenberg F, Ardelt A. Practice variability in brain death determination: a call to action. Neurology. 2013;81(23):2009–14.
22. Braksick SA, Robinson CP, Gronseth GS, Hocker S, Wijdicks EFM, Rabinstein AA. Variability in reported physician practices for brain death determination. Neurology. 2019;92(9):e888–e94.
23. Chen PM, Trando A, LaBuzetta JN. Simulation-based training improves fellows' competence in brain death discussion and declaration. Neurologist. 2021;27(1):6–10.

24. Busl KM, Lewis A, Varelas PN. Apnea testing for the determination of brain death: a systematic scoping review. Neurocrit Care. 2020;34:608.
25. Migdady I, Stephens RS, Price C, Geocadin RG, Whitman G, Cho SM. The use of apnea test and brain death determination in patients on extracorporeal membrane oxygenation: a systematic review. J Thorac Cardiovasc Surg. 2020;48:364.
26. Shah SK, Kasper K, Miller FG. A narrative review of the empirical evidence on public attitudes on brain death and vital organ transplantation: the need for better data to inform policy. J Med Ethics. 2015;41(4):291–6.
27. Siminoff LA, Mercer MB, Arnold R. Families' understanding of brain death. Prog Transplant. 2003;13(3):218–24.
28. Siminoff LA, Burant C, Youngner SJ. Death and organ procurement: public beliefs and attitudes. Kennedy Inst Ethics J. 2004;14(3):217–34.
29. Seifi A, Lacci JV, Godoy DA. Incidence of brain death in the United States. Clin Neurol Neurosurg. 2020;195:105885.
30. Jones AH, Dizon ZB, October TW. Investigation of public perception of brain death using the internet. Chest. 2018;154(2):286–92.
31. Lewis A, Lord AS, Czeisler BM, Caplan A. Public education and misinformation on brain death in mainstream media. Clin Transpl. 2016;30(9):1082–9.
32. Lewis A, Weaver J, Caplan A. Portrayal of brain death in film and television. Am J Transplant. 2017;17(3):761–9.
33. Yang Q, Miller G. East-west differences in perception of brain death. Review of history, current understandings, and directions for future research. J Bioeth Inq. 2015;12(2):211–25.
34. Terunuma Y, Mathis BJ. Cultural sensitivity in brain death determination: a necessity in end-of-life decisions in Japan. BMC Med Ethics. 2021;22(1):58.
35. Miller AC, Ziad-Miller A, Elamin EM. Brain death and Islam: the interface of religion, culture, history, law, and modern medicine. Chest. 2014;146(4):1092–101.
36. Yanke G, Rady MY, Verheijde JL. When brain death belies belief. J Relig Health. 2016;55(6):2199–213.
37. Gabbay E, Fins JJ. Go in peace: brain death, reasonable accommodation and Jewish mourning rituals. J Relig Health. 2019;58(5):1672–86.
38. Morrison WE, Kirschen MP. A taxonomy of objections to brain death determination. Neurocrit Care. 2022;37(2):369–71.
39. https://law.justia.com/cases/arizona/supreme-court/1979/4271-2.html.
40. https://law.justia.com/codes/arizona/2015/title-14/section-14-1107/.
41. https://www.ncleg.gov/EnactedLegislation/Statutes/HTML/BySection/Chapter_90/GS_90-323.html#:~:text=%C2%A7%2090%2D323accepted%20standards%20of%20medical%20practice.
42. https://law.justia.com/codes/georgia/2010/title-31/chapter-10/31-10-16/.
43. Lewis A, Greer D. Current controversies in brain death determination. Nat Rev Neurol. 2017;13(8):505–9.
44. https://codes.findlaw.com/ca/health-and-safety-code/hsc-sect-1254-4.html.
45. Pope T. Brain death and the law: hard cases and legal challenges. Hast Cent Rep. 2018;48(Suppl 4):S46–S8.
46. Lewis A, Scheyer O. Legal objections to use of neurologic criteria to declare death in the United States: 1968 to 2017. Chest. 2019;155(6):1234–45.
47. https://law.justia.com/cases/nevada/supreme-court/2015/68531.html.
48. Bjelland S, Jones K. A systematic review on improving the family experience after consent for deceased organ donation. Prog Transplant. 2022;32(2):152–66.
49. Ma J, Zeng L, Li T, Tian X, Wang L. Experiences of families following organ donation consent: a qualitative systematic review. Transplant Proc. 2021;53(2):501–12.
50. Knihs NDS, Schuantes-Paim SM, Bellaguarda MLDR, Treviso P, Pessoa JLE, Magalhães ALP, et al. Family interview evaluation for organ donation: communication of death and information about organ donation. Transplant Proc. 2022;54(5):1202–7.

51. Meyfroidt G, Gunst J, Martin-Loeches I, Smith M, Robba C, Taccone FS, et al. Management of the brain-dead donor in the ICU: general and specific therapy to improve transplantable organ quality. Intensive Care Med. 2019;45(3):343–53.
52. Martin-Loeches I, Sandiumenge A, Charpentier J, Kellum JA, Gaffney AM, Procaccio F, et al. Management of donation after brain death (DBD) in the ICU: the potential donor is identified, what's next? Intensive Care Med. 2019;45(3):322–30.
53. Robinson K. New drafting and study committees to be appointed. 2020; https://www.uniformlaws.org/committees/community-home/digestviewer/viewthread?MessageKey=a71e3d9d-4cf9-4529-9169-a08acf5edde6&CommunityKey=d4b8f588-4c2f-4db1-90e9-48b1184ca39a&tab=digestviewer.
54. Omelianchuk A, Bernat J, Caplan A, Greer D, Lazaridis C, Lewis A, et al. Revise the uniform determination of death act to align the law with practice through neurorespiratory criteria. Neurology. 2022;98(13):532–6.
55. Bioethics BotPCfC. Proposal for revising the uniform determination of death act. 2022; https://www.thehastingscenter.org/defining-brain-death/.
56. Manara AR. All human death is brain death: the legacy of the harvard criteria. Resuscitation. 2019;138:210–2.

Long-Term Outcome and the Role of Neurorehabilitation After Severe Traumatic Brain Injury

32

Oleksandr Strelko and Anthony M. DiGiorgio

32.1 Progression and Outcomes of Severe TBI

Patients suffering from TBI initially present to primary care clinics or hospital emergency departments (ED). For severe TBI (initial GCS ≤8) it is almost universally an ED presentation. From the ED, they may get admitted to the floor or the intensive care unit (ICU). Approximately 10% of all TBI injuries can be classified as severe, with an average mortality of 39% in patients suffering from severe TBI [1]. Unfavorable short-term recovery outcomes for victims of severe TBI are reportedly common at 60% [2]. When measuring longer-term outcomes using the Glasgow Outcome Scale-Extended (GOSE), a little over 12% of patients with severe TBI had favorable outcomes (GOSE 4–8) 2 weeks after injury, with the favorable outcome rate reaching 52% 12 months after injury. Disability rates resulting from severe TBI also improve over time. Whereas more than 90% of patients with severe TBI suffered from moderate disability (DRS scores ≥4) 2 weeks post-injury, 19% of patients had no disability and only 13.9% of patients with severe TBI had a mild disability 12 months after the initial injury. Out of patients who were in a vegetative state induced by severe TBI at 2 weeks, 78% were able to regain consciousness and 25% regained orientation at 12 months after injury. However, even with cognitive and functional improvements seen over time, at least 1 in 4 patients who experienced severe TBI still suffer from a number of problems and deficits such as headaches, dizziness, noise sensitivity, sleep

O. Strelko
Loyola University Chicago Stritch School of Medicine, Maywood, IL, USA

Department of Neurological Surgery, University of California, San Francisco, San Francisco, CA, USA

A. M. DiGiorgio (✉)
Department of Neurological Surgery, University of California, San Francisco, San Francisco, CA, USA
e-mail: anthony.digiorgio@ucsf.edu

E. Brogi et al. (eds.), *Traumatic Brain Injury*, Hot Topics in Acute Care Surgery and Trauma, https://doi.org/10.1007/978-3-031-50117-3_32

disturbances, fatigue, irritability, depression, memory problems, difficulties concentrating, blurred vision, and restlessness [3, 4]. Of the above-mentioned deficits, memory impairment, slowness, problems concentrating or multitasking, chronic fatigue, and irritability were observed in over 60% of patients as long as 8 years following the original hospitalization resulting from severe TBI. Many patients are unable to return to work and normal daily function, resulting in unemployment and dependence on others for day-to-day tasks [5]. Although this chapter focuses on severe TBI, even in patients with mild, computed tomography (CT) negative TBI, 17% are unable to return to work 1 year after their injury [6].

32.1.1 Using Biomarkers for Predicting Outcomes

In the context of clinical care, molecular biomarkers are generally utilized as indicators of specific clinically induced biological states and can be measured using samples derived from tissue or peripheral body fluids. Some markers can be altered by changes in protein expression, enzymatic activity, post-translational modification, alterations in expressions of genes and proteins, or a combination of the above. Blood and cerebrospinal fluid (CSF) based biomarkers specific to TBI can be classified into 4 unique groups: protein biomarkers, inflammatory markers, small molecule biomarkers, and lipid metabolite biomarkers (Table 32.1).

Molecular biomarkers, abundant in CSF and serum, are relatively easy to access and demonstrate high utility for use as an additional diagnostic tool in the setting of early TBI assessment to determine TBI severity [24]. In addition, increased initial serum levels of many biomarkers have been linked with poor outcomes 6 months after injury [7, 25]. Based on these findings, longitudinal biomarker trajectory assessments may identify ongoing injury and predict patient deterioration before clinical symptoms develop and thus help guide therapeutic interventions.

32.1.2 Imaging Diagnostic Methods for Severe TBI

Diagnostic imaging biomarkers are also extensively used in the context of TBI. In addition to widely used CT and magnetic resonance imaging (MRI), more novel prognostic imaging methods have been developed to assess the extent and morbidity of TBI more accurately. One of these methods, diffusion-tensor imaging (DTI), has allowed detection of microstructural white tract (axonal) injuries associated with TBI [26]. When compared to healthy controls, TBI patients showed more damage to the white matter tracts on DTI. Global damage has also been found to be associated with worse 6-month recovery when controlling for other injury characteristics [27].

Table 32.1 TBI biomarkers

Biomarker group	Biomarker name	Biomarker description	Importance	References
Protein	1. S100B	1. Calcium binding protein expressed by astrocytes. Found in CSF and/or serum	1. Increase is correlated with increased TBI morbidity and mortality	[7, 8]
	2. Glial fibrillary acidic protein (GFAP)	2. Astrocyte derived monomeric intermediate filament	2. Increase is correlated with increased TBI morbidity and mortality	[7, 9]
	3. Neuron specific enolase (NSE)	3. Isoenzyme of enolase. Found in neurons, glial cells, erythrocytes, and thrombocytes	3. Increase is correlated with injury severity and increase in mortality	[7, 10, 11]
	4. Myelin basic protein (MBP)	4. Protein component of myelin. Found in CSF and serum after white matter injury	4. Increase in serum MBP levels correlates with worse outcomes	[12]
	5. Fatty acid binding proteins (FABPs)	5. Brain specific FABPs have recently been discovered	5. Increase in serum brain FABP levels is correlated with presence of TBI	[13, 14]
	6. Phosphorylated neurofilament (NF-H)	6. Neuron specific filament	6. Early increase in serum levels is correlated with brain injury in an animal model of TBI	[15]
Inflammatory marker	1. Interleukin-1 (IL-1)	1. Contributes to formation of glial scars after brain injury	1. Peak IL-1 CSF levels have been found to be correlated with 3-month outcomes in patients with severe TBI	[16, 17]
	2. Tumor necrosis factor (TNF)-α	2. Pro-inflammatory factor that plays a role in neutrophil and monocyte recruitment to the site of injury	2. Increased serum and CSF levels of TNF-α have been found to be correlated with severe TBI	[18, 19]
Small molecule biomarker	1. Norepinephrine	1. Neurotransmitter	1. Increase in serum levels has been correlated with moderate-severe TBI	[20]
	2. Serotonin	2. Neurotransmitter	2. Increase in CSF levels has been found to be correlated with TBI	[21, 22]
Lipid metabolite biomarkers	1. F2-isoprostane	1. Prostaglandin-like compound synthesized as a result of peroxidation of arachidonic acid	1. Increased levels have been observed in patients with severe TBI	[23]

32.2 Targets of Care

Improving care for patients who experience TBI is divided into acute care, immediate post-acute care, and chronic care. While treatment of the immediate injury is paramount in the acute phase of TBI, treatment during the post-acute phase is also crucial to prevent detrimental long-term effects. Depending on how soon rehabilitation therapy is initiated after TBI, the focus of care should not only be focused on medical care, but also improvement of the patient's everyday life post-TBI. Resuming activities of daily living is the first goal of TBI rehabilitation. Establishing goals and realistic targets of neurorehabilitative care is one of the key primary segments of TBI recovery.

For many patients, ranging from those with mild to severe TBI, finding focused neurorehabilitative care is difficult to achieve. Primary care providers are often uncomfortable or lack the appropriate level of training necessary for post-TBI care. Specialized clinics are uncommon.

Patients who experience a TBI may present to an ED or through a primary care provider (Fig. 32.1). For those presenting to the ED, they often receive imaging and may be admitted to the hospital, either to the ICU or an inpatient floor. The severity of the TBI and acute recovery will determine the intensity of the post-acute care needs.

The patient's post-acute care needs can range from dealing with assistance in returning to pre-injury baseline to requiring around-the-clock care. For those that require more intensive post-acute care, the care team and family should focus on identifying and addressing any complications that may arise, assessing any functional deficits that may have an immediate, disproportionate impact on the patient, and educating family/close community members on administering appropriate

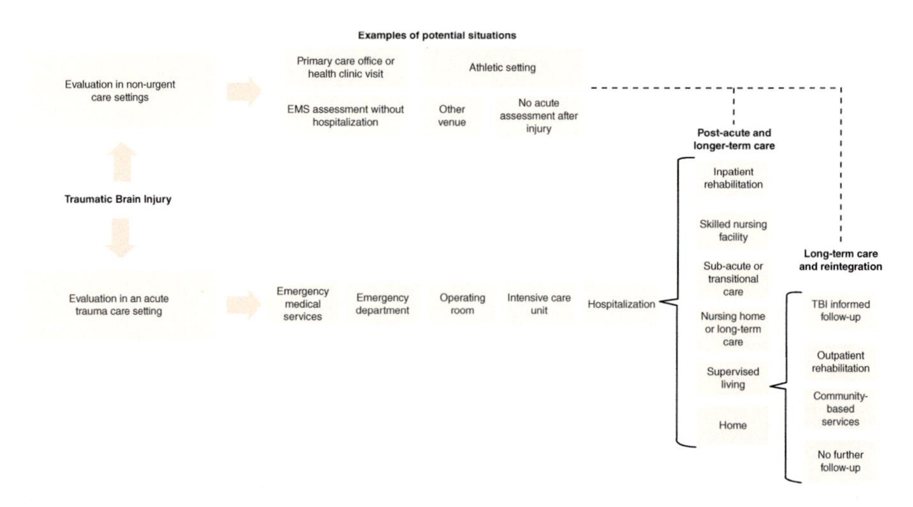

Fig. 32.1 Avenues of acute and post-acute management of TBI. (Adopted from National Academies of Sciences, Engineering, and Medicine. *Traumatic Brain Injury: A Roadmap for Accelerating Progress.* Washington, DC: The National Academies Press. 2022, ch. 5 [28])

assistance for the patient. For TBI patients who have gone through the majority of rehabilitation, there are several ways to adjust to a new lifestyle post-rehabilitation: employer assistance with adjustments to their current job, exploring new vocations tailored for their condition, seeking a support system in their journey, assessing any new cognitive deficits that may arise post-rehabilitation that need to be addressed, being aware of any accessible resources for further treatment, maximizing self-efficacy and life satisfaction, and being cognizant of behavior that can be detrimental to their recovery. For patients who have developed chronic symptoms, it is important to maintain a consistent course of recovery in the patient's physical health, mental health, and their aspirations. Although it is ideal for TBI patients to undergo rehabilitative therapy right after injury, some patients may not have the means to start right away. However, patients and their families can be assured that making progress in therapy is beneficial for TBI recovery.

32.3 Neurorehabilitation

Once the patient is medically stable in the acute care setting, they are transferred to post-acute care, where individuals suffering from severe TBI are provided intermediate care and some acute rehabilitation. More specifically, based on clinical experience Greenwald and colleagues [29] define the following criteria for inpatient neurorehabilitation: (1) acute disability experienced by the patient that requires in-hospital stay; (2) medical or surgical conditions are stable enough to allow implementation of rehabilitative therapies; (3) patient has the ability to partake in at least 1 h of therapy at least two times a day; (4) patient demonstrates the ability to make discernible progress in the setting of acute care therapies; and, finally, (5) the patient is able to rely on a social support system at home that will allow them to leave the hospital after a clinically significant improvement of function. In summary, neurorehabilitative therapy should be recommended if the patient is stable enough and will likely benefit from the implementation of such therapy. A more detailed breakdown of eligibility criteria can be seen in Fig. 32.2.

The first 3 months following injury are most crucial for recovery, capitalizing on the need to provide quality rehabilitation during this period [30]. Thankfully, there are multiple types of rehabilitation available to TBI patients, including: acute inpatient rehabilitation, post-acute inpatient, and post-acute outpatient rehabilitation (Figs. 32.1 and 32.2). When available, acute inpatient rehabilitation is introduced, exposing patients with severe TBI to physical, occupational, and speech therapy while an admitted patient is still in the hospital. More specifically, an acute rehabilitation team would assist the patient in recovering activities of daily living such as independent eating, dressing, using the bathroom, ambulating, and speaking while in an inpatient setting.

Following the initial stage of acute TBI care focused on sustaining life, stabilizing the patient, and minimizing injury to the brain, post-acute care focuses on the optimization of a patient's daily independent function and the ability to return to activities of daily living (ADLs). In addition, post-acute treatment aids in minimizing physical and

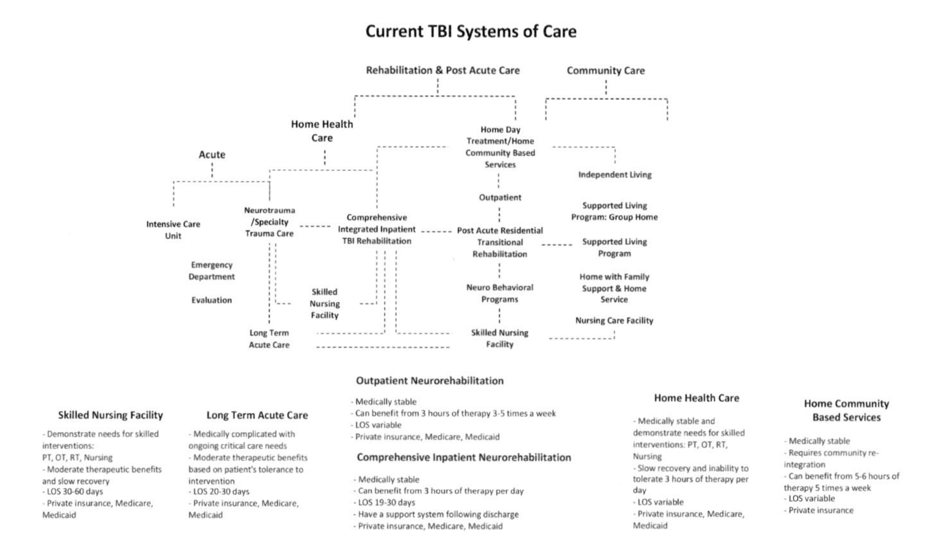

Fig. 32.2 Integrated model of TBI care based on general eligibility criteria. (Adopted from Massachusetts General Hospital. *Rehabilitation access and outcome after severe traumatic brain injury.* Boston, MA. 2022)

neurocognitive complications as well as the development of new and compounding of pre-existing comorbidities following occurrences of severe TBI. Outpatient neurorehabilitation offers quite a variety of services aimed at improving the efficacy and rate of physical, neurocognitive, and occupational components of recovery from severe TBI. Some of the outpatient rehabilitative destinations patients are usually discharged to are skilled nursing facilities, long- and short-term care hospitals, supervised living facilities, and specialized rehabilitative centers. Patients are also often discharged home for self or assisted care. However, access to neurorehabilitative care is not uniform among all patients suffering from severe TBI and is dependent on several factors, including but not limited to the individual needs of the patient and/or the family, referral patterns and biases among care providers, space, geographic proximity, and sufficient financial resources or appropriate insurance type. Any one of these factors can delay the delivery of care or preclude the delivery of services altogether, thereby negatively impacting the trajectory and extent of recovery and, ultimately, the long-term outcome from brain injury [31].

32.3.1 Mechanisms of Neurorehabilitation

One of the main goals of neurorehabilitation is to provide an enriching environment (EE) to the patient. For the past 50 years, translational and clinical research has empirically demonstrated that an EE can significantly benefit the behavioral and physiological outcomes of an individual who has experienced a traumatic brain injury or any clinically significant insult to the central nervous system. First investigated by Donald Hebb in the 1940s, a consensus established by a plethora of scientific publications describes the benefits of EE in the context of TBI recovery and its positive effects on neuroplasticity.

Similar to other regions of the body, injuries to the brain often lead to cell death and remodeling of the cerebral cytoarchitecture [32–34]. The above-mentioned process of neuroplasticity is the ability of the nervous system to recover and reorganize itself in response to intrinsic and extrinsic stimuli by reorganizing its structure, function, and synaptic networks [35]. First demonstrated in animal studies, introduction of an EE [36], task-specific training and repetitive exercise are key factors in promoting synaptogenesis and neuroplasticity following insult to the CNS [37]. Acquisition and adaptation of skills can be achieved more effectively by incorporating relevant, task-specific activities as opposed to unspecific, repetitive exercise and passive modalities [38]. Of essence are the amount and timing of neurorehabilitative therapy. Animal models demonstrate that earlier post-injury intervention is more effective than delayed intervention [39]. The likely mechanism of rewiring is theorized to be mediated by promotion of long-term potentiation (LTP) and by inhibition of long-term depression (LTD) [40] and has been shown to be achieved through stimulation of electrical activity in the brain utilizing changes in the neuronal resting membrane potential in order to affect cortical excitability. Animal studies using transcranial direct current stimulation (tDCS) to manipulate cortical excitability have demonstrated its utility in the context of TBI recovery, highlighting the importance of inducing cortical firing to promote recovery from CNS injury [41, 42]. Taken together, this evidence points to the importance of early, targeted neurorehabilitative intervention aimed at inducing cortical activity to promote rewiring of injured cortex and gain of functionality after severe TBI.

32.4 Disparities in Long-Term TBI Care

32.4.1 Disparities in Neurorehabilitation

While it is ideal for all patients with severe TBI to have access to quality care, the reality is that there are certain patient populations that do not have the same access to proper neurorehabilitation. Several socioeconomic factors have been shown to contribute to disparities in access to neurorehabilitation. Patients in rural areas do not get the same quality care as do patients in urban areas. For instance, a study from Johnstone et al. [43] found that post-TBI patients who lived in urban areas had better financial assistance to attend the vocational rehabilitation program and more transportation support, even when both urban and rural TBI patients had similar injury severity and neuropsychological scores. Compared to urban trauma care that has more resources and uniformity, trauma care in rural areas tends to be variable, with worse outcomes for rural patients [44]. Lack of health insurance also plays a big role in contributing to disparities in neurorehabilitation, with one study showing that TBI patients who did not have health insurance were more likely to not seek post-hospital care [45]. Without health insurance, patients are discouraged from seeking further care, which can exacerbate symptoms in the future, although insurance alone does not guarantee access. Medicaid beneficiaries and patients belonging to racial minority groups are more likely to have worse outcomes and less likely to receive high quality longitudinal neurorehabilitative care when compared to patients with private insurance [46, 47]. This lack of access to post-acute care for Medicaid patients also translates into longer length of stay in the acute care setting [48].

32.4.2 Addressing Disparities

With geographic location being one of the biggest factors in disparities of neurorehabilitation, one potential solution to reach out to patients in rural areas who have limited access to care is via telehealth, or telerehabilitation. Follow-up with patients becomes crucial to ensure they adhere to appropriate long-term care. Tsaousides et al. [49] demonstrated the feasibility of delivering group therapy by videoconferencing to improve emotion regulation in persons with TBI. Ng and colleagues (2013) found it feasible to deliver the cognitive orientation to daily occupational performance (CO-OP) approach, a metacognitive intervention, via videoconferencing to adults with TBI, and observed trends toward increased community integration and fewer symptoms of cognitive dysfunction with its use. A study by De Luca and colleagues (2020) supports the feasibility and usability of a virtual reality rehabilitation system for cognitive rehabilitation for patients with severe TBI and their caregivers during the patient's hospitalization, suggesting its potential therapeutic use at home. Telehealth rehabilitation serves as a possible method to reduce disparities for patients in areas that lack the proper service for TBI patients. There are many regulatory hurdles to this, notably allowing practice of medicine across state lines and appropriate reimbursement. Another viable option for addressing disparities in TBI care is physician advocacy groups. Neurosurgeons, neurologists, psychiatrists, PM&R physicians, and other healthcare professionals involved in the care for patients with severe TBI may form powerful groups to highlight disparities in TBI care and advocate for their patients to receive better and longitudinal neurorehabilitative care after they are discharged from the hospital. Lastly, of course, payment parity between insurers is necessary for equal access to post-acute care services.

References

1. Rosenfeld JV, Maas AI, Bragge P, Morganti-Kossmann MC, Manley GT, Gruen RL. Early management of severe traumatic brain injury. Lancet. 2012;380(9847):1088–98. https://doi.org/10.1016/S0140-6736(12)60864-2.
2. Maasdorp SD, Swanepoel C, Gunter L. Outcomes of severe traumatic brain injury at time of discharge from tertiary academic hospitals in Bloemfontein. Afr J Thorac Crit Care Med. 2020;26(2):32. https://doi.org/10.7196/AJTCCM.2020.v26i2.057; Published 2020 Jun 15.
3. Ponsford JL, Downing MG, Olver J, Ponsford M, Acher R, Carty M, et al. Longitudinal follow-up of patients with traumatic brain injury: outcome at two, five, and ten years post-injury. J Neurotrauma. 2014;31:64–77. https://doi.org/10.1089/neu.2013.2997.

4. McCrea MA, Giacino JT, Barber J, et al. Functional outcomes over the first year after moderate to severe traumatic brain injury in the prospective, longitudinal TRACK-TBI study. JAMA Neurol. 2021;78(8):982–92. https://doi.org/10.1001/jamaneurol.2021.2043.
5. Ruet A, Bayen E, Jourdan C, et al. A detailed overview of long-term outcomes in severe traumatic brain injury eight years post-injury. Front Neurol. 2019;10:120. https://doi.org/10.3389/fneur.2019.00120; Published 2019 Feb 21.
6. Gaudette É, Seabury SA, Temkin N, et al. Employment and economic outcomes of participants with mild traumatic brain injury in the TRACK-TBI study. JAMA Netw Open. 2022;5(6):e2219444. https://doi.org/10.1001/jamanetworkopen.2022.19444; Published 2022 Jun 1.
7. Vos PE, Lamers KJ, Hendriks JC, et al. Glial and neuronal proteins in serum predict outcome after severe traumatic brain injury. Neurology. 2004;62(8):1303–10. https://doi.org/10.1212/01.wnl.0000120550.00643.dc.
8. Savola O, Pyhtinen J, Leino TK, Siitonen S, Niemelä O, Hillbom M. Effects of head and extracranial injuries on serum protein S100B levels in trauma patients. J Trauma. 2004;56(6):1229–34. https://doi.org/10.1097/01.ta.0000096644.08735.72.
9. Pelinka LE, Kroepfl A, Schmidhammer R, et al. Glial fibrillary acidic protein in serum after traumatic brain injury and multiple trauma. J Trauma. 2004;57(5):1006–12. https://doi.org/10.1097/01.ta.0000108998.48026.c3.
10. Ross SA, Cunningham RT, Johnston CF, Rowlands BJ. Neuron-specific enolase as an aid to outcome prediction in head injury. Br J Neurosurg. 1996;10(5):471–6. https://doi.org/10.1080/02688699647104.
11. Skogseid IM, Nordby HK, Urdal P, Paus E, Lilleaas F. Increased serum creatine kinase BB and neuron specific enolase following head injury indicates brain damage. Acta Neurochir. 1992;115(3–4):106–11. https://doi.org/10.1007/BF01406367.
12. Berger RP, Adelson PD, Pierce MC, Dulani T, Cassidy LD, Kochanek PM. Serum neuron-specific enolase, S100B, and myelin basic protein concentrations after inflicted and noninflicted traumatic brain injury in children. J Neurosurg. 2005;103(1 Suppl):61–8. https://doi.org/10.3171/ped.2005.103.1.0061.
13. Glatz JF, van der Vusse GJ. Cellular fatty acid-binding proteins: their function and physiological significance. Prog Lipid Res. 1996;35(3):243–82. https://doi.org/10.1016/s0163-7827(96)00006-9.
14. Pelsers MM, Hanhoff T, Van der Voort D, et al. Brain- and heart-type fatty acid-binding proteins in the brain: tissue distribution and clinical utility. Clin Chem. 2004;50:1568–75.
15. Anderson KJ, Scheff SW, Miller KM, et al. The phosphorylated axonal form of the neurofilament subunit NF-H (pNF-H) as a blood biomarker of traumatic brain injury. J Neurotrauma. 2008;25:1079–85.
16. Giulian D, Lachman LB. Interleukin-1 stimulation of astroglial proliferation after brain injury. Science. 1985;228:497–9.
17. Singhal A, Baker AJ, Hare GM, Reinders FX, Schlichter LC, Moulton RJ. Association between cerebrospinal fluid interleukin-6 concentrations and outcome after severe human traumatic brain injury. J Neurotrauma. 2002;19:929–37.
18. Crespo AR, Da Rocha AB, Jotz GP, et al. Increased serum sFas and TNFalpha following isolated severe head injury in males. Brain Inj. 2007;21:441–7.
19. Goodman JC, Robertson CS, Grossman RG, Narayan RK. Elevation of tumor necrosis factor in head injury. J Neuroimmunol. 1990;30:213–7.
20. Clifton GL, Ziegler MG, Grossman RG. Circulating catecholamines and sympathetic activity after head injury. Neurosurgery. 1981;8:10–4.
21. Porta M, Bareggi SR, Collice M, et al. Homovanillic acid and 5-hydroxyindole-acetic acid in the csf of patients after a severe head injury. II. Ventricular csf concentrations in acute brain posttraumatic syndromes. Eur Neurol. 1975;13:545–54.
22. Inagawa T, Ishikawa S, Uozumi T. Homovanillic acid and 5-hydroxyindoleacetic acid in the ventricular CSF of comatose patients with obstructive hydrocephalus. J Neurosurg. 1980;52:635–41.

23. Varma S, Janesko KL, Wisniewski SR, et al. F2-isoprostane and neuron-specific enolase in cerebrospinal fluid after severe traumatic brain injury in infants and children. J Neurotrauma. 2003;20:781–6.
24. Shahim P, Politis A, van der Merwe A, Moore B, Chou YY, Pham DL, Butman JA, Diaz-Arrastia R, Gill JM, Brody DL, Zetterberg H, Blennow K, Chan L. Neurofilament light as a biomarker in traumatic brain injury. Neurology. 2020;95:e610–22.
25. Liliang PC, Liang CL, Weng HC, et al. Tau proteins in serum predict outcome after severe traumatic brain injury. J Surg Res. 2009;160(2):302.
26. Niogi SN, Mukherjee P. Diffusion tensor imaging of mild traumatic brain injury. J Head Trauma Rehabil. 2010;25(4):241–55.
27. Palacios EM, Yuh EL, Mac Donald CL, et al. Diffusion tensor imaging reveals elevated diffusivity of white matter microstructure that is independently associated with long-term outcome after mild traumatic brain injury: a TRACK-TBI study. J Neurotrauma. 2022;39(19–20):1318–28. https://doi.org/10.1089/neu.2021.0408.
28. National Academies of Sciences, Engineering, and Medicine. Traumatic brain injury: a roadmap for accelerating progress. Washington, DC: The National Academies Press; 2022. https://doi.org/10.17226/25394.
29. Greenwald BD, Rigg JL. Neurorehabilitation in traumatic brain injury: does it make a difference? Mt Sinai J Med. 2009;76:182–9.
30. Barnes MP. Rehabilitation after traumatic brain injury. Br Med Bull. 1999;55(4):927–43. https://doi.org/10.1258/0007142991902727.
31. Cioe N, Seale G, Marquez de la Plata C, Groff A, Gutierrez D, Ashley M, Connors SH. Brain injury rehabilitation outcomes. Vienna, VA: Brain Injury Association of America; 2016.
32. Lowenstein DH, Thomas MJ, Smith DH, McIntosh TK. Selective vulnerability of dentate hilar neurons following traumatic brain injury: a potential mechanistic link between head trauma and disorders of the hippocampus. J Neurosci. 1992;12(12):4846–53. https://doi.org/10.1523/JNEUROSCI.12-12-04846.1992.
33. King JB, Lopez-Larson MP, Yurgelun-Todd DA. Mean cortical curvature reflects cytoarchitecture restructuring in mild traumatic brain injury. Neuroimage Clin. 2016;11:81–9. https://doi.org/10.1016/j.nicl.2016.01.003; Published 2016 Jan 6.
34. McKee AC, Cantu RC, Nowinski CJ, et al. Chronic traumatic encephalopathy in athletes: progressive tauopathy after repetitive head injury. J Neuropathol Exp Neurol. 2009;68(7):709–35. https://doi.org/10.1097/NEN.0b013e3181a9d503.
35. Cramer SC, Sur M, Dobkin BH, et al. Harnessing neuroplasticity for clinical applications. Brain. 2011;134(Pt 6):1591–609. https://doi.org/10.1093/brain/awr039.
36. Hoffman AN, Malena RR, Westergom BP, et al. Environmental enrichment-mediated functional improvement after experimental traumatic brain injury is contingent on task-specific neurobehavioral experience. Neurosci Lett. 2008;431(3):226–30. https://doi.org/10.1016/j.neulet.2007.11.042.
37. Plautz EJ, Milliken GW, Nudo RJ. Effects of repetitive motor training on movement representations in adult squirrel monkeys: role of use versus learning. Neurobiol Learn Mem. 2000;74(1):27–55. https://doi.org/10.1006/nlme.1999.3934.
38. Krakauer JW. Arm function after stroke: from physiology to recovery. Semin Neurol. 2005;25(4):384–95. https://doi.org/10.1055/s-2005-923533.
39. Krakauer JW, Carmichael ST, Corbett D, Wittenberg GF. Getting neurorehabilitation right: what can be learned from animal models? Neurorehabil Neural Repair. 2012;26(8):923–31. https://doi.org/10.1177/1545968312440745.
40. Kleim JA, Jones TA. Principles of experience-dependent neural plasticity: implications for rehabilitation after brain damage. J Speech Lang Hear Res. 2008;51(1):S225–39. https://doi.org/10.1044/1092-4388(2008/018).
41. Kim HJ, Han SJ. Anodal transcranial direct current stimulation provokes neuroplasticity in repetitive mild traumatic brain injury in rats. Neural Plast. 2017;2017:1372946. https://doi.org/10.1155/2017/1372946.

42. Yoon KJ, Lee YT, Chae SW, Park CR, Kim DY. Effects of anodal transcranial direct current stimulation (tDCS) on behavioral and spatial memory during the early stage of traumatic brain injury in the rats. J Neurol Sci. 2016;362:314–20. https://doi.org/10.1016/j.jns.2016.02.005.
43. Johnstone B, Price T, Bounds T, Schopp L, Schootman M, Schumate D. Rural/urban differences in vocational outcomes for state vocational rehabilitation clients with TBI. NeuroRehabilitation. 2003;18(3):197–203.
44. Haider AH, Weygandt PL, Bentley JM, Monn MF, Rehman KA, Zarzaur BL, Crandall ML, Cornwell EE, Cooper LA. Disparities in trauma care and outcomes in the United States: a systematic review and meta-analysis. J Trauma Acute Care Surg. 2013;74(5):1195–205.
45. Gao S, Kumar R, Wisniewski S, Fabio A. Disparities in health care utilization of adults with traumatic brain injuries are related to insurance, race and ethnicity: a systematic review. J Head Trauma Rehabil. 2018;33(3):e40–50.
46. Asemota AO, George BP, Cumpsty-Fowler CJ, Haider AH, Schneider EB. Race and insurance disparities in discharge to rehabilitation for patients with traumatic brain injury. J Neurotrauma. 2013;30(24):2057–65. https://doi.org/10.1089/neu.2013.3091.
47. McQuistion K, Zens T, Jung HS, et al. Insurance status and race affect treatment and outcome of traumatic brain injury. J Surg Res. 2016;205(2):261–71. https://doi.org/10.1016/j.jss.2016.06.087.
48. Yue JK, Krishnan N, Chyall L, et al. Predictors of extreme hospital length of stay after traumatic brain injury [published online ahead of print, 2022 Sep 1]. World Neurosurg. 2022;S1878-8750(22):01232–3. https://doi.org/10.1016/j.wneu.2022.08.122.
49. Tsaousides T, D'Antonio E, Varbanova V, Spielman L. Delivering group treatment via videoconference to individuals with traumatic brain injury: a feasibility study. Neuropsychol Rehabil. 2014;24(5):784–803.

Printed in the United States
by Baker & Taylor Publisher Services